EPIDEMIOLOGY OF LUNG CANCER

LUNG BIOLOGY IN HEALTH AND DISEASE

Executive Editor

Claude Lenfant
Director, National Heart, Lung and Blood Institute
National Institutes of Health
Bethesda, Maryland

1. Immunologic and Infectious Reactions in the Lung, *edited by Charles H. Kirkpatrick and Herbert Y. Reynolds*
2. The Biochemical Basis of Pulmonary Function, *edited by Ronald G. Crystal*
3. Bioengineering Aspects of the Lung, *edited by John B. West*
4. Metabolic Functions of the Lung, *edited by Y. S. Bakhle and John R. Vane*
5. Respiratory Defense Mechanisms (in two parts), *edited by Joseph D. Brain, Donald F. Proctor, and Lynne M. Reid*
6. Development of the Lung, *edited by W. Alan Hodson*
7. Lung Water and Solute Exchange, *edited by Norman C. Staub*
8. Extrapulmonary Manifestations of Respiratory Disease, *edited by Eugene Debs Robin*
9. Chronic Obstructive Pulmonary Disease, *edited by Thomas L. Petty*
10. Pathogenesis and Therapy of Lung Cancer, *edited by Curtis C. Harris*
11. Genetic Determinants of Pulmonary Disease, *edited by Stephen D. Litwin*
12. The Lung in the Transition Between Health and Disease, *edited by Peter T. Macklem and Solbert Permutt*
13. Evolution of Respiratory Processes: A Comparative Approach, *edited by Stephen C. Wood and Claude Lenfant*
14. Pulmonary Vascular Diseases, *edited by Kenneth M. Moser*
15. Physiology and Pharmacology of the Airways, *edited by Jay A. Nadel*
16. Diagnostic Techniques in Pulmonary Disease (in two parts), *edited by Marvin A. Sackner*
17. Regulation of Breathing (in two parts), *edited by Thomas F. Hornbein*
18. Occupational Lung Diseases: Research Approaches and Methods, *edited by Hans Weill and Margaret Turner-Warwick*
19. Immunopharmacology of the Lung, *edited by Harold H. Newball*
20. Sarcoidosis and Other Granulomatous Diseases of the Lung, *edited by Barry L. Fanburg*
21. Sleep and Breathing, *edited by Nicholas A. Saunders and Colin E. Sullivan*
22. *Pneumocystis carinii* Pneumonia: Pathogenesis, Diagnosis, and Treatment, *edited by Lowell S. Young*

23. Pulmonary Nuclear Medicine: Techniques in Diagnosis of Lung Disease, *edited by Harold L. Atkins*
24. Acute Respiratory Failure, *edited by Warren M. Zapol and Konrad J. Falke*
25. Gas Mixing and Distribution in the Lung, *edited by Ludwig A. Engel and Manuel Paiva*
26. High-Frequency Ventilation in Intensive Care and During Surgery, *edited by Graziano Carlon and William S. Howland*
27. Pulmonary Development: Transition from Intrauterine to Extrauterine Life, *edited by George H. Nelson*
28. Chronic Obstructive Pulmonary Disease: Second Edition, Revised and Expanded, *edited by Thomas L. Petty*
29. The Thorax (in two parts), *edited by Charis Roussos and Peter T. Macklem*
30. The Pleura in Health and Disease, *edited by Jacques Chrétien, Jean Bignon, and Albert Hirsch*
31. Drug Therapy for Asthma: Research and Clinical Practice, *edited by John W. Jenne and Shirley Murphy*
32. Pulmonary Endothelium in Health and Disease, *edited by Una S. Ryan*
33. The Airways: Neural Control in Health and Disease, *edited by Michael A. Kaliner and Peter J. Barnes*
34. Pathophysiology and Treatment of Inhalation Injuries, *edited by Jacob Loke*
35. Respiratory Function of the Upper Airway, *edited by Oommen P. Mathew and Giuseppe Sant'Ambrogio*
36. Chronic Obstructive Pulmonary Disease: A Behavioral Perspective, *edited by A. John McSweeny and Igor Grant*
37. Biology of Lung Cancer: Diagnosis and Treatment, *edited by Steven T. Rosen, James L. Mulshine, Frank Cuttitta, and Paul G. Abrams*
38. Pulmonary Vascular Physiology and Pathophysiology, *edited by E. Kenneth Weir and John T. Reeves*
39. Comparative Pulmonary Physiology: Current Concepts, *edited by Stephen C. Wood*
40. Respiratory Physiology: An Analytical Approach, *edited by H. K. Chang and Manuel Paiva*
41. Lung Cell Biology, *edited by Donald Massaro*
42. Heart–Lung Interactions in Health and Disease, *edited by Steven M. Scharf and Sharon S. Cassidy*
43. Clinical Epidemiology of Chronic Obstructive Pulmonary Disease, *edited by Michael J. Hensley and Nicholas A. Saunders*
44. Surgical Pathology of Lung Neoplasms, *edited by Alberto M. Marchevsky*
45. The Lung in Rheumatic Diseases, *edited by Grant W. Cannon and Guy A. Zimmerman*
46. Diagnostic Imaging of the Lung, *edited by Charles E. Putman*
47. Models of Lung Disease: Microscopy and Structural Methods, *edited by Joan Gil*

48. Electron Microscopy of the Lung, *edited by Dean E. Schraufnagel*
49. Asthma: Its Pathology and Treatment, *edited by Michael A. Kaliner, Peter J. Barnes, and Carl G. A. Persson*
50. Acute Respiratory Failure: Second Edition, *edited by Warren M. Zapol and Francois Lemaire*
51. Lung Disease in the Tropics, *edited by Om P. Sharma*
52. Exercise: Pulmonary Physiology and Pathophysiology, *edited by Brian J. Whipp and Karlman Wasserman*
53. Developmental Neurobiology of Breathing, *edited by Gabriel G. Haddad and Jay P. Farber*
54. Mediators of Pulmonary Inflammation, *edited by Michael A. Bray and Wayne H. Anderson*
55. The Airway Epithelium, *edited by Stephen G. Farmer and Douglas Hay*
56. Physiological Adaptations in Vertebrates: Respiration, Circulation, and Metabolism, *edited by Stephen C. Wood, Roy E. Weber, Alan R. Hargens, and Ronald W. Millard*
57. The Bronchial Circulation, *edited by John Butler*
58. Lung Cancer Differentiation: Implications for Diagnosis and Treatment, *edited by Samuel D. Bernal and Paul J. Hesketh*
59. Pulmonary Complications of Systemic Disease, *edited by John F. Murray*
60. Lung Vascular Injury: Molecular and Cellular Response, *edited by Arnold Johnson and Thomas J. Ferro*
61. Cytokines of the Lung, *edited by Jason Kelley*
62. The Mast Cell in Health and Disease, *edited by Michael A. Kaliner and Dean D. Metcalfe*
63. Pulmonary Disease in the Elderly Patient, *edited by Donald A. Mahler*
64. Cystic Fibrosis, *edited by Pamela B. Davis*
65. Signal Transduction in Lung Cells, *edited by Jerome S. Brody, David M. Center, and Vsevolod A. Tkachuk*
66. Tuberculosis: A Comprehensive International Approach, *edited by Lee B. Reichman and Earl S. Hershfield*
67. Pharmacology of the Respiratory Tract: Experimental and Clinical Research, *edited by K. Fan Chung and Peter J. Barnes*
68. Prevention of Respiratory Diseases, *edited by Albert Hirsch, Marcel Goldberg, Jean-Pierre Martin, and Roland Masse*
69. *Pneumocystis carinii* Pneumonia: Second Edition, Revised and Expanded, *edited by Peter D. Walzer*
70. Fluid and Solute Transport in the Airspaces of the Lungs, *edited by Richard M. Effros and H. K. Chang*
71. Sleep and Breathing: Second Edition, Revised and Expanded, *edited by Nicholas A. Saunders and Colin E. Sullivan*
72. Airway Secretion: Physiological Bases for the Control of Mucous Hypersecretion, *edited by Tamotsu Takishima and Sanae Shimura*
73. Sarcoidosis and Other Granulomatous Disorders, *edited by D. Geraint James*
74. Epidemiology of Lung Cancer, *edited by Jonathan M. Samet*

75. Pulmonary Embolism, *edited by Mario Morpurgo*

ADDITIONAL VOLUMES IN PREPARATION

Sports and Exercise Medicine, *edited by Stephen C. Wood and Robert C. Roach*

Endotoxin and the Lungs, *edited by Kenneth L. Brigham*

Regulation of Breathing: Second Edition, Revised and Expanded, *edited by Jerome A. Dempsey and Allan I. Pack*

Mesothelial Cell and Mesothelioma, *edited by Jean Bignon and Marie-Claude Jaurand*

EPIDEMIOLOGY OF LUNG CANCER

Edited by

Jonathan M. Samet

University of New Mexico School of Medicine
and the New Mexico Tumor Registry
Albuquerque, New Mexico

Marcel Dekker, Inc. **New York • Basel • Hong Kong**

Library of Congress Cataloging-in-Publication Data

Epidemiology of lung cancer / edited by Jonathan M. Samet.
p. cm. -- (Lung biology in health and disease; 74)
Includes bibliographical references and index.
ISBN 0-8247-8853-2 (alk. paper)
1. Lungs--Cancer--Epidemiology. I. Samet, Jonathan M. II. Series: Lung biology in health and disease; v. 74.
[DNLM: 1. Lung Neoplasms--epidemiology. W1 LU62 v.74 1994 / WF 658 E64 1994]
RC280.L8E65 1994
614.5'999--dc20
DNLM/DLC
for Library of Congress 93-46314
CIP

The publisher offers discounts on this book when ordered in bulk quantities. For more information, write to Special Sales/Professional Marketing at the address below.

This book is printed on acid-free paper.

Marcel Dekker, Inc.
270 Madison Avenue, New York, New York 10016

Current printing (last digit):
10 9 8 7 6 5 4 3 2 1

PRINTED IN THE UNITED STATES OF AMERICA

INTRODUCTION

Undoubtedly, the readers of the *Lung Biology in Health and Disease* series have noted that many volumes address lung cancer, either specifically or indirectly. While one may ask, "Why so many books on the same subject?", it is clear that over the last two or three decades we have come to recognize the extreme importance of lung cancer as a public health problem. Its increased incidence is driving the mortality rate upward, particularly in women. As a consequence, a huge research effort is in progress to find ways to prevent the disease. This effort spans the entire biomedical research spectrum, from subcellular, cellular, clinical, and demonstration research to research on education to augment the public realization that lung cancer is a preventable condition and that we are in charge, but not in control, when it comes to this disease. The sheer abundance of this research has prompted the inclusion of so much on lung cancer in this series.

Although the pioneering observation that carcinoma of the lung appeared to be the consequence of smoking was first published in 1941 (Ochsner and DeBakey, 1941), the authors of this landmark publication had inklings of that relationship in the early to mid-1930s. Not long after their publication, two masterful epidemiological studies (Wynder and Graham, 1950 and Doll and Hill, 1950) clearly established that "tobacco smoking was an etiologic factor in bronchogenic carcinoma." In a significant way, these studies demonstrated the power of epidemiological research. Since that time, much work has been pursued on the epidemiology of lung cancer, and this work has taught us a great deal. Most important, we have learned that although tobacco smoking is by far the most significant factor, it is only one of the many factors that can injure the lung and initiate a neoplastic differentiation. Indeed, while the deleterious effect of cigarette smoking has been demonstrated time and again, other causes of lung cancer also have been identified.

This volume, edited by the distinguished epidemiologist Jonathan M. Samet, is a comprehensive, perhaps even unique, treatise on the epidemiology of lung cancer. It assembles a roster of well-known contributors who have devoted years of scholarly work to one aspect or another of the epidemiology of this disease. Of course, all will note that the first chapter, titled "Introduction and Overview," is written by Sir Richard Doll, who published one of the 1950s reports cited above. Elsewhere, Sir Richard wrote "cast out one devil and seven others may enter." That is what has happened in the elucidation of the causes of lung cancer. This book tells the story of all those devils, but it also provides the ammunition that will help us to eliminate them . . . that is, if we only listen!

I am grateful to Dr. Samet and his colleagues for this very valuable contribution to the series of monographs *Lung Biology in Health and Disease*.

Claude Lenfant
Bethesda, Maryland

References

Doll, R., and Hill, A. B. (1950). Smoking and carcinoma of the lung. *Br. Med. J.* 2:739.

Ochsner, A., and DeBakey, M. (1941). Carcinoma of the lung. *Arch. Surg.* 42:209–258.

Wynder, E. L., and Graham, E. A. (1950). Tobacco smoking as a possible etiologic factor in bronchogenic carcinoma. *JAMA* 143:329–336.

PREFACE

Lung cancer, a rare malignancy at the start of the 20th century, has become a leading cause of death throughout the world. Epidemiological studies initiated during the 1940s and 1950s in response to evidence of a lung cancer "epidemic" quickly and convincingly established cigarette smoking as a potent causal factor. However, lung cancer has causes other than cigarette smoking: Exposure to arsenic, asbestos, chloromethyl ethers, radon progeny, and other agents in the workplace; outdoor air that has been contaminated by carcinogens generated by power plants, industry, and vehicles; indoor environments, such as homes, schools, and businesses, where radon is omnipresent, have all been linked to increased lung cancer risks. Even nonsmokers inhaling the smoke generated by active smoking are at some increased risk of lung cancer.

Environmental causes of lung cancer have been identified, but little is known about individual determinants of susceptibility. Cigarette smoking has been shown to interact synergistically with some occupational exposures; a family history of lung cancer is likewise associated with increased risk. Some factors may actually modify risks for smokers, including dietary intake of beta-carotene and other nutrients. New investigational techniques are providing insights into respiratory carcinogenesis and its underlying genetic mechanisms.

Thus, although epidemiological investigations have identified causes of lung cancer and provided sufficient data for potentially preventing the majority of cases, many research questions remain unanswered. Factors determining susceptibility to cigarette smoking have not been adequately characterized and the risks of some agents to which large numbers of people are exposed have not been described with sufficient certainty.

This book reviews the extensive epidemiological literature on lung cancer. Its chapters address each of the causes and the factors that may influence susceptibility. The resulting synthesis should serve those concerned with lung cancer from research, clinical, public health, and regulatory perspectives.

Chapter 1 traces the evolution of our understanding of the causes of lung cancer. The phenomenon of cigarette smoking and the toxicologic effects of tobacco smoke are described in Chapter 2, which includes an extensive new description of cigarette smoking in the United States. The emergence of lung cancer as a major public health problem is chronicled in Chapter 3. Chapter 4 selectively reviews the voluminous evidence on cigarette smoking and lung cancer.

Indoor and outdoor air pollution have also been linked to lung cancer. Environmental tobacco smoke, an indoor pollutant of great concern in developed countries, is covered in Chapter 5. Chapter 6 reviews more recent evidence on outdoor air pollution, a persistent concern in both developed and developing countries. Chapter 7 is devoted to a wide array of evidence on indoor air pollution and lung cancer in developing countries.

A series of chapters covers specific causal agents. Occupational agents that cause lung cancer include arsenic (Chap. 9), asbestos (Chap. 8), and radon (Chap. 10). Silica, a suspect occupational factor, is covered in Chapter 11. Chapter 12 is devoted to other agents.

Both environmental and host factors may influence lung cancer risk. Chapter 13 reviews the evidence on diet and lung cancer. The rapidly expanding information on the cellular and molecular biology of lung cancer is summarized in Chapter 14. Chapter 15 addresses the role of chronic lung disease as a risk factor. The cellular origins of lung cancer, the histologic classification of lung cancer, and the implications of histologic type for epidemiological research are covered in Chapter 16. Epidemiological information has guided the development of programs for control of lung cancer. Chapter 17 describes approaches to lung cancer prevention through smoking prevention and control. In conclusion, Chapter 18 discusses the complex interactions of tobacco smoking with other causes of lung cancer.

These chapters effectively cover the broad range of epidemiological information that is now available on lung cancer. The book should serve as a comprehensive source for researchers and everyone concerned with lung cancer prevention.

Jonathan M. Samet

CONTRIBUTORS

William J. Blot, Ph.D. Chief, Biostatistics Branch, National Cancer Institute, National Institutes of Health, Bethesda, Maryland

Paolo Boffetta, M.D., M.P.H. Unit of Analytical Epidemiology, International Agency for Research on Cancer, Lyon, France

David M. Burns, M.D. Professor of Medicine, Department of Medicine, Division of Pulmonary and Critical Care Medicine, University of California Medical Center, San Diego, California

Tim Byers, M.D., M.P.H. Chief, Chronic Disease Prevention, Division of Nutrition, National Center for Chronic Disease Prevention, Centers for Disease Control, Atlanta, Georgia

Andrew Churg, M.D., Ph.D. Professor, Department of Pathology, University of British Columbia, Vancouver, British Columbia, Canada

David B. Coultas, M.D. Associate Professor of Medicine, Pulmonary and

Critical Care Division, University of New Mexico School of Medicine, and the New Mexico Tumor Registry, Albuquerque, New Mexico

Sarah C. Darby, Ph.D. Staff Scientist, Cancer Epidemiology Unit, Imperial Cancer Research Fund, University of Oxford, Oxford, United Kingdom

Richard Doll, D.M., F.R.C.P., F.R.S. Professor, Imperial Cancer Research Fund, Cancer Studies Unit, University of Oxford, Oxford, United Kingdom

Peter Economou, M.D. Pulmonary Fellow, Department of Medicine, Pulmonary and Critical Care Division, University of New Mexico School of Medicine, Albuquerque, New Mexico

Joseph F. Fraumeni, Jr., M.D. Associate Director for Epidemiology and Biostatistics, National Cancer Institute, National Institutes of Health, Bethesda, Maryland

David F. Goldsmith, M.S.P.H., Ph.D. Senior Research Associate, Western Consortium for Public Health, Berkeley, California

Marianne Haenlein, Ph.D. Program Director, Data-Based Intervention Research Program, Division of Cancer Prevention and Control, National Cancer Institute, National Institutes of Health, Bethesda, Maryland

Janet M. Hughes, Ph.D. Professor, Biostatistics and Epidemiology, Tulane University School of Public Health and Tropical Medicine, New Orleans, Louisiana

John F. Lechner, Ph.D. Assistant Director, Molecular and Cellular Toxicology Group, Inhalation Toxicology Research Institute, Albuquerque, New Mexico

Youcheng Liu, M.E.H. Department of Environmental Health, Harvard School of Public Health, Boston, Massachusetts

Thomas J. Mason, Ph.D. Director, Epidemiologic Research, Division of Population Science, Fox Chase Cancer Center, Philadelphia, Pennsylvania

Göran Pershagen, M.D., Ph.D. Professor, Department of Epidemiology, Institute of Environmental Medicine, Karolinska Institute, Stockholm, Sweden

Jonathan M. Samet, M.D. Professor of Medicine, and Chief, Pulmonary and Critical Care Division, Department of Medicine, University of New Mexico

School of Medicine, and the New Mexico Tumor Registry, Albuquerque, New Mexico

Rodolfo Saracci, M.D. Chief, Unit of Analytical Epidemiology, International Agency for Research on Cancer, Lyon, France

Donald R. Shopland Coordinator, Smoking and Tobacco Control Program, National Cancer Institute, National Institutes of Health, Bethesda, Maryland

Kirk R. Smith, M.P.H., Ph.D. Senior Fellow, Program on Environment, East–West Center, Honolulu, Hawaii

Frank E. Speizer, M.D. Professor, Channing Laboratory, Department of Medicine, Brigham and Women's Hospital and Harvard Medical School, Boston, Massachusetts

Melvyn S. Tockman, M.D., Ph.D. Associate Professor, Environmental Health Sciences, The Johns Hopkins University School of Hygiene and Public Health, Baltimore, Maryland

Hans Weill, M.D. Professor of Medicine, Director, Center for Bioenvironmental Research, Department of Medicine, Section of Bioenvironmental Research, Tulane University Medical Center, New Orleans, Louisiana

Anna H. Wu-Williams, Ph.D. Associate Professor in Research, Preventive Medicine, University of Southern California School of Medicine, Los Angeles, California

CONTENTS

1

Introduction and Overview

SIR RICHARD DOLL

University of Oxford
Oxford, United Kingdom

Study of the epidemiology of lung cancer has been one of the most rewarding aspects of medical research in the past 40 years. It has shown how a disease that has become the most common type of cancer throughout the world (except, perhaps, for the easily treated nonmelanomatous cancers of the skin) (1) can be made to become relatively rare.

Few deaths were attributed to the disease until the 1920s, when it was noticed that in Europe and North America the numbers were beginning to increase, even after allowance was made for the increase in the proportion of people who lived to an age when cancers were likely to occur. But whether this was due to improved methods of diagnosis and the discovery of cases that would previously have been missed or to a genuine increase in the incidence of the disease at each specific age (or perhaps to both in combination) proved to be a source of controversy until after World War II. That this should have been so is easy enough to understand. Specialist chest clinics had only just begun to be established, and new methods of diagnosis were being rapidly introduced. Chest x-rays came into common use in the 1920s and bronchograms 10 years later, while bronchoscopy became widespread only when the flexible bronchoscope was introduced in the 1950s, and open chest surgery became generally practicable only when anesthesia was improved during World War II. More important still, pneumonia used to kill many people in the early stages of the disease, when it was difficult to diagnose clinically, before the introduction of sulfapyradine (the first effective antipneumococcal drug) in 1938 and tuberculosis was so common that it tended to be diagnosed whenever a patient presented with serious chest disease that was not obviously due to some other cause. Two factors, however, argued in favor of the increase being real: that the rate of increase was faster in men than in women and that in the autopsy records of many pathology departments increases were found in the proportion of cancers that had originated in the bronchi. To some investigators, such as Hoffman (2,3), a statistician employed by the Metropolitan Life Insurance Company in the United States, the evidence for a real increase was compelling, as it was for some chest surgeons. Pathologists, however, tended to be more skeptical (5–7), and in 1947, when the British Medical Research Council held a conference to consider the reasons for the increase, it was able to decide that research ought to be undertaken to seek for external causes, only on the grounds that it would be unwise to assume that the increase was wholly spurious (8).

I. Smoking

By this time, two ideas about the possible causes for a real increase in the incidence of the disease were current: increased smoking and increased atmospheric pollution.

That the disease might be caused by tobacco was suggested by Rottman in 1898 (9) to account for a cluster of cases that he had observed among tobacco workers in Leipzig, and it was mentioned again a decade later in Adler's monograph (10) on the disease. In the next 30 years, it was occasionally repeated by physicians (11–13) and surgeons (4,14) on the basis of their personal series, by pathologists (15) because of the tarry material in the smoke, and by statisticians (3) because of the contemporaneous increase in cigarette smoking and the mortality from the disease. Concrete evidence to support the idea was, however, weak. Roffo (16), in Argentina, had produced cancers on rabbit skin with tobacco tar as early as 1931 and had subsequently shown that the tar contained benzo(*a*)pyrene (17). His findings were, however, generally discounted on the grounds that the tar was obtained by distillation at temperatures well above those that occurred during smoking and the only other positive experimental findings were the production of isolated cancers on the skin of laboratory animals with tar from tobacco burned as in pipe smoking by Cooper et al. (18), Sugiura (19), and Flory (20). No remotely scientific human evidence was available until Müller (21) reported substantial differences between the smoking habits of people with and without the disease in Germany and Schairer and Schöniger (22) confirmed them.

Little notice was taken of these early epidemiological findings, or of Wassink's findings (23) in the Netherlands, and it was not until 1950, when five more case-control studies were reported in Britain and the United States, that the possibility that cigarette smoking might cause a substantial proportion of all lung cancers became a serious scientific issue. The principal results of these eight studies are listed in Table 1. Two of the studies carried particular weight, partly because so many cases were studied and partly because of the detailed methodology and the consideration given to other possible explanations of the results. One had been started by Wynder while still a medical student, because of "the knowledge that the burning of tobacco in pipes, or as cigars or cigarettes, could lead to the formation of cancer-causing chemicals" (29), and this led to the conclusion that "excessive and prolonged use of tobacco, especially cigarettes, seems to be an important factor in the induction of bronchogenic carcinoma" (27). The other had been instigated by the British Medical Research Council, with the support of Percy Stocks and Sir Ernest Kennaway (who thought, respectively, that the principal cause was likely to be atmospheric pollution and cigarette smoke), and this led to the conclusion that "smoking is a factor, and an important factor, in the production of carcinoma of the lung" (28).

These conclusions about the carcinogenicity of tobacco smoke were not based solely on the simple quantitative association shown in Table 1, but on a detailed consideration of the total evidence along the lines subsequently set out by Hill (30) in his Cutter lecture. The results, it was shown, could not easily be explained by bias or by confounding with some other factor likely to cause the disease. The relative risk associated with heavy smoking was very high (more than 25-fold compared with that in lifelong nonsmokers in both studies); there were plausible biological relationships between the relative risk of developing the disease and the individual's smoking habits (amount smoked, method of smoking, age at starting to smoke, and age at stopping), and the ecological evidence showed

Table 1 Smoking and Lung Cancer: Early Case-Control Studies

No. of men		Percent of nonsmokers		Percent of heavy smokers		
with lung cancer	without lung cancer	with lung cancer	without lung cancer	with lung cancer	without lung cancer	Ref.
86	86	3.5	16.3	65	36	21
93	270	3.2	15.9	52	27	22
134	100	4.5	19.0	55	19	23
82	522	14.6	23.9	18	9	24
444	430	7	31	—	—	25
236	481	15.3	21.7	—	—	26
605	780	1.3	14.6	51	19	27
649	649	0.3	4.2	26	13	28

clear correlations between the number of cigarettes smoked and sex, place, and time.

Even so, the conclusions were initially controversial. That smoking was an important cause of the disease was accepted immediately by Sir Harold Himsworth, then Secretary of the British Medical Research Council (31), and formally by the Council itself in 1957 (32), but it was not for several more years that it became widely accepted by physicians and by government departments (e.g., Refs. 33, 34). By this time, the results of the case-control studies had been reproduced in several other countries, and results were also available from studies of a different type designed to test the prediction that the risk of the disease increased *pari passu* with the amount smoked by obtaining smoking histories from large numbers of men and women and then following them up to see who died of the disease. These provided quantitatively almost identical results (35–38) and convinced most scientists, apart from Berkson and Sir Ronald Fisher, of the validity of the conclusion.

Berkson, the most eminent medical statistician in the United States, argued that you could draw no conclusions from case-control studies of patients admitted to the hospital or from the early cohort studies. The first were invalidated because the risk of admission might be increased if the putative causal factor was also present, and the second by the failure to recruit a truly random population. The volunteers who did respond might, he thought, include a disproportionate number of heavy smokers who were already suffering from the early effects of the disease (39). Such a bias would, of course, wear off in a few years; but in fact the converse happened, and the quantitative relationship with the amount smoked became stronger as the cohort study was prolonged.

Fisher was the leading theoretical statistician of his day, and he was unwilling to accept the conclusion because of the lack of a relationship with inhaling, which in his opinion was a biological necessity if smoking caused the disease (see Ref. 40). He noted that monozygous twins tended to have similar smoking habits and consequently suggested that genetic factors caused an individual both to want to smoke and to be unusually susceptible to the disease. His criticisms of the epidemiological findings ignored all but the first report by Doll and Hill (28) and failed to recognize that self-reported inhaling was very imprecise and that, without knowledge of the size of the droplet that carried the carcinogen at different stages of respiration, nothing could be said about the effect that alteration in the rate and depth of respiration might have on the extent and rate of its deposition (41,42). As it turned out, inhaling was subsequently found to be associated with an increased risk of peripheral tumors and a deceased risk of central tumors (43), and deep inhaling was shown to cause the bronchi to be relatively spared (44). Eventually, too, Fisher's unattractive hypothesis was disproved by a follow-up study of twins with different smoking habits, which showed that the differences in risk between smokers and nonsmokers and between heavy and light smokers were much the same in monozygous twins as in dizygous twins and in the general population—based, however, on very small numbers (45).

No one would suggest that observational data alone could provide proof of causation in the strict logical sense. They can, however, provide proof beyond a reasonable doubt and consequently grounds for assuming for all practical purposes that the observed relationship is causal. Experiments that show that the agent can cause cancer in animals strengthen the evidence, as happened when Wynder et al. (46) showed that tar obtained from the smoke of cigarettes burned at the temperatures that occur in normal smoking caused cancer of the skin when painted on the skin of mice; they do not, however, alter it qualitatively. The conclusion still must be tested in practice by reducing exposure to the agent and seeing if the risk of the disease is correspondingly reduced, something that was soon shown to happen in British doctors (47) and later in whole national populations.

II. Atmospheric Pollution

The alternative explanation that was most favored as a possible reason for the increase in lung cancer was that it was due to atmospheric pollution, principally coal smoke but also possibly the pollution caused by the exhaust fumes of lorries and cars. This alternative idea was supported by the common finding that the disease was more prevalent in towns than in the countryside and that the mortality in towns increased *pari passu* with the size of their population (48), the range varying from one and a half to four times in different countries. That coal smoke might be the principal cause was an attractive idea, as smoke was visible, plentiful, and unpleasant and, moreover, was known to contain many polycyclic hydrocarbons, which were the first chemicals to be shown to be carcinogenic in animal experiments. The idea was not, however, attractive epidemiologically for three reasons. First, the amount of coal burned had increased only slightly since 1900 and an increasing proportion was being burned more efficiently and with less smoke production than in domestic grates by an increasing tendency to burn it in large plants to provide gas and electricity for domestic use. Second, there was no evident reason why men should be more affected by general atmospheric pollution than women. Third, the increase in the disease was not limited to smoky areas, but was also marked in countries like Switzerland where smoke pollution was relatively slight. Pollution caused by the exhaust fumes of cars and the tarring of roads fitted better the temporal trend in mortality, but the idea that it might be the principal cause of the disease was not supported when men whose occupation kept them mostly on the roads failed to show any excess risk (49).

Once the strong relationship with smoking had been observed, the question then arose whether the urban excess could be accounted for by differences in the rate of spread of cigarette smoking in urban and rural areas. Early studies quickly showed that urban populations certainly smoked more than rural ones and that differences in risk between urban and rural residents who currently smoked the same amounts were relatively small. All were consistent with the idea that atmospheric pollution and cigarette smoking might act synergistically to increase the other's effects, but none showed any major difference in the incidence of the disease in nonsmokers (50,51), and it was clear that of the two suspect agents only tobacco had any major effect when acting on its own. In these circumstances, it was impossible to be sure about the quantitative effect of atmospheric pollution and indeed about whether it would have any detectable effect in the absence of smoking, because of the impossibility of allowing adequately for the totality of an individual's smoking history, including in particular the amount likely to have been smoked early in life.

An alternative approach to estimating the effect of atmospheric pollution was to extrapolate from the experience of men who were exposed to large amounts of polycyclic hydrocarbons in the course of their work, on the assumption that the risk of developing lung cancer produced by the combustion products of fossil fuels was proportional to the amount of (say) benzo(*a*)pyrene in those products to which they were exposed. With this method Pike et al. (52) estimated that 1 ng benzo(*a*)pyrene/m^3 in city air might result in the annual production of 4 cases per 10^{-6} men aged 40–70 years with average British smoking habits, again on the assumption that the polycyclic hydrocarbons in city air act synergistically with tobacco smoke. Since as much as 30–40 ng of benzo(*a*)pyrene/m^3 had been commonly present in the air of big cities, this implied that atmospheric pollution might have contributed to some 10% of the lung cancers from which their populations suffered, and a very similar conclusion was reached by the International Task Group on Air Pollution and Cancer (53): namely, that "combustion products of fossil fuels in ambient air, probably acting together with cigarette smoke, have been responsible for cases of lung cancer in large urban areas, the number produced being of the order of 5–10 cases per 100,000 males per year (European Standard Population)." Both these estimates related to times when the average concentration of benzo(*a*)pyrene in city air was an order of magnitude greater than it has been in Western Europe and North America for the last 20 years and estimates of the current risk would, therefore, be much smaller.

Whether such extrapolation is justifiable is a matter of debate, as the biological activity of polycyclic hydrocarbons in the hot fumes to which industrial workers may be exposed could be quite different from that of the hydrocarbons attached to smoke particles in urban air. Difficult though it is to make direct epidemiological observations on people exposed to the types of pollution that actually occur in towns or—as now appears to be a greater hazard—from the combustion of fuel in unventilated houses in some developing countries (54), there may be no better way of establishing its effect.

III. Occupational Hazards

The local pollution that is liable to cause an occupational hazard was, and is, a very different matter. By 1950, when the definitive studies on smoking were completed, a hazard of lung cancer had been established only in the cobalt mines of Schneeberg and Jachymov, where the hazard from radon had been so great that some 50% of all the miners died from the disease (Ref. 55, for review). Hazards had, however, been suspected from the manufacture of coal gas (56), exposure to asbestos (57) and arsenic (58,59), the manufacture of chromates (60), and the refining of nickel (61), and all these hazards were shown to be causes of the disease within the next few years (62–68).

Since then many other agents have come under suspicion, but relatively few have been shown unequivocally to cause the disease. Those that have, like five of the six hazards that were established or suspected before 1950, have been detected either because the risk was so great that a cluster of cases attracted clinical attention or because the agent to which the workers were exposed was already known to cause cancer in humans in another organ or to cause the disease in animals. The one exception, asbestos, was thought to be a likely cause of the disease because of the autopsy finding that lung cancer was more commonly associated with asbestosis than with any other form of pneumoconiosis. None of the established causes can be said to have been discovered specifically by epidemiological enquiry, although it has on rare occasions drawn attention to a situation where a known hazard was subsequently found to occur, as in the fluorspar mines of Newfoundland, which were found to have high concentrations of radon in their air. What epidemiology has done is to establish that some of the suspected agents do, in fact, cause lung cancer and to show that the methods subsequently adopted to prevent the disease have been successful. Often, too, it has shown that other agents either do not cause the disease or cause it so infrequently that the risk is too small to be detected.

This last conclusion may, however, be very unsatisfactory when the background risk from smoking is so high that quite material risks in absolute terms can fail to be detected unless large numbers at risk have been observed for many years. The need to detect real risks that may be relatively small in comparison with a high background risk in the general population has, in consequence, been a powerful stimulus to improve epidemiological techniques for relating risk quantitatively to measures of exposure (by, for example, the use of nested case-control studies) and to encourage international collaboration so as to increase the numbers of workers under observation and to reduce the relative importance of random variation. Even so, the verdict, in relation to several agents that have been found to cause cancer experimentally in animals, continues to remain open.

IV. Ionizing Radiation

Sometimes, as when attempts have been made to assess the effects of general atmospheric pollution, measures of the risk of exposure to occupational hazards have been used to deduce the effects of the much smaller doses of the same agents to which the population may be exposed in the general environment. Estimates have been made in this way of the effects of the minute amounts of arsenic and asbestos that are commonly found in city air and to the effects of the more common polycyclic hydrocarbons, and recently the same method has been extended to estimate the effect of the relatively much greater amounts of radon to which, it is now realized, many people may be exposed in their homes.

Minute amounts of radon are liberated to the atmosphere from the combustion of coal, and substantial increases in radioactivity were observed under the weather conditions that caused both coal smoke and the radon associated with it, together with that diffusing from buildings and the soil, to be retained near the surface of the earth. Under these conditions, Anderson et al. (69) found the concentration of radon on the first day of the great London smog of December 1952 to be 400 times that previously recorded on a clear sunny day. It is hardly surprising, therefore, that even the very crude estimate of risk associated with the Schneeberg and Jachymov mines that was available in 1950 could lead to the conclusion that in Britain radon might "be a significant cause of lung cancer" (70).

With the disappearance of coal smoke from the cities of much of the developed world, the discovery that the natural radon that is trapped in houses may vary more than 100-fold, and the realization that the average dose received at home is about twice as great as had previously been assumed, interest in the effects of radon on the general population has shifted from the effects of urban pollution to the effects of natural radon in the home, and renewed attempts have been made to estimate its effects by extrapolation from the experience of those occupationally exposed in mines.

Much more data are now available for exposed miners than was the case in the 1950s, but even so the process of extrapolation requires many assumptions about the nature of the observed risk for which the epidemiological evidence is still extremely weak. The assumptions made by the U.S. National Research Council (71) have led to the conclusion that natural radon in houses may be responsible for about 10% of all cases of lung cancer in the United States and 6% in Britain, where the average level in houses is substantially lower; in both countries on the assumption that it acts mainly in conjunction with cigarette smoking. Many of the

Research Council's assumptions are, however, open to question, including, for example, the relative tissue doses from the same concentrations of radon in the dusty air of mines and at home, the relative doses with the different rates of breathing at work and at home, the linearity of the dose-response relationship over the wide range of doses and dose rates observed, the relative effects of exposure at different ages and at different times after exposure has ceased, and the extent to which radon and tobacco smoke modify one another's reactions.

New evidence is leading to assumptions in which we can have progressively greater confidence (72,73), but it is unlikely to close completely the gap between the conditions in mines and those at home, and we can hope to be confident about the effects of natural radon under the conditions to which people are normally exposed only by direct observation of the relative risk of residence in different houses, such as is now being sought in many epidemiological enquiries.

V. Other Factors

Of lung cancer it might be said, as it used to be said of syphilis, that anyone who knew all about it knew medicine. Clinically the disease can present in so many ways that its differential diagnosis includes an immense number of other diseases, and epidemiologically an equally wide variety of risk factors has, at one time or another, been associated with its causation or prevention. These risk factors have included, apart from the many referred to earlier, previous respiratory disease (the scars left by tuberculosis and productive cough), viral infection (an increased risk in butchers and the owners of parrots), genetic susceptibility, and diet.

Genetic susceptibility was from the earliest days recognized to be a factor that might influence the risk of developing the disease—it was even suggested that a hereditary factor concentrated by in-breeding might account for the enormously high incidence in the miners of Schneeberg and Jachymov—but it clearly could not explain the geographical and temporal variation that had come to be observed in the first half of this century. Nor was there any reason to think that people could be divided sharply into two classes: those who were liable to develop the disease and those who were not. Had this been so, some evidence of attenuation of the population at risk should have been seen with increasing age in heavy smokers, whereas the incidence continued to rise steadily at least to 75 years of age, by which time 30% of heavy smokers were estimated to develop it in the absence of other causes of death (74). This did not mean that differences in genetic susceptibility did not occur, but only that there was no evidence of a simple dichotomy that would encourage the belief that the great majority of people could regard themselves as immune—something that was commonly suggested because "only" 10% or so of cigarette smokers died of the disease. That one person dies of lung cancer at 50 years of age while another exposed to the same environment develops it at 70 and a third lives on to 90 without developing it at all is no more an indication of genetic differences in susceptibility than the fact that a cancer does not appear in the left lung for 20 years after a successful pneumonectomy for cancer in the right. Luck accounts for the difference in outcome in the two lungs by determining the concatenation of events that brings about the required number of specific changes in an individual cell at a particular time, and it may similarly account for much of the difference in the age of onset in different people.

Demonstration of genetic differences that affect individual susceptibility has not been easy, partly because of the difficulty of separating the hereditary and social factors that cause members of the same family to have similar smoking habits and partly because of the effect that smoking itself may have on the induction of enzymes that affect the metabolism of carcinogens and procarcinogens in vivo. Progress in unraveling these differences has, however, recently been made, and there can be no doubt that some differences exist in individual susceptibility to the induction of the disease.

Diet, by contrast, was not suspected of playing any part until Bjelke (75) reported that the risk of lung cancer in a Norwegian cohort varied with an index of consumption of vitamin A irrespective of the amount smoked. This seminal observation stimulated interest in the role of micronutrients in human cancer in general, but, as so often happens, continued observation showed that the difference observed between different categories was much less than was originally reported (76). Vitamin A, too, seems less likely to be a protective factor than beta-carotene, which is partly converted to vitamin A in vivo and was, in Bjelke's first study, included within his vitamin A index. Whether beta-carotene itself or some other micronutrient with which it is associated in food is the active agent can, perhaps, be determined only by means of the sort of controlled trial with random allocation of treatments that Hennekens and Eberlein (77) are now carrying out with the collaboration of 20,000 U.S. physicians. There is, however, no doubt that some components of the diet associated with beta-carotene, if not beta-carotene itself, can have a material effect in reducing the incidence of the disease.

VI. Conclusion

Epidemiology, as a subject, has had its ups and downs. From being the favored and indeed almost the only technique available for discovering the causes of disease, it was thought to have been relegated to the scrapbook of history by the development of laboratory science and the brilliant discoveries of biochemistry, microbiology, and experimental pathology. Epidemiology is certainly a poor tool for learning about the mechanism by which a disease is produced, but it has the tremendous advantage that it focuses on the diseases and the deaths that actually occur, and experience has shown that it continues to be second to none as a means of discovering links in the chain of causation that are capable of being broken. For no disease has this been more evident than for cancer of the lung. A great deal still remains to be learned about the cellular changes that lead to the appearance of malignant bronchial clone and about the quantitative effect of small amounts of agents that clearly cause the disease when the amounts are large. Epidemiology has, however, already taught us enough for it to be possible to ensure that lung cancer ceases to be the most common form of fatal cancer throughout the world and that it returns to the place it occupied in the nineteenth century among the least common human cancers, if society is prepared to act on the knowledge obtained.

References

1. Parkin, D. M., Läärä, E., and Muir, C. S. (1988) Estimates of the worldwide frequency of sixteen major cancers in 1980. *Int. J. Cancer* 41:184–197.
2. Hoffman, F. L. (1928). Cancer of the lungs. *Am. Rev. Tuberc.* 19:392–406.
3. Hoffman, F. L. (1931). Cancer and smoking habits. *Ann. Surg.* 32:50–67.
4. Ochsner, A., and De Bakey, M. (1939). Symposium on cancer. Primary pulmonary malignancy. Treatment by total pneumonectomy: Analyses of 79 collected cases and presentation of 7 personal cases. *Surg. Gyn. Obst.* 68:435–451.
5. Steiner, P. E. (1944). Incidence of primary carcinoma of lung with special reference to its increase. *Arch. Path.* 37:185.
6. Willis, R. A. (1948). *Pathology of Tumours*. London, Butterworth.
7. Rigdon, R. H., and Kirchoff, H. (1952). Consideration of some of the theories relative to etiology and incidence of lung cancer. *Texas Rep. Biol. Med.* 10:76–91.
8. Cuthbertson, D. (1967). Historical notes on the origin of the association between lung cancer and smoking. *J. Physicians Coll.* 2:191–196.
9. Rottman, H. (1898). *Über primäre Lungencarcinoma*. Inaugural dissertation, Universität Würzburg.
10. Adler, I. (1912). *Primary Malignant Growths of the Lung and Bronchi*. London, Longmans Green & Co.
11. Tylecote, F. E. (1927). Cancer of the lung. *Lancet* 2:256–257.
12. Lickint, F. (1930). Tabak und Tabakrauch als ätiologischer Faktor des Carcinoms. *Z. Krebsforsch* 30:349–365.
13. Arkin, A., and Wagner, D. H. (1936). Primary carcinoma of the lung. *JAMA* 106:587–591.
14. Ochsner, A., and De Bakey, M. (1941). Carcinoma of the lung. *Ann. Surg.* 42:209–258.
15. McNally, W. D. (1932). The tar in cigarette smoke audits possible effects. *Am. J. Cancer* 63:1114.
16. Roffo, A. H. (1937). Der Tabak als krebserzeugende Agens. *Dtsch. Med. Wochnschr.* 63:1267–1271.
17. Roffo, A. H., (1939). Krebseizeugendes Benzpyren gewonnen aus Tabakteer. *Z. Krebsforsch.* 49:588–597.
18. Cooper, E. A., Lamb, F. W. M., Sanders, E., and Hirst, E. L. (1932). The role of tobacco-smoking in the production of cancer. *J. Hyg. Lond.* 32:293–300.

19. Sugiura, K. (1940). Observations on animals painted with tobacco tars. *Am. J. Cancer* 38:41.
20. Flory, C. M. (1941). Production of tumors by tobacco tars. *Cancer Res.* 1:262–276.
21. Müller, F. H. (1939). Tabakmissbrauch und Lungencarcinom. *Z. Krebsforsch.* 49: 57–85.
22. Schairer, E., and Schöniger, E. (1943). Lungenkrebs und Tabakverbrauch. *Z. Krebsforsch.* 54:261–269.
23. Wassink, W. F. (1948). Onstaansvoorwasrden voor Longkanker. *Med. Tijdschr. Geneesk.* 92:3732–3747.
24. Schrek, R., Baker, L. A., Ballard, G. P., and Dolgoff, S. (1950). Tobacco smoking as an etiologic factor in disease: Cancer. *Cancer Res.* 10:49–58.
25. Mills, C. A., and Porter, M. M. (1950). Tobacco smoking habits and cancer of the mouth and respiratory system. *Cancer Res.* 10:539–542.
26. Levin, M. L., Goldstein, H., and Gerhardt, P. R. (1950). Cancer and tobacco smoking. *JAMA* 143:336–338.
27. Wynder, E. L., and Graham, E. A. (1950). Tobacco smoking as a possible etiologic factor in bronchogenic carcinoma. *JAMA* 143:329–336.
28. Doll, R., and Hill, A. B. (1950). Smoking and carcinoma of the lung. *Br. Med. J. 2:739.*
29. *Wynder, E. L. (1988). Tobacco and health: A review of the history and suggestions for public health policy. Public Health* 103:8–17.
30. Hill, A. B. (1953). Observation and experiment. *N. Engl. J. Med.* 248:995–1001.
31. Webster, C. (1984). Tobacco smoking addiction: A challenge to the National Health Service. *Br. J. Addict.* 79:7–16.
32. Medical Research Council. (1957). Tobacco smoking and cancer of the lung. *B. Med. J.* 1:1523.
33. Royal College of Physicians. (1962). *Smoking and Health.* London, Pitman Medical Publishing Co. Ltd.
34. Advisory Committee to the Surgeon General of the U.S. Public Health Service (1964). *Smoking and Health.* Washington, DC, Public Health Service Publication No. 1103, U.S. Government Printing Office.
35. Doll, R., and Hill, A. B. (1954). The mortality of doctors in relation to their smoking habits. A preliminary report. *Br. Med. J.* 1:1451–1455.
36. Doll, R., and Hill, A. B. (1956). Lung cancer and other causes of death in relation to smoking. *Br. Med. J.* 2:1071–1076.
37. Hammond, E. C., and Horn, D. (1954). The relationship between human smoking habits and death rates: A follow-up study of 187,766 men. *JAMA* 154:1316–1328.
38. Hammond, E. C., and Horn, D. (1958). Smoking and death rates: Report on forty four months of follow-up of 187,783 men. *JAMA* 166:1159–1172, 1294–1308.
39. Berkson, J. (1955). The statistical study of association between smoking and lung cancer. *Proc. Staff Meetings Mayo Clin.* 30:319–348.
40. Stolley, P. D. (1991). When genius errs; RA Fisher and the lung cancer controversy. *Am. J. Epidemiol.* 133:416–425.
41. Davies, C. N. (1949). Inhalation risk and particle size in dust and mist. *Br. J. Ind. Med.* 6:245.

42. Davies, C. N. (1957). Dangers of cigarette smoking. *Br. Med. J.* 2:410.
43. Doll, R., and Hill, A. B. (1952). A study of the aetiology of carcinoma of the lung. *Br. Med. J.* 2:1271–1286.
44. Wald, N. J., Boreham, J., and Bailey, A. (1984) Relative intakes of tar, nicotine and carbon monoxide from cigarettes of different yields. *Thorax* 39:361–364.
45. Floderus, B., Cederlöf, R., and Friberg, L. (1988). Smoking and mortality: A 21 year follow-up based on the Swedish Twin Registry. *Int. J. Epidemiol.* 17:332–340.
46. Wynder, E. L., Graham, E. A., and Croninger, A. B. (1955). Experimental production of carcinoma with cigarette tar. *Cancer Res.* 15:445.
47. Doll, R., and Hill, A. B. (1964). Mortality in relation to smoking: Ten years' observations of British doctors. *Br. Med. J.* 1:1399–1414, 1460–1467.
48. Stocks, P. (1952). Epidemiology of cancer of lung in England and Wales. *Br. J. Cancer* 6:99.
49. Doll, R. (1953). Bronchial carcinoma: Incidence and aetiology. *Br. Med. J.* 2:521–527, 585–590.
50. Doll, R. (1978). Atmospheric pollution and lung cancer. *Environ. Health Perspect.* 22:23–31.
51. Friberg, L., and Cederlöf, R. (1978). Late effects of air pollution with special reference to lung cancer. *Environ. Health Perspect.* 22:45.
52. Pike, M. C., Gordon, R. J., Henderson, B. E., Menck, H. R., and Soohoo, J. (1975). Air pollution. In *Persons at High Risk of Cancer: An Approach to Cancer Etiology and Control*. Edited by J. F. Fraumeni. New York, Academic Press.
53. International Task Group on Air Pollution and Cancer. (1978). Air pollution and cancer: Risk assessment methodology and epidemiological evidence. *Environ. Health Perspect.* 22:1–12.
54. Chen, B. H., Hong, C. J., Pandey, M. R., and Smith, K. R. (1990). Indoor air pollution in developing countries. *World Health Stat. Q.* 43:127–138.
55. Lorenz, E. (1944). Radioactivity and lung cancer: Critical review of lung cancer in miners of Schneeberg and Joachimstaal. *JNCI* 5:1–15.
56. Kennaway, E. L., and Kennaway, N. M. (1947). A further study of the incidence of cancer of the lung and larynx. *Br. J Cancer* 1:260.
57. Merewether, E. R. A. (1949). *Annual Report of the Chief Inspector of Factories for the Year 1947*. London, Her Majesty's Stationery Office, p. 45.
58. Hill, A. B., and Faning, E. L. (1948). Studies in the incidence of cancer in a factory handling inorganic compounds of arsenic: I. Mortality experience in the factory. *Br. J. Ind. Med.* 5:1–7.
59. Perry, K., Bowler, R. G., Buckell, H. M., Druett, H. A., and Schilling, R. S. F. (1948). Studies in the incidence of cancer in a factory handling inorganic compounds of arsenic. II. Clinical and environmental investigations. *Br. J. Ind. Med.* 5:7–15.
60. Machle, W., and Gregorius, F. (1948). Cancer of the respiratory tract in the United States chromate producing industry. *Public Health Rep. (Wash.)* 63:1114.
61. Amor, A. J. (1939). *Bericht über den VIII internationalen Kongress für Unfallmedizin und Berufskrankheiten*. Frankfurt am Main, September 1938. Leipzig, Thieme.
62. Gloyne, S. R. (1951). Pneumoconiosis: Historical survey of necropsy material in 1205 cases. *Lancet* 1:810–814.

63. Doll, R. (1952). The causes of death among gasworkers with special reference to cancers of the lung. *Br. J. Ind. Med.* 9:180.
64. Doll, R. (1955a). Mortality from lung cancer in asbestos workers. *Br. J. Ind. Med.* 12: 81–86.
65. Doll, R. (1958). Cancer of the lung and nose in nickel workers. *Br. J. Ind. Med.* 15: 217–223.
66. Brinton, H. P., Frasier, F. S., and Koven, A. L. (1952). Morbidity and mortality experience among chromate workers. *Public Health Rep. (Wash.)* 67:835.
67. Morgan, J. G. (1958). Some observations on the incidence of respiratory cancer in nickel workers. *Br. J. Ind. Med.* 15:224–234.
68. Lee, A. M., and Fraumeni, J. F. (1969). Arsenic and respiratory cancer in men: An occupational study. *JNCI* 42:1046–1052.
69. Anderson, W., Mayneord, W. V., and Turner, R. C. (1954). The radon content of the atmosphere. *Nature* 174:424.
70. Doll, R. (1955b). Etiology of lung cancer. In *Advances in Cancer Research*, Vol. 3. Edited by J. P. Greenstein and A. Haddow. New York: Academic Press Inc., pp. 1–50.
71. National Research Council. (1988). *Health Risks of Radon and Other Internally Deposited Alpha-Emitters. BEIR IV.* Washington, D.C., National Academy Press.
72. National Research Council. (1991). *Comparative Dosimetry of Radon in Mines and Homes*. Washington, D.C., National Academy Press.
73. Darby, S., and Doll, R. (1991).Radon in houses: How big is the risk? *Radiat. Prot. Aust.* (in press).
74. Pike, M. C., and Doll, R. (1965). Age at onset of lung cancer: Significance in relation to effect of smoking. *Lancet* 1:665–668.
75. Bjelke, E. (1975). Dietary vitamin A and human lung cancer. *Int. J. Cancer* 15: 561–565.
76. Kvåle, G., Bjelke, E., and Gart, J. J. (1983). Dietary habits and lung cancer risk. *Int. J. Cancer* 31:397–405.
77. Hennekens, C. H., and Eberlein, K. A. (1985). A randomized trial of aspirin and beta-carotene among U.S. physicians. *Prev. Med.* 14:165–168.

2

Tobacco Smoking

DAVID M. BURNS

University of California Medical Center
San Diego, California

I. Introduction

Tobacco use in the Americas predates the arrival of Columbus (1) in the new world, but the social context of its use among native Americans was largely ceremonial and religious in contrast to the regular and continuous use that characterizes current cigarette smoking. A substantial European market for American tobacco developed following the colonization of the new world. Tobacco was a major cash crop for the new American colonies and a major component of the economy of the United States after it became independent. In Europe and the American colonies, tobacco use was incorporated into daily life in a pattern of regular and relatively continuous use throughout the day, distinct from the pattern of use by native Americans. However, the forms of tobacco being used were largely snuff, chewing tobacco, pipes, and cigars. Tobacco has been consumed as cigarettes primarily during the twentieth century. In the United States during 1870, 102 million pounds of tobacco were used in producing chewing tobacco and snuff and 1.18 billion cigars were manufactured, in contrast to only 16 million cigarettes (1). By the turn of the century, some 30 years later, the production of chewing tobacco and snuff had tripled and the production of cigars had increased fivefold, whereas the production of cigarettes had increased 300-fold, setting the stage for the explosive growth of cigarette smoking that occurred in the current century.

The development of a machine in 1881 that could manufacture cigarettes, along with the invention of safety matches, allowed the convenient use of tobacco as cigarettes and provided the technology to introduce cigarettes to the marketplace. However, it was the introduction of mass marketing techniques on a national level that led to the dramatic rise in cigarette consumption during the first two decades of this century (2) (Fig. 1).

Coincident with this growth in cigarette use, the type and processing of the tobacco used in cigarettes changed. Initially cigarette tobacco was simply cigar tobacco cut more finely. Around the turn of the century, a milder tobacco leaf that was flue cured became the predominant product used in cigarettes. This change in the characteristics of the tobacco in cigarettes caused a marked increase in the disease risks that result from smoking. Tobacco smoke produced by the tobaccos in pipes and cigars is both harsher and more alkaline than that produced by cigarettes; thus, pipe and cigar smokers are less likely to inhale smoke into the lung (3). The lower pH of cigarette smoke also decreases the absorption of nicotine, the active addictive agent in tobacco smoke, across the oral mucosa so that inhalation of the smoke into the lung is required to facilitate the absorption of nicotine (4). Along with nicotine, a large number of other toxic and carcinogenic compounds in cigarette smoke are inhaled, deposited in the airways and alveoli, and absorbed into the body. It is this increased deposition and absorp-

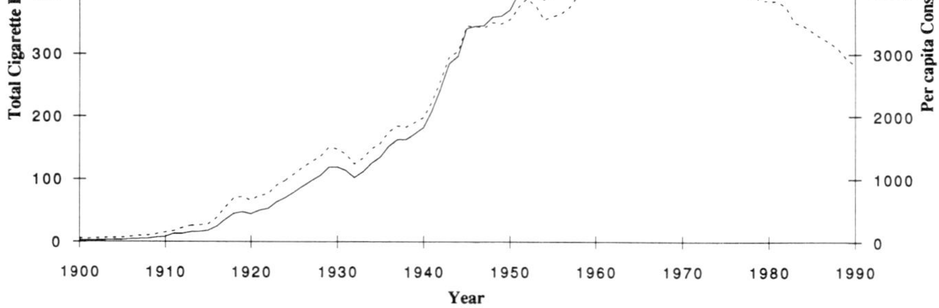

Figure 1 Total and per capita cigarette consumption in the United States, 1900–1990.

tion in the lung of disease-causing agents that makes the use of cigarettes significantly more hazardous than pipes or cigars.

II. Tobacco Leaf and Cigarette Manufacture

The tobacco plant used in U.S. cigarettes is *Nicotiana tabacum*. Tobacco plants are sprayed with "casing," a sauce composed of sugars, humectants, and flavoring agents, prior to harvesting and are then "cured" by air drying (burley) or, more commonly, by using artificial heat (flue curing) (5). The tobacco leaf is then processed into sheets, mixed with a variety of additives to improve the taste, burn rate, and other characteristics of the tobacco, and chopped to make cigarettes. The specific additives used by each manufacturer are considered proprietary secrets and are neither generally known nor publicly evaluated for their potential toxicity.

The tobacco is wrapped in a tube of paper and a filter of cellulose acetate is often attached to the end. The filter may contain other materials such as charcoal and may be designed with air channels or holes to entrain air. The location and size of these air channels may alter the tar yield of the cigarette under different conditions of smoking. The machine-measured tar yield (see Sec. III) reported by the Federal Trade Commission is measured with these channels open, but smokers may crush or occlude the channels with their lips resulting in markedly higher tar yields (6). In comparison with nonfiltered cigarettes, filtered cigarettes have less tar and nicotine, but may have the same or higher yield of carbon monoxide (7).

III. Cigarette Smoke Chemistry

Cigarette smoke is a complex aerosol classified as mainstream or sidestream smoke that is made up of the distillation and combustion products from the burning of tobacco. Mainstream smoke is produced at a high temperature (up to 950°C) as air is drawn through the column of tobacco in the cigarette (5). It is the predominant source of smoke exposure for the active smoker. Sidestream smoke, produced at lower temperatures (350°C) (8) during the smoldering of the cigarette between puffs, is the major source of environmental tobacco smoke, the smoke inhaled during passive smoking. For analytic purposes, the particulate and gas phases of the smoke are mostly commonly separated using a glass-fiber filter pad stabilized with an organic binder (Cambridge filter method) (5). This filter removes 99.7% of those particles 0.1 μm in diameter or larger, but does not completely separate solid and gaseous components of smoke, as some gases are retained with the precipitated particles (9). Tar is the total particulate matter of the smoke after nicotine and water have been removed. The compounds remaining after removal of the particulate phase constitute the vapor phase of smoke.

The most widely used approach for measuring the tar yield of cigarettes is that of the Federal Trade Commission (10). This approach uses a machine to draw a 35-ml puff from the cigarette over 2 s with a bell-shape flow profile. The cigarettes are puffed once every 2 min and are smoked to a butt length of 23 mm (nonfiltered cigarettes) or 3 mm longer than the filter overwrap (filter-tipped cigarettes). These parameters were established in 1967 when the majority of cigarettes were predominantly nonfiltered and of relatively uniform construction (10). Since then, a variety of changes have been made in the cigarette-manufacturing process that probably changed the validity of machine-measured tar yields as an indicator of the actual yield received during active smoking. Changes in the length of the cigarette, the porosity of the paper, the design of the filter, and the length of the overwrap can all change the measured tar yield, even if the tobacco used in the cigarette is unchanged. There are substantial differences among different brands of cigarettes in these characteristics, and the characteristics of specific brands have frequently changed over time. Information on these changes is maintained only by the cigarette manufactures.

The chemical composition of mainstream smoke and the ratios of the concentrations of constituents in mainstream to sidestream smoke can vary substantially from one cigarette to another (11) and with the pattern of smoking (12). One overall measure of mainstream smoke characteristics—the machine-measured tar yield of U.S. cigarettes—has declined from a sales-weighted average of 35 mg in 1957 to the current yield of approximately 13 mg (13). The sales-weighted tar yield decline has resulted from both a reduction in tar yields of particular brands of cigarettes over time and a shift in the market share of individual brands to favor those with lower tar yield. There has been little further decline in sales-weighted tar yields since 1980. This decline in sales-weighted tar and nicotine content of U.S. cigarettes over time is the result of technical changes in the manufacturing process, such as the addition of filters in the early 1950s, as well as reductions in the amount of tobacco contained in each cigarette. The changes during the mid-1950s and early 1960s were often the result of putting less tobacco leaf in each cigarette by including stems and by "puffing" the reconstituted tobacco sheets used to make cigarettes (12). These changes may have reduced the actual tar exposures of individuals smoking these cigarettes. However, more recent changes have been designed to lower the machine-measured yields without necessarily reducing the tar received by the smoker. Cigarettes with machine-measured yields of 0.01 mg tar (essentially no mainstream smoke) have been manufactured using holes and channels in the filter that allow air to be drawn in during machine smoking, but which are occluded when smoked by the smoker (6). When these cigarettes are smoked by a machine, smoke is not drawn through the filter in any substantial amount and nearly smoke-free air is measured as the tar yield of the cigarette. Since the smoker smokes to obtain the tobacco smoke, not simply air, the smoker inhales more deeply and more rapidly. This pattern of inhalation leads to a substantially higher yield of tar from the cigarette than would be predicted by the machine-measured value. In addition, the larger volume of the inhaled puff precludes holding the smoke in the mouth for a moment before inhaling the smoke into the lung. This direct inhalation without a pause may increase exposure of the lung to those constituents of smoke that have short half-lives.

More than 4000 individual chemical constituents of cigarette smoke have been identified (13); it is estimated that 2550 of these come from processed unadulterated tobacco, with the remainder representing additives, pesticides, and other organic and metallic compounds (9, 14). Table 1 lists some of the constituents of the particulate and vapor phases of mainstream smoke and the ratio of concentrations in mainstream and sidestream smoke. The chemical composition of smoke and the distribution of constituents between the particulate and vapor phases of the smoke changes as the smoke cools, ages, and mixes with air. Highly reactive free radicals in the vapor phase disappear quickly, and exposure of alveolar structures to these compounds may be diminished in smokers who hold the smoke in their mouths prior to inhaling. In contrast, relatively stable, free radicals in the particulate phase, principally a quinone/hydroquinone complex, remain able to reduce molecular oxygen to superoxide and eventually hydrogen peroxide and hydroxyl radicals (15, 16). The production of smoke in relatively oxygen-deficient environments such as the burning cone of tobacco results in a reducing capacity for mainstream smoke that increases with number of puffs, but disappears rapidly as the smoke ages (17).

The water content of the smoke particles changes with the relative humidity of the environment in the respiratory tract, with a resultant change in particle size (18). Nicotine, which is contained largely in the particulate phase in fresh smoke, volatilizes into the gas phase as the smoke ages and is a vapor phase constituent of environmental tobacco smoke (19).

Radioactive constituents are also present in both tobacco and tobacco smoke. They include radon and its decay products, as well as lead (Pb-210), bismuth (Bi-210), and polonium (Po-210) (20). These alpha-emitting radioisotopes may contribute to the carcinogenicity of cigarette smoke (21–24). The absorption of Po-210 from the lung into the bloodstream has been demonstrated (25). The radiation dose from Po-210 in cigarettes has been variously estimated at 1 rad per year (26), 8 rem per year (27), and 80–100 rad per lifetime (28).

The concentrations of many of the toxic constituents present in mainstream cigarette smoke are above levels that would be rapidly fatal with uninterrupted exposure. For example, carbon monoxide is present at concentrations similar to that found in automobile exhaust. It is the dilution of the smoke with room air and the intermittency of smoke inhalation that prevents cigarette smoking from being immediately lethal. For these reasons, it is often difficult to translate the concentrations of agents found in smoke directly into dosage received by the smoker.

Table 1 Toxic and Tumorigenic Agents of Cigarette Smoke, Ratio of Sidestream Smoke (SS) to Mainstream Smoke (MS)

	Amount per cigarette	SS/MS
A. Gas phase		
Carbon dioxide	10–80 mg	8.1[a]
Carbon monoxide	0.5–26 mg	2.5[a]
Nitrogen oxides (NO_x)	16–600 μg	4.7–5.8
Ammonia	10–130 μg	44–73
Hydrogen cyanide	280–550 μg	0.17–0.37
Hydrazine	32 μg	3
Formaldehyde	20–90 μg	51
Acetone	100–940 μg	2.5–3.2
Acrolein	10–140 μg	12
Acetonitrile	60–160 μg	10
Pyridine	32 μg	10
3-Vinylpyridine	23 μg	28
N-Nitrosodimethylamine	4–180 ng	10–830
N-Nitrosoethylmethylamine	1.0–40 ng	5–12
N-Nitrosodiethylamine	0.1–28 ng	4–25
N-Nitrosopyrrolidine	0–110 ng	3–76
B. Particulate phase		
Total particulate phase	0.1–40 mg	1.3–1.9[a]
Nicotine	0.06–2.3 mg	2.6–3.3[a]
Toluene	108 μg	5.6
Phenol	20–150 μg	2.6
Catechol	40–280 μg	0.7
Stigmasterol	53 μg	0.8
Total phytosterols	130 μg	0.8
Naphthalene	2.8 μg	16
1-methylnaphthalene	1.2 μg	26
2-Methylnaphthalene	1.0 μg	29
Phenanthrene	2.0–80 ng	2.1
Benz(*a*)anthracene	10–70 ng	2.7
Pyrene	15–90 ng	1.9–3.6
Benzo(*a*)pyrene	8–40 ng	2.7–3.4
Quinoline	1.7 μg	11
Methylquinoline	6.7 μg	11
Harmane	1.1–3.1 μg	0.7–2.7
Norharmane	3.2–8.1 μg	1.4–4.3
Aniline	100–1,200 ng	30
o-Toluidine	32 ng	19
1-Naphthylamine	1.0–22 ng	39
2-Naphthylamine	4.3–27 ng	39

Table 1 Continued

	Amount per cigarette	SS/MS
4-Aminobiphenyl	2.4–4.6 ng	31
N′-Nitrosonornicotine	0.2–3.7 μg	1–5
NNK[b]	0.12–0.44 μg	1–8
N′-Nitrosoanatabine	0.15–4.6 μg	1–7
N-Nitrosodiethanolamine	0–40 ng	1.2

[a]In cigarettes with perforated filter tips the SS/MS ratio rises with increasing air dilution. In the case of smoke diluton with air to 17%, the SS/MS ratios for TPM rise to 2.14, CO_2 36.5, CO 23.5, and nicotine 13.1.
[b]NNK = 4-(Methylnitrosamino)-1-(3-pyridyl)-1-butanone.

Dosage received by the smoker depends on both the concentrations in the smoke and the pattern of smoking.

IV. Deposition and Absorption of Smoke

As mainstream cigarette smoke emerges from the cigarette, it has approximately 10^9–10^{10} particles per ml; the particles range in size from 0.1 to 1.0 μm, with a mean of 0.2 μm (29). After being inhaled, the particle size may change with the increased humidity in the airway and with aggregation of the particles due to their high concentration (30). The aerodynamic diameter of the particle determines the sites of deposition in the airways and alveolar regions of the lung (31). The fraction of the smoke retained by the smoker varies markedly with the pattern of inhalation. Smokers who hold the smoke in their mouth without inhaling retain only a small fraction of the smoke, whereas smokers who inhale deeply and hold their inhalation may retain up to 90% of the smoke (32, 33). Cigarette smoke is still in a stage of rapid chemical evolution as it emerges from the butt of the cigarette, and the exposure of the upper airway to short-lived constituents of smoke, such as free radicals, may vary markedly with patterns of smoking that include holding the smoke in the mouth briefly prior to inhaling.

The absorption of constituents from the gas phase of the smoke varies markedly with the solubility and other characteristics of the compounds. Highly soluble compounds tend to be absorbed efficiently in the upper airways and reach the alveoli in much lower concentrations than are present in the smoke as it exists at the end of the cigarette. Carbon monoxide, because it is bound to hemoglobin and is absorbed largely at the alveolar level, is a marker for the extent of smoke inhalation. Biologic markers of absorption of smoke constituents include nicotine and cotinine in the blood, saliva, or urine; carboxyhemoglobin in the blood and expired air; the cyanate in the blood, saliva, or urine; and globin-adducts of nitrogen oxides, ethylene, and tobacco-specific nitrosamines (13).

Once deposited, the smoke particles are subject to clearance by the normal clearance mechanisms of the lung: alveolar macrophages and mucociliary transport. However, the acute and chronic inhalation of smoke can alter these clearance mechanisms as well. The acute inhalation of cigarette smoke results in ciliostasis, paralysis of the cilia (34), and reduced rate of mucociliary clearance (35, 36). Chronic inhalation of smoke alters clearance by converting ciliated epithelium to nonciliated epithelium by altering the amount and character of the mucus produced and by inflammatory narrowing of the airway and loss of elastic recoil of the lung (37).

V. Toxicity and Carcinogenicity of Cigarette Smoke

Cigarette smoke contains irritants, oxidants, free radicals and a variety of other toxins and carcinogens. The full range of toxicity of cigarette smoke is reviewed in the reports of the Surgeon General (12, 13, 20, 37–44) and will not be discussed in detail. Cigarette smoking produces disease through diverse mechanisms. For example, cigarette smoke causes the influx of activated cells into the lung, oxidizes antiprotease in the blood, interferes with oxygen transport, increases platelet aggregation, alters drug metabolism, and causes bronchoconstriction. In general, these mechanisms can be grouped by their effects: acute and chronic irritation and inflammation, activation of cellular and biochemical processes, blockage of normal biological and metabolic functions, toxic injury to cellular and biochemical elements, alteration of immune response, and carcinogenesis. These effects, singly and in combination, lead to the structural damage that we define as disease states caused by smoking.

A. Carcinogenicity

Exfoliative cytology in populations of smokers at high risk of developing lung cancer shows a progression of changes in the cells over time from dysplasia through metaplasia to frank carcinoma in situ; with cessation, these changes revert toward normal. Pathologic studies of smokers' lungs show that the extent of these changes are closely correlated with the number of cigarettes smoked per day and the duration of smoking (45).

Cigarette smoking also causes cancers in nonrespiratory tract sites including the pancreas and urinary bladder. Carcinogens in tobacco smoke are absorbed into the blood, and some are excreted unchanged or as active metabolites through the urinary tract. Cigarette smoking leads to activation of several microsomal enzyme systems, including the cytochrome P-450–dependent microsomal monooxygenases (5) that can facilitate metabolic activation of precarcinogens. The urine of cigarette smokers is strongly mutagenic in bacterial test systems (46).

The bulk of the carcinogenic activity of tobacco smoke is contained in the particulate phase. Table 2 lists the tumorigenic agents in cigarette smoke and the status of the evidence that characterizes them as carcinogens (5 40). Additionally, cells are considered to be most susceptible to carcinogenic transformation during cell replication, and the irritant and inflammatory effects of tobacco smoke lead to increased cell turnover as well as interference with the normal barrier and clearance mechanisms of the lung.

B. Models Relating Tobacco Dose to Carcinogenesis

The epidemiologic evidence establishing the strength of the relationship between cigarette smoking and lung cancer is presented in Chapter 4 and clearly establishes that the risk of lung cancer increases with increasing the number of cigarettes smoked per day and with longer duration of smoking. Mathematical modeling approaches have been used to link our understanding of the biologic mechanisms of carcinogenesis reviewed in Chapter 14 with the observed lung cancer mortality experience of smokers.

Two biological models have led to mathematical models for predicting lung cancer death rates from smoking dosage data.

The Multistage Model

This model (47) suggests that multiple inheritable changes in the cell are required to result in malignant transformation. Successive stages in the transformation of one cell may be separated from each other by several years, and the factors influencing early stages may be different from those influencing later stages. Extracellular influences may also influence the number of cells transformed and the rate of cell growth, particularly for a process as complex as cigarette smoking (48). In its simplest form, incidence I of lung cancer at age x is a constant times age raised to a power ($I_x = bKX^{k-1}$). Since 90% of the occurrence of lung cancer is related to cigarette smoking, the equation has been formulated $I_x = bNK(x - w)^{k-1}$, where N is the number of cigarettes smoked per day and w is the age of initiation of regular smoking. The terms b and k are the fitting parameters for the model. Doll and Peto (58) have presented a formulation of this model developed from a prospective mortality study of British physicians in the form: Incidence $= C(\#\text{cig per day} + 6)^2(\text{age} - 22.5)^{4 \text{ or } 5}$. The term (age − 22.5) was derived by assuming a uniform age of smoking uptake of 19 years and a 3.5-year latency from carcinogenic transformation of the cell to death from lung cancer. This term becomes duration of smoking prior to carcinogenic transformation.

Variations of this model have been used by a number of investigators to

Table 2 Tumorigenic Agents in Tobacco and Tobacco Smoke

Compounds	Processed tobacco (per gram)	Mainstream smoke (per cigarette)	Evidence for IARC evaluation of carcinogenicity: In lab animals	In humans
PAH				
Benz(*a*)anthracene		2–70 ng	Sufficient	NA
Benzo(*b*)fluoranthene		4–22 ng	Sufficient	NA
Benzo(*j*)fluoranthene		6–21 ng	Sufficient	NA
Benzo(*k*)fluoranthene		6–12 ng	Sufficient	NA
Benzo(*a*)pyrene	0.1–90 ng	20–40 ng	Sufficient	Probable
Chrysene		40–60 ng	Sufficient	NA
Dibenz(*a*,*h*)anthracene		4 ng	Sufficient	NA
Dibenz(*a*,*i*)pyrene		1.7–3.2 ng	Sufficient	NA
Dibenzo(*a*,*l*)pyrene		Present	Sufficient	NA
Indeno(1,2,3-*c*,*d*)pyrene		4–20 ng	Sufficient	NA
5-Methylchrysene		0.6 ng	Sufficient	NA
Aza-arenes				
Quinoline		1– μg	NA	NA
Dibenz(*a*,*h*)acridine		0.1 ng	Sufficient	NA
Dibenz(*a*,*j*)acridine		3–10 ng	Sufficient	NA
7H-Dibenzo(*c*,*g*)carbazole		0.7 ng	Sufficient	NA
N-Nitrosamines				
N-Nitrosodimethylamine	ND-215 ng	0.1–180 ng	Sufficient	NA
N-Nitrosoethylmethylamine		3–13 ng	Sufficient	NA
N-Nitrosodiethylamine		ND-25 ng	Sufficient	NA
N-Nitrosopyrrolidine	ND-360 ng	1.5–110 ng	Sufficient	NA
N-Nitrosodiethanolamine	ND-6,900 ng	ND-36 ng	Sufficient	NA
N′-Nitrosonornicotine	0.3–89 μg	0.12–3.7 μg	Sufficient	NA
4-(methylnitrosamino)-1-(3-pyridyl)-1-butanone	0.2–7 μg	0.08–0.77 μg	Sufficient	NA
N′-Nitrosoanabasine	0.01–1.9 μg	0.14–4.6 μg	Limited	NA
N-Nitrosomorpholine	ND-690 ng		Sufficient	NA
Aromatic amines				
2-Toluidine		30–200 ng	Sufficient	Inadequate
2-naphthylamine		1–22 ng	Sufficient	Sufficient
4-Aminobiophenyl		2–5 ng	Sufficient	Sufficient
Aldehydes				
Formaldehyde[a]	1.6–7.4 μg	70–100 μg[a]	Sufficient	NA
Acetaldehyde[a]	1.4–7.4 mg	18–1,400 mg[a]	Sufficient	NA
Crotonaldehyde	0.2–2.4 μg	10–20 μg	NA	NA

Table 2 Continued

Compounds	Processed tobacco (per gram)	Mainstream smoke (per cigarette)	Evidence for IARC evaluation of carcinogenicity: In lab animals	In humans
Miscellaneous organic compounds				
Benzene		12–48 μg	Sufficient	Sufficient
Acrylonitrile		3.2–15 μg	Sufficient	Limited
1,1-Dimethylhydrazine	60–147 μg		Sufficient	NA
2-Nitropropane		0.73–1.21 μg	Sufficient	NA
Ethylcarbamate	310–375 ng	20–38 ng	Sufficient	NA
Vinyl chloride		1–16 ng	Sufficient	Sufficient
Inorganic compounds				
Hydrazine	14–51 ng	24–43 ng	Sufficient	Inadequate
Arsenic	500–900 ng	40–120 ng	Inadequate	Sufficient
Nickel	2,000–6,000 ng	0–600 ng	Sufficient	Limited
Chromium	1,000–2,000 ng	4–70 ng	Sufficient	Sufficient
Cadmium	1,300–1,600 ng	41–62 ng	Sufficient	Limited
Lead	8–10 μg		Sufficient	Inadequate
Polonium-210	0.2–1.2 pCi	0.03–1.0 pCi	NA	NA

Note: ND, no data; NA, evaluation has not been done by IARC.
[a]The Fourth Report of the Independent Scientific Committee on "Smoking and Health" (1988) published values for the 14 leading U.K. cigarettes in 1986 (51.4% of the market) of 20–105 μg/cigarette (mean, 59 μg) for formaldehyde and 550–1150 μg/cigarette (mean, 910 μg) for acetaldehyde.

match British national smoking prevalence data with British lung cancer death rates. Stevens and Moolgavkar (49, 50) used birth cohort data on tobacco prevalence and birth cohort–specific cumulative tar–weighted cigarette consumption to construct a model that fits British birth cohort lung cancer death rate data. Their model summed the risks for nonsmoking and ever-smoking members of a birth cohort, with the risks for the nonsmokers being a function of age to the fourth power and the risks in smokers being equal to the risk in nonsmokers multiplied by 10 raised to the power of the cumulative cigarette consumption expressed in 20-pack-year units. This model assumed a single age of initiation and a single number of cigarettes smoked per day for all smokers as well as a simple linear relationship between tar yield of a cigarette and its carcinogenic risk.

Townsend (51) expanded the basic multistage model to include birth cohort–

specific duration of exposure and number of cigarettes per day. This model used the prevalence of smoking estimated at 5-calendar-year increments to divide each birth cohort into fractions with different durations of smoking. A weighted mean of the number of cigarettes smoked per day at each age was used as the dosage term with the weighting such that recent smoking was more important than past smoking. The number of cigarettes was also adjusted by assuming that filtered cigarettes were 40% less carcinogenic and that the carcinogenic risk of a cigarette was directly proportional to the tar content of the cigarette. The estimated lung cancer occurrence for each of the fractions with different durations of exposure was summed and added to the nonsmoker risk to predict the lung cancer death rate for the birth cohort. Nonsmoker death rates were taken from the American Cancer Society prospective mortality study of 1 million men and women (52). She also included a term for pipe and cigar smoking, but this term was found to have little effect on the estimation of death rates. To test this model she varied the constants in the model over a range and found the values that resulted in the best fit of the model to the British age-specific lung cancer mortality data. When the exponent for the duration of exposure term was set at 5 (the best fit value), the model explained 98% of the variation in excess mortality in the male birth cohorts but only 84.8% of the variation in women. The adjustment for filters and tar content of the cigarette in this study reduced the predicted risk of cigarettes by almost 40% from 1946 to 1966, and this adjustment is clearly overly generous for British cigarettes and invalid for U.S. cigarettes (12). This overadjustment for the decline in tar content of cigarettes may have led to an underestimate of the effect of duration of smoking.

The Two-Mutation Model

This "recessive oncogenesis" model suggests that there are two rate-limiting steps in the development of a carcinogenic cell. These steps are mutations that lead to homozygous loss of antioncogene function (53). This mechanism has been established in some tumors (54) and suggested for lung cancer (55, 56). Moolgavkar and colleagues (57) have developed a mathematical expression of this model and used the lung cancer data from the British physicians study to fit the model. The data fit the two-mutation model at least as well as the multistage model proposed by Doll and Peto (58). The simplified formulation of this model derived from the British physicians study is:

$$h(t,d) = (c_0 + c_2 d)\left\{c_0 \exp[bd(t - t_0)] \int_0^{t_0} X(s) \exp[a(t - s)]ds + (c_0 + c_1 d) \times \int_{t_0}^{t} X(s) \exp[(a + bd)(t - s)]ds\right\}.$$

The term $h(t,d)$ is the lung cancer incidence at the time t in someone who smoked d cigarettes per day. The terms $(c_0 + c_2 d)$ and $(c_0 + c_1 d)$ are the first and second mutation rates (per cell per year) among smokers of d cigarettes per day, and $(a + bd)$ is the net proliferation rate of intermediate cells. $X(s)$ is the mean number of susceptible cells at age s, and t_0 is the age of initiation.

There are important differences between these two models in their prediction of lung cancer risks. The multistage model implies that the risk from smoking is determined by cumulative dose of smoking regardless of when that smoking occurred, that is, smoking 30 cigarettes per day early in life and 10 cigarettes per day late in life is the same as smoking 10 cigarettes per day early, and 30 late. The two-mutation model suggests that early smoking is much more important in determining lung cancer risk. The multistage model uses duration of exposure as the sole age-related measure determining risk, whereas the two-mutation model implies that age of initiation has an effect independent of its effect on duration of exposure.

None of the models using duration of exposure have been applied to the U.S. data. However, Brown and Kessler (59) have used a multistage model to predict U.S. lung cancer death rates to the year 2025. This model incorporates terms for calendar year effects and a term for cohort effects and uses a tar-weighted consumption measure for number of cigarettes smoked per day. This model assumes a linear relationship between tar content and lung cancer risk and uses a single cohort term to model the complex effects of differences in age of initiation and duration of exposure that occur across cohorts. These limitations result in a model that predicts that lung cancer death rates in men will change very little between 1985 and 2010. This projection clashes with the decline in age-specific lung cancer death rates among white men under the age of 55 that has already occurred as of 1985, and which should reduce overall lung cancer death rates as these birth cohorts replace older, higher-risk cohorts. The characteristics of smoking behavior that can be used to fit these models for the U.S. population are presented later in this chapter.

VI. Tobacco Use in the United States

A. Current Tobacco Use

The prevalence of cigarette smoking in the United States was 29.1% of the population over the age of 20 in 1987 (13), with 31.7% of the men and 26.8% of the women smoking. Smoking has been declining for the last 25 years, and if past trends continue, smoking prevalence is expected to be about 27% in 1991. The prevalence among blacks is higher than among whites, although blacks tend to smoke fewer cigarettes per day (13). Blue-collar workers have a higher prevalence of smoking than white-collar workers (42).

Cigarette use is not uniformly distributed across the U.S. population. All the major demographic and socioeconomic measures can be linked to smoking behavior. Age, race, ethnicity, gender, level of education, level of income, and year of birth have all been associated with smoking behavior. The interrelationships between smoking prevalence, age, and year of birth are particularly complex; misinterpretation of trends in smoking and disease occurrence may result without appropriate consideration of these relationships. The major indicators of risk for most of the diseases related to smoking are smoking status, duration of smoking, age of initiation, and number of cigarettes smoked per day. With the exception of number of cigarettes per day, these phenomena are best presented as birth cohort analyses of smoking prevalence across calendar year.

Several birth cohort analyses of smoking prevalence have been published (42, 60–62) based on one or two of the National Health Interview Study (NHIS) data sets on tobacco use. The limited sample sizes of these data sets reduce the precision of estimates of smoking behavior, particularly for the earlier birth cohorts. We have generated a single data set that combines all of the NHIS surveys that recorded data on smoking behavior and have generated race- and gender-specific 5-year birth cohort estimates of those cigarette smoking measures that are most strongly predictive of lung cancer risk: smoking prevalence, age of initiation, age of cessation, and duration of smoking.

The NCHS, through the NHIS, has collected health information since 1964 from a probability sample of the civilian noninstitutionalized population of the United States. From 1965 on, there has been a section on tobacco use included in the survey. In each of these surveys, ever-smokers were defined by the question, "Have you ever smoked 100 cigarettes?" and current smokers by the question, "Do you smoke cigarettes now?" The data presented in this chapter are preliminary estimates of smoking behavior from this data set, which have not been adjusted for the differential mortality associated with smoking and its effect on the ratio of ever-smokers to never-smokers in the population. However, these estimates offer a much better description of smoking behavior in the U.S. population over time than does examination of multiple cross-sectional samples.

B. Generation of Birth Cohort Analyses from the Combined NHIS Survey Data Set

We have combined the basic demographic data and smoking data for the NHIS Survey data sets for the years 1965, 1966, 1970, 1974, 1976, 1977, 1978, 1979, 1980, 1983, 1985, 1987, and 1988. All variables were recoded to a common coding scheme. When smoking variables were not available for a given survey, they were either left blank or coded as missing depending on the smoking status of the respondent.

This combined file has 518,376 records and provides a convenient format for analyzing age cohorts across survey years. The prevalence of smoking by age and calendar year has been constructed for each 5-year race and gender-specific birth cohort from 1900 to 1964 (see Figs. 2–9). Since the data available for a number of survey years did not contain information on age of initiation, and some years did not contain information on the age of cessation for former smokers, it was necessary to construct the prevalence curves for each birth cohort by combining separately derived initiation and cessation curves. The prevalence curve for each birth cohort was constructed by subtracting from the fraction of the cohort that had begun to smoke in a given year (age) the fraction that had quit by that year (age). The fraction of the birth cohort that had initiated smoking by a specific age or year was generated by performing a survival analysis for the entire birth cohort subgroup (age 20+) censoring each individual at his or her age (year) at the time of the survey. Similarly, a survival curve for the entire birth cohort subgroup was run for all ever-smokers (age 20+) censoring each individual at his or her age (year) at the time of the survey to develop the curves for the fraction of the birth cohort that quit at any specific age (year). The prevalence at any given age or year can then be calculated by multiplying the fraction of the cohort that initiated at that age or year by the fraction of the ever-smokers that quit by that age or year.

The validity of this approach for calculating prevalence was examined by comparing the estimated prevalence using the above approach with the point prevalences for the birth cohort in each of the years in which a survey was conducted. There were 13 survey years in which a point prevalence and a calculated prevalence could be compared for those cohorts born before 1940, with fewer points for later cohorts. This comparison was made for each of the 13 birth cohorts in each of the 4 race and gender groups (52 birth cohorts) with excellent results. In only 149 of 620 comparisons did the calculated prevalence fall outside the 95% confidence limit of the point prevalence estimate.

We have also examined the potential effect of differential mortality among smokers who initiated smoking at different ages on the distribution of age of initiation reported for older birth cohorts. Those who begin smoking early in life have higher overall mortality rates than those who initiate later in life, and we were concerned that this effect might result in a shift in the distribution of the age of initiation toward older ages among the oldest birth cohorts. To examine this potential bias, we compared the distributions of age of initiation for each of the six oldest 5-year birth cohorts obtained from three separate NHIS surveys (1970, 1970, and 1987). The distribution of age of initiation for each birth cohort across five fixed age categories was examined for a shift in the distribution of age of initiation across the 17-year period represented by the three surveys, but no shift was identified.

Once a birth cohort ages beyond 45–50 years, the excess mortality of smokers begins to alter the proportion of ever-smokers in the population, and sequential cross-sectional measurements of smoking behavior over time show a decline in the fraction of ever-smokers among the remaining members of the cohort. Thus, the surviving members of the cohort are disproportionately never-

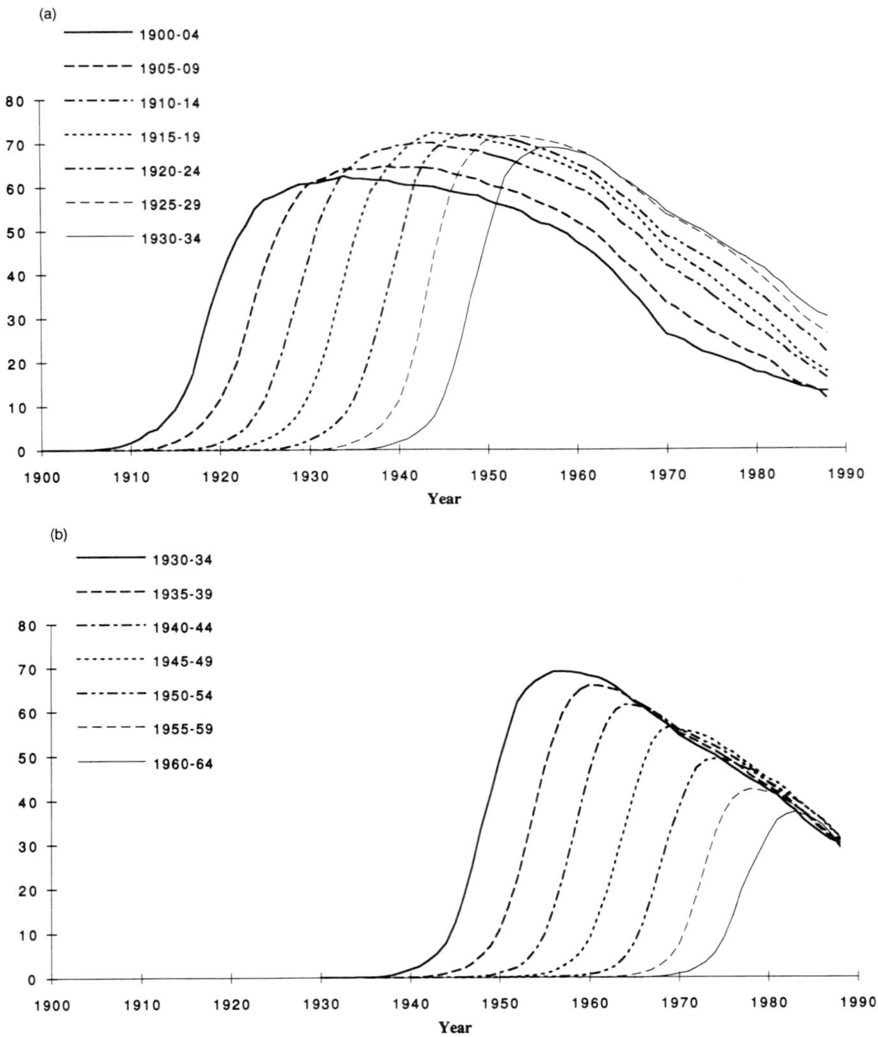

Figure 2 White male smoking prevalence by year for 5-year birth cohorts: (a) 1900–1934; (b) 1934–1964.

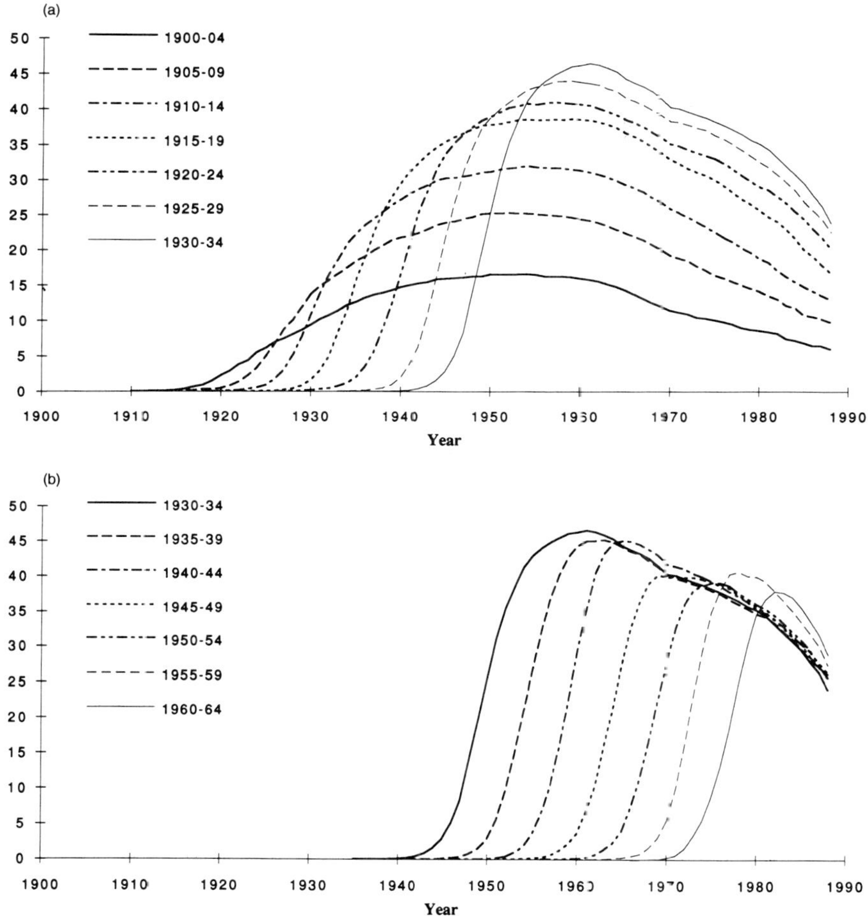

Figure 3 White female smoking prevalence by year for 5-year birth cohorts: (a) 1900–1934; (b) 1934–1964.

smokers. Consequently, smoking prevalence estimates for earlier birth cohorts should be corrected for this differential mortality if estimates of the true smoking prevalence for the first half of the century are to be made. It is necessary to correct for the decline in the fraction of ever-smokers in a birth cohort as the cohort ages past age 50. The effect of differential mortality on the prevalence of smoking estimates, however, is small because of the small fraction of ever-smokers who have not quit at these older ages. The effect on the prevalence of former smokers

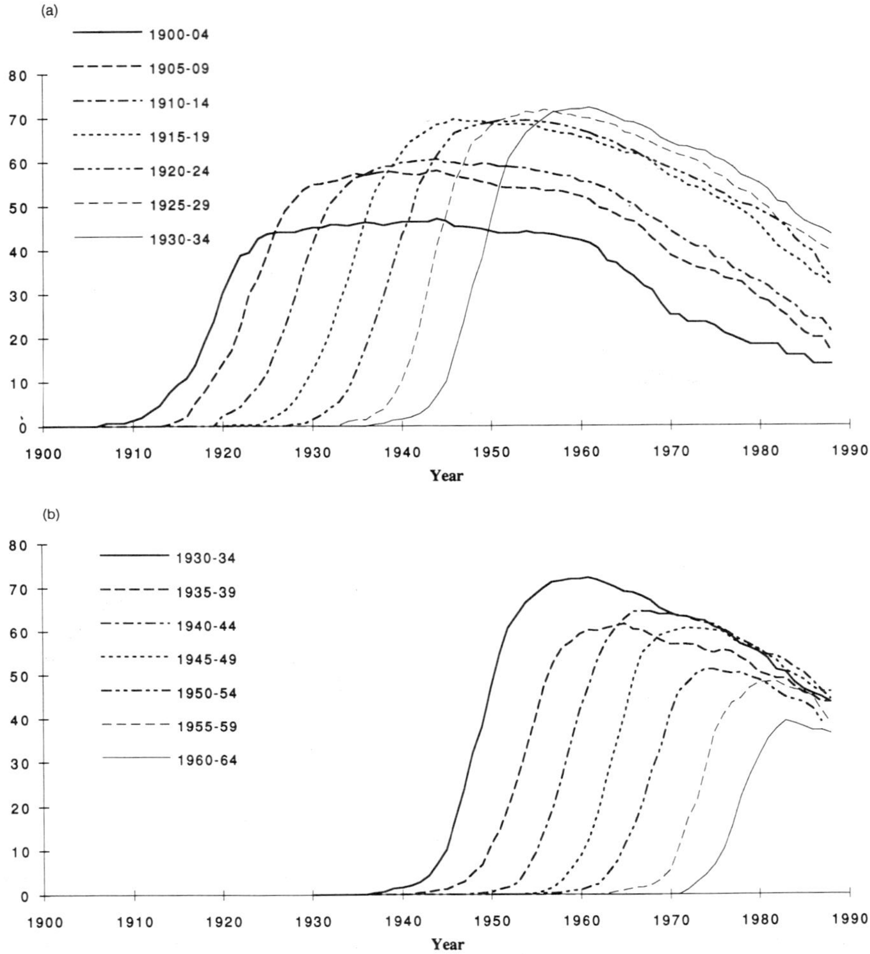

Figure 4 Black male smoking prevalence by year for 5-year birth cohorts: (a) 1900–1934; (b) 1934–1964.

is proportionately larger and should be corrected prior to estimating the prevalence of the former smokers in the cohort.

C. Smoking Prevalence by Birth Cohort

Figures 2–5 present the prevalence of current smoking by calendar year for 5-year birth cohorts born between 1900 and 1964. Figures 6–9 present the smoking prevalence for the same cohorts with the data presented by age instead of calendar

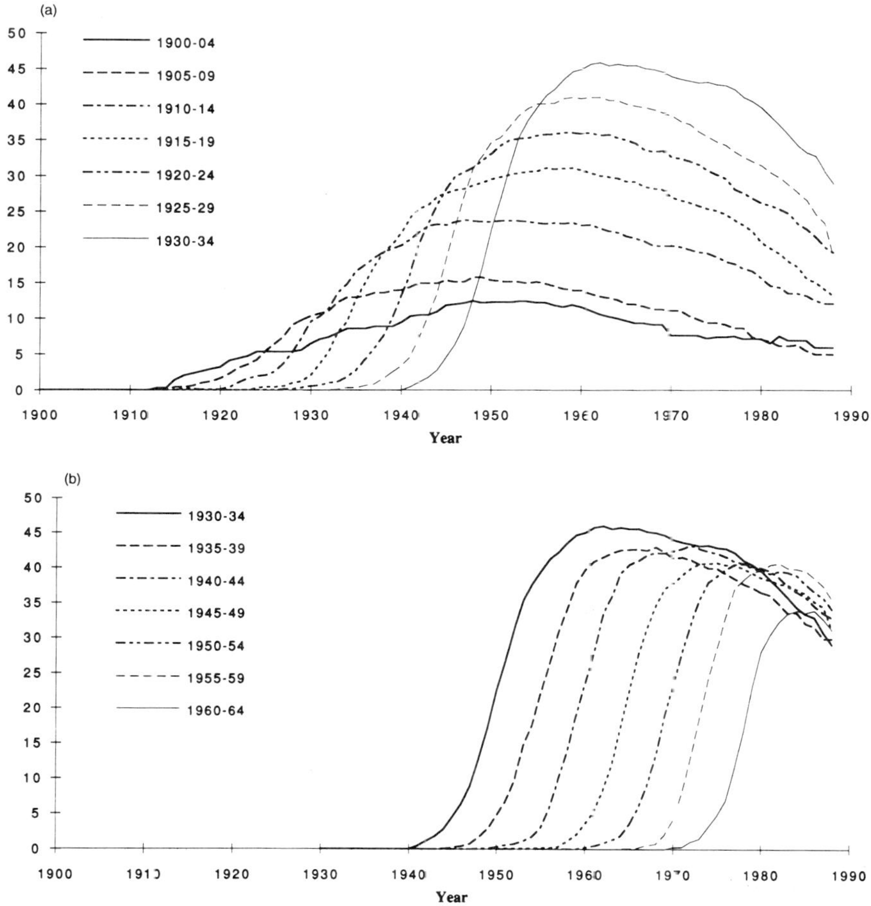

Figure 5 Black female smoking prevalence by year for 5-year birth cohorts: (a) 1900–1934; (b) 1934–1964.

year. Examination of these figures shows clearly that it would be impossible to characterize the life experience with smoking by a single measure that would define the risk across the different race/gender/birth cohorts. Therefore, it is useful to examine the differences in smoking through a set of separate measures.

Peak Prevalence of Smoking

The fraction of any cohort that smokes varies with age; the initiation of smoking occurs in adolescence and is largely complete in young adulthood. The major

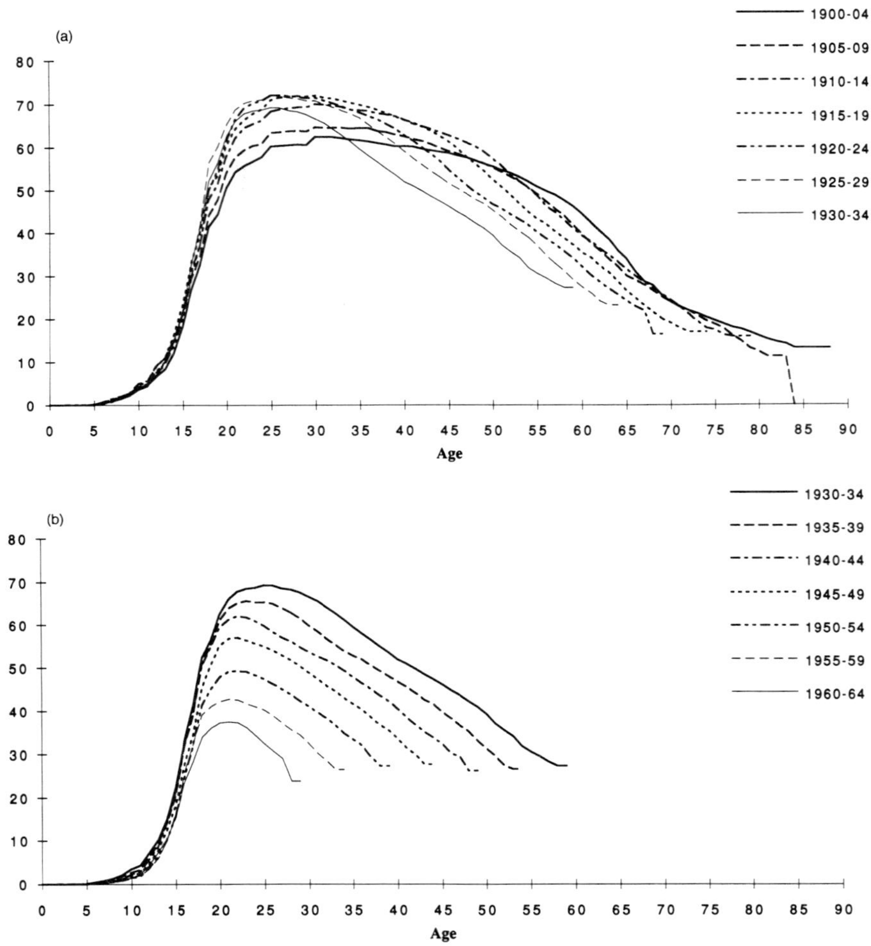

Figure 6 White male smoking prevalence by age for 5-year birth cohorts: (a) 1900–1934; (b) 1934–1964.

change in smoking behavior that occurs after age 25 is cessation, particularly for the cohorts born after 1925. Consequently, the prevalence of smoking typically peaks in young adulthood and then declines. Thus, the peak prevalence offers one measure of the fraction of a birth cohort that had exposure to smoking, which is close to the fraction of ever-smokers in the cohort.

The peak prevalence of smoking for white males increased with each succeeding cohort from 1900 to 1929 and then declined steadily among later birth

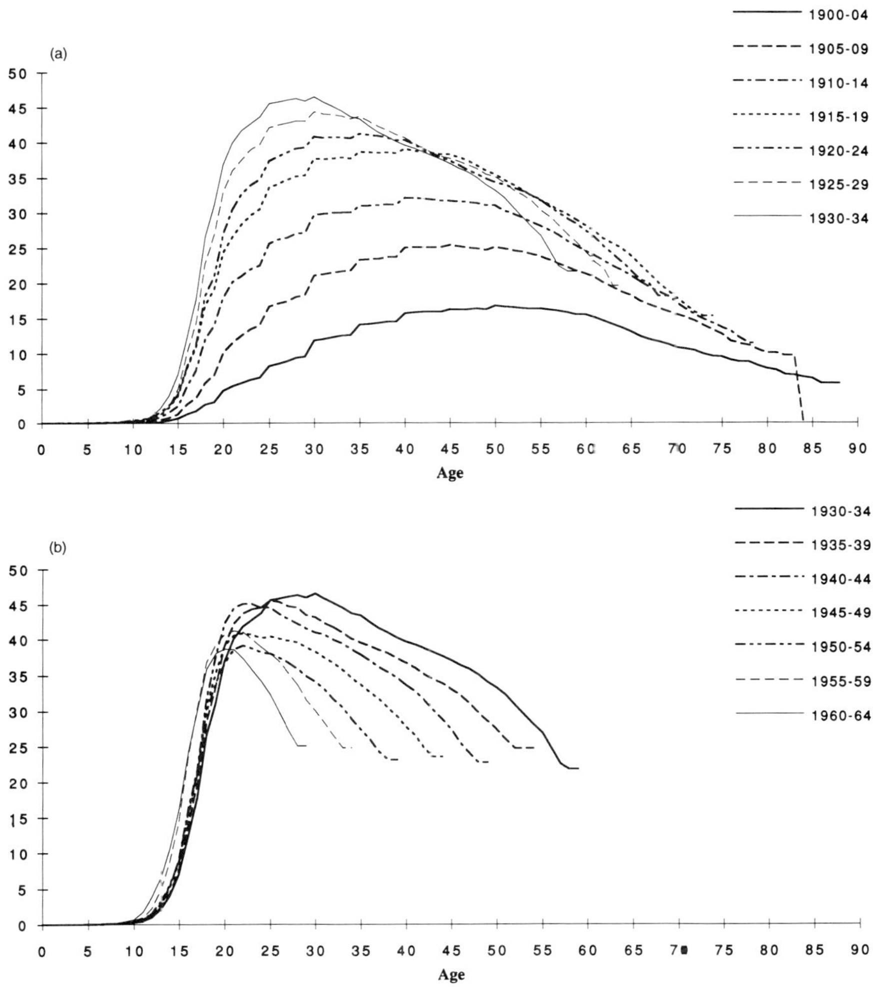

Figure 7 White female smoking prevalence by age for 5-year birth cohorts: (a) 1900–1934; (b) 1934–1964.

cohorts. The peak prevalences of smoking among cohorts of white women were much lower than among white males for all but the last two birth cohorts, which had similar peak prevalences. The differences in peak prevalences were larger for earlier birth cohorts, reflecting the temporal pattern of women not beginning to smoke in large numbers until much later in the century than males. The peak

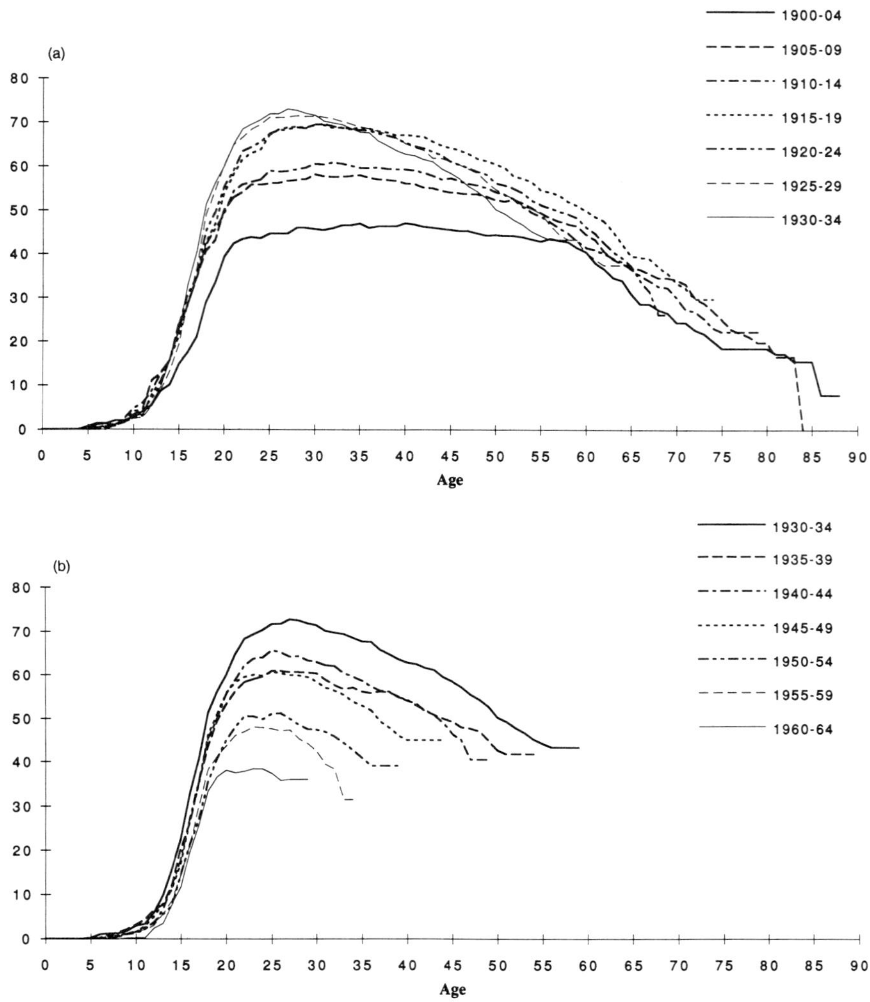

Figure 8 Black male smoking prevalence by age for 5-year birth cohorts: (a) 1900–1934; (b) 1934–1964.

prevalences among birth cohorts of white women increased with each successive cohort up to those born in 1940 through 1944 before declining in later cohorts.

The patterns of peak prevalence among birth cohorts of black males and females are similar to those for whites with the exception that the earliest cohorts of black males were less likely to smoke and the most recent cohorts more likely to smoke.

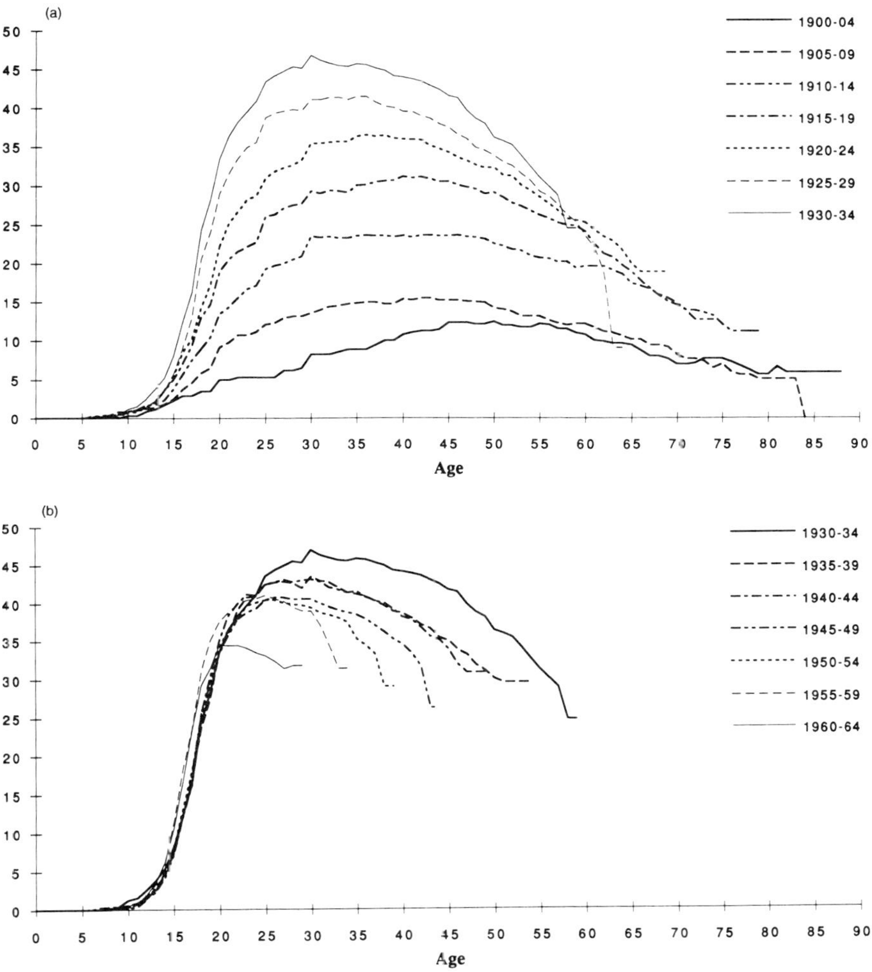

Figure 9 Black female smoking prevalence by age for 5-year birth cohorts: (a) 1900–1934; (b) 1934–1964.

Age of Initiation

Age of initiation is a strong determinant of the age-specific risks of smokers. Earlier age of initiation increases the duration of smoking and possibly the exposure of developing lungs or other organs is particularly hazardous. Figure 10 presents the age of initiation for ever-smokers by birth cohort for white males and demonstrates that the starting of smoking among white males is largely complete

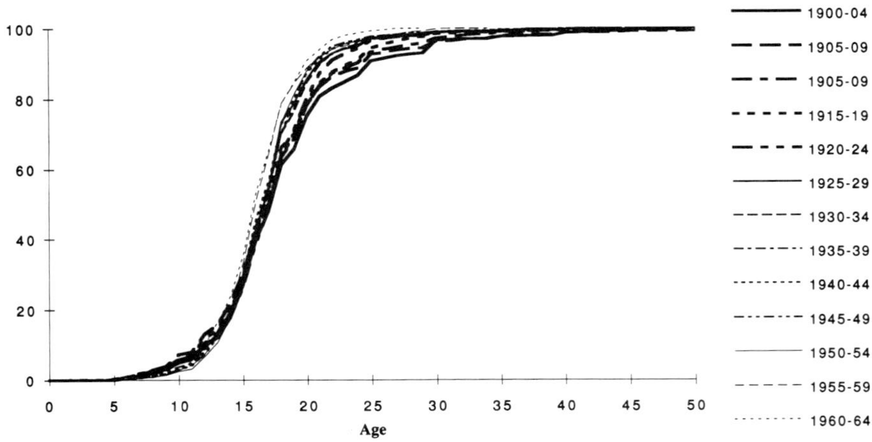

Figure 10 White male initiation by age as a percentage of ever-smokers.

by age 25 for all cohorts. There has perhaps been a small shift toward younger ages of initiation among more recent cohorts, but overall the pattern is very similar across all of the century's birth cohorts.

The pattern of age of initiation for white women across cohorts is quite different (Fig. 11), however, with initiation of smoking continuing into the thirties and forties in the earliest birth cohorts. In more recent cohorts, there is a clear and progressive shift to earlier ages of initiation.

The pattern of age of initiation among blacks is similar to that among whites of the same gender, with perhaps a slightly later age of initiation among blacks.

Age of Cessation

The initiation of smoking is largely confined to those under age 25 among males in all birth cohorts and among females who began to smoke after the mid-1950s. Consequently, the major influence on smoking prevalence after that age is smoking cessation. Figure 12 presents the prevalence of smoking for the six oldest birth cohorts of white males. Cursory examination of the data for any of these cohorts could lead to the conclusion that the decline of smoking cessation is determined by age, and that age is, therefore, a major influence on smoking cessation. However, a more careful examination of the temporal patterns of prevalence for the different cohorts suggests that cessation may be more strongly influenced by calendar year than by the attained age of the cohort. The initiation lines clearly parallel in each 5-year cohort showing a rapid rise 5 years later than the previous one. The declines reflecting smoking cessation do not show the same parallel

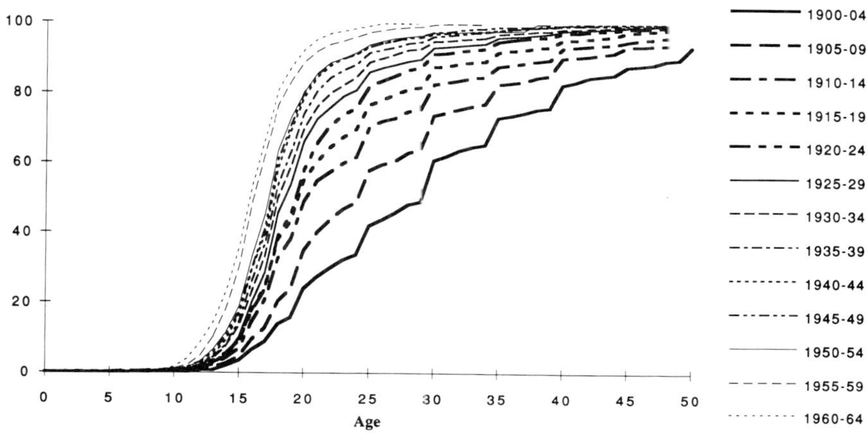

Figure 11 White female initiation by age as a percentage of ever-smokers.

5-year spacing. Instead, the declines for all cohorts appear to begin in the mid-1950s and decline rapidly in the late 1960s. This pattern suggests that cessation may be more influenced by calendar year than by age and, thus, more responsive to environmental stimuli than to age itself.

Figure 13 provides further evidence in support of the importance of calendar year rather than age in determining cessation. It plots the annual changes in the

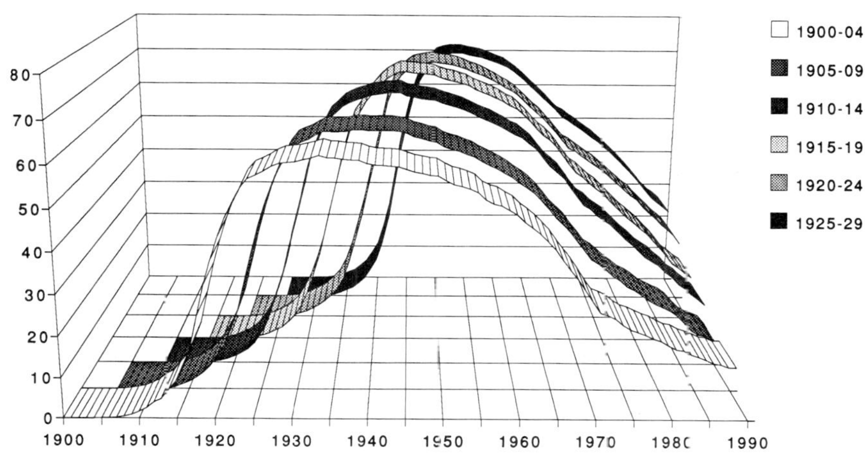

Figure 12 Prevalence of smoking among birth cohorts of white males born 1900–1929.

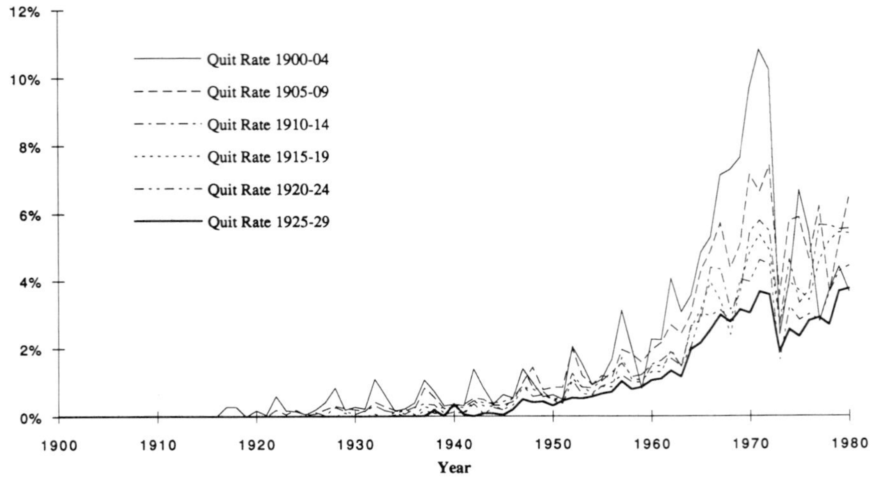

Figure 13 One-year quit rates for 5-year birth cohorts of white males born 1900–1929.

percentages of the cohorts that were former smokers with the prevalence of smoking in that cohort for the previous year as the denominator. This percentage describes the fraction of the population that has successfully quit in that year and is labeled "Quit Rate" on the chart. While age has some influence on the quit rate, Figure 13 shows that all of the cohorts experienced a major change synchronous by calendar year. The quit rates peak around 1970 in all of the cohorts with a subsequent decline. This peak occurred around the time that antismoking messages were present in large numbers on television to counter cigarette advertising under the Fairness Doctrine. When cigarette advertising was banned from television in 1970, these antismoking spots were also removed.

The cessation of cigarette smoking is often treated as a single definable event in epidemiological studies, when in reality it is a complex phenomenon with substantial short- and long-term rates of relapse to smoking and multiple attempts to quit prior to long-term success (44). The prevalence of smoking recorded in any given cross-sectional survey will underestimate the true prevalence of smoking for a birth cohort over time because the instantaneous prevalence at the time of the interview includes those who have quit only recently and are likely to relapse in large numbers. National surveys have indicated that approximately one-third of smokers attempt to quit each year (63). A recent survey in California revealed that 11.3% of those who had been smoking 12 months prior to the survey were nonsmokers at the time of the survey, and 3.6% had maintained cessation for less than 3 months (64).

Duration of Smoking

The duration of smoking is one of the most powerful predictors of disease risk for smokers, reflecting the age when smoking was initiated and the attained age of the smoker. For any given cohort the cumulative duration of exposure can be approximated by the area under the prevalence curve in Figures 2–9. The differences between male and female cohorts in duration of smoking, therefore, include both the differences in peak prevalences and the differences in age of initiation. The differences in both peak prevalences and ages of initiation for similar birth cohorts of males and females dramatically accentuate the difference in duration of exposure that occurred between males and females among the older birth cohorts. These older cohorts provided most of the lung cancer deaths in the early prospective mortality studies of smoking, and the large difference between the smoking-related mortality ratios for males and females in these studies is explained primarily by this difference in duration of exposure (13).

D. Effects of Education on Smoking Prevalence

The prevalence of smoking varies with a variety of measures of socioeconomic status including income and job classification (13). Recent data from California show an extremely strong relationship with years of formal education achieved. Figure 14 shows smoking status by level of education; it is clear that both current

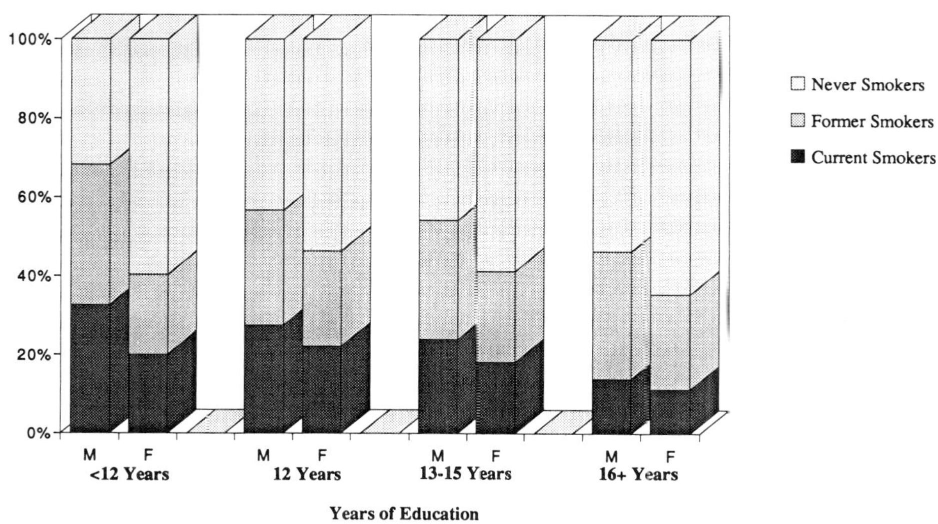

Figure 14 Smoking status of those with different years of education.

smoking status decreases and never-smoking status increases as level of education increases. Those with higher levels of education included fewer ever-smokers and more quitters. Since most of the initiation of cigarette smoking occurs prior to the age at which education is complete, this association with education reflects the environmental factors that influence both educational achievement and nonsmoking status. The gradient in smoking status with socioeconomic status demonstrated for adults is even more evident for adolescents. College freshmen have smoking prevalence rates of less than 10%, whereas Job Core applicants of the same age have smoking prevalence rates of over 60%.

E. Racial and Ethnic Differences

There are significant differences in smoking prevalence across racial, ethnic, and gender groupings. Blacks of both genders have higher smoking prevalences than whites (63). Hispanic smokers, particularly Hispanic women, have lower rates of smoking. Data from California in 1991–92 are presented to compare the differ-

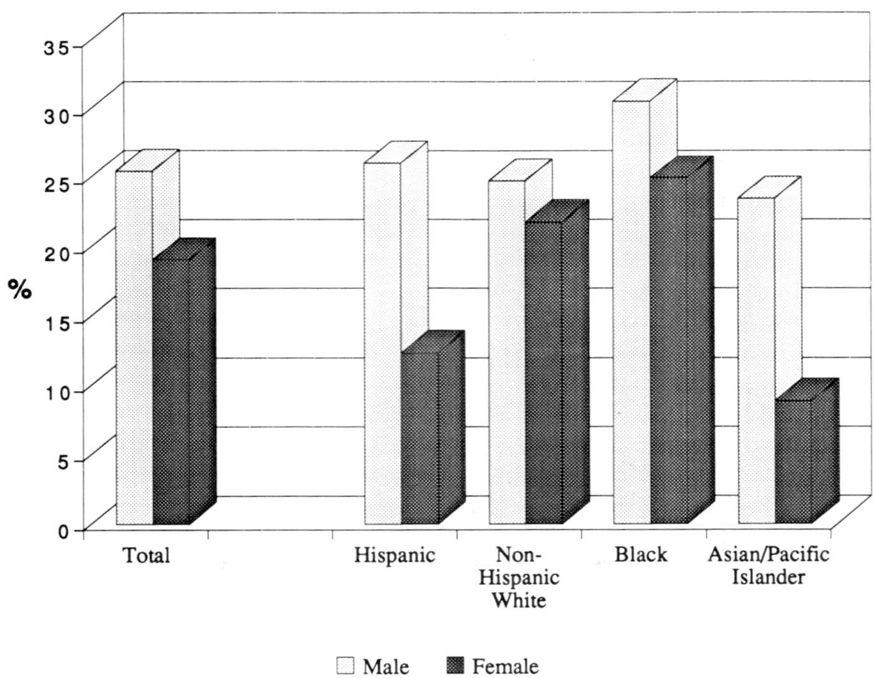

Figure 15 Prevalence of smoking among Californians of different racial and ethnic backgrounds (1900–1991 data).

ences across the groups (Fig. 15) (64). Substantially lower rates were observed for Hispanic and Asian women.

VII. Smoking Prevalence in Other Countries

Smoking prevalence for males and females in various countries are presented in Table 3. The data sources used to estimate prevalence in many of these countries are less extensive and often less representative of the overall population than those used to describe U.S. smoking behavior earlier in this chapter. However, they do offer a number of insights into smoking behavior outside the United States.

In general, the prevalence of smoking is higher among males compared to females and the differences are larger for Asian countries and less developed countries. For many of these countries the pattern of smoking is similar to that of the United States in the 1940s, that is, smoking is predominantly a male behavior, but women are beginning to smoke in large numbers, particularly younger women. This pattern suggests that many countries may see acceleration of their lung cancer death rates in the future, particularly among women.

VIII. Summary

Tobacco use was a widespread social phenomenon even prior to Columbus' voyage to the New World. It is, however, only in the last century that the use of tobacco as cigarettes has been prevalent. The milder tobacco and more acidic smoke of cigarettes leads to the deeper inhalation of tobacco into the lung with resultant deposition and absorption of the toxic and carcinogenic components of the smoke. More than 4000 individual constituents have been identified in cigarette smoke, and the relative concentrations of these constituents vary widely between brands of cigarettes. Tar, a measure of the total particulate matter of the smoke, varies markedly with characteristics of the cigarette manufacture and with the pattern of inhalation. As a result, tar is not a good measure of the dose of toxic or carcinogenic agents received by the individual smoker.

The particle size of cigarette smoke is in the range that will lead to deposition in the airways and alveoli of the lung, and many of the gas phase constituents are absorbed across the alveolar capillary membrane. The irritant agents in the smoke lead to acute and chronic changes in lung structure and function that may lead to the greater retention of carcinogens within the lung and increased vulnerability of the lung to the effects of these carcinogens. Carcinogens and other constituents present in cigarette smoke are also absorbed into the blood and metabolized to active forms through microsomal enzyme systems induced by cigarette smoke. The cellular influx of neutrophils and alveolar macrophages that is part of the inflammatory response may be the precursor of the alveolar wall destruction that results in emphysema.

Table 3 Percentage of Adult Male and Female Smokers in Various Countries

Country or territory	Comment	Year of survey	% of total who smoke: Male	% of total who smoke: Female
South America				
Bolivia	Urban La Paz	1986	46	29
Colombia	Nationwide	1988	37	18
Ecuador	Urban areas	1988	39	16
Peru	Towns >2,500	1989	42	13
Venezuela	Urban areas	1988	32	23
Argentina	Urban areas	1988	43	27
Chile	Three communities	1987	35	32
Paraguay	Physicians nationwide	1989	35	24
Uruguay	Urban areas	1988	44	23
Brazil	Twelve state capitals	1988	45	33
Central America				
Costa Rica	Nationwide	1988	35	20
El Salvador	Nationwide, urban	1988	38	12
Guatemala	Urban areas	1989	38	18
Honduras	Urban areas	1988	36	11
Nicaragua	Employed persons	1988	51	6
Panama	Nationwide	1983	56	20
Latin Caribbean				
Cuba	Nationwide	1988	48	26
Dominican Republic	Nationwide	1989	66	14
Puerto Rico	San Juan	1989	23	11
Selected Caribbean countries				
Anguilla	Islandwide	1989	10	2
Bahamas	Areawide	1989	19	4
Jamaica	Household	1987	25	6
Aruba and Netherlands Antilles	Random sample 1% population	1989	32	13
Trinidad and Tobago	St. James	1981	42	8
U.S. Virgin Islands	Household	1989	15	9
North America				
Canada	National	1983	41	32
Mexico	Urban areas	1988	37	17
USA	National	1980	38	30
Australia	National	1983	37	30
Bangladesh	Dhaka urban	1984	70	20
Brunei	Tutong urban	1979	20	7
China	Hunan	1981	56	1
	Shanghai county	1981	44	3
	Ghanzhou urban	1984	95	—

Table 3 Continued

Country or territory	Comment	Year of survey	% of total who smoke: Male	Female
Egypt	National	1982	40	1
France	National	1978	47	20
Germany	National	1980	40	29
Guatemala	Urban	1972	36	10
Hawaii				
Caucasians	Statewide	1979	51	50
Hawaiians	Statewide	1979	57	47
Chinese	Statewide	1979	37	18
Filipinos	Statewide	1979	48	28
Japanese	Statewide	1979	53	26
Hong Kong	National	1984	33	4
India	Goa urban	1984	29	3
	Goa rural	1984	61	7
Indonesia	Various sites	1984	61	5
Ireland	National	1980	49	36
Israel	National	1983	44	30
Italy	National	1981	54	32
Ivory Coast	Abidjan	1981	24	0.8
Japan	National	1980	70	14
Kuwait	National	1980	52	12
Malaysia		1983	18	2
Nepal	Urban	1980	84	14
New Zealand	National	1981	35	29
Norway	National	1982	40	34
Pakistan	Karachi	1982	44	6
Papua New Guinea	Highlands	1981	77	80
	Southcoast	1981	85	76
Poland	National	1980	63	29
Romania	Urban, Rural	1970	52	9
Singapore	National	1975	51	8.3
Sri Lanka	Kandy urban	1968	48	2
Sweden	National	1982	30	30
Switzerland	Zurich county	1980	50	26
Thailand	Urban nationwide	1981	51	4
	Rural	1981	70	40
Tunisia	Tunis urban	1984	58	6
UK	National	1982	38	33
USSR	Moscow	1981	44	10
Zambia	Lusaka urban	1984	63	56

Source: Ref. 5.

The prevalence of smoking is not uniformly distributed across the population. Men began smoking in large numbers very early in the century, but women only began to smoke in large numbers at the time of World War II. More recent birth cohorts of males and females are less likely to take up smoking than older cohorts, and the pattern of smoking uptake and cessation is similar for males and females in the most recent cohorts. Blacks are more likely to smoke than whites, and Asian and Hispanic women are less likely to smoke than white women. The prevalence of smoking is currently declining in both men and women.

References

1. U.S. Dept. of Health and Human Services. (1992). Smoking and Health in the Americas. Public Health Service, Centers for Disease Control, Office on Smoking and Health. DHHS Publication No. (CDC) 92–8419.
2. Burrough, B., Helyar, J. (1990). *Barbarians at the Gate: The Fall of RJR Nabisco*. New York, Harper & Row.
3. Brunnemann, K. D., and Hoffman, D. (1974). The pH of tobacco smoke. *Food Cosmetics Toxicol.* 12:115–124.
4. Gori, G. B., Benowitz, N. L., and Lynch, C. J. (1986). Mouth versus deep airways absorption of nicotine in cigarette smokers. *Pharmacol. Biochem. Behav.* 25:1181–1184.
5. International Agency for Research on Cancer (IARC). (1986). Tobacco smoking. IARC Monographs on the Evaluation of Carcinogenic Risk of Chemicals to Humans, Vol. 38. Lyon, IARC.
6. Kozlowski, L. T., Frecker, R. C., Khouw, V., and Pope, M. A. (1980). The misuses of "less hazardous" cigarettes and its detection: Hole-blocking of ventilated filters. *Am. J. Public Health* 70:1202–1203.
7. Wald, N. J., Howard, S., and Evans, J. (1976). Smoking tables for carbon monoxide? *Br. Med. J.* I:434–435.
8. Baker, R. R. (1984). The effect of ventilation on cigarette combustion mechanisms. *Recent Adv. Tobacco Sci.* 10:88–150.
9. Dube, M. F., and Green, C. R. (1984). Methods of collection of smoke for analytical purposes. *Recent Adv. Tobacco Sci.* 8:42–102.
10. Pillsbury, H. C., Bright, C. C., O'Connor, K. J., and Irish, F. W. (1969). Tar and nicotine in cigarette smoke. *J. Assoc. Off. Anal. Chem.* 52:458–462.
11. Adams, J. D., O'Mara-Adams, K. J., and Hoffman, D. (1985). On the mainstream-sidestream distribution of cigarette smoke components. Paper presented at the 39th Tobacco Chemists' Research Conference, Montreal, Canada, Oct. 2–5.
12. DHHS. (1981). The health consequences of smoking: The changing cigarette. U.S. Department of Health and Human Services, Public Health Service, Office of the Assistant Secretary for Health, Office on Smoking and Health. DHHS Publication No. (PHS) 81-50156.
13. DHHS. (1989). The health consequences of smoking: 25 years of progress. U.S. Department of Health and Human Services, Public Health Service, Centers for

Disease Control, Office on Smoking and Health. DHHS Publication No. (CDC) 89-8411.

14. Wynder, E. L., and Hoffman, D. (1967) *Tobacco and Tobacco Smoke. Studies in Experimental Carcinogenesis.* New York, Academic Press.
15. Nakayama, T., Kodama, M., and Nagata, C. (1984). Generation of hydrogen peroxide and superoxide anion radical from cigarette smoke. *Jpn. J. Cancer Res.* 75:95–98.
16. Church, D. F., and Pryor, W. A. (1985). Free-radical chemistry of cigarette smoke and its toxicologicological implications. *Environ. Health Perspect.* 64:111–126.
17. Schmeltz, I., Tosk, J., Jacobs, Z. G., and Hoffmann, D. (1977). Redox potential and quinone content of cigarette smoke. *Anal. Chem.* 49:1924–1929.
18. Muir, D. C. F. (1974). Tobacco smoke inhalation. *Scand. J. Resp. Dis.* 91(Suppl.):44–46.
19. Eudy, L. W., Green, C. R., Heavor, D. L., Ingebrethsen, B. J., and Thorne, F. A. (1985). Studies on the vapor-particulate phase distribution of environmental nicotine by selective trapping and detection methods. Presented at the 39th Tobacco Chemists' Research Conference, Montreal, Oct. 2–5.
20. DHHS. (1986). The health consequences of smoking: Involuntary smoking. U.S. Department of Health and Human Services, Public Health Service, Office of the Assistant Secretary for Health, Office on Smoking and Health. DHHS Publication No. (PHS) 87-8398.
21. Radford, E. P., and Hunt, V. R. (1964). Polonium-210 A volatile radioelement in cigarettes. *Science* 14:247–249.
22. Black, S. C., and Bretthaauer, E. W. (1968). Polonium-210 in tobacco. *Radiol. Health Data Rep.* 9:145–149.
23. Radford, E. P. (1982). Radioactivity in cigarette smoke (letter). *N. Engl. J. Med.* 307: 1449–1450.
24. Cross, F. T. (1984). Radioactivity in cigarette smoke issue. *Health Phys.* 46:205–208.
25. Little, J. B., and McGandy, R. B. (1968). Systemic absorption of polonium-210 inhaled in cigarette smoke. *Arch. Environ. Health* 17:693–696.
26. Cohen, B. S., Eisenbud, M., and Harley, N. H. (1980). Alpha radioactivity in cigarette smoke. *Radiat. Res.* 83:190–196.
27. Steinfeld, A. D. (1980). Environmental radiation hazards. *Am. Fam. Physician* 22: 95–99.
28. Martell, E. A. (1983). Alpha radiation dose at bronchial bifurcations of smokers from indoor exposure to radon progeny. *Proc. Natl. Acad. Sci.* 80:1285–1289.
29. Ingebrethsen, B. J. (1986). Aerosol studies of cigarette smoke. *Recent Adv. Tobacco Sci.* 12:54–142.
30. Hinds, W. C. (1982). *Aerosol Technology.* New York, John Wiley and Sons.
31. International Committee on Radiation Protection (ICRP), Task Group on Lung Dynamics. (1966). Deposition and retention models for internal dosimetry of the human respiratory tract. *Health Phys.* 12:173–207.
32. Mitchell, R. I. (1962). Controlled measurement of smoke-particle retention in the respiratory tract. *Am. Rev. Resp. Dis.* 85:526–533.
33. Hinds, W. C., First, M. W., Huber, G. I., and Shea, J. W. (1983). A method for measuring respiratory deposition of cigarette smoke during smoking. *Am. Ind. Hyg. J.* 44:113–118.

34. Donnelly, G. M., McKean, H. E., Heird, C. S., and Green, J. (1981). Bioassay of a cigarette smoke fraction. I. Examination of dose-response relations and dilution bioassay assumptions in a ciliostasis system. *J. Toxicol. Environ. Health* 7:405–417.
35. Hilding, A. C. (1956). On cigarette smoking, bronchial carcinoma and ciliary action. II. Experimental study on the filtering action of cow's lungs, the deposition of tar in the bronchial tree and removal by ciliary action. *N. Engl. J. Med.* 254:1150–1160.
36. Dalhamn, T. (1959). The effect of cigarette smoke in the ciliary activity of the upper respiratory tract. *Arch. Otolaryngol.* 70:166–168.
37. DHHS. (1984). The health consequences of smoking: Chronic obstructive lung disease. U.S. Department of Health and Human Services, Public Health Service, Office of the Assistant Secretary for Health, Office on Smoking and Health. DHHS Publication No. (PHS) 84–50205.
38. U.S. Public Health Service (USPHS). (1964). Smoking and health: A report of the advisory committee to the Surgeon General of the Public Health Service. U.S. Department of Health, Education and Welfare, Public Health Service, Center for Disease Control, PHS Publication #1103.
39. DHEW. (1979). The health consequences of smoking: A report of the Surgeon General. U.S. Department of Health and Human Services, Public Health Service, Office of the Assistant Secretary for Health, Office on Smoking and Health. Publication No. (PHS) 79-50066.
40. DHHS. (1982). The health consequences of smoking: Cancer. U.S. Department of Health and Human Services, Public Health Service, Office of the Assistant Secretary for Health, Office on Smoking and Health. DHHS Publication No. (PHS) 82-50179.
41. DHHS. (1983). The health consequences of smoking: Cardiovascular disease. U.S. Department of Health and Human Services, Public Health Service, Office of the Assistant Secretary for Health, Office on Smoking and Health. DHHS Publication No. (PHS) 84-50204.
42. DHHS. (1985). The health consequences of smoking: Cancer and chronic lung disease in the workplace. U.S. Department of Health and Human Services, Public Health Service, Office of the Assistant Secretary for Health, Office on Smoking and Health. DHHS Publication No. (PHS) 85-50207.
43. DHHS. (1988). The health consequences of smoking: Nicotine addiction. U.S. Department of Health and Human Services, Public Health Service, Centers for Disease Control, Office on Smoking and Health. DHHS Publication No. (CDC) 88-8406.
44. DHHS. (1990). The health benefits of smoking cessation. U.S. Department of Health and Human Services, Public Health Service, Centers for Disease Control, Office on Smoking and Health. DHHS Publication No. (CDC) 90-8416.
45. Auerbach, O., Hammond, E. C., and Garfinkel, L. (1979). Changes in the bronchial epithelium in relation to cigarette smoking, 1955–1960 vs 1970–1977. *N. Engl. J. Med.* 300:381–386.
46. Yamasaki, E., and Ames, B. N. (1977). Concentration of mutagens from urine by absorption with the nonpolar resin XAD–2: Cigarette smokers have mutagenic urine. *Proc. Natl. Acad. Sci.* 74:3555–3559.
47. Armitage, P., and Doll, R. (1961). Stochastic models for carcinogenesis. *Proceedings*

of the Fourth Berkeley Symposium on Mathematical Statistics and Probability, University of California Press, Berkeley, pp. 19–38.

48. Burns, D., Frionds, J., and Jarvik, M. (1988). Biologic interactions between smoking and occupational exposures. *Am. J. Ind. Med.* 13:169–179.
49. Stevens, R., and Moolgavkar, S. (1979). Estimation of relative risk from vital data: Smoking and cancers of the lung and bladder. *JNCI* 63:1351–1357.
50. Stevens, R., and Moolgavkar, S. (1984). A cohort analysis of lung cancer and smoking in British males. *Am. J. Epidemiol.* 119:624–641.
51. Townsend, J. (1978). Smoking and lung cancer: A cohort study of men and women in England and Wales 1935–70. *J. R. Statis. Soc.* A 141 (part 1):95–107.
52. Hammond, E. C. (1966). Smoking in relation to the death rates of one million men and women. *Natl. Cancer Inst. Monogr.* 19:127–204.
53. Knudson, A. (1985). Hereditary cancer, oncogenes and antioncogenes. *Cancer Res.* 45:1437–1443.
54. Cavanee, W., Dryja, T., Philips, R., et al. (1983). Expression of recessive alleles by chromosomal mechanisms in retinoblastoma. *Nature* 305:779–784.
55. Harbour, J., Lai, S., Whang-Peng, J., et al. (1988). Abnormalities in structure and expression of the human retinoblastoma gene in SCLC. *Science* 241:353–357.
56. Birrer, M., and Minna, J. (1988). Molecular genetics of lung cancer. *Semin. Oncol.* 15:226–235.
57. Moolgavkar, S., Dewanji, A., and Luebek, G. (1989). Cigarette smoking and lung cancer: Reanalysis of the British doctors' data. *JNCI* 81:415–420.
58. Doll, R., and Peto, R. (1978). Cigarette smoking and bronchial carcinoma: Dose and time relationships among regular smokers and lifelong non-smokers. *J. Epidemiol. Comm. Health* 32:303–313.
59. Brown, C., and Kessler, L. (1988). Projections of lung cancer mortality in the United States: 1985–2025. *JNCI* 80:43–51.
60. DHHS. (1980). The health consequences of smoking for women. U.S. Department of Health and Human Services, Public Health Service, Office of the Assistant Secretary for Health, Office of Smoking and Health.
61. Harris, J. (1983). Cigarette smoking among successive birth cohorts of men and women in the United States during 1900–80. *JNCI* 71:473–479.
62. Crane, L., Herman-Shipley, N., and Tolley, D. (1992) Smoking prevalences and lung cancer death rates. In *Tobacco Control Monograph No. 1: Comprehensive Approaches to Tobacco Control*. Edited by D. Burns, J. Samet, and E. Gritz. U.S. Department of Health and Human Services, Public Health Service, National Cancer Institute.
63. Pierce, J., and Hatziandreu, E. (1989). Report of the 1986 adult use of tobacco survey. U.S. Department of Health and Human Services, Public Health Service, Centers for Disease Control, Office on Smoking and Health, U.S. Government Printing Office OM 90-2004.
64. Burns, D., and Pierce, J. (1992). Tobacco use in California 1990–1991. California Department of Health Services.

3

The Descriptive Epidemiology of Lung Cancer

THOMAS J. MASON

Fox Chase Cancer Center
Philadelphia, Pennsylvania

I. Background

Descriptive epidemiology facilitates the (1) identification of problems, (2) development of hypotheses for risk factors, and (3) monitoring consequences of intervention. This chapter will provide insights on recent contributions to the literature that have attempted to identify and better characterize etiologic determinants of lung cancer from the perspective of its descriptive epidemiology. Emphasis is given to differences in exposure(s) and response between males and females. Similarities and differences between the United States and other countries at the national and regional level, when available, are presented.

During the 1980s considerable progress was made in understanding the multiple factor etiology (1) of lung cancer. The literature is replete with studies that have identified specific agents causally associated with the epidemic rise of lung cancer. It has been recognized for some time now that the dynamics of rate change over time, however, have differed markedly between the sexes (2). Of initial concern was what was known about demographic factors that could aid in our understanding (3). The patterns for the association between income and education and lung cancer were consistent with the predicted inverse relation for males, but counter-intuitive for females with a positive association between income and education and lung cancer rates (predominantly attributable to white females) (4). In the mid-1980s, data were obtained on smoking practices as part of the Current Population Survey under the direction of the U.S. Bureau of the Census, which were used to estimate smoking-attributable mortality and years of potential life lost (5). Cullen emphasized the dramatic differences between rates of decline of smoking prevalence between the sexes (males twice as likely as females to stop smoking since the mid-1960s, 37% vs. 18%) and that females were starting to smoke at younger ages (6).

II. Geography and Age

In the mid-1970s, the first two in the series of atlases of cancer mortality for the U.S. were published (7,8). For the 20-year period (1950–1969) provocative patterns of geographic and temporal distribution were found for lung cancer among males, which prompted a series of analytic field studies (9). With the publication of the most recent atlases in this series (10,11) in the late 1980s, geographic patterns for males became even more pronounced, whereas distinct patterns emerged for females who had previously not shown striking heterogeneity. Tabular material is provided in these atlases for individual decades, which serve to highlight the differences between the sexes. Age-adjusted rates among females, for both whites and nonwhites, more than doubled between the 1960s and 1970s. Table 1 presents the percent change of the average annual age-specific rates for lung cancer among U.S. females for the time periods from the cancer atlases (1950–1969 vs. 1970–1980). The age-specific differences between whites and nonwhites suggest that secular differences between the two groups on exposure(s) may have played some role in the emergent epidemic rise of lung cancer among women (12).

Recent publications have found that the differences between the sexes have

Table 1 Percent Change in Age-Specific Lung Cancer Mortality Rates per 100,000 Among U.S. Females 1970–1980 vs. 1950–1969

	Percent change			Percent change	
Age group (y)	Whites	Nonwhites	Age group (y)	Whites	Nonwhites
35–39	+66.9	+53.7	60–64	+203.4	+141.2
40–44	+103.2	+92.6	65–69	+180.1	+133.6
45–49	+142.3	+161.1	70–74	+126.9	+155.0
50–54	+170.5	+162.5	75–84	+86.1	+131.1
55–59	+194.5	+157.9	+85	+82.5	+144.7

persisted to the extent that rates of lung cancer among U.S. males plateaued in the late 1970s and started to decrease between 1982 and 1983 (13). Extending the time period through 1986, declining rates for lung cancer mortality among young men and women have been found (14,15). Rates of decline were greatest among young (35–44-year-old) white males (28.7%) and least among white females of the same age (5.3%) (15). Changes in age-specific incidence rates were found to differ even more dramatically between white and black males and females. For black females there is no indication of declining rates, and the rates of increase are the greatest.

A comparison of temporal changes in U.S. and Swedish lung cancer between 1950 and 1982 by Manton et al. (16) concluded that the magnitude and change of cohort differentials between the United States and Sweden support the conjecture that most of the differences may be attributed to differences in smoking habits. The mean age at death from lung cancer among U.S. females declined over the first two decades (1950–1970) and was followed by a compensating increase in 1980.

National comparisons by Mizuno et al. (17) have also contrasted lung cancer risk among male smokers in a Japanese cohort and the British physicians cohort. Hakulinen et al. (18) compared lung cancer incidence among males in Finland and Norway. In both instances, differences were concluded to be attributable to smoking habits. Specifically, adjustment for effective duration of cigarette smoking (latency) resulted in comparable risks for the low-incidence-rate areas (Japan and Norway) as compared to those for the higher-rate regions.

This conclusion, however, has not been universal in all such studies. A study that compared incidence rates by histologic type in northwest England (a high-incidence area) with Osaka, Japan (a low-incidence area), is notable in this regard (19). The authors suggested that causal factors other than smoking may exist for adenocarcinoma for both males and females in Japan.

Within-country (defined geographic area) differences have been reported by the Pannonian Tumor Epidemiology Group (20) in neighboring regions of Hungary, Austria, Yugoslavia, and Czechoslovakia. Zaridze and Gurevicius (21) published data from five of the former Soviet republics. In the first instance, the regions are contiguous and have had cancer registries in place since the 1950s with the exception of Austria, which commenced in 1970. Data were analyzed for three time periods—1969–1972, 1973–1976, and, 1977–1980. Among males, lung cancer incidence increased significantly in Hungary and Czechoslovakia. Among females, rates significantly declined in Hungary and Yugoslavia and remained constant in the other regions.

Incidence data for five former Soviet republics—Byelorussia, Estonia, Georgia, Moldavia, and Lithuania—were analyzed for the time period 1971–1982. Increases were found among men for all ages. Among women, significant increases in age-specific rates were found in Georgia among 40- to 49-year-olds and in Lithuania among 50- to 59-year-olds. The authors suggest that regional differences in smoking are the most likely explanation.

III. Smoking

Between 1989 and 1991 data from U.S. national surveys document an overall decline in the prevalence of smoking with a number of implications for prevention of smoking-related lung cancer. Data from the National Health Interview Surveys, from 1974 to 1985, were used to project that a larger proportion of women in the United States will be smokers than men after 1995 (22) and that almost half (44%) of young women who did not proceed beyond high school were smokers in 1985 (23). This pattern in women contrasts with a decline among young men in this age group. Data from the 1985 Current Population Survey collected by the Census Bureau provide additional evidence of disparate patterns of smoking for males and females (24). The authors emphasize the "complexity and potential danger of extrapolating national patterns of smoking prevalence (by demographic subgroups) to specific regions, divisions and states." Later sections present data on national and regional histologic distributions which support this concern.

Most recently (August 1991), data were analyzed from the American Cancer Society (ACS) prospective study of 1.2 million men and women (25). This assessment of smoking-attributable cancer mortality found that "slightly more than 90% of male and 78% of female lung cancer deaths are directly attributed to cigarette smoking." This finding does not diminish the need for research activities dedicated to minimizing the initiation of smoking or maximizing its cessation, but rather encourages research into the role(s) that factors other than smoking play in contributing to the unprecedented increase of lung cancer among women.

A case-control study among French women examined the effects of different smoking habits on lung cancer (26). Significant increases in matched relative risks were found for the usually suspect variables: starting smoking at a young age, number of cigarettes smoked daily, duration frequency of inhalation, use of dark tobacco, and use of nonfilter cigarettes. More than half of the cases were squamous cell carcinomas. Also worthy of note in this series is the fact that 52% of all cases were in nonsmokers and 71% of those with adenocarcinoma were in nonsmokers.

The Saskatchewan Cancer Foundation, a population-based registry, was recently used to assess all primary lung cancer cases between 1979 and 1983 (27). Women developed primary lung cancer at an earlier age than men while smoking fewer cigarettes for a shorter time than men. There were more lifetime nonsmokers among women than men (23% vs. 3.7%). Among smokers, a higher percentage of women compared to men smoked to a lesser extent as measured by pack-years. The authors suggest that "unknown endogenous, distinctly female factors as well as exogenous factors may contribute to the development of primary lung cancer in women."

Lest the reader suspect that insufficient attention is given to lung cancer among males, two recent articles have given occasion to reflect on our body of knowledge. A case-control study (28) on cigarette smoking and male lung cancer in Glasgow and western Scotland, an area with "the highest recorded incidence in the world," found a steep increase in the relative risk of lung cancer in western Scotland smokers among low daily cigarette consumers (1–14 cigarettes) and moderate consumers (15–24 cigarettes). They did not, however, detect the usually observed steady increase at the higher levels of smoking. Data from a prospective cohort study (29) of cardiorespiratory health and disease were used to test whether the observations from the case-control study could be supported. Comparison of the lung cancer rates for this cohort with those observed in other cohort studies suggested that rates of lung cancer among residents in western Scotland were substantially higher at all levels of cigarette exposure. One conclusion drawn by the authors is that the rates of lung cancer among nonsmokers in this region must be higher than in other studies for there to be high absolute levels of risk and low relative levels. Increased rates among both smokers and nonsmokers could be the result of a factor or factors unrelated to smoking. Regional differences in the consumption of fresh fruits and vegetables are suggested. Survey data have consistently shown a lower consumption of fresh fruit (25% less) and fresh green vegetables (50% less) in Scotland as compared with England. No obvious explanation is offered for the flattening of the dose-response relation, although the existence of a dose-incidence threshold is suggested.

IV. Histology

A. Smoking Effect and Secular Trends

Given the differences between the sexes for a number of factors related to lung cancer and the possibility that histologic classification of lung cancer provides clues in understanding its complex multifactor etiology (1), a number of recent publications are noteworthy.

In 1984, Lubin and Blot (30) reported on patterns of risk by histologic type from a large (7804 cases and 15,207 controls) hospital-based case-control study conducted in western Europe between 1970 and 1980. Because of the numbers of persons included in this study, cigarette smoking was identified as a risk factor for not only Kreyberg I cell types, but also for adenocarcinoma. Risks for adenocarcinoma among current smokers were 3.5 for males and 1.8 for females. They also found risk for squamous cell among males to overshadow that for small cell (20.9 vs. 10.5). Risks for these two types among females were almost identical (6.8 for squamous cell vs. 7.4 for small cell). Of particular relevance to the developing awareness of the epidemic rise of lung cancer among women, Lubin and Blot (30) found sex differences for lung cancer that could not be explained by smoking and encouraged research initiatives to identify sex-related factors (e.g., potential exposures), which may explain these findings.

In 1985, Andrews et al. (31) reported on 1752 patients whose lung cancers were diagnosed from 1957 through 1980. Their study suggested that for all cell types of lung cancer in women smoking was a major causal factor, in contrast to the preponderance of Kreyberg I tumors among men who smoke. This disparity led the authors to conclude that there remained "unanswered questions concerning the causes of lung cancer among women."

Subsequent studies have documented secular trends in histologic types of lung cancer. Wu et al. (32) reported on a 10-year period (1972–1981) in Los Angeles County, California. Rates of annual increase were greatest for adenocarcinoma among males (29%) and small-cell carcinoma among females (55%). A similarly dramatic rise for small-cell carcinoma among women was also found among non-Hispanic white females in New Mexico. Rates more than doubled when comparisons were made between 1980–81 and 1970–72 (33).

Beard et al. (34) addressed the basic concern of the effects of time-dependent changes in classification schemes on secular trends of histologic types of lung cancer. They reported on 50-year trends in lung cancer incidence where one pathologist reviewed all the slides and used the same classification scheme throughout. They found the rise in the proportion of adenocarcinoma was greater among men than among women.

A comparable increase of adenocarcinoma among men was found in a large series (3398 cases) of lung cancer histologically ascertained in 1973–1984 in Italy (35). Cases were divided into two periods of 6 years each. For the first period (1973–1978) the percentages by major type were: among males—60% squamous, 23% small cell, and 11% adeno; among females—30% squamous, 25% small cell, and 31% adeno. During the later period (1979–1984) the greatest increase among men was to 16% adeno and increases among women to 35% adeno and 33% squamous. Not only did the histologic-type distribution change, but there was also a demonstrable shift in the age distribution among women to increases at younger ages for both adenocarcinoma and squamous cell carcinomas.

This phenomenon of detecting adenocarcinomas at an earlier age has been reported among males and females in many settings (19,26,27). Over a 10-year period (1975–1985), lung cancer in young patients seen at a U.S. Army medical center has been reported (36). Among the 800 cases seen, 11 were under the age of 40. Nine were males. There was one case of squamous cell carcinoma, one case of oat cell carcinoma, five cases (45%) of adenocarcinoma, and four cases of large cell carcinoma. The authors concluded that "the disease is probably not more aggressive in younger patients, but, instead is further advanced when the patient is originally seen since the disease is not suspected in patients of this age." The smoking history for these patients was extensive, with a mean pack-year per patient of 43 years.

Another series of 29 cases of lung cancer among men aged 40 or less was examined at autopsy (37). The histologic type of lung cancer among these young men—squamous (28%), small cell (28%), adeno (24%), and large cell (14%)—is comparable to that among patients of all ages studied at autopsy.

Charts for all patients 40 years of age and younger with lung cancer seen at UCLA Hospital between 1956 and 1976 have been reviewed (38). An attempt was made to perform an additional review of the diagnostic histologic specimen of each patient. The diagnoses at review were: among males—adenocarcinoma (41%), squamous (5%), and small cell (22%); among females—adenocarcinoma (52%), squamous (13%), and small cell (10%).

B. U.S. Trends

The publication of the latest in the NCI's Cancer Statistics Review (39) provides an opportunity to reflect on changes in the percent distribution by major histologic type for lung cancer. This publication is the first in this series to present histology. Table 2 presents the total number of cases and percentages by major histologic type of lung cancer for cases identified and meeting criteria of the NCI's SEER program (1983–87) (39) and its predecessor, the Third National Cancer Survey

Table 2 Percent Distribution by Major Histologic Type for Cancer of the Lung and Bronchus

	1969–1971[a]			1983–1987[b]		
Histology	All races (n = 4077)	White (n = 3695)	Black (n = 340)	All races (n = 20867)	White (n = 18303)	Black (n = 1795)
Females						
Small-cell carcinoma	14.5	14.6	13.5	20.2	21.0	16.5
Squamous cell, other and unspecified	21.5	21.1	26.7	18.9	18.6	23.2
Adenocarcinoma, NOS	23.1	22.8	23.5	29.7	29.4	28.6
	All races (n = 16078)	White (n = 14199)	Black (n = 1735)	All races (n = 39653)	White (n = 33316)	Black (n = 4588)
Males						
Small-cell carcinoma	13.4	13.9	9.7	16.6	17.3	11.6
Squamous cell, other and unspecified	38.3	37.7	43.5	31.3	30.8	35.9
Adenocarcinoma, NOS	12.9	12.9	13.5	22.7	22.5	22.7

[a]From Ref. 40.
[b]From Ref. 39.

(1969–71) (40). The histologic classification of these cases is based on pathology reports from hospitals and thus subject to trends of reporting practices and observer variation. Among females, small-cell carcinoma and adenocarcinoma increased over this time period. The increase of small-cell carcinoma among white females was the largest. Among males, an approximate 70% increase in adenocarcinoma is seen for both blacks and whites.

C. High-Rate Areas of the United States

As mentioned above, the most recent atlases of cancer mortality identified patterns of high rate areas in the United States which differ markedly between the sexes. Table 3 presents the histologic distribution that was found when analytic field studies were carried out in Louisiana (41) and New Jersey (42,43) as well as a study that utilized Florida's statewide population-based registry (44).

In comparison to the distribution of histologic types from the SEER data (39) (Table 2, 1983–87), a number of differences are evident. Among females in

Table 3 Histologic Distribution of Lung Cancer Observed in High-Rate Areas

	Louisiana[a] (1979–1982)		New Jersey[a] (1982–1983)	Florida[b] (1981–1985)	
Histology	White (*n* = 212)	Black (*n* = 75)	White (*n* = 994)	White (*n* = 11686)	Nonwhite (*n* = 554)
Females					
Small-cell carcinoma	24.5	24.0	22.1	21.2	14.4
Squamous cell, other and unspecified	25.9	32.0	27.0	23.2	24.2
Adenocarcinoma	22.7	21.3	29.2	35.6	37.4
	(1979–1982)		1980–1981	(1981–1985)	
	White (*n* = 655)	Black (*n* = 311)	White (*n* = 741)	White (*n* = 21048)	Nonwhite (*n* = 1895)
Males					
Small-cell carcinoma	15.4	12.9	15.2	16.4	10.6
Squamous cell, other and unspecified	41.2	51.8	49.1	35.9	40.9
Adenocarcinoma	18.9	16.4	15.9	25.8	25.8

[a]From Refs. 41–43.
[b]From Ref. 44.

both Louisiana and New Jersey, there is more small-cell and squamous cell carcinoma. Among males only the percent of squamous cell carcinoma is greater for these two areas. For both males and females in Florida, the percent of cases of squamous cell carcinoma and adenocarcinoma exceed those from the SEER areas. The greatest difference is seen for adenocarcinoma among women.

In 1982, Mayo et al. (45) reported on a series of 307 cases of lung cancer among women in Kentucky from 1956 through 1979 for whom tissue biopsies confirmed the diagnosis. The histologic type distribution was 15% small cell carcinoma, 36% squamous cell, and 35% adenocarcinoma. Their prediction that lung cancer mortality among women would exceed that for breast cancer within 3 years was borne out (46).

A larger series of 648 cases of lung cancer among women seen at one hospital in Pittsburgh between 1958 and 1988 has recently been reported (47). Several characteristics of the series are noteworthy: 435 (67%) of the lung cancers were epidermoid and 66% of the total "admitted to smoking cigarettes and to being indirectly affected by passive smoking and other atmospheric contaminants in the workplace."

All female cases of pathologically verified primary carcinoma of the lung diagnosed between 1969 and 1977 at northern California Kaiser hospitals were identified from hospital discharge records and records of the California Tumor Registry (48). The pathology distribution for cases who smoked was markedly different in comparison to that of never-smokers. Among smokers, 33% were adenocarcinomas, 22% small cell, and 19% squamous. Among nonsmokers, 67% were adenocarcinomas, 3% were squamous, and no person was found to have small-cell carcinoma.

V. Etiologic Implications

It has been recognized for quite some time now that smoking-related risks for the major histologic types of lung cancer are highly variable. Depending upon the setting of the study (geography and gender), squamous and/or small-cell carcinomas of the lung have the highest smoking-related risks, and adenocarcinoma of the lung has had the lowest risk. From the materials presented in Table 3, among male cases included in case-control studies in Louisiana and New Jersey, squamous cell carcinoma was the predominant type. Among females in these geographic areas, the distribution is much more homogeneous. The quantification of smoking-related attributable risks for lung cancer in excess of 90% among males but less than 80% among females are consistent with these disparate percent distributions, as well as the recent increase of adenocarcinoma among males and small-cell carcinoma among females. Additional support comes from the observations that smoking rates among U.S. females are approaching rates for males and, specifically, cessation rates among females are considerably lower than cessation rates among males. One is reminded that throughout the recent past (primarily the 1980s) there have been repeated findings in the literature that support the need for further research to identify factors other than smoking that are related to the dynamic changes in lung cancer (1,2,5,12,25,30,31,49). The most recent addition by Shopland (49) provides extensive analyses of smoking behaviors by sex, race, calendar period, and birth cohort. His analyses suggest lung cancer risk(s) among females not attributable to smoking. Two candidates are factors related to the endocrine system and occupational exposures.

Support for the role of the endocrine system in lung cancer among women derives in large part from studies of lung cancer among Japanese, Chinese, and Hawaiian women (50–53). Gao et al. (53) demonstrated an increased risk for adenocarcinoma, which was associated with short irregular menstrual cycles. The working causal hypothesis in this setting, where women rarely smoke, is that exposures such as volatiles from oils used in traditional cooking are selective for initiating adenocarcinoma, and the short irregular menstrual cycles result in increased exposure to growth-promoting estrogens.

Support for the role of selective occupational exposures among females derives in part from the following: When one compares age-specific rates of lung cancer among white and nonwhite females marked differences in the rates of change between the two groups are observed (see Table 1). These percent changes for white females are consistent with a cohort effect among white females that appears to be working through the population. Age-specific rates among white females more than double among relatively young women and then decline with increasing age. The pattern for nonwhite females is distinctly different in that age-specific rates show an all but constant percent change across all age categories. These differences in percent change suggest certain cohorts to be at distinctly different risks for the subsequent development of lung cancer.

Andrews et al. (31) conjectured that a "change that may have contributed to early lung cancer in women was the large influx of women entering the job force during World War II." He and his colleagues are not the first to express this concern, but as has been the case previously, no specifics were provided.

Prompted by their comments, I have attempted to find specifics for this phenomenon. The data in Table 4 present the numbers of women in the U.S. labor force (in thousands) by age before, during, and after World War II (54). The greatest changes are seen among adolescent females (age 16–19): the number employed more than doubled from 1940 to 1944 and then decreased dramatically. Not only did the absolute numbers increase, but "the war manufacturing industries (metal, chemical, and rubber) showed an enormous net gain in woman employment from 1940 to 1944 of more than 460 percent, and this produced a large gain in the total manufacturing employment of women" (55).

Table 4 Women in the U.S. Labor Force in Thousands by Age Before, During, and After World War II

Year	Total	Age Group (y) 16–19	20–24	25–44	45–64
1940	13,077	1,396	2,698	6,081	2,554
1943	18,830	2,930	3,180	8,260	3,970
1944	19,390	2,900	3,340	8,330	4,320
1945	19,304	2,270	3,310	8,370	4,410
1950	16,443	1,331	2,251	7,666	4,416
	Percent Change				
Avg (1943–1945) vs. 1940	+47	+104	+21	+37	+66
1950 vs. Avg (1943–1945)	−14	−53	−23	−8	+4

Source: Ref. 54.

An earlier publication from the Women's Bureau of the U.S. Department of Labor (56) provides a wealth of detail on what the working conditions were like in the summer of 1942. A survey was performed which included women workers from a cross section of industries in New Jersey. A total of 137 plants were included. In each plant at least 50% of the production was devoted to war contract work. This bulletin, specific to the New Jersey experience (56) also provides information on the potential for differential exposures to white and black women in the workforce.

> It is the expressed policy in only a few firms not to employ Negro women on productive work. In most cases there were no such restrictions, though in a substantial proportion no Negro women actually were employed except in maintenance or service capacities, and the data in general show that Negro women were not doing factory work in significant numbers except in rare instances. (p. 13)

The appendix includes excerpts from this bulletin that characterize the working environment as it relates to the health of the women workers. Specific sections on exposures to cutting oils and mica are included. These are followed by characterizations of exposure to harmful dusts and the status of ventilation. The reader is encouraged to consider these specifics in light of what is now known about a number of these conditions/exposures and the development of lung cancer, as well as the fact that females aged 16–19 in 1944 were 47–50 years old in 1975.

The appendix indicates the wealth of information available in the bulletins of the Women's Bureau, which provide an assessment of working conditions coincident with exposure and, thus, not subject to selective recall; the detail provided did not, in my opinion, lend itself to summarization, but rather should serve to promote subsequent investigations that can add to our understanding of determinants of lung cancer.

VI. Summary

The materials presented have attempted to address three objectives of descriptive epidemiology. The plateauing of age-specific rates for lung cancer among males is consistent with the reported success of smoking cessation programs among men. The continued rise of rates among women, unfortunately, identifies a problem area. Given the epidemic rise of lung cancer among women, targeted programs for young women to influence their rates of starting smoking, as well as facilitate their stopping, are indicated. Geographic patterns for lung cancer in the United States as well as in many other countries worldwide continue to suggest regions where additional study is highly likely to identify previously unrecognized causal determinants. In the United States, a number of high-rate areas for lung cancer have been identified (7,8,10,11). Studies in these areas have suggested a number of testable hypotheses (9).

Today's society has become sensitized to the fact that a number of issues related to women's health need to be addressed. With regard to lung cancer, there can be no question that the magnitude of the problem is of epidemic proportions. All of the materials presented suggest that lung cancer among males is primarily caused by active smoking. That this is not the case among women suggests that greater than 20% of this dramatically increasing disease is due to other causes. The appendix supports the contention that "today's woman" is what Miller referred to as a "prepared host" (2) for whom lung cancer is caused by a number of different interacting factors. These factors are also addressed in subsequent chapters dealing with such diverse issues as occupational determinants, residential exposures, and diet.

Acknowledgments

The assistance of Harriett Harper, Chief, Division of Statistical and Economic Analysis, Women's Bureau, U.S. Department of Labor, is gratefully acknowledged. She provided access to historic materials which characterize the working environment of American women during World War II. I would like to also thank Jonathan Samet for his guidance and understanding. Alicia D. Blake and Marion Horn facilitated the synthesis of the materials and provided much appreciated editorial support.

Appendix*

Exposure of Women to Health Hazards

Effect of War Conditions on Industrial Health

The increasing diversity of women's work in the war program has implications not only for greater opportunity to use talents and to secure better wages than in more customary women's employment; it also brings about the exposure of women to toxic materials to which they rarely have been exposed in modern American industry.

In the plants surveyed in New Jersey women were at work on a great variety of occupations exposing them to diverse hazards. Not only had the number of hazards and the number of exposed women increased, but exposures themselves were found to be intensified by many factors: (1) Longer hours, (2) shortened lunch periods, (3) pressure for increased production, (4) overcrowding of workers, (5) use of makeshift washing facilities, (6) allowing too little time for washing and cleaning up before leaving work, and (7) increased fatigue because of constant standing, reaching, standing on concrete floors, sitting on backless stools or chairs of the kitchen-chair variety.

Fatigue always lowers resistance to occupational poisons as it does to other diseases. The longer the hours the longer the exposure to the poisons. If washing is not adequate the worker may be exposed for 24 hours a day through her contaminated skin or clothing. The poison may even be ingested with food if hands and nails have not been adequately washed. Doubling and trebling the number of people in the same working space may mean that ventilation adequate for the smaller number needs retesting for the larger number. A final factor is equally important—the difficulty of providing adequate medical care, including physical examinations, coupled with the increasing percentage of applicants who are physically below par.

A great many more or less unfamiliar industrial poisons have come into use with the necessity for accelerated production of explosives, synthetic rubber, and all the numerous articles of Army and Navy ordinance as well as substitutes for civilian consumption. (p. 28)

Potential Exposures of Women

The industries surveyed in New Jersey expose women to a number of harmful materials or conditions. These may be classified as follows:

Skin irritants:

Benzol (see also under systemic)	Glass Silk
Tetryl	Materials used in manufacture of plastics
Mercury fulminate	Dyes of various kinds
Mica Dust	Cutting oils and compounds
Pyranol	

---

*All materials quoted from Ref. 56.

Systemic poisoning:

Lead oxides	Tetryl
Benzol	Mercury
Radium	Carbon monoxide

Respiratory diseases: Silica dust; steel dust; mica dust.
Acid burns—Nitric acid
X-ray burns—X-ray
Heat prostration—Excessive heat (p. 28)

Cutting oils.—A number of metal manufacturing companies reported cutting oils and compounds as the principal dermatitis exposures to their women employees on machine work. Control of these infections as described to the agents consisted in adding an antiseptic to the oil in one plant; in another to medical check and transfer of affected workers, as well as choice of applicants for such work who have no skin lesions.

Cutting oils are the most frequent cause of dermatitis among metal workers, according to reports of United States Public Health Service. Prevention among women workers merits much attention because of the great increase in woman employment in metal industries. New employees not selected on the basis of susceptibility naturally show a high rate of cases.

The dermatitis may begin with comedones of the hands and arms. Folliculitis of arms and thighs is the common type. Infected follicles may develop into boils and even carbuncles, and infection of wounds of the skin caused by metallic slivers may cause the development of boils. The defatting action of cutting oils on the skin may cause drying, cracking, and fissuring. The open fissures are subject to secondary infection. Dry skins are most likely to be affected in this way. Some of the oils may contain chlorine compounds, the dermatitis taking the forms of a typical chloracne. Allergic eczemas occasionally occur from contact with machine oils. The addition of strong antiseptics to the oil may itself be the cause of such skin infection.

Briefly summarized, prevention should include (1) provision of facilities and time for personal cleanliness, (2) clean work clothes and impervious sleeves and aprons to protect arms and thighs, (3) provision of clean towels for wiping hands, (4) removal of metal slivers from oil, (5) change of oil at least once a week. Re-used oil should be screened to remove metal, sterilized, and neutralized. Of these, personal cleanliness is the most important item. (pp. 30–31)

Mica.—Exposure to mica dust noted in another plant was stated to have caused skin irritation. They tried transferring these girls to other work for 2 weeks, after which it might be 2 months before the rash appeared again. Gloves were furnished by the company.

Mica dust exercises an irritant mechanical action on the skin, the eyes, and the respiratory passages. Authorities refer to cases of eczema and ulcerative lesions among workers making micanite.

It is also said to enter the respiratory and digestive passages, which it impregnates, giving rise to a disease rare in this country, designated as "silicosis universalis." Mica dust should not enter the breathing area of workers but should be controlled by systems of ventilation. (p. 31)

Respiratory Diseases

In a number of instances women were found needlessly exposed to harmful dusts. In one the women were fettling small porcelain parts without adequate exhaust ventilation. That this operation may cause dangerous concentrations of silica dust is shown by the 1939 study of the pottery industry made by the United States Public Health Service. The study also shows how harmful concentrations can be controlled by down-draft ventilation. (p. 31)

Plant Conditions and Facilities: Ventilation

Ventilation was a problem in every type of industry, but it was more serious in some than in others. Heat and moisture were reported as excessive and overpowering in many departments of cotton and woolen mills and several employees attributed their repeated illnesses to this condition. Wraps hanging on wall pegs near humidifiers were very damp at the end of the day. Undue dust was reported in some grinding operations, and in ceramic plants also there was unusual exposure to powder and dust. In the use of rubber, in welding, in soldering there was exposure to fumes, and in a number of instances no really effective measures had been taken to reduce what amounted to hazards in various workrooms. (pp. 32–33)

Conditions in some of the ceramic departments elicited many comments:
The dust is everywhere.
Powder makes the throat dry.
Many quit after working 1 or 2 days in the powder-filled air.
Girls from other departments refuse to be transferred here.
We suffocate if we wear those masks.
The heat from the ovens is terrific.
We asked for fans but never got them.
The girls near the ovens say they'll quit unless something is done about the heat.

Skylights, only one of which opened, were the only ventilation for fettlers working in the dust near the ovens. (p. 33)

From interviews with women employed at one plant:

Nothing to blow out the air. Small windows on one side and only a few will open.

The heat was terrible. I work next to the ovens. (Had fainted.)

It is hot to work there. A fan is brought back and forth; sometimes we have it and sometimes we don't. It doesn't belong to us.

The taste of paint is in your throat all the time. (One of the few spray painters. Solderers also complained of fumes.) (p. 41)

References

1. Frank, A. L. (1982). The epidemiology and etiology of lung cancer. *Clin. Chest Med.* 3(2):219–228.

2. Miller, A. B. (1983). Trends in cancer mortality and epidemiology. *Cancer* 51:2413–2418.
3. Oleske, D. M. (1987). The epidemiology of lung cancer: An overview. *Semin. Oncol. Nurs.* 3(3):165–173.
4. Devesa, S. S., and Diamond, E. L. (1983). Socioeconomic and racial differences in lung cancer incidence. *Am. J. Epidemiol.* 118(6):818–831.
5. Cullen, J. W. (1989). The impact of prophylactic methods in the control of lung cancer in the U.S.A. In: *Basic and Clinical Concepts of Lung Cancer*. Edited by H. H. Hansen. Boston, Kluwer Academic Publishers, pp. 15–33.
6. Lung cancer among women. Leads from the MMWR. *JAMA* 252(20):2806, 1984.
7. Mason, T. J., McKay, F. W., Hoover, R., Blot, W. J., and Fraumeni, J. F., Jr. (1975). *Atlas of Cancer Mortality for U. S. Counties: 1950–1969*. Washington, D.C., U.S. Government Printing Office, DHEW Publication No. (NIH)75-780, 1975.
8. Mason, T. J., McKay, F. W., Hoover, R., Blot, W. J., and Fraumeni, J. F., Jr. (1975). *Atlas of Cancer Mortality Among U. S. Nonwhites: 1950–1969*. Washington, D.C., U.S. Government Printing Office, DHEW Publication No. (NIH)76-1204, 1976.
9. Fraumeni, J. F., Jr. (1988). Etiologic insights from cancer mapping. In: *Unusual Occurrences as Clues to Cancer Etiology*. Edited by R. W. Miller et al., Tokyo, Japan Sci. Soc. Press, 13–25.
10. Pickle, L. W., Mason, T. J., Howard, N., Hoover, R., and Fraumeni, J. F., Jr. (1987). *Atlas of U. S. Cancer Mortality Among Whites, 1950–1980*. Washington, D. C., U.S. Government Printing Office, DHHS Publ. No. (NIH)87-2900.
11. Pickle, L. W., Mason, T. J., Howard, N., Hoover, R., and Fraumeni, J. F., Jr. (1990). *Atlas of U. S. Cancer Mortality Among Nonwhites: 1950–1980*. Washington, D. C., U.S. Government Printing Office, DHHS Publ. No. (NIH)90-1258.
12. Mason, T. J. (1992). Age-specific cancer mortality in the United States among persons over 55 years of age. In: *Geriatric Oncology*, Philadelphia, J.B. Lippincott Press, pp. 35–41.
13. Horm, J. W., and Kessler, L. G. (1986). Falling rates of lung cancer in men in the United States. *Lancet* (February 22), pp. 425–426.
14. Division of Cancer Prevention and Control, National Cancer Institute. (1989). *Annual Cancer Statistics Review 1973–1986. Including a Report on the Status of Cancer Control*. Washington, D.C., U.S. Government Printing Office, DHHS Publ. No. (PHS)89-2789.
15. Devesa, S. S., Blot, W. J., and Fraumeni, J. F., Jr. (1989). Declining lung cancer rates among young men and women in the United States: A cohort analysis. *JNCI* 81:1568–1571.
16. Manton, K. G., Malker, H., and Malker, B. (1986). Comparison of temporal changes in U.S. and Swedish lung cancer, 1950–51 to 1981–82. *JNCI* 77(3):665–675.
17. Mizuno, S., Akiba, S., and Hirayama, T. (1989). Lung cancer risk comparison among male smokers between the "six-prefecture cohort" in Japan and the British physicians' cohort. *Jpn. J. Cancer Res.* 80:1165–1170.
18. Hakulinen, T., Magnus, K., and Tenkanen, L. (1987). Is smoking sufficient to explain the large difference in lung cancer incidence between Finland and Norway? *Scand. J. Soc. Med.* 15(1):3–10.

19. Hanai, A., Benn, T., Fujimoto, I., and Muir, C. S. (1988). Comparison of lung cancer incidence rates by histological type in high and low incidence countries, with reference to the limited role of smoking. *Jpn. J. Cancer Res.* 79(4):445–452.
20. Pannonian Tumor Epidemiology Study Group. Comparative study on cancer incidence in neighboring regions of Hungary, Austria, Yugoslavia, and Czechoslovakia in 1969–1980. *Neoplasma* 36(4):377–386.
21. Zaridze, D. G., and Gurevicius, R. (1986). Lung cancer in the USSR: Patterns and trends. *IARC Sci. Publications* 74:87–101.
22. Pierce, J. P., Fiore, M. C., Novotny, T. E., Hatziandreu, E. J., and Davis, R. M. (1989). Trends in cigarette smoking in the United States: Projections to the year 2000. *JAMA* 261(1):61–65.
23. Pierce, J. P., Fiore, M. C., Novotny, T. E., Hatziandreu, E. J., and Davis, R. M. (1989). Trends in cigarette smoking in the United States: Educational differences are increasing. *JAMA* 261:56–60.
24. Marcus, A. C., Shopland, D. R., Crane, L. A., and Lynn, W. R. (1989). Prevalence of cigarette smoking in the United States: Estimates from the 1985 current population survey. *JNCI* 81(6):409–414.
25. Shopland, D. R., Eyre, H. J., and Pechacek, T. F. (1991). Smoking-attributable cancer mortality in 1991: Is lung cancer now the leading cause of death among smokers in the United States? *JNCI* 83:1142–1148.
26. Benhamou, E., Benhamou, S., and Flamant, R. (1987). Lung cancer and women: Results of a French case-control study. *Br. J. Cancer* 55(1):91–95.
27. McDuffie, H. H., Klaassen, D. J., and Dosman, J. A. (1987). Female-male differences in patients with primary lung cancer. *Cancer* 59(10):1825–1830.
28. Gillis, C. R, Hole, D. J., and Boyle, P. (1988). Cigarette smoking and male lung cancer in an area of very high incidence. I. Report of a case-control study in the West of Scotland. *J. Epidemiol. Commun. Health* 42(1):38–43.
29. Gillis, C. R., Hole, D. J., and Hawthorne, V. M. (1988). Cigarette smoking and male lung cancer in an area of very high incidence. II. Report of a general population cohort study in the West of Scotland. *J. Epidemiol. Commun. Health* 42(1):44–48.
30. Lubin, J. H., and Blot, W. J. (1984). Assessment of lung cancer risk factors by histologic category. *JNCI* 73:383–389.
31. Andrews, J. L., Jr., Bloom, S., Balogh, K., and Beamis, J. F., Jr. (1985). Lung cancer in women. Lahey clinic experience, 1957–1980. *Cancer* 55:2894–2898.
32. Wu, A. H., Henderson, B. E., Thomas, D. C., and Mack, T. M. (1986). Secular trends in histologic types of lung cancer. *JNCI* 77(1):53–56.
33. Butler, C., Samet, J. M., Humble, C. G., and Sweeney, E. S. (1987). Histopathology of lung cancer in New Mexico, 1970–72 and 1980–81. *JNCI* 78(1):85–90.
34. Beard, C. M., Jedd, M. B., Woolner, L. B., Richardson, R. L., Bergstralh, E. J., and Melton, L. J., III. (1988). Fifty-year trend in incidence rates of bronchogenic carcinoma by cell type in Olmsted County, Minnesota. *JNCI* 80:1404–1407.
35. Galietti, F., Giorgis, G. E., Toffola, A. D., Ciotta, D., Moschini, M. T., Oliaro, A., Barberis, S., and Ardizzi, A. (1988). Epidemiological study of 3,398 cases of lung cancer histologically ascertained in 1973–84. *Panminerva Medica* 30(1):16–22.
36. Cavanaugh, D. G., Gomez, A. C., and Cabellon, S., Jr. (1987). Lung cancer in young

patients: A ten-year experience at William Beaumont Army Medical Center. *Milit. Med.* 152(6):326.
37. Sarma, D. P., and Byers, V. J. (1986). Lung cancer in men aged 40 or younger. *J. Surg. Oncol.* 33(2):124–125.
38. Ganz, P. A., Vernon, S. E., Preston, D., and Coulson, W. F. (1980). Lung cancer in younger patients. *West. J. Med.* 133(5):373–378.
39. Division of Cancer Prevention and Control, National Cancer Institute. (1991). *Cancer Statistics Review, 1973–1988*, Washington, D.C., U.S. Government Printing Office, DHHS Publ. No. (NIH)91-2789.
40. Cutler, S. J., and Young, J. L., Jr. (Eds.) (1975). Third National Cancer Survey's Incidence Data. Monograph 41. Washington, D.C., U.S. Government Printing Office, DHEW Publ. No. (NIH)75-787, 1975.
41. Fontham, E. T. H., Pickle, L. W., Haenszel, W., Correa, P., Lin, Y., and Falk, R. T. (1988). Dietary vitamins A and C and lung cancer risk in Louisiana. *Cancer* 62: 2267–2273.
42. Ziegler, R. G., Mason, T. J., Stemhagen, A., Hoover, R., Schoenberg, J. B., Gridley, G., Virgo, P. W., Altman, V. R., and Fraumeni, J. F., Jr. (1984). Dietary carotene and vitamin A and risk of lung cancer among white men in New Jersey. *JNCI* 73(6):1429–1435.
43. Schoenberg, J. B., Wilcox, H. B., Mason, T. J., Bill, J., and Stemhagen, A. (1989). Variation in smoking-related lung cancer risk among New Jersey women. *Am. J. Epidemiol.* 130(4):688–695.
44. Stockwell, H. G., Armstrong, A. W., and Leaverton, P. E. (1990). Histopathology of lung cancers among smokers and nonsmokers in Florida. *Int. J. Epidemiol.* 19(3): S48–S52.
45. Mayo, P., Saha, S. P., and Jernigan, C. M. (1982). Lung cancer in women: A twenty-five year review. *J. Ky. Med. Assoc.* 80(5):275.
46. Division of Epidemiology, Kentucky Department of Health Services. (1983). The rising epidemic of lung cancer among Kentucky women. *Ky. Epidemiol. Notes Rep.* 1811:1–2.
47. Smith, E. B. (1989). Primary cancer of the lung in women. *J. Natl. Med. Assoc.* 81(9):945–948.
48. Osann, K. E. (1991). Lung cancer in women: The importance of smoking, family history of cancer, and medical history of respiratory disease. *Cancer Res.* 51:4893–4897.
49. Shopland, D. R. (1991). Smoking prevalence and lung cancer death rates. In: *Smoking and Tobacco Control Monograph No. 1: Strategies to Control Tobacco Use in the U. S.*, Washington, D.C., U.S. Government Printing Office, DHHS Publ. 92-3316, Dec. 1991.
50. MacLennan, R., DaCosea, J., Day, N. E., Law, C. H., Ng, Y. K., Lee, J., and Shan-Mugarainam, K. (1977). Risk factors for lung cancer in Singapore Chinese: A population with high female incidence rates. *Int. J. Cancer* 20(85):854–860.
51. Chan, W. C., Colbourne, M. J., Fung, S. C., and Ho, H. C. (1979). Bronchial cancer in Hong Kong. *Br. J. Cancer* 39:182–192.
52. Hinds, H. W., Stemmerman, G. N., Yang, H. Y., Kolonel, L. N., Lee, J., and Wegner,

F. (1981). Differences in lung cancer risk from smoking among Japanese, Chinese and Hawaiian women in Hawaii. *Int. J. Cancer* 27:297–302.

53. Gao, Y. T., Blot, W. J., Zheng, W., Ershow, A. G., Hsu, C. W., Levin, L. I., Zhang, R., and Fraumeni, J. F., Jr. (1987). Lung cancer among Chinese women. *Int. J. Cancer* 40:604–609.
54. *Historical Statistics of the United States: Colonial Times to 1970 (Bicentennial Edition)*, Part 1. U.S. Department of Commerce, Bureau of the Census, Washington, D.C., U.S. Government Printing Office, 1975.
55. *Changes in Women's Employment During the War.* Special Bulletin No. 20 of the Women's Bureau, U.S. Department of Labor, Washington, D.C., U.S. Government Printing Office, 1944.
56. *Women Workers in Some Expanding Wartime Industries: New Jersey, 1942*. Bulletin of the Women's Bureau, No. 197, U.S. Department of Labor, Washington, D.C., U.S. Government Printing Office, 1943.

4

Lung Cancer and Cigarette Smoking

ANNA H. WU-WILLIAMS

University of Southern California
School of Medicine
Los Angeles, California

JONATHAN M. SAMET

University of New Mexico School
of Medicine
and the New Mexico Tumor Registry
Albuquerque, New Mexico

I. The Evolution of the Evidence on Tobacco Smoking and Lung Cancer

The causal relationship between smoking and lung cancer was clearly established in cohort and case-control studies reported in the 1950s and 1960s. Many of the studies conducted in the last two decades have further refined description of the relationship between tobacco smoking and lung cancer while reaffirming the causal nature of this association. Results from these studies show that differences in various aspects of smoking behavior affect lung cancer risk and can account for most observed differences in lung cancer rates among population groups. These newer studies considered such aspects of smoking behavior as age at starting to smoke, numbers of cigarettes smoked, types of cigarettes smoked, and inhalation pattern.

These studies also provide data on the risk of smoking as cigarettes have changed with the addition of filters and other modifications designed to reduce the amount of tar and nicotine delivered to the smoker. The results of the studies conducted during the 1970s and 1980s have clear public health implications as they have addressed these newer, purportedly lower-risk products.

II. The Risk of Lung Cancer in Cigarette Smokers

As data on the health risks of smoking were collected, it quickly became apparent that cigarette smoking was associated with lung cancer. The initial evidence, based primarily on hospital-based case-control studies, was soon followed by confirmatory findings from a number of large prospective studies. In this section we review the evidence on the overall risks of lung cancer associated with cigarette smoking as derived from case-control and cohort studies. Of necessity this review is selective; the studies considered are either illustrative or among the larger investigations conducted.

The risk of lung cancer in cigarette smokers depends on various aspects of smoking behavior including age at starting, number of cigarettes smoked, the products smoked, and inhaling pattern (see subsequent sections). The overall risk estimates presented in this section thus integrate these distinct dimensions of smoking behavior for the subjects in each study. Changes in overall patterns of risk in broad smoking groups (i.e., never smoker, former smoker, current smoker) may reflect changes in one or more of these dimensions. Nevertheless, the overall risk estimates provide a useful measure of the risk of smoking for public health purposes.

A. Case-Control Studies

Although several studies published through the 1940s had indicated an association between cigarette smoking and lung cancer, three hospital-based case-control studies published during the early 1950s provided evidence that is now regarded as conclusively establishing the link between cigarette smoking and lung cancer. Doll and Hill (1) compared the smoking habits of lung cancer patients from London and nearby counties with those of patients admitted with cancer at another site or with a disease other than cancer. The initial report described the findings for the London patients (2), whereas a later report provided results for patients from additional communities. Wynder and Graham (3) used a similar design, obtaining cases from throughout the United States and controls primarily in St. Louis. Levin and colleagues (4) compared smoking habits of male lung cancer patients with those of persons with other cancers or with a disease other than cancer. A significantly greater proportion of the lung cancer patients were smokers.

For men, the initial studies showed a strong effect of cigarette smoking on lung cancer risk (Table 1). Subsequent studies have continued to show about the same level of risk associated with ever being a regular cigarette smoker. The later studies have also shown the reduced risk associated with cessation of smoking. For women, the initial studies showed much lower odds ratios in comparison to the findings among men (Table 2). These lower odds ratios are compatible with the temporal pattern of differences in the smoking patterns of men and women up to

Table 1 Results of Selected Case-Control Studies of Smoking and Lung Cancer in Men

Location/Years	Odds ratios[a]			Ref.
	Ever smoked	Current smokers	Former smokers	
U.S., before 1950	12.8	—	—	3
U.K., 1948–1951	9.1	—	—	2
U.S., 1966–1969	9.7	—	—	17
Western Europe, 1976–1980	9.0	—	—	22
Sweden, 1972–1977	7.3	10		79
U.S., 1977–1984	11.2	16.0	6.9	77
New Mexico, 1980–1982	10.8	17.3	6.2	24

[a]Calculated as crude odds ratios from data provided or extracted from tables or figures.

Table 2 Results of Selected Case-Control Studies of Smoking and Lung Cancer in Women

Location/Years	Odds ratios[a]			Ref.
	Ever smoked	Current smokers	Former smokers	
U.K., 1948–1951	2.1	—	—	2
U.S., 1953–1955	4.3	—	—	104
U.S., 1955–1957	2.4	—	—	105
U.S., 1966–1969	3.1	—	—	17
Western Europe, 1976–1980	3.9	—	—	22
U.S., 1977–1984	7.8	10.9	4.0	77
New Mexico, 1980–1982	9.4	12.3	5.5	24
Los Angeles, 1981–1982		4.1[b]	1.2[b]	106
		35.3[c]	7.7[c]	
New Jersey, 1982–1983	8.5			36

[a]Calculated as crude odds ratios from data provided or extracted from unpublished tables and figures.
[b]For adenocarcinoma of the lung.
[c]For squamous-cell carcinomas.

that time; women had tended to start smoking at an older age and less often to be heavy smokers (5). The case-control studies show a strong temporal trend of increasing lung cancer risk among women in studies covering the 1970s and 1980s, presumably reflecting the changing patterns of cigarette smoking among women.

B. Cohort Studies

In the 1950s several large cohort (longitudinal) studies of mortality and cigarette smoking were undertaken in the United States, the United Kingdom, and other countries (Table 3). Complete descriptions of the major studies are included in the 1986 monograph on tobacco smoking prepared by the International Agency for Research on Cancer (6). These studies examined mortality from lung cancer and other diseases within strata defined by use of cigarettes and other tobacco products. Strengths of this approach include the prospective assessment of tobacco use and the capability of examining multiple disease endpoints. Weaknesses include the difficulty of following large populations, the inability to establish

Table 3 Cohort Studies of Lung Cancer Mortality in Men

			Mortality rate (10^{-5})		
Population	Years	Mortality ratio[a]	Never smokers	Cigarette smokers	Ref.
Men in 9 states, ages 50–69 years, American Cancer Society	1952–1955	10.7	12.8	127.2	107
Men in 25 states, ages 35–84 years, American Cancer Society	1959–1963	9.2	12	111	7
U.S. veterans	1954–1969	12.1	—	—	108
Men in 50 states, ⩾35 years, American Cancer Society	1982–1986	22.4[b]	—	—	5
		9.4[c]	—	—	
British physicians	1951–1971	8.3	10	83	30
Sample of Swedes, ages 18–66 years	1963–1979	7.4	19.6	—	82
Sample of Japanese, ⩾40 years	1966–1982	4.5	24.1	107.3	9

[a]Ratio of mortality in cigarette smokers to never smokers by authors' definitions: regular cigarette smokers (Ref. 107); cigarette only (Ref. 7); regular or current smoker at enrollment (Ref. 108); current or former smokers (Ref. 30); cigarettes only at enrollment (Ref. 82); daily cigarette smokers on enrollment (Ref. 9).

[b]Smoking at enrollment (Ref. 5).

[c]Stopped at enrollment (Ref. 5).

changes in smoking practices unless cohort members are resurveyed, and the limitations of classifying cause of death on the basis of death certificates.

The cohort studies have primarily addressed the risks of smoking in men (see Table 3). The studies implemented during the 1950s generally showed mortality ratios, comparing smokers to never smokers, that were compatible with the odds ratios in contemporaneous case-control studies (see Table 1). The three studies initiated in the United States during the 1950s, the American Cancer Society's 9-state and 25-state studies (now known as Cancer Prevention Study I), and the study of U.S. Veterans provided closely agreeing estimates of overall risk of ever being a smoker. The later nationwide study conducted by the American Cancer Society (Cancer Prevention Study II) showed higher levels of risk. Comparing current smokers on enrollment with never smokers, the estimated relative risks for males aged 35 years and older were 11.4 in the older 25-state study and 22.4 in the newer study (5). Other large cohort studies have included British physicians, a population sample in Sweden, and a population sample in Japan (see Table 3). The levels of risk associated with smoking in the British and Swedish studies were somewhat lower than in the studies in the United States at the same time. The mortality ratio in the study in Japan is much lower, although the background rate of lung cancer was the highest reported.

Less evidence is available from cohort studies on the risk of smoking in women. In the American Cancer Society's 25-state study, the mortality rate from lung cancer was 7 per 100,000 in never smokers and 16 per 100,000 in women with a history of cigarette smoking (7). The study of British physicians also included 6194 females (8). The annual death rate from lung cancer was 7 per 100,000 in never smokers; it increased progressively with amount of smoking in current smokers and was 23 per 100,000 in former smokers. In the Japanese study, the relative risk for death from lung cancer was 2.3, comparing daily smokers with nonsmokers (9). Extensive, recent information is available for U.S. women from the nationwide study of the American Cancer Society (10). The cohort included 619,225 women followed over a 4-year period (1982–1986). The standardized mortality ratio was 12.7 for current smokers on enrollment and 4.8 for former smokers. As for men, there has been a substantial increase in lung cancer risk from the 1950s through the 1980s. For females 35 years of age and older, the relative risk for current smokers in the earlier 25-state study was estimated as 2.7, whereas the newer study provided a value of 11.9 (5).

III. Determinants of Lung Cancer Risk in Cigarette Smokers

This section considers factors influencing the level of risk in individual smokers, as investigated in epidemiological studies. Emphasis is placed on the quantitative aspects of cigarette smoking including duration of smoking, the numbers of cigarettes smoked, age at starting to smoke, the types of cigarettes smoked, and depth of inhalation. Risks of lung cancer by gender, ethnicity, and histologic type of lung cancer are also considered. Information on many of these factors has been readily obtained by questionnaires in cohort and case-control studies. These questionnaire measures are subject to misclassification, and such variables as duration of smoking, number of cigarettes smoked, and depth of inhalation are only crude indexes of the dose of biologically relevant smoke components delivered to target sites in the lung (11). Nevertheless, the resulting data have been analyzed descriptively and with complex modeling approaches to assess predictors of risk. These analyses have provided significant insights into the process of respiratory carcinogenesis and a biological basis for programs to control lung cancer caused by cigarette smoking. Future research that combines the rapidly advancing techniques of cellular and molecular biology with epidemiology can be anticipated to provide further advances in our understanding of determinants of individual susceptibility.

A. Duration of Cigarette Smoking

In smokers who continue to smoke regularly after starting, the risk of lung cancer depends strongly on the duration of smoking (6,11,12). Table 4 shows representative findings from the American Cancer Society's CPS-II study of 619,225 women followed over the 4-year period from 1982 to 1986 (10). Comparing the shortest duration with the longest duration, the risk of lung cancer is approximately doubled. This relation between duration of smoking and lung cancer risk has been consistently demonstrated in numerous cohort and case-control studies.

Doll and Peto (12) have conducted an extensive analysis of the effect and duration in regular cigarette smokers in the study of British male doctors. In this cohort, the incidence of lung cancer increased in an exponential fashion with the

Table 4 Standardized Mortality Ratios for Lung Cancer in Women Participants in the American Cancer Society's CPS-II Study by Duration of Smoking and Number of Cigarettes Smoked, Current Smokers Only

Duration of smoking (y)	Cigarettes per day				
	1–10	11–19	20	21–30	31+
21–30	2.9	6.7	13.6	18.4	18.9
31–40	7.9	19.2	19.2	26.5	25.3
41–70	10.0	17.0	25.1	34.3	38.8

Source: Ref. 10.

duration of smoking (Fig. 1). As discussed subsequently, the linear relation observed in this log–log plot is consistent with a multistage process of respiratory carcinogenesis. A model to predict lung cancer incidence was fit to the data; incidence was found to increase approximately with the fourth power of the duration of smoking.

Table 5 provides the effects of various durations of smoking on annual excess incidence as estimated by this model. The steep increase with increasing duration is apparent. The timing of this increase is consistent with patterns of age-specific lung cancer mortality in many countries, which rise steeply from the fifth decade on (6,11).

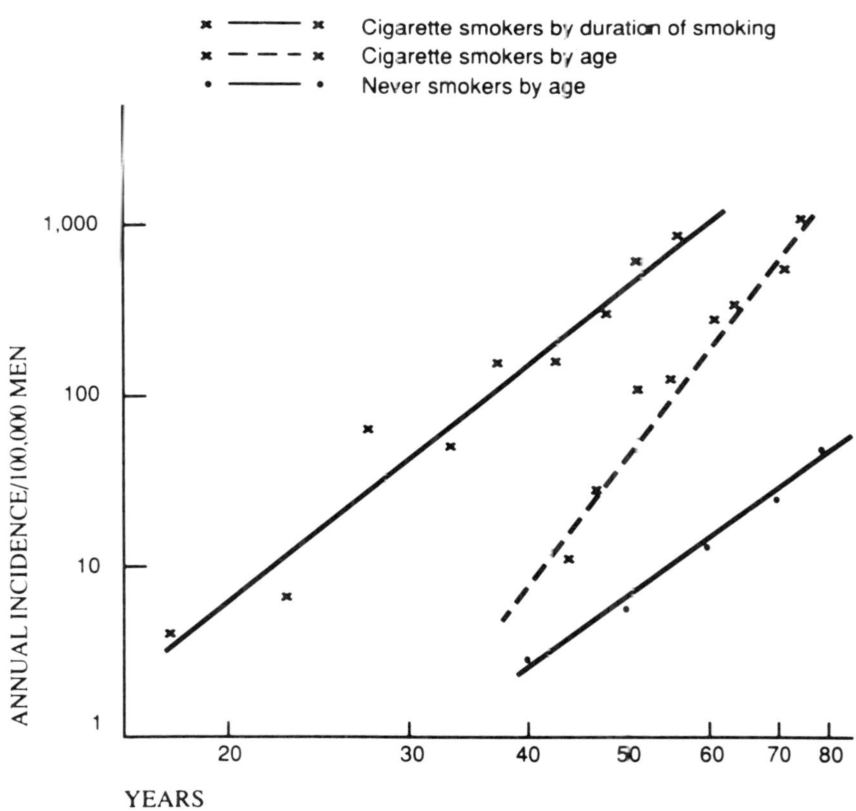

Figure 1 Incidence of bronchial carcinoma in continuing cigarette smokers in relation to age and duration of smoking and in nonsmokers in relation to age: double logarithmic scale. (From Ref. 86, reprinted with permission.)

Table 5 Effect of Duration of Cigarette Smoking on Annual Excess Incidence of Lung Cancer, Based on Study of British Male Doctors

	Annual excess incidence	
Years of smoking	Moderate smokers	Heavy smokers
15	0.005 (%)	0.01 (%)
30	0.1	0.2
45	0.5	1

Source: Ref. 6.

B. Age at Initiation of Smoking

Age at starting to smoke is tightly linked to duration of smoking. For persons who have smoked regularly since any particular age, those who have smoked the longest started at the youngest age. Thus, separating the potential effect of age at starting to smoke from the effect of duration of smoking is problematic (6). Age at starting to smoke could plausibly modify the risk of smoking because of differential susceptibility of the lung as growth and development are completed across the teenage years and young adulthood. However, while the risk of lung cancer increases rapidly with younger age at starting to smoke if duration of smoking is uncontrolled, an effect of age at starting to smoke independent of duration of smoking has not been demonstrated (6,13,14).

C. Quantity of Cigarettes Smoked

Dose–response relationships between the number of cigarettes smoked and the relative risk of lung cancer have been consistently found in epidemiological studies. In fact, this dose–response relationship meets one of the criteria for causality applied in interpreting epidemiological data; it was considered as important evidence in support of a causal relationship between smoking and lung cancer in the 1964 Surgeon General's Report (15).

Representative data from selected cohort studies are provided in Table 6. A consistent pattern is evident across the studies. Differences in the values of relative risk between males and females probably reflect differences in duration of smoking, whereas differences among the studies may be the consequence of differing durations of smoking and types of products smoked. In individual studies, an effect of numbers of cigarettes is evident within strata defined by numbers of years smoked (see Table 4).

The analysis of data from British male physicians indicated a lesser dependence of risk on number of cigarettes smoked than on duration (12). In the model

Table 6 Lung Cancer Mortality Ratios for Men and Women by Number of Cigarettes Smoked Per Day—Cohort Studies

	Men		Women	
Study	Cigarettes per day	Ratio	Cigarettes per day	Ratio
ACS CPS-I	Never smoker	1.0	Never smoker	1.0
	1–9	4.6	1–9	1.3
	10–19	8.6	10–19	2.4
	20–30	14.7	20–39	4.9
	40+	18.7	40+	7.5
British physicians	Never smoker	1.0	Never smoker	
	1–14	7.8	1–14	1.3
	15–24	12.7	15–24	6.4
	25+	25.1	25+	29.7
Swedish study	Never smoker	1.0	Never smoker	1.0
	1–7	2.3	1–7	1.8
	8–15	8.8	8–15	11.3
	16+	13.7		
Japanese study	Never smoker	1.0	Never smoker	1.0
	1–9	2.1	1–9	2.3
	10–19	4.0	10–19	2.6
	20+	6.2	20+	4.5

Source: Refs. 9, 13.

for incidence of lung cancer in current smokers, incidence was estimated to increase with approximately the square of the number of cigarettes smoked versus the fourth power for duration of smoking.

D. Filter Type and Tar Content of Cigarettes

One objective of the nearly continuous effort since the 1950s to modify commercial cigarettes has been to reduce the tar yield of cigarettes. The tar content of both filter and nonfilter cigarettes has decreased over the last three decades (Fig. 2). The average tar yield of nonfilter cigarettes decreased from about 35 mg in the 1950s to about 20 mg in the 1980s, and the tar of filter cigarettes dropped from about 25 mg in the 1960s to about 10 mg in the 1980s (6). These yields are determined using a cigarette-smoking machine operated in a pattern thought to be reflective of human smoking. The tar yield is the weight of matter deposited on a filter.

Studies conducted in the 1960s and 1970s (16–21) reported that filter smokers compared with nonfilter smokers showed a lower risk of lung cancer. However, because filter use was not common until the late 1950s, these studies included mostly smokers who had used filters on a short-term basis, and there-

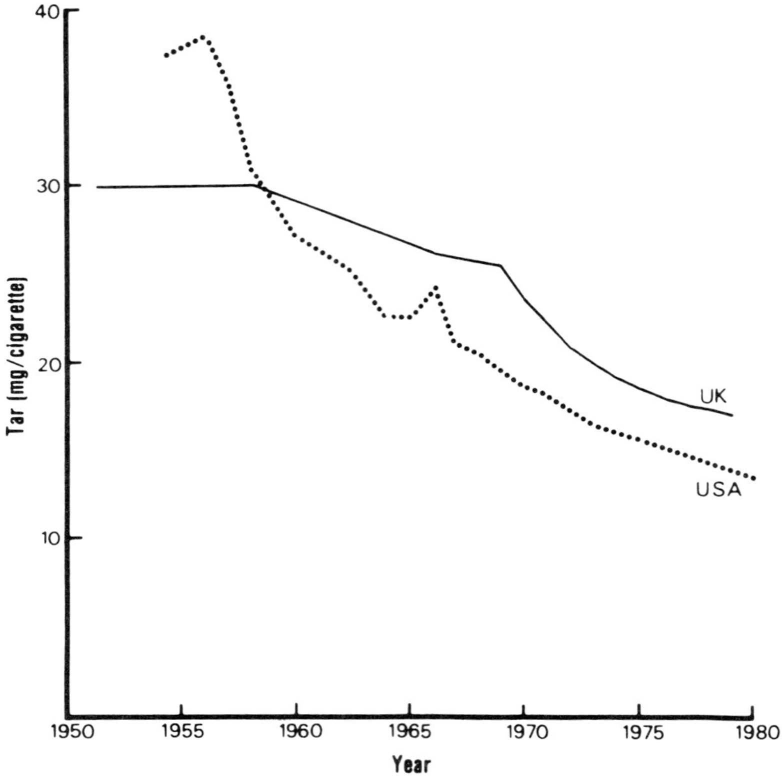

Figure 2 Sales-weighted average tar yields of U. K. and U. S. cigarettes by year of manufacture. (From Ref. 6, reprinted with permission.)

fore the studies could not adequately evaluate the risk of lung cancer associated with long-term or exclusive use of filter or low-tar cigarettes.

Table 7 presents more recent studies, which give information on lifetime filter smokers or smokers of low-tar cigarettes. Similar to findings of earlier studies, filter smokers generally showed lower risk of lung cancer than nonfilter smokers (22,23) (Table 7A). Several investigators attempted to refine the measure of lung cancer risk among filter smokers by calculating the proportion of years filter cigarettes were smoked or by estimating the average lifetime exposure to tar from cigarettes. In these studies, information on lifetime smoking habits was obtained by asking about all commercial filter and nonfilter cigarettes smoked (24), the brands of cigarettes smoked, the specific years in which each brand/filter type was smoked, and the number of cigarettes of each brand/filter type smoked (22,25–27) (Table 7B,C). In these studies, risk of lung cancer was higher among lifetime nonfilter smokers than among lifetime filter smokers, but there was not a smooth trend of increasing risk with increasing proportion of years that nonfilter cigarettes were smoked (22,24). In the study by Joly et al. (25), there was not a consistent trend of increasing risk with increasing tar content when years of smoking and number of cigarettes smoked were accounted for. Wilcox et al. (26) found an increasing risk with increasing lifetime cigarette tar level smoked, but this dose trend was attenuated when intensity and duration of smoking were accounted for. In the study by Kaufman et al. (27), smokers with the highest tar intake showed a higher risk of lung cancer, but the tar level of the lowest "tar" group in this study (<22 mg/cigarette) was considerably higher than levels in other studies (18,26).

In two of these studies, the smoking behavior of smokers after they switched from nonfilter to filter cigarettes was controlled for in the analysis. Using the study population of current smokers in the report by Wynder and Kabat (23), Augustine et al. (28) reported that over 50% of those who switched from nonfilter to filter cigarettes compensated for the lower tar intake per cigarette by increasing the number of cigarettes smoked per day. Those with lung cancer tended to have compensated more than controls. Compared to switchers who smoked the same number of cigarettes per day before and after the switch of filter type, there was a linear increase in risk with increasing number of filter cigarettes smoked per day after switching to filters. In fact, switchers who smoked an additional 20 or more cigarettes after switching showed a higher risk of lung cancer than those who remained as nonfilter smokers only. Similarly, in Wilcox et al.'s study (26) cases were more likely than controls to increase the number of cigarettes smoked after switching to cigarettes labeled as low-tar cigarettes. Thus the more recent studies emphasize that any reduction of risk from smoking filter or lower-tar cigarettes may be negligible if smokers compensate for the lower tar/nicotine by increasing the number of cigarettes smoked per day or by altering the manner of smoking (e.g., puff frequency or duration).

E. Inhalation

Inhalation of smoke into the lungs is the principal route by which lung tissue is exposed to the carcinogens that ultimately produce lung cancer. Biomarkers are available for estimating the degree of tobacco smoke inhalation, such as carboxyhemoglobin level, end-tidal concentration of carbon monoxide level, and nicotine or cotinine. These methods for measuring inhalation have not been applied in epidemiological studies of lung cancer mortality. In most studies, smokers were asked to report subjectively about their inhalation practices. Several prospective

Table 7 Risk of Lung Cancer by Filter Type and Tar Level of Cigarette

A. By filter type of cigarette (F = filter, NF = nonfilters)

	F only	F, 10+ y	F, 1–9 y	NF only[a]
Kreyberg I, M	0.69	0.66[b]	0.83	1.00
Kreyberg I, F	0.64	0.74	0.99	1.00
Kreyberg II, M	0.87	0.79	0.96	1.00
Kreyberg II, F	0.96	0.99		1.00

B. By proportion of years filters or nonfilters were smoked

	Proportion of years smoked nonfilters					
	0% NF	1–49%	50–69%	70–83%	84–99%	100% NF[c]
M	1.0	1.5	1.4	1.7	1.7	1.7[d]
F	1.0	1.8	1.7	1.9	2.1	2.0[d]

	Proportion of years smoked filters				
	100% F	67–99%	34–66%	1–33%	0% F
Non-Hispanic white, M	0.80	0.71	0.58	0.83	1.00
Hispanic white, M	0.04[b]	0.26[b]	0.39	0.56	1.00

C. By tar exposure

	Lifetime tar exposure (mg)		
Males only	<15,640	15,640–24,079	≥24,080
Adj. y smoked	1.0	1.1	1.2
Adj. # cig/day	1.0	1.3	1.2

	Tar level (mg/cigarette)			
Males only	≤14.0	14.1–17.5	17.6–21.0	21.1–28.0
Unadj.	0.53	0.86	1.04	1.00
Adj. # cig/day	0.61	1.01	1.16	1.00
Adj. y smoked	0.58	0.89	1.05	1.00

Table 7 Continued

	Tar level (mg/cigarette)		
	<22	22–28	>29
M	1.0	3.6[b]	4.0[b]
F	1.0	1.8	4.7[b]

[a]Adjusted for inhalation, age, years of education, and number of cigarettes per day.
[b]95% confidence interval excludes 1.0.
[c]Adjusted for years of smoking and number of cigarettes per day.
[d]Test of linear trend, $p < 0.01$.
Sources: Refs. 22–27.

studies (7,29) have shown higher risk of lung cancer among smokers who reported inhaling deeply or frequently (Table 8). The effect of depth of inhalation is observed for men and women with lung cancer, for all histologic types of lung cancer, and for different filter types of cigarettes smoked (see Table 8). However, there is some suggestion that the effect of inhalation may be more apparent for light than for heavy smokers. In a study of British physicians, men smoking 25–40 cigarettes/day who reported inhaling showed a lower risk of lung cancer than those smoking the same amount but not inhaling (30). In two other studies, the effect of inhalation was more apparent among light smokers (1–9 cigarettes/day) than among heavier smokers (22,31). There are no satisfactory explanations for these observations. Questions on inhalation are subjective and may be inaccurate, but we are unaware of any data suggesting that heavier smokers are less truthful about their inhaling habits. Doll and Peto (12) proposed that with deep inhalation, smoke particles may be carried well past the upper part of the bronchi, a common site of lung tumors, to another location before the particles are deposited. However, it is not clear why location of deposition would be affected by number of cigarettes smoked per day. An alternative explanation suggested by Wald et al. (32) is that light and heavy smokers may differ in the way they inhale. If slow inhalation is more common among light smokers and rapid inhalation is more common among heavier smokers, the walls of the larger bronchi of slow inhalers may have more exposure to cancer-causing substances than those of rapid inhalers.

F. Gender

Differences in lung cancer risk, comparing male and female smokers, might reflect smoking practice, other environmental exposures, or a biologically determined effect of gender, perhaps mediated hormonally. Cohort and case-control studies conducted in the United States and the United Kingdom (or western countries) in the 1950s and 1960s generally showed two- to fourfold lower lung

Table 8 Effect of Inhalation and Risk of Lung Cancer

By degree of inhalation	Degree of inhalation: None	Slight	Moderate	Deep	Ref.
Males	8.0[a]	8.9	13.1	17.0	7
Females	1.8[a]		3.7		
Females	6.9[a]	15.2	18.5	31.9	10
Males	3.7[a]		7.8	9.2	29
Females			7.2[a]	1.9	

By inhalation and other parameters of smoke exposure	Depth of inhalation	Filter type: Filter	Mixed	Nonfilter	Ref.
Males	Slight/never	1.0	1.0	1.0	22
	Moderate	1.5	1.3	1.4	
	Deeply	2.1	1.9	1.7	
Females	Slight/never	1.0	1.0	1.0	
	Moderate	1.5	2.2	2.9	
	Deeply	2.6	4.5	2.5	

	Inhalation	# cigarettes/day: 1–9	10–19	≥20	Ref.
Males	No	3.8[a]	8.8	15.1	31
	Yes	4.4	9.0	10.7	

	Depth of inhalation	# cigarettes/day: 1–9	10–19	20–39	40+	Ref.
Males	Slight/never	1.0[a]	2.5	3.5	4.8	22
	Moderate	1.6	2.5	4.5	4.6	
	Deeply	2.2	3.3	4.3	6.3	

[a]Compared to never smoker.

cancer risk ratios for women than for men for comparable levels of tobacco smoke exposure (e.g., by number of cigarettes smoked) (13). These early male–female risk differences reflect in part differences in the smoking patterns of males and females. Historically, a high proportion of males began to smoke at the time of World War I, whereas females began to smoke in larger numbers about 20–25 years later, during the World War II era (13). Moreover, women usually started smoking at a later age, smoked fewer cigarettes per day than men, and inhaled less deeply than men. The smoking pattern of U.S. females has converged toward the pattern in males in more recent cohorts (5). The changes in smoking practices among females have been accompanied by concurrent changes in lung cancer risk patterns (33,34).

In cohort and case-control studies conducted in the last two decades, males and females included in the same study generally showed little or no difference in their risk of lung cancer in association with comparable levels of tobacco smoke exposure, as measured by number of cigarettes smoked per day, duration of smoking, age started smoking, and amount and duration of smoking (Table 9). These results were obtained for men and women in case-control studies conducted in western and eastern countries, in studies that used hospital controls (22,23), and in studies that used population-based controls (35,36,69). Thus, the epidemiological evidence indicates no effect of gender alone on lung cancer risk; men and women have an equally high risk of lung cancer for comparable levels of tobacco exposure.

Table 9 Risk of Lung Cancer in Men and Women by Different Parameters of Tobacco Smoke Exposure

		Current smoker (cigarettes/day)	
	Ex-smoker	⩾20	>20
M	7.2	9.2	24.7
F	6.5	19.2	26.0

	# cigarettes/day and years of smoking				
	Any cigarettes	⩽20/d ⩽35 yr	20+/d 35+ yr	⩽20/d ⩽35 yr	20+/d 35+ yr
M	11.6	2.8	7.3	11.3	17.9
F	8.2	3.0	6.1	7.8	15.8

	Age started smoking		
	10–19	20–29	30+ years
M	5.1	4.7	1.2[a]
F	5.6	3.8	2.0

[a]95% confidence interval includes 1.0.
Sources: 35, 36, 69.

G. Histologic Type of Lung Cancer

The most common histologic types of lung cancer are squamous cell, small-oat cell, adenocarcinoma, and large-cell tumors. For usual clinical purposes and in most epidemiological studies, the determination of histologic type is made on the basis of a light microscopic examination by a pathologist. This classification is subject to substantial intra- and interobserver variation as well as variation between institutions (37). The method for obtaining lung cancer patients may also affect the distribution of histologic types. In most clinical practice, central tumors, which tend to be small cell or squamous cell carcinomas, are more often diagnosed by cytology or bronchoscopy. Surgical series of patients would tend to overpresent squamous cell carcinoma and adenocarcinoma; surgery is rarely performed for small-cell carcinoma. The biological relevance of histologic type of lung cancer remains uncertain. Few specific associations between histologic type and specific risk factors have been identified, and different cellular origins for the principal types have not been identified (38).

Smoking habits, ethnicity, and gender have been related to the distribution of histologic types of lung cancer. Kreyberg first suggested that the association between lung cancer and smoking may differ among the histologic types of lung cancer (39). In particular, Kreyberg proposed classification of lung cancer into two groups determined largely by epidemiological characteristics of the different cell types. The Group I (or Kreyberg I) tumors included squamous and small-cell carcinomas, usually located centrally in the respiratory tract. The Group II (or Kreyberg II) tumors consisted of adenocarcinomas, bronchioloalveolar carcinomas, and large-cell carcinomas, found primarily in the periphery of the lung. The histologic cell type distribution has been different for men and women. A study in New Mexico comparing 1970–72 with 1980–81 cases showed a declining proportion of adenocarcinoma in women as the proportion of small-cell carcinoma increased (40). Squamous cell carcinoma is the predominant cell type among men, whereas adenocarcinoma is the predominant cell type among women (40–43). The distribution of histologic types of lung cancer also differs for smokers and nonsmokers. In nonsmokers, adenocarcinoma is the predominate cell type accounting for about 75% of lung cancers, whereas squamous cell and small-cell carcinoma are the predominate cell types among smokers (44–46).

The association between smoking and lung cancer by histologic type was reviewed recently by IARC (6); 12 studies published prior to 1984 were included. Most of these studies had small numbers, ranging from 2 to 64, of adenocarcinoma cases. In about half of the studies, only the prevalence of smoking by histologic type of lung cancer was presented. This limited review suggested that the association between smoking and lung cancer appeared to be stronger for squamous/oat cell cancer (or Kreyberg I) than for adenocarcinoma of the lung (or Kreyberg II).

Table 10 summarizes some recent studies that offer additional information on histologic type of lung cancer. The more recent studies included larger sample sizes, particularly of adenocarcinoma of the lung, and provided more stable estimates of risks by histologic type of lung tumor. In addition, they allowed a more thorough investigation of how different parameters of tobacco smoke exposure may influence risk of different histologic types of lung cancer. Data for males and females were presented separately for various studies conducted in the United States, western Europe, and China. In each of the studies, higher relative risks (RRs) were observed for squamous/small- or oat cell cancers (or Kreyberg I) than for adenocarcinomas (or Kreyberg II). These findings were observed in males and females and for different parameters of tobacco smoke exposure including numbers of cigarettes smoked (23,47), years of smoking (47), and amount and duration of tobacco smoke exposure (36,47,48) (see Table 10). On the other hand, differences in RRs by histologic type are less clear for other parameters of tobacco smoke exposure, including years of smoking cessation, inhalation pattern, and filter types, in the one study with data on these measures (47) (Table 11). In the European case-control study, Lubin and Blot (47) found a decline in RR with cessation of smoking that was more apparent for squamous/small- or oat cell cancers than for adenocarcinoma of the lung. The RR for adenocarcinoma of the lung equaled or exceeded the corresponding RR for squamous cell cancers when frequency and depth of inhalation were considered in the analysis (47). In two studies, the reduction of risk associated with smoking filter compared with nonfilter cigarettes was more apparent for squamous/small- or oat cell cancer than for adenocarcinoma of the lung (23,47).

Interpretation of these findings in a biologically based framework is presently difficult. Although it is certain that cigarette smoking increases the risk of the major histologic types of lung cancer, the factors that determine the development of specific histologic types of tumors have not been identified (38).

H. Ethnic Differences

It is generally assumed that differences in rates of lung cancer can be explained by the different levels of cigarette smoking. In particular, several ethnic groups have been investigated because of suspected differences in the smoking and lung cancer relationship compared to that in Caucasians. In the United States, incidence rates of lung cancer in men are highest in blacks, intermediate in whites, and lowest in Hispanics (49). Based on 1978–81 data from the Surveillance, Epidemiology, and End Results Program (SEER), a group of cancer registries that covers about 10% of the U.S. population, the average annual age-adjusted lung cancer incidence rates per 100,000 were 119.0, 81.0, and 34.3, respectively, for black, white, and Hispanic men (49).

Blacks. The SEER data show that incidence rates of lung cancer in blacks are 47% higher than in whites. The extent to which the black–white difference in lung cancer rates can be explained by differences in smoking habits is unclear.

However, a consistent picture has emerged showing differences in smoking habits between U.S. black and white males since the 1960s. Compared with white males, black males have a higher percentage of current and a lower percentage of former smokers (Table 12). Black male smokers also smoke cigarettes with greater tar and nicotine yields than whites, and prefer to smoke menthol cigarettes, which may promote deeper inhalation of cigarette smoke (50). However, among smokers,

Table 10 Risk of Lung Cancer by Histologic Type in Association with Dose and Duration of Tobacco Smoke Exposure

	Number of cigarettes smoked per day					
	0	1–10	11–20	21–30	31–40	40+
Males						
Kreyberg I[a] (n = 676)	1.0	13.3	15.8	29.6	37.7	64.1
Kreyberg II (n = 475)	1.0	2.4	8.4	15.4	11.1	28.4
Females						
Kreyberg I (n = 401)	1.0	6.6	18.2	26.5	95.2	88.7
Kreyberg II (n = 384)	1.0	3.1	4.5	9.4	13.8	20.7

	Years of smoking[c]			
	1–29	30–39	40–49	≥50
Males				
Squamous (n = 3708)	1.0	2.3	3.3	4.0
Small-, oat cell (n = 1172)	1.0	1.8	2.2	2.4
Adenocarcinoma (n = 716)	1.0	1.5	1.8	1.5
Females				
Squamous (n = 272)	1.0	2.4	2.5	5.1
Small-, oat cell (n = 199)	1.0	2.1	1.6	4.7
Adenocarcinoma (n = 223)	1.0	2.0	1.8	3.3

		Years of smoking[d]		
Males	# cig/day	1–29	30–39	40+
Squamous/oat (n = 396)	1–19	2.3	2.9	5.0
	20–29	2.6	3.9	10.4
	30+	7.7	8.3	31.2
Adenocarcinoma (n = 163)	1–19	1.4[f]	2.2	2.6
	20–29	0.7[f]	1.5[f]	3.6
	30+	5.4	3.2	11.8

Table 10 Continued

	Dose and duration of tobacco smoking[e]				
	Any cigarettes	<20 <35	20+ <35	<20 35+	20+ cig/day 35+ year
Males					
Squamous[b]	18.9	4.8	12.4	18.0	29.0
Small-cell	22.9	4.1	16.5	20.4	35.8
Adenocarcinoma	4.8	1.1[f]	2.8	5.2	7.4
Females					
Squamous	10.6	2.5	7.1	10.9	21.1
Small-cell	59.0	18.0	36.8	57.6	132.0
Adenocarcinoma	3.6	1.8	3.0	3.6	6.4

[a]Kreyberg I included squamous cell, large cell, and oat cell cancers; Kreyberg II included adenocarcinoma, bronchiolar, and alveolar cell carcinoma. From Ref. 23.
[b]Sample size for males and females combined: squamous (n = 269), small-cell (n = 220), adenocarcinoma (n = 290).
[c]From Ref. 22
[d]From Ref. 48.
[e]From Ref. 36.
[f]p value > 0.05.

black males smoke fewer cigarettes per day and start smoking at a slightly later age than whites (see Table 12). In addition to differences in smoking habits, a recent study found higher cotinine levels in young black than in young white smokers; the difference could not be explained by reporting bias or differences in nicotine yields of the cigarettes smoked. While not yet confirmed, these findings suggest that there may also be differences between blacks and whites in the metabolism of nicotine or excretion of cotinine (51).

Smoking patterns have been associated with socioeconomic status in the United States and other countries. A recent ecologic study using incidence data from SEER and corresponding census-tract data on population density suggested that all of the black–white differences in lung cancer rates can be accounted for by differences in socioeconomic status between the two groups (52). However, this study is limited in that data on smoking habits were not available.

Hispanics. Based on the SEER data, rates of lung cancer are 58% lower in Hispanics than in non-Hispanic whites (49). The percent of current smokers is comparable for Hispanic and white males, but the percent of ex-smokers is lower among Hispanics compared to whites (see Table 12). Hispanic males also tend to be lighter smokers; on average, they smoke about half as many cigarettes per day as non-Hispanic white males, and start smoking at a slightly later age (see Table

Table 11 Risk of Lung Cancer by Histologic Type in Association with Other Measures of Tobacco Smoke Exposure

	Years since smoking cessation					
Males	0	1–4	5–9	10–14	15–19	20+
Squamous	1.0	1.1	0.7	0.6	0.4	0.4
Small-/Oat cell	1.0	0.9	0.6	0.5	0.2	0.2
Adenocarcinoma	1.0	1.0	0.8	0.6	0.6	0.5
Females	0	1–4	5–9	10–14	15–19	20+
Squamous	1.0	1.1	0.9	0.4	0.4	0.3
Small-/Oat cell	1.0	1.1	0.3	0.1	—	0.1
Adenocarcinoma	1.0	0.7	1.0	0.4	1.2	0.3

	Filter type		
	Filters only	Mixed	Nonfilters only
Males			
Squamous	1.0	1.6	1.9
Small-/Oat cell	1.0	1.5	1.3
Adenocarcinoma	1.0	1.5	1.4
Females			
Squamous	1.0	1.8	6.7
Small-/Oat cell	1.0	2.0	1.4
Adenocarcinoma	1.0	3.0	2.2

	Depth of inhalation		
	Slight	Moderate	Deep
Males			
Squamous	1.0	1.3	1.6
Small-/Oat cell	1.0	1.4	1.4
Adenocarcinoma	1.0	2.1	2.4
Females			
Squamous	1.0	1.2	2.9
Small-/Oat cell	1.0	2.4	3.1
Adenocarcinoma	1.0	2.0	5.3

Source: Ref. 22.

Table 12 Smoking Pattern Among Black, White, and Hispanic Males in the United States

Source of data	Smoking status	Prevalence of smoking (%)			Ref.
		Black	White	Hispanic	
BRFS[a] 1981–83	Current smoker	39.7	35.3	31.5	109
NHIS[b] 1974–85	Current smoker (1974)	54.6	42.3	—	110
	Current smoker (1985)	40.6	32.1	—	
CPS[c] 1985	Current smoker	37.2	30.7	30.9	111
NHIS[d] 1979–80	Never smoked	39.2	33.8	42.1	112
	Ex-smoker	16.6	27.7	16.9	
	Current smoker	44.1	38.4	41.1	
	# cig/day[d]	15.3	23.8	12.8	
	Age started to smoke[d]	17.6	17.2	17.5	

[a]Behavioral Risk Factor Survey, 22,236 individuals were surveyed.
[b]National Health Interview Survey, used data collected in 1974, 1976, 1978, 1979, 1980, 1983, and 1985.
[c]Current Population Survey; about 60,000 households were surveyed.
[d]National Health Interview Survey; 17,385 individuals were surveyed: number of cigarettes smoked per day, age started to smoke among smokers.

12). The smoking behavior of Hispanics in the United States is influenced by country of origin. Data from the Hispanic Health and Nutrition Examination Survey (1982–1983) showed that current rates of smoking, number of cigarettes smoked per day, and secular pattern of change in smoking rates differed for Mexican, Cuban, and Puerto Rican Hispanic males and females by place of origin (53–55). Although there is some suggestion that smoking rates of Hispanics may be related to their degree of acculturation in the United States (56), this has not been shown in other studies (57,58).

In a case-control study conducted in New Mexico where most of the Hispanics are born in the United States, the effects of smoking on lung cancer risk were similar for Hispanic and non-Hispanic white males (24,35). This finding suggests that the lower lung cancer incidence among U.S. Hispanics compared with whites may be explained by differences in smoking patterns of these two groups.

Chinese. The high rates of lung cancer among Chinese females have been a focus for research because the prevalence of smoking is low among Chinese females (59). Such high rates have been observed for Chinese females residing in Asia and in western countries (60–62). Investigations of these populations have been prompted by the opportunity to identify some aspect of being Chinese that strongly modifies the risk of smoking or particularly strong environmental risk factors other than smoking, perhaps indoor air pollution from cooking and heating.

Results from recent studies conducted in Hong Kong (63–65), Singapore (66), Xuanwei County, Yunnan Province (67,68), Shanghai (69), and north China (48,70) have helped to clarify the role of cigarette smoking as well as other risk factors in the etiology of lung cancer among Chinese females. Chinese female smokers have been shown to have a two- to fourfold increased risk of lung cancer compared to never smokers (Table 13). The attributable risk for lung cancer associated with smoking ranged from about 25% in Shanghai to about 40% in Hong Kong and northern China (70,71). The lower attributable risk associated with smoking among Chinese females compared with Caucasian females is due to the lower percent of Chinese females who have ever smoked. In these studies, 22–56% of cases versus 16–42% of controls have ever smoked (see Table 13). Compared with female controls in Los Angeles County, the percent of female controls who have ever smoked is lower among Chinese (54% ever smoked in Los Angeles, 37% in north China). Among smokers, Chinese females smoked fewer cigarettes (6.1 cigarettes/day in China, 22.6 in Los Angeles County) and started smoking at a later age (24.0 years in north China, 21.0 years in Los Angeles County) (70). Nevertheless, heavy smokers (i.e., smoked >40 years and >20 cigarettes/day) in Shanghai and north China showed levels of risk of lung cancer that closely resembled those reported for women in western countries (69,70). Thus, the effect of cigarette smoking on lung cancer risk among Chinese females is qualitatively and quantitatively similar to its effect on lung cancer risk in women in other parts of the world. In addition to tobacco smoking, a number of other risk factors have

Table 13 Prevalence of Smoking and Risk of Lung Cancer in Association with Smoking Among Chinese Females

	% ever smoked			
Area	Cases	Controls	Relative risks	Ref.
Singapore	54	42[a]	1.6	62
	48	20[b]	3.6[c]	
Hong Kong	56	26	3.8[c]	63
Hawaii	22	16	1.8	113
Hong Kong	56	31	2.8[c]	64
Hong Kong	55	24	3.8[c]	65
Shanghai	35	18	3.3[c]	69
North China	56	37	2.3[c]	70

[a]Cantonese-speaking.
[b]Non-Cantonese-speaking.
[c]$p < 0.05$

emerged, which may explain in part the high rates of lung cancer in Chinese females. These risk factors include personal and family history of lung diseases (70,72) and exposure to various sources of indoor air pollution, including prolonged exposure to oil volatiles from cooking (70,72) and coal-burning devices (48,70).

IV. Smoking Cessation

As suggested by Doll and Peto (12), the lung cancer rate among former smokers is assumed to be a combination of the background rate (such as in nonsmokers), which depends on age, and the excess rate, which depends on duration of exposure. After smoking ceases, the absolute excess risk of lung cancer stays approximately constant, and the risk compared with that of continuing smokers decreases over time.

The 1990 Report of the U.S. Surgeon General provides a comprehensive review of the evidence on smoking cessation and lung cancer (11). Numerous cohort and case-control studies conducted in different countries have documented a 20–90% reduction in risk among former smokers compared with current smokers (Table 14). These studies generally show a similar pattern of risk reduction for males and females for all histologic types of lung cancer and for different types of tobacco smoked.

An important modifier of the pattern of risk reduction is the number of years of abstinence. Based on reanalysis of data from the large European case-control study conducted by Lubin et al. (73), Brown and Chu (90) showed that the RR of lung cancer among ex-smokers decreases sharply with increasing years of abstinence. However, because duration of smoking is negatively correlated with time since stopping smoking, the decline in risk with years since stopping plateaued when duration of smoking is accounted for (Fig. 3). In the first few years after smoking stops, risks of lung cancer among former smokers may be higher than among current smokers because some former smokers may have stopped smoking because of illness or early symptoms related to their lung cancer. In most studies, the benefit of cessation becomes apparent approximately 5 years after quitting, and increases as the duration of abstinence lengthens. However, the risk of lung cancer among former smokers remains elevated above the risk among never-smokers, even in the longest periods of abstinence evaluated (11).

In addition, characteristics of active smoking history prior to smoking cessation may also influence the risk of lung cancer after cessation (11). The collective evidence suggests that the magnitude of risk reduction among ex-smokers is considerably less among heavy smokers than light smokers. In the study of Lubin et al. (73), there appeared to be a greater reduction in risk among those who had smoked fewer cigarettes per day (1–9) than among those who had smoked more (30 or more), although this finding was not observed in other studies (7,10). The decline in risk associated with stopping is greater for those who had

Table 14 Effect of Smoking Cessation on Risk of Lung Cancer

By years stopped smoking[a]

# years stopped	Males	Females
1–4	1.1	0.9
5–9	0.7	0.7
10–14	0.6	0.4
15–19	0.4	0.5
20–24	0.4	0.5
25+	0.3	0.3
Current smoker	1.0	1.0

By histologic type of lung cancer[b]

Years since stopped smoking	Males—Kreyberg type I	Males—Kreyberg type II	Females—Kreyberg type I	Females—Kreyberg type II
1–3	53.8	14.2	13.6	6.7
4–6	24.9	5.9	6.3	3.6
7–10	17.2	6.6	5.1	4.1
11–15	13.7	5.4	8.8	5.6
16+	5.0	1.2	—	0.9
Current	32.3	10.7	10.5	4.4
Never smoker	1.0	1.0	1.0	1.0

By types of tobacco products smoked[c]

Tobacco product	Smoking status: Never	Ex	Current
Cigarettes only	1.0	6.9	16.0
Cigars only	1.0	2.5	3.1
Pipes only	1.0	0.7	1.9
Cigars and pipes	1.0	2.4	2.5
Mixed smokers	1.0	5.1	10.5

[a]From Ref. 22.
[b]From Ref. 114.
[c]From Ref. 77.

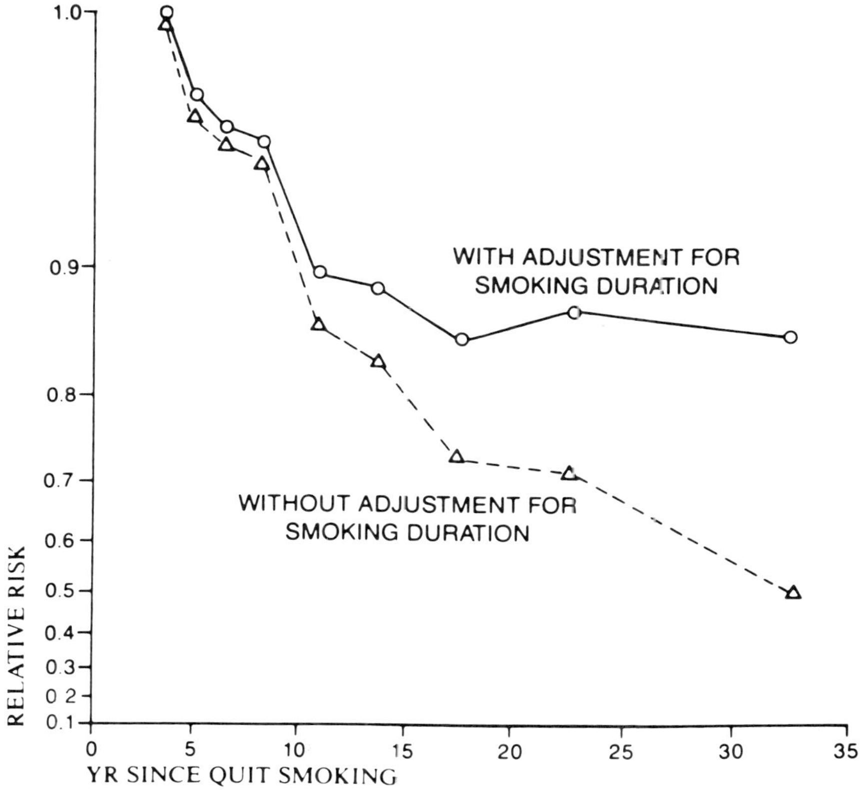

Figure 3 Relative risk of lung cancer among ex-smokers compared with continuing smokers as a function of time since stopped smoking, estimated from logistic regression model, pattern adjusted for smoking duration compared with pattern unadjusted for duration. Reprinted with permission from *Journal of Chronic Diseases*, 40 (Suppl. 2), C. C. Brown and K. C. Chu, "Lung Cancer and Cigarette Smoking, ©1987, Pergamon Press, Ltd.

smoked for shorter periods than for ex-smokers who had smoked for longer periods (73,74). Data from one study also suggest that ex-smokers who had inhaled less often or less deeply showed a greater reduction in risk (73). Since there are now a large number of ex-smokers, future studies will be able to examine the pattern of declining risk more fully as duration of abstinence lengthens.

V. Other Types of Tobacco Products

Most studies suggest that smokers of only pipes and cigars experience some increase in risk of lung cancer compared with never smokers, although the magnitude of the increase in risk has varied in different studies, depending mainly on the amount smoked and the inhaling pattern. In areas such as the United States, Canada, western Europe, and the United Kingdom where the percentages of pipe and cigar smokers are low (i.e., less than 5%), the risks of lung cancer among cigar-only and pipe-only smokers are only slightly higher than those among nonsmokers. Risk of lung cancer among exclusively pipe or cigar smokers compared with never smokers varied from no increased risk in some studies (7,75) to about an approximately twofold higher risk in other studies (76,77) (Table 15). There is good agreement in these studies that the risk of lung cancer among exclusively pipe/cigar smokers is considerably lower than that among exclusively cigarette smokers or among smokers of a combination of tobacco products.

On the other hand, in countries such as Sweden (78,79), Switzerland (80), and the Netherlands (81), where pipe or cigar smoking is nearly as common as cigarette smoking, risks of lung cancer among exclusively pipe or cigar smokers (78,79,82) are as high as those experienced by cigarette smokers (see Table 15).

Differences in the manner in which pipes and cigars are smoked in different countries may explain some of the differences in risks. The small increased risk observed in some countries may reflect low consumption of pipe or cigar tobacco or limited inhaling. Although the tobacco smoke of cigars and pipes has carcinogenic activity resembling that of cigarettes, pipe/cigar smokers are less likely to inhale when they smoke than cigarette smokers, probably because of the greater alkalinity of the smoke of pipes/cigars (83). The percent of exclusive cigar/pipe smokers who report inhaling deeply or all the time was much lower than that of exclusive cigarette smokers in several studies (25,76). Mixed cigar/pipe and cigarette smokers tended to inhale cigarette smoke less frequently and less deeply than cigarette-only smokers, but they inhaled cigar/pipe smoke more deeply than exclusive cigars/pipe smokers. In fact, even in studies conducted in countries with a low rate of cigar/pipe smoking (25,76,77), risks of lung cancer among the very small number of deep inhalers or heavy smokers of pipe and cigars approached the risks observed in studies conducted in countries with a high rate of cigar/pipe smoking.

VI. Modeling Approach

Model fitting allows one to formally test whether a specified mathematical relationship between disease risk and predictor variables gives a good fit to the data. Models have been widely applied to lung cancer and cigarette smoking. This association lends itself to mathematical modeling because smoking can be described by a few parameters and it is generally the most powerful determinant of lung cancer risk. Models have been used to test theoretical constructs of the underlying biological mechanism of lung cancer and tobacco smoking (see Table 16).

Table 15 Risk of Lung Cancer[a] by Type of Tobacco Smoked, in Males

	Type of tobacco product					
Study/Location	Cigarettes only	Cigars only	Pipes only	Cigars/ pipes only	Mixed	Cigarettes and cigars/pipes
Hammond/United States (1966)	8.5	NA[b]	NA	3.2	NA	NA
Higgins/United States (1988)	11.2	2.8	1.3	2.4	7.6	7.9
Lubin/western Europe (1984)	9.0	2.9	2.5	4.6	7.4	7.5
Benhamou/France (1986)	13.3	5.6	1.6	3.2	NA	9.3
Alderson/England (1985)	NA	NA	NA	3.8	NA	9.1
Joly/Cuba (1983)	NA	NA	NA	4.4	NA	15.0
Cartensen/ Sweden (1987)	7.4	7.6	7.2	NA	NA	NA
Damber/Sweden (1986)	7.0	6.9	NA	NA	NA	NA

[a]Compared to nonusers of any tobacco, in males.
[b]Not available.

Mathematical models have also been used to predict trends in smoking-related lung cancer rates as a basis for health planning and cancer control activities.

The most extensively used model in studies of lung cancer and smoking is the multistage model proposed by Armitage and Doll (84). Underlying all multistage models is the postulate that cancer arises from a single cell line undergoing a series of distinct, heritable changes in a particular sequence. Support for the multistage model derives from many cancer age-incidence curves, which show that incidence increases with time or age to the fourth or fifth power (85). Using data from the British Physicians Study, Doll (86) plotted the incidence of lung cancer in cigarette smokers against duration of smoking. He made several observations: (1) incidence increased approximately in proportion to the fourth power of duration, in agreement with the relationship between lung cancer incidence and age in nonsmokers; (2) the excess incidence rate of lung cancer in ex-smokers seemed to remain constant after smoking stopped; and (3) lung cancer incidence appeared to be related linearly to the amount smoked. Thus, a first-stage effect was implicated because the excess lung cancer risk among smokers increased with the same power of duration of smoking as the risk with age among never-smokers. Armitage (87) noted that the stabilization of excess lung cancer

Table 16 Summary of Selected Biologic Models on Lung Cancer and Smoking

Data set	Method	Findings	Ref.
British physician	Reanalyzed data using finer categories of amount and years of smoking; excluded those over 80 years	Supports Armitage-Doll model. Incidence rate proportional to between the 4th and 5th power of smoking duration and linear in amount smoked. The power relationship between lung cancer incidence rate of smokers and smoking duration is comparable to that between nonsmokers and age.	88
British physician	Evaluated mortality rate among ex-smokers: a) as a proportion of the rate expected if they had continued smoking; b) as a proportion of the rate among nonsmokers of the same age	Supports Armitage-Doll model. Decrease in incidence among ex-smokers is consistent with removal of a penultimate-stage carcinogen. Mortality rate remains about constant at the level reached when smoking stopped.	89
European multi-center case-control study of lung cancer	Fitted two separate logistic regression models to estimate the effects of smoking on the first and penultimate stages	Supports Armitage-Doll model. Smoking affects two stages—may have a much greater effect on late than early stage events.	90
British physician	Evaluated the fit of two functions to describe tobacco smoke exposure:	Supports Armitage-Doll model. Both functions fit British data equally well; higher smoking-specific death rates using British than U.S. data.	91
U.S. veterans study	a) pack function: excess death rate depends linearly on cumulative amount smoked;	Neither function fit U.S. veterans data—may be due to wrong assumptions about subject's smoking history.	
Case-control study of lung cancer in New Mexico	b) multistage function: smoking affects transition to first and penultimate stage	Multistage function fitted New Mexico data better than pack function; both functions overpredicted death rates among ex-smokers. The effect on penultimate stage is double that of the first stage.	

		Questions whether multistage model is correct; excess lung cancer incidence among ex-smokers declined instead of stabilized.	92
British physician	Fitted multistage models with 3–9 stages, included 25–84 years old	Models with 5–8 stages fitted best; 1 or 2 stages sensitive (first, penultimate, or last); results differed for ex- and current smokers.	
U.S. veterans from Dorns study	Fitted models to combined cohorts	Model did not fit data for non-, ex-, or current smokers.	
ACS volunteers	Fitted models separately for males and females	Model with 6 and 5 stages fitted best for current male and female smokers, respectively; results differed for ex- and current smokers.	
British physician	Fitted excess risk to those smoking at least 10 cigarettes/day; the incidence in each age-smoking-level category was not used	Not consistent with Armitage-Doll model for first and penultimate stage; for models with 6 stages or less. Model did not fit smokers and ex-smokers simultaneously. Proposed using a 2-stage model with clonal growth.	93
British physician	Restricted analysis to men aged 40–79, used two-mutation model	Model fit data well; consistent with various interpretations about daily amount and duration of smoking.	94

risk at the level when smoking stopped suggested that smoking also affected a late stage, namely, the penultimate stage in the carcinogenic process. Thus the Armitage–Doll approach specified the number of stages as a parameter to be estimated from the observed data.

Several investigators have further analyzed the data from the British Physician study or have fitted the Armitage–Doll multistage model to other data sets on lung cancer and smoking (88–94) (see Table 16). Results from some studies are supportive of the Armitage–Doll model (88,90,91) and suggest that the relative magnitude of the effect of smoking on early and late stages of the carcinogenic process is critical in the determination of subsequent risk following cessation of smoking (89–91). On the other hand, others have questioned the fit of the multistage model (92) and have proposed alternative models, including the clonal growth model (93) and the two-mutation recessive oncogenesis model (94). The Moolgavkar approach does not estimate the number of stages. Instead, the number of stages is assumed based on experimental and observational cancer data. Thus, the two-mutation model incorporates the transition of target stem cells into cancer cells via an intermediate stage and accounts for growth and differentiation of normal target and intermediate cells.

On the other hand, different forms of regression models have been used to predict incidence and mortality patterns for lung cancer. The age-period-cohort modeling approach has been widely used to describe changes in lung cancer incidence and mortality over time as a result of the complex changes in smoking behavior. Hakulinen and Pukkala (95) used an age-period-cohort simulation model to estimate lung cancer incidence in Finland during the period 1980–2000 under various assumptions of rates of smoking cessation and prevalence of smoking (95). Day and Charney (96) simultaneously fitted both cohort and cross-sectional parameters with an age effect to lung cancer incidence data from Finland and Slovenia. These investigators assumed that the cohort parameters are represented by the typical smoking pattern of a cohort (i.e., by number and type of cigarettes smoked). On the other hand, the cross-sectional parameters are reflected by changes in smoking prevalence as a result of antismoking campaigns or changing tar content of cigarettes. In other studies, data on lung cancer rates and on smoking rates from the same population were modeled. Stevens and Moolgavkar (97) developed a statistical model to predict lung cancer rates in England and Wales using data on proportion of smokers and cumulative cigarette consumption in these study areas. They modeled lung cancer rates as a function of age, cohort, and cigarette consumption by assuming that lung cancer risk is proportional to the cumulative cigarette consumption for the given cohort for the given year. Brown and Kessler (98) extended the use of age-period-cohort models from description of time-trend data on lung cancer to projections of lung cancer mortality rates in the United States for 1985 to 2025. In their model, Brown and Kessler projected lung cancer mortality rates by assuming that rates of lung cancer are proportional to the product of an age, a cohort, and a year parameter. In another version of their model, total cigarette consumption and tar content of cigarettes were incorporated as the period factor. A factor to account for the time elapsed between a smoking pattern and its impact on lung cancer was also considered. A further modification of the Brown and Kessler model was recently published (99). This cohort-specific, smoking-duration–based model adjusted for competing risks of deaths and used mortality risk as a function of smoking initiation and cessation rates based on the Markov assumption. Usefulness in addition to limitations of mathematical modeling approaches were discussed by investigators of these studies (96–102). A major concern is that these models may not be biologically based.

These studies show that different models can be fitted to different data sets, and it is unlikely that any one model will satisfactorily describe lung cancer incidence in relation to all aspects of tobacco smoke exposure, including current and past exposure and dose and duration of exposure. Thomas (103) advocates that "because many competing models will give essentially equivalent fits to the data, it is important not to conclude that a well-fitting model represents the truth. Rather, the usefulness of a model lies in its falsifiability."

VII. Conclusions

In this review we have attempted to provide a summary of the evolution of the evidence on tobacco smoking and lung cancer. Early studies in the 1950s suggested the association between smoking and lung cancer, accumulating evidence in the 1960s firmly established the causal relationship, and studies in the 1970s and 1980s refined our understanding of the relationship between lung cancer and different parameters of tobacco exposure.

References

1. Doll, R., and Hill, A. B. (1952). A study of the aetiology of carcinoma of the lung. *Br. Med. J.* 2:1271–1286.
2. Doll, R., and Hill, A. B. (1950). A study of the aetiology of carcinoma of the lung. *Br. Med. J.* 2:740–748.
3. Wynder, E. L., and Graham, E. A. (1950). Tobacco smoking as a possible etiologic factor in bronchiogenic carcinoma. A study of six hundred and eighty-four proved cases. *JAMA* 143:329–346.
4. Levin, M. L., Goldstein, H., and Gerhardt, P. R. (1950). Cancer and tobacco smoking. A preliminary report. *JAMA* 143:336–338.
5. U.S. Department of Health and Human Services. (1989). Reducing the health consequences of smoking: 25 years of progress. A report of the surgeon general. DHHS Publication No. (CDC)89-8411. Washington, D.C., U.S. Government Printing Office.

6. International Agency for Research on Cancer. (1986). IARC monographs on the evaluation of the carcinogenic risk of chemicals to humans: Tobacco smoking, Vol. 38. Lyon, France: World Health Organization, IARC.
7. Hammond, E. C. (1966). Smoking in relation to the death rates of one million men and women. *Natl. Cancer Inst. Monogr.* 19:127–204.
8. Doll, R., Gray, R., Hafner, B., and Peto, R. (1980). Mortality in relation to smoking: 22 years' observations on female British doctors. *Br. Med. J.* 2:967–971.
9. Hirayama, T. (1990). *Life-Style and Mortality. A Large-Scale Census-Based Cohort Study in Japan*. Basel, Karger.
10. Garfinkel, L., and Stellman, S. D. (1988). Smoking and lung cancer in women: Findings in a prospective study. *Cancer Res.* 48:6951–6955.
11. U. S. Department of Health and Human Services. (1990). The health benefits of smoking cessation. A report of the Surgeon General. DHHS Publication No. (CDC)90-8416.
12. Doll, R., and Peto, R. (1978). Cigarette smoking and bronchial carcinoma: Dose and time relationships among regular smokers and life-long non-smokers. *J. Epidemiol. Commun. Health* 32:303–313.
13. U. S. Department of Health and Human Services. (1982). The health consequences of smoking: cancer. A report of the Surgeon General. DHHS Publication No. (PHS)82-50179, Washington, D. C., U. S. Government Printing Office.
14. Peto, R., Parish, S. E., and Gray, R. G. (1985). There is no such thing as aging, and cancer is not related to it. In: *Age-Related Factors in Carcinogenesis*. Edited by A. Likhachev, V. Anisimov, and R. Montesano. IARC Scientific Publication No. 58, Lyon, International Research on Cancer, pp. 43–53.
15. U. S. Public Health Service. (1964). Smoking and health. Report of the advisory committee to the Surgeon General of the Public Health Service. DHEW Publication No. (PHS)1103, Washington, D. C., U. S. Government Printing Office.
16. Bross, I. D., and Gibson, R. (1968). Risks of lung cancer in smokers who switch to filter cigarettes. *Am. J. Public Health* 58:1396–1403.
17. Wynder, E. L., Mabuchi, K., and Beattie, E. J. (1970). The epidemiology of lung cancer. *JAMA* 213:2221–2228.
18. Hammond, E. C., Garfinkel, L., Seidman, H., and Lew, E. A. (1976). "Tar" and nicotine content of cigarette smoke in relation to death rates. *Environ. Res.* 12:263–274.
19. Dean, G., Lee, P. N., Todd, G. F., and Wicken, A. J. (1977). Report on a second retrospective mortality study in northeast England. Part I: Factors related to mortality from lung cancer, bronchitis, heart disease and stroke in Cleveland County with particular emphasis on the relative risks associated with filter and plain cigarettes. Tobacco Research Council Research Paper No. 14, Part I. London, Tobacco Research Council.
20. Hawthorne, V. M., and Fry, J. S. (1978). Smoking and health: Cardiorespiratory disease and mortality, and smoking behaviour in West Central Scotland. *Epidemiol. Commun. Health* 2:260–266.
21. Rimington, J. (1981). The effects of filters on the incidence of lung cancer in cigarette smokers. *Environ. Res.* 24:162–166.
22. Lubin, J. H., Blot, W. J., Berrino, F., Flamant, R., Gillis, C. R., Kunze, M.,

Schmahl, D., and Visco, G. (1984). Patterns of lung cancer risk according to type of cigarette smoked. *Int. J. Cancer* 33:569–576.
23. Wynder, E. L., and Kabat, G. C. (1988). The effect of low-yield cigarette smoking on lung cancer risk. *Cancer* 62:1223–1230.
24. Pathak, D. R., Samet, J. M., Humble, C. G., and Skipper, B. J. (1986). Determinants of lung cancer risk in cigarette smokers in New Mexico. *JNCI* 76:597–604.
25. Joly, O. G., Lubin, J. H. and Caraballoso M. (1983). Dark tobacco and lung cancer in Cuba. *JNCI* 70:1033–1039.
26. Wilcox, H. B., Schoenberg, J. B., Mason, T. J., Bill, J. S., and Stemhagen, A. (1988). Smoking and lung cancer: Risk as a function of cigarette tar content. *Prev. Med.* 17:263–272.
27. Kaufman, D. W., Palmer, J. R., Rosenberg, L., Stolley, P., Warshauer, E., and Shapiro, S. (1989). Tar content of cigarettes in relation to lung cancer. *Am. J. Epidemiol.* 129:703–711.
28. Augustine, A., Harris, R. E., and Wynder, E. L. (1989). Compensation as a risk factor to lung cancer in smokers who switch from nonfilter to filter cigarettes. *Am. J. Public Health* 79:188–191.
29. Cederlof, R., Friberg, L., Hrubec, Z., and Lorich, U. (1975). The relationship of smoking and smoke social covariables to mortality and cancer morbidity. A ten year follow-up in a probability sample of 55000 Swedish subjects age 18 to 69, Part 1 and Part 2. Stockholm, Department of Environmental Hygiene, The Karolinska Institute.
30. Doll, R., and Peto, R. (1976). Mortality in relation to smoking: 20 years' observation on male British doctors. *Br. Med. J.* 2:1525–1536.
31. Higenbottam, T., Shipley, M. J., and Geoffrey, R. (1982). Cigarettes, lung cancer, and coronary heart disease: The effects of inhalation and tar yield. *J. Epidemiol. Commun. Health* 36:113–117.
32. Wald, N. J., Idle, M., Boreham, J., and Bailey, A. (1983). Inhaling and lung cancer: An anomaly explained. *Br. Med. J.* 287:1273–1275.
33. Harris, J. E. (1983). Cigarette smoking among successive birth cohorts of men and women in the United States during 1900–80. *JNCI* 71:473–479.
34. Devesa, S. S., Blot, W. J., and Fraumeni, J. F. (1989). Declining lung cancer rates among young men and women in the United States: A cohort analysis. *JNCI* 81:1568–1571.
35. Humble, C. G., Samet, J. M., Pathak, D. R., and Skipper, B. J. (1985). Cigarette smoking and lung cancer in "Hispanic" whites and other whites in New Mexico. *Am. J. Public Health* 75:145–148.
36. Schoenberg, J. B., Wilcox, H. B., Mason, T. J., Bill, J., and Stemhagen, A. (1989). Variation in smoking-related lung cancer risk among New Jersey women. *Am. J. Epidemiol.* 130:688–695.
37. Ives, J. C., Buffler, P. A., and Greenberg, S. D. (1983). Environmental associations and histopathologic patterns of carcinoma of the lung: The challenge and dilemma in epidemiologic studies. *Am. Rev. Respir. Dis.* 128:195–209.
38. National Research Council, Panel on Dosimetric Assumptions Affecting the Application of Radon Risk Estimates. (1991). *Comparative Dosimetry of Radon in Mines*

and Homes. Companion to BEIR IV Report. Washington, D. C., National Academy Press.
39. Kreyberg, L. (1962). Histological lung cancer types: A morphological and biological correlation. *Acta Pathol. Microbiol. Immunol. Scand.* 157(Suppl.):11–90.
40. Butler, C., Samet, J. M., Humble, C. G., et al. (1987). Histopathology of lung cancer in New Mexico, 1970–72 and 1980–81. *JNCI* 78:85–90.
41. Greenberg, R. E., Jorson, R., Baker, J., Barrett, J., Baron, J. A., and Yates, J. (1984). Incidence of lung cancer by cell type: A population-based study in New Hampshire and Vermont. *JNCI* 72:599–603.
42. Dobbs, L., Davis, S., and Polissar, L. (1986). A population based study of lung cancer incidence trends by histologic type, 1974–81. *JNCI* 76:21–29.
43. Wu, A. H., Henderson, B. E., Thomas, D., and Mack, T. (1986). Secular trends in histologic types of lung cancer. *JNCI* 77:53–56.
44. Rosenow, E. C., and Carr, D. T. (1979). Bronchogenic carcinoma. *CA* 29:243–245.
45. Kabat, G. C., and Wynder, E. L. (1984). Lung cancer in nonsmokers. *Cancer* 53:1214–1221.
46. Fontham, E. T. H., Correa, P., Wu-Williams, A., Reynolds, P., Greenberg, R. S., Buffler, P. A., Chen, V. W., Boyd, P., Alterman, T., Austin, D. F., Liff, J., and Greenberg, D. S. (1991). Lung cancer in nonsmoking women: A multicenter case-control study. *Cancer Epidemiol. Biol. Prev.* 1:35–43.
47. Lubin, J. H., and Blot, W. J. (1984). Assessment of lung cancer risk factors by histologic category. *JNCI* 73:383–389.
48. Xu, Z. Y., Blot, W. J., Xiao, H. P., Wu, A., Feng, Y. P., Stone, B. J., Sun, J., Ershow, A. G., Henderson, B. E., and Fraumeni, J. F., Jr. (1989). Smoking, air pollution and high rates of lung cancer in Shenyang, China. *JNCI* 81:1800–1806.
49. Baquet, C. R., Ringen, K., Pollack, E. S., Young, J. L., Horm, J. W., Gloeckler Ries, L. A. (1986). Cancer among blacks and other minorities: Statistical profiles. NIH Publication No. 86-2785. Bethesda, MD, National Cancer Institute.
50. Cummings, K. M., Giovino, G., and Mendicino, G. (1987). Cigarette advertising and black-white differences in brand preference. *Public Health Rep.* 102:698–701.
51. Wagenknecht, L. E., Cutter, G. R., Haley, N. H., Sidney, D. S., Manolio, T. A., Hughes, G. H., and Jacobs, D. R. (1990). Racial differences in serum cotinine levels among smokers in the coronary artery risk development in (young) adults study. *Am. J. Public Health* 80:1053–1056.
52. Baquet, C. R., Horm, J. W., Gibbs, T., and Greenwald, P. (1991). Socioeconomic factors and cancer incidence among blacks and whites. *JNCI* 83:551–557.
53. Marcus, A. C., and Crane, L. A. (1985). Smoking behavior among U. S. Latinos: An emerging challenge for public health. *Am. J. Public Health* 75:169–172.
54. Escobedo, L. G., and Remington, P. L. (1989). Birth cohort analysis of prevalence of cigarette smoking among Hispanics in the United States. *JAMA* 261:66–96.
55. Haynes, S. G., Harvey, C., Montes, H., Nickens, H., and Cohen, B. H. (1990). Patterns of cigarette smoking among Hispanics in the United States: Results from HHNANES 1982–84. *Am. J. Public Health* 80(Suppl.):47–54.
56. Marin, G., Perez-Stable, E. J., and Marin, B. V. (1989). Cigarette smoking among

San Francisco Hispanics: The role of acculturation and gender. *Am. J. Public Health* 79:196–199.
57. Markides, K. S., Coreil, J., and Ray, L. A. (1987). Smoking among Mexican Americans: A three generation study. *Am. J. Public Health* 77:708–711.
58. Samet, J. M., Howard, C. A., Coultas, D. B., and Skipper, B. J. Acculturation, education, and income as determinants of cigarette smoking in New Mexico. *Cancer Causes and Control* (in press).
59. Gao, Y. T. (1986). Smoking and lung cancer in Shanghai. In: *Tobacco: A Major International Health Hazard*. Edited by D. G. Zaridze and R. Peto. IARC Scientific Publication No. 74:604-9. Lyon, IARC.
60. Fraumeni, J. F., Jr., and Mason, T. J. (1974). Cancer mortality among Chinese Americans, 1950–69. *JNCI* 52:659–665.
61. Law, C. H., Day, N. E., and Chanmugaratnam, K. (1976). Incidence rates of specific histological types of lung cancer in Singapore Chinese dialect groups, and their aetiological significance. *Int. J. Cancer* 17:304–309.
62. Chan, W. C., and MacLennan, R. (1977). Lung cancer in Hong Kong Chinese: Mortality and histological types, 1960–1972. *Br. J. Cancer* 35:226–231.
63. Chan, W. C., Colbuorne, M. J., Fung, S. C., and Ho, H. C. (1979). Bronchial cancer in Hong Kong 1976–1977. *Br. J. Cancer* 39:182–192.
64. Koo, L. C., Ho, J. H., and Lee, N. (1985). An analysis of some risk factors for lung cancer in Hong Kong. *Int. J. Cancer* 35:149–155.
65. Lam, T. H., Kung, I. T. M., Wong, C. M., Lam, J. W., Kleevens, L., Saw, D., Hsu, C., Seneviratne, S., Lam, S. Y., Lo, K. K., and Chan, W. C. (1987). Smoking, passive smoking and histological types in lung cancer in Hong Kong Chinese women. *Br. J. Cancer* 56:673–678.
66. MacLennan, R., Da Costa, J., Day, N. E., Law, C. H., Ng, Y. K., and Shanmugaratnam, K. (1977). Risk factors for lung cancer in Singapore Chinese, a population with high female incidence rates. *Int. J. Cancer* 20 854–860.
67. Mumford, J. L., Hw, X. Z., Chapman, R. S., et al. (1987). Lung cancer and indoor air pollution in Xuan Wei, China. *Science* 235:217–220.
68. Liu, Z., He, X., and Chapman, R. (1991). Smoking and other risk factors for lung cancer in Xuanwei, China. *Int. J. Epidemiol.* 20:25–31.
69. Gao, Y. T., Blot, W. J., Zheng, W., Fraumeni, J. F., Jr., and Hsu, C. W. (1988). Lung cancer and smoking in Shanghai. *Int. J. Epidemiol.* 17:277–280.
70. Wu-Williams, A. H., Dai, D. X., Blot, W., Xu, Z. Y., Xiao, H. P., Stond, B. J., Yu, S. F., Feng, Y. P., Ershow, A. G., Sun, J., Fraumeni, J. F., and Henderson, B. (1990). Lung cancer among women in northeast China. *Br. J. Cancer* 62:982–987.
71. Shimizu, H., Wu, A. H., Koo, L. C., Gao, Y. T., Kolonel, L. N. (1985). Lung cancer in women living in the Pacific Basin area. *Natl. Cancer Inst. Monogr.* 69: 197–201.
72. Gao, Y. T., Blot, W. J., Zheng, W., Ershow, A. G., Hsu, C. W., Levin, L. I., Zhang, R., Fraumeni, J. F., Jr. (1987). Lung cancer among Chinese women. *Int. J. Cancer* 40:604–609.
73. Lubin, J. H., Blot, W. J., Berrino, F., Flamant, R., Gillis, C. R., Kunze, M.,

Schmahl, D., and Visco, G. (1984). Modifying risk of developing lung cancer by changing habits of cigarette smoking. *Br. Med. J.* 288:1953–1956.
74. Graham, S., and Levin, M. L. (1971). Smoking withdrawal in the reduction of risk of lung cancer. *Cancer* 27:865–871.
75. Kahn, H. A. The Dorn study of smoking and mortality among U. S. veterans: Report on eight and one-half years of observations. In *Epidemiological Approaches to the Study of Cancer and Other Chronic Diseases*. Washington, D. C., National Cancer Institute, Monograph No. 19, pp. 71–126.
76. Lubin, J. H., Richter, B. S., and Blot, W. J. (1984). Lung cancer risk with cigar and pipe use. *JNCI* 73:377–381.
77. Higgins, I. T. T., Mahan, C. M., and Wynder, E. L. (1988). Lung cancer among cigar and pipe smokers. *Prev. Med.* 17:116–128.
78. Cedelorf, R., Friberg, L., Hrubec, Z., and Lorich, U. (1975). The relationship of smoking and smoke covariables to mortality and cancer morbidity. A ten year follow-up in a probability sample of 55000 Swedish subjects age 18 to 69, Part 1 and Part 2. Stockholm, The Karolinska Institute.
79. Damber, L. A., and Larsson, L. G. (1986). Smoking and lung cancer with special regard to type of smoking and type of cancer. A case-control study in north Sweden. *Br. J. Cancer* 53:673–681.
80. Abelin, T., and Gsell, O. R. (1967). Relative risk of pulmonary cancer in cigar and pipe smokers. *Cancer* 20:1288–1296.
81. Gsell, O. R., and Abelin, T. (1972). Cigar and pipe smoking in relation to lung cancer and excess mortality. *JNCI* 48:1795–1803.
82. Cartersen, J. M., Pershagen, G., and Eklund, G. (1987). Mortality in relation to cigarette and pipe smoking: 16 years' observation of 25000 Swedish men. *J. Epidemiol. Commun. Health* 41:166–172.
83. Bailey, A. (1984). The epidemiology of bronchial carcinoma. In *Bronchial Carcinoma*. Edited by M. Bates. Berlin, Springer-Verlag, pp. 11–22.
84. Armitage, P., and Doll, R. (1954). The age distribution of cancer and a multistage theory of carcinogenesis. *Br. J. Cancer* 8:1–11.
85. Cook, P., Doll, R., and Fellingham, S. (1969). A mathematical model of the age distribution of cancer in man. *Int. J. Cancer* 4:92.
86. Doll, R. (1971). The age distribution of cancer: Implications for models of carcinogenesis. *J.R.Stat.Soc.* A134:133–166.
87. Armitage, P. (1971). Discussion on a paper by R. Doll. *J.R.Stat.Soc.* A134:155.
88. Whittemore, A., and Altshuler, B. (1976). Lung cancer incidence in cigarette smokers: Further analysis of Doll and Hill's data for British physicians. *Biometrics* 32:805–816.
89. Day, N. E., and Brown, C. C. (1980). Multistage models and primary prevention of cancer. *JNCI* 64:977–989.
90. Brown, C., and Chu, K. C. (1987). Use of multistage models to infer stage affected by carcinogenic exposure: Example of lung cancer and cigarette smoking. *J. Chron. Dis.* 40(Suppl. 2):171s–179s.
91. Whittemore, A. (1988). Effect of cigarette smoking in epidemiological studies of lung cancer. *Stat. Med.* 7:223–238.

92. Freedman, D. A., and Navidi, W. C. (1989). Multistage models for carcinogenesis. *Environ. Health Perspect.* 81:169–188.
93. Gaffney, M., and Altshuler, B. (1988). Examination of the role of cigarette smoke in lung carcinogenesis using multistage models. *JNCI* 80:925–931.
94. Moolgavkar, S. H., Dewanji, A., and Luebeck, G. (1989). Cigarette smoking and lung cancer: Reanalysis of the British doctors' data. *JNCI* 81:415–420.
95. Hakulinen, T., and Pukkala, E. (1982). Prediction of cancer incidence by utilization of risk factors and the effect of intervention. In *Trends in Cancer Incidence*. Edited by K. Magnus. Washington, D. C., Hemisphere, pp. 111–123.
96. Day, N. E., and Charney, B. (1982). Time trends, cohort effects and aging as influence on cancer incidence. In *Trends in Cancer Incidence*. Washington, D. C., Hemisphere, pp. 51–65.
97. Stevens, R. G., and Moolgavkar, S. H. (1984). A cohort analysis of lung cancer and smoking in British males. *Am. J. Epidemiol.* 119:624–641.
98. Brown, C., and Kessler, L. G. (1988). Projections of lung cancer mortality in the United States: 1985–2025. *JNCI* 80:43–51.
99. U. S. Department of Health and Human Services. (1991). Strategies to control tobacco use in the United States: A blueprint for public health action in the 1990's. NIH Publication No. 92-3316. Washington, D. C., U. S. Government Printing Office.
100. Kupper, L. L., Janis, J. M., Karmous, A., and Greenberg, B. G. (1985). Statistical age-period-cohort analysis: A review and critique. *J. Chron. Dis.* 38:811–830.
101. Holford, T. R. (1985). An alternative approach to statistical age-period-cohort analysis. *J. Chron. Dis.* 38:831–836.
102. Mattson, M. E., and Kessler, L. G. (1987). The use of time-related epidemiologic data on smoking for planning cancer control programs. *J. Chron. Dis.* 40(Suppl.): 25–38.
103. Thomas, D. C. (1988). Models for exposure-time-response relationships with applications to cancer epidemiology. *Ann. Rev. Public Health* 9:451–482.
104. Wynder, E. L., Bross, I. J., Cornfield, J., and O'Donnell, W. E. (1956). Lung cancer in women. A study of environmental factors. *N. Engl. J. Med.* 255(24):1111–1121.
105. Haenszel, W., Shimkin, M. B., and Mantel, N. (1958). A retrospective study of lung cancer in women. *JNCI* 21(5):825–842.
106. Wu, A. H., Henderson, B. E., Pike, M. C., and Yu, M.C. (1985). Smoking and other risk factors for lung cancer in women. *JNCI* 74:747–751.
107. Hammond, E. C., and Horn, D. (1958). Smoking and death rates—Report on forty-four months of follow-up of 187,783 men. II. Death rates by cause. *JAMA* 166(11): 1294–1308.
108. Rogot, E., and Murray, J. L. (1980). Smoking and causes of death among U.S. veterans: 16 years of observation. *Publ. Health Rep.* 95:213–222.
109. Remington, P. L., Forman, M. R., Gentry, E. M., Marks, J. S., Hogelin, G. C., and Trowbridge, F. L. (1985). Current smoking trends in the United States. The 1981–1983 behavioral risk factor survey. *JAMA* 253:2975–2978.
110. Fiore, M. C., Novotny, T. E., Pierce, J. P., Hatziandreu, E. J., Patel, K. M., and Davis, R. M. (1989). Trends in cigarette smoking in the United States. The changing influence of gender and race. *JAMA* 261:49–55.

111. Marcus, A. C., Shopland, D. R., Crane, L. A., and Lynn, W. R. (1989). Prevalence of cigarette smoking in the United States: Estimates from the 1985 current population survey. *JNCI* 81:409–414.
112. Rogers, R. G., and Crank, J. (1988). Ethnic differences in smoking patterns: Findings from NHIS. *Publ. Health Rep.* 103:387–393.
113. Hinds, M. W., Stemmermann, G. N., Yang, H. Y., Kolonel, L. N., Lee, J., and Wegner, E. (1981). *Int. J. Cancer* 27:297–302.
114. Wynder, E. L., and Stellman, S. D. (1979). Impact of long-term filter cigarette usage on lung and larynx cancer risk: A case-control study. *JNCI* 62:471–477.

5

Passive Smoking and Lung Cancer

GÖRAN PERSHAGEN

Karolinska Institute
Stockholm, Sweden

I. Introduction

Tobacco smoking is the dominant cause of lung cancer, and tobacco smoke contains a number of recognized human carcinogens. These compounds are also present in environmental tobacco smoke (ETS), which raises the possibility of passive smoking as a cause of lung cancer in nonsmokers. Since the publication in 1981 of the first reports on increased lung cancer risks in nonsmokers married to smokers, there has been a growing interest in the health effects of ETS, both in the scientific community and among the general public. Although cancer induction is probably not the most significant effect of ETS from a public health point of view, there is no doubt that the potential for such effects has had a great impact on the attitudes towards passive smoking and constituted an important incentive for measures to restrict the exposure.

This review focuses on the epidemiological evidence regarding passive smoking and lung cancer. Exposure to ETS is discussed initially, especially in relation to doses received by smokers. After summarizing the data on ETS and lung cancer, bias and methodological aspects of importance for the assessment of causal relationships are highlighted. Comparisons are also made of exposure–response relationships in passive smokers and smokers. Extensive reviews of the health consequences of ETS, including cancer risks, have been performed by the National Research Council (1) and the Surgeon General of the United States (2) and more recently by Pershagen (3) and Samet (4).

II. Exposure to ETS

In many countries about half of the male adult population and more than 25% of the women are daily smokers (5). This implies that large segments of the population are also exposed to ETS, and that health effects resulting from this exposure will be of public health significance. ETS may also be an important occupational hazard, for example, among people working in bars and restaurants. Furthermore, the often involuntary nature of the exposure should be kept in mind, such as in children of smokers.

Tobacco smoke contains more than 40 carcinogenic agents (5). In addition, a large number of other components may be of importance as effect modifiers, including many irritants. The complex composition of tobacco smoke and the lack of knowledge of the role of its specific components in the cancer induction make it difficult to identify suitable, single indicators of the carcinogenic potential of tobacco smoke.

Environmental tobacco smoke is produced from the sidestream smoke (SS) released from the burning tobacco product and mainstream smoke (MS) exhaled by the smoker. There are substantial differences in the composition of mainstream and sidestream smoke (1). As a rule the amounts emitted from a cigarette are greater in the sidestream smoke. For example, more than 50 times higher amounts of some nitrosamines are emitted in the sidestream smoke, but the SS/MS ratio is around 2–5 for most components.

ETS is predominantly an indoor problem, and the exposure levels depend on the intensity of smoking, room size, and air exchange. It is evident that ETS is a major component of indoor suspended particulate. In homes of smokers monthly average particulate concentrations exceeding 100 $\mu g/m^3$ have been measured (6,7). Short-term concentrations of several hundred $\mu g/m^3$ are seen in very smoky environments, such as bars and nightclubs (8,9). Particulate matter in ETS occurs mainly in the aerodynamic size range 0.2–0.4 μm, suggesting a deposition in the respiratory tract of about 10–30% (2).

Some of the carcinogens in ETS are mainly found in the particulate phase, such as polyaromatic hydrocarbons and metals (1). ETS contributes significantly to indoor airborne particulate mutagenicity (10). Radon daughters attach to ETS particles, and radon daughter levels in smoky environments may increase by reducing plate out on other surfaces (11). However, the increased carcinogenic potency of the ETS particles is counterbalanced by a lower fraction of unattached daughters, reducing the estimated radiation dose to the bronchial epithelium (12).

Vapor phase constituents in ETS of interest for carcinogenicity include

Table 1 Exposure to Some Constituents in Mainstream Smoke (MS) of One Cigarette and Environmental Tobacco Smoke (ETS) in Polluted Environments

Constituent	Amount in MS of one cigarette	ETS concentration in indoor environments	Inhaled ETS during 1 h
Acrolein	60–100 μg	6–50 ppb	8–72 μg
Benzo[*a*]pyrene	20–40 ng	0.0002–0.04 ppb	1.7–460 ng
CO	10–23 mg	1–18.5 ppm	1.2–22 mg
Dimethylnitrosamine	10–40 ng	0.003–0.072 ppb	6–140 ng
Nicotine	1–2.5 mg	0.15–7.5 ppb	0.6–30 μg

Source: Ref. 2.

benzene, ethene, and different nitrosamines (5). Sidestream smoke contains relatively more free nicotine in the vapor phase than mainstream smoke from cigarettes because of pH differences (13). Nicotine levels have been shown to decrease more rapidly than ETS particles in smoke-filled rooms, probably through condensation on other surfaces (14). On the other hand, the concentration of some tobacco-generated gases, such as CO, decreases only slowly in poorly ventilated rooms after smoking has ceased. Differences in removal rates may thus complicate the use of single components as markers of ETS exposure.

The exposure to some constituents in tobacco smoke among smokers and passive smokers is compared in Table 1. It is evident that large differences in the relative exposure for active and passive smokers may occur between certain constituents. For some gaseous components, such as dimethylnitrosamine, the inhalation of ETS during 1 h can yield a dose several times higher than received from the mainstream smoke of one cigarette. For other agents such as nicotine the inhaled amounts during 1 h of passive smoking may be less than 1% of the MS content of a cigarette. It should be pointed out that actual absorbed doses are also dependent on other factors, such as breathing patterns and particle size, which may differ for active and passive smoking. Furthermore, the time spent in different locations with varying degrees of ETS contamination determines the total exposure. The term "cigarette equivalent" has often been misused for quantifying ETS exposure, and a minimum requirement is that the component of interest is specified and that time activity patterns are considered.

III. Biologic Markers of ETS Exposure

Exposure to ETS can be estimated with biological markers. Nicotine and its metabolite cotinine are two sensitive and specific markers, which may be measured in saliva, serum, and urine. Cotinine has some advantages in comparison with nicotine, including a longer biological half-life. The half-life of cotinine in serum, saliva, and urine is in the order of 15–30 h (15–17), which implies that a spot sample is influenced by exposure during the last few days prior to sampling. There is some evidence of a longer half-life in nonsmokers than in smokers (16,18), which may be due to induction of metabolizing systems in smokers.

Cotinine concentrations in urine of nonsmokers and smokers are compared in Table 2. The levels of nonsmokers reporting ETS exposure range from about one-half to a few percent of those in regular smokers. The two studies in the table reporting the highest cotinine concentrations in nonsmokers included subjects who had been exposed in heavily polluted bars and nightclubs. Similarly high urinary cotinine concentrations have also been reported in children with smoking parents, indicating a substantial exposure to ETS (24–26).

There are major problems in using cotinine as a biological marker of ETS exposure (27). Nicotine is only one of several thousand compounds in tobacco smoke, and its representativeness for estimating carcinogenic or other toxic activities of ETS is questionable. Other sources of nicotine intake must be controlled, such as snuff and nicotine gums, and to a lesser extent certain food items. Individual differences in metabolism also have to be considered. In epidemiological studies, which often try to estimate exposures over years or decades, a spot sample may be of limited value if exposure is highly variable (28).

Some other markers have been used for assessment of ETS exposure, including carboxyhemoglobin and thiocyanate in body fluids and urinary mutagenicity (20,22). These are generally less sensitive and specific than cotinine, but can be used to distinguish smokers and nonsmokers. A combination of markers may be particularly useful for separating heavily exposed passive smokers from light smokers.

Table 2 Mean Cotinine Concentrations in Urine (μg/L) of Adult Nonsmokers and Smokers

Nonsmokers				
No ETS exposure	ETS exposure	Smokers	ETS exposure/ Smokers (%)	Ref.
4.8	12.9	1448	0.9	19
2	8	1391	0.6	20
2	6	1474	0.4[a]	21
8	56	1578	3.5	22
6	9	1017	0.9	23

[a]Concentrations represent median values; ETS/smoker ratio is 1.5% using mean values (34).

IV. Epidemiological Evidence on ETS and Lung Cancer

Lung cancer in nonsmokers is a very rare disease, with a yearly incidence of only about 5–10 cases per 100,000 (29–31). In some populations, such as Cantonese women, the rates may be higher (32). No clear time trends in lung cancer mortality among nonsmokers were evident in a U.S. study (30). However, it is difficult to assess such trends using mortality registry information, because death certificates tend to overreport lung cancer in nonsmokers, particularly for women (30,33). Changes in diagnostic criteria and quality over time may influence observed time trends, and such data should be interpreted with caution.

The design of the analytic epidemiological studies on ETS and lung cancer based on 27 different study groups is presented in Table 3. The table presents only information regarding nonsmokers, although studies also sometimes included smokers. A total of almost 3000 nonsmoking lung cancer cases have been included, suggesting a total study base in the order of 40 million person–years under observation. Most of the studies were of case-control design, and only three were cohort studies (30,31,42). The studies come from six countries (China with Hong Kong, Greece, Japan, Sweden, United Kingdom, and United States) and include predominantly women (more than 90% of the cases).

Face-to-face interview with the study subjects was the most common source of the exposure information: however, a few studies employed self-administered questionnaires. In view of the short survival time for lung cancer patients, it is not surprising that almost half of the case-control studies used information provided by next of kin for some subjects. As a rule no validation of the exposure data was attempted. A thorough discussion of design issues and consequences of some aspects of poor data quality is included in the next section.

For various reasons a few studies reporting data on passive smoking and lung cancer have not been included in the table or in the subsequent evaluation (63–67). Some of the reasons for not including these studies were that nonsmokers could not be separated from smokers, that the number of study subjects was unspecified or too small for any meaningful analyses, that the data were included in other studies, and that no controls were used. The results of these studies were not inconsistent with the other epidemiological evidence, and the exclusions have no consequence for the overall evaluation.

Exposure to ETS was defined in different ways in the epidemiologic studies. A common measure used in most studies based the exposure classification on smoking habits of spouses. Although this still implies substantial differences within and between studies regarding actual exposure to components in ETS, there is a possibility to directly compare the results with regard to consistency as well as to combine the data to increase statistical power. In Figures 1–4, lung cancer risks in nonsmokers in relation to smoking habits of spouses are depicted for Europe, the United States, China, and Japan separately to facilitate the comparison of

Table 3 Epidemiologic Studies on Passive Smoking and Lung Cancer

Nonsmoking study subjects	Location	Source of exposure information	Controlled variables[a] (besides age and sex)	Ref.
176,739 women followed 1960–72 and including 153 lung cancer deaths	1121 counties in 25 U.S. states	Questionnaire	Education Husband's occupation Race Residence	30
91,540 women and 20,289 men followed 1966–81 including 200 and 64 deaths from lung cancer, respectively	29 health districts in Japan	Interview	Diet (green-yellow vegetables) Husband's occupation Husband's drinking habits	31, 35
77 women with lung cancer other than adeno- and terminal-bronchial carcinoma diagnosed 1978–82 and 225 controls with orthopedic diseases	3 hospitals in Athens, Greece	Interview	—	36, 37
84 women with lung cancer diagnosed 1967–77 and 139 orthopedic patients	Hong Kong, China	Interview	—	38
22 women and 8 men with lung cancer except bronchioalveolar carcinomas; 72 female and 154 male hospital controls	Louisiana	Interview (surrogate: 24 and 11% of cases and controls, respectively)[b]	Race	39
41 and 11 white women and men with lung cancer diagnosed 1976–80; 90 male and 196 female population controls	6 counties in Texas	Interview (surrogate: 84 and 81% of cases and controls, respectively)	Area Race Vital status	40
1784 women and 671 men followed 1972(76)–85, including 6 and 3 lung cancer deaths respectively	2 towns in the West of Scotland	Questionnaire	Social class	41, 42
53 female and 25 male lung cancer cases diagnosed 1971–80; same number of hospital controls with diseases not related to tobacco	U.S. cities, predominantly New York	Interview	Hospital Race	43

88 women with lung cancer diagnosed 1981–83; 137 population controls	Hong Kong, China	Interview	Area Education Housing type Number of livebirths	44, 45
134 women with lung and 402 controls with colorectal cancer identified 1971–81	3 hospitals in New Jersey, 1 in Ohio	Interview (surrogate: 88% of cases, no data for controls)	Hospital Socioeconomic status Year of diagnosis	46
29 women with adenocarcinoma of the lung and 2 with squamous carcinoma identified 1981–82; 92 neighborhood controls	Los Angeles County, California	Interview	—	47
94 women and 19 men with lung cancer diagnosed 1971–80 in cohort of atomic bomb survivors; 270 female and 110 male controls from the cohort	Hiroshima and Nagasaki, Japan	Interview (surrogate: 87%)	City Occupation Radiation exposure Vital status	48
32 female and 15 male lung cancer patients identified 1979–82; 66 female and 30 male hospital controls	4 hospital regions in England	Interview (surrogate: 38%)	Dusty job Hospital ward and region Time of interview	49
19 white women with adenocarcinoma diagnosed 1979–82; hospital controls with cancer of colon or bone marrow	Denver, Colorado	Interview (surrogate: 69 and 39% of cases and controls, respectively)	Income Occupation	50
246 women with lung cancer diagnosed 1984–86; 375 population controls	Shanghai, China	Interview	Education	51
20 women and 8 men with lung cancer diagnosed 1980–84; 162 and 130 female and male population controls	New Mexico	Interview (surrogate: 52 and 2% of cases and controls respectively)**	Race	52
199 women with lung cancer identified 1983–86; 335 neighborhood controls	Hong Kong, China	Interview	—	53
67 women with lung cancer identified 1961–80 in 2 cohorts; 347 controls from the same cohorts	Sweden	Mailed questionnaire (surrogate: 95 and 64% of cases and controls, respectively)	Residential radon Urban residence	33

Table 3 Continued

Nonsmoking study subjects	Location	Source of exposure information	Controlled variables[a] (besides age and sex)	Ref.
54 women with lung cancer diagnosed 1983–84 and 93 population controls	Tianjin, China	Interview	Marital status Race	54
29 women who died from lung cancer 1973–83 and 54 controls who died from cerebrovascular disease	2 cities in Kanagawa prefecture, Japan	Interview (probably mostly with surrogates)	District Year of death	55
90 women with lung cancer identified 1982–85; 163 hospital controls	4 hospitals in Nagoya, Japan	Questionnaire	Hospital Occupational exposure	56
34 women with lung cancer identified 1983–85; 120 population and 54 hospital controls	3 hospitals in Stockholm, Sweden	Interview	Diet (carotene) Occupation Residential radon	57
146 female and 45 male lung cancer patients diagnosed 1982–84; same numbers of population controls	New York state	Interview (surrogate: 32%)	County Source of exposure information	58
91 women with lung cancer identified 1987–89; 120 hospital controls with orthopedic diseases	7 hospitals in Athens, Greece	Interview	Diet Interviewer Years of schooling	59
120 women with lung cancer diagnosed 1986–89; 519 hospital controls	8 hospitals in Osaka, Japan	Questionnaire	Cooking fuel	60
417 women with lung cancer diagnosed 1985–87; 602 population controls	Shenyang and Harbin, China	Interview	Area Education	61
124 women with lung cancer; 241 population controls	Florida	[c]	[c]	62

[a]Variables considered in the design and/or analysis of the studies, particularly in relation to assessment of the ETS/lung cancer association.
[b]Based also on smoking lung cancer cases and controls included in the study.
[c]Information not provided (only abstract available).

results under similar cultural circumstances. In general the information was taken directly from the published material, but 95% confidence intervals were sometimes estimated according to the test-based method (68). Methods for estimation of pooled relative risks and confidence intervals were described by the National Research Council (1).

Figure 1 summarizes the findings on spousal smoking and lung cancer for the six European studies. The cohort study by Hole et al. based the exposure classification on smoking habits of a "cohabitee" at the time of initial survey, presumably often the spouse. The relative risks range from about 1.0 to 3.5 for nonsmokers married to smokers; however, statistically significant increases in risk were seen only in three of the studies. The data primarily pertain to nonsmoking women, who were married to smokers in about 40–70% according to data in the cohorts and control groups. The overall relative risk associated with marriage to a smoker combining the data for men and women was 1.47 with a 95% confidence interval (CI) of 1.12–1.92. This estimate was based on a dichotomous exposure classification in each of the studies (spouse smoker/spouse nonsmoker or unmarried) and separating the data for men and women.

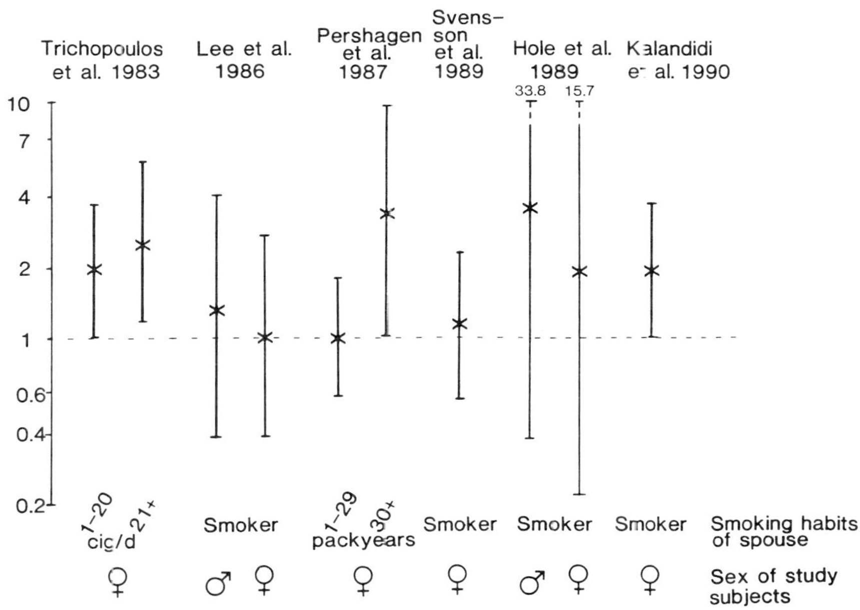

Figure 1 Relative risk of lung cancer for nonsmokers according to smoking habits of spouses in epidemiological studies from Europe (bars indicate 95% confidence intervals).

The corresponding results in the eight studies from the United States are shown in Figure 2. Relative risks associated with marriage to a smoker ranged from about 0.4 to 3 in the different studies, and positive trends in relation to husband's smoking were seen in two out of three studies. Between 46 and 72% of the nonsmoking women in the different studies had been married to smokers. Pooling the data gives a relative risk in nonsmokers living with smokers of 1.23 (1.02–1.49). The number of study subjects in different exposure categories was not given in three of the studies, and the variance of the relative risk estimates was calculated from the confidence intervals (47,58,62). Two studies in which the smoking habits of spouses could not be separated in the ETS exposure measures were not included in the figure (40,50).

Figure 3 shows relative risks for lung cancer in female nonsmokers according to smoking of spouses for six studies from China. No data were available for men. It should be noted that the "unexposed" reference category in the study by Gao et al. included women who had lived with a smoker less than 20 years. Excluding this study, between 50 and 60% of the women were married to smokers. Four of the studies indicate increased relative risks, which were positively related to husband's smoking in two. A recent larger study from two heavily polluted cities in northeast China showed a significant decrease in risk for women with smoking spouses, which was not consistent for the two cities (61). The pooled

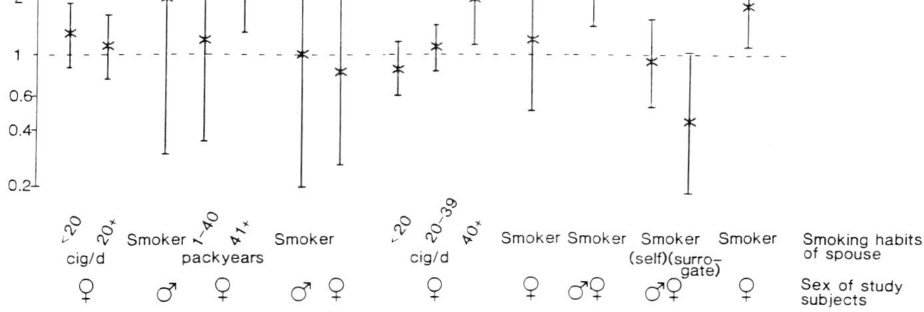

Figure 2 Relative risk of lung cancer for nonsmokers according to smoking habits of spouses in epidemiological studies from the United States (bars indicate 95% confidence intervals).

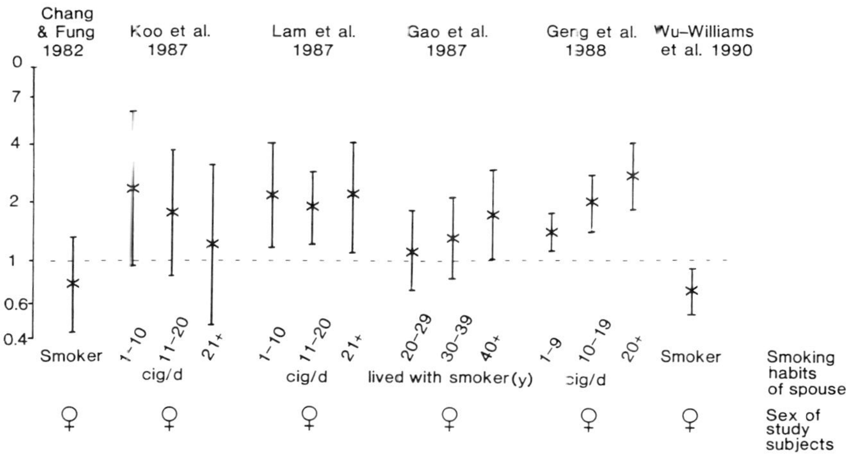

Figure 3 Relative risk of lung cancer for nonsmokers according to smoking habits of spouses in epidemiological studies from China (bars indicate 95% confidence intervals).

relative risk for all studies was 1.10 (0.94–1.28). This estimate is heavily influenced by the recent larger study, and excluding that gives an estimate of 1.36 (1.11–1.66).

For Japan the data appear somewhat more consistent (Fig. 4). Three of the five studies included women only. All three studies providing information on lung cancer risks in relation to detailed smoking habits of spouses gave evidence of positive trends. Between 56 and 76% of the nonsmoking women in the different studies had been married to smokers. Combining all studies, the pooled relative risk was 1.32 (1.08–1.61) associated with marriage to a smoker.

Combining the results of the studies in Figures 1–4 gives a pooled relative risk of lung cancer in nonsmoking women and men living with smokers of 1.23 (1.11–1.36) and 1.82 (0.98–3.37), respectively. The studies by Humble et al. (52) and Janerich et al. (58) have been excluded from these calculations because results were not provided separately for men and women. The pooled relative risk for both sexes taken together is 1.23 (1.12–1.35). Excluding the study by Humble et al. (1987), which probably contains some smokers, reduces this estimate to 1.21 (1.10–1.34). If the large Chinese study by Wu-Williams et al. (61), the only study showing a statistically significant decrease of lung cancer in nonsmokers married to smokers, is excluded, the pooled relative risk becomes 1.33 (1.20–1.48).

Many of the studies also used measures of ETS exposure during adulthood other than smoking habits of spouses, for example, ETS exposure at work or from other household members. Two studies suggested an excess lung cancer risk in

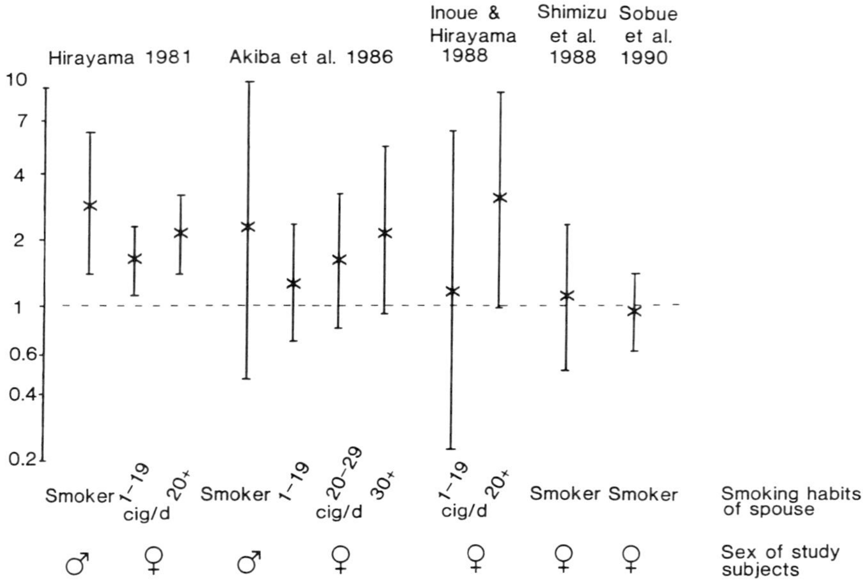

Figure 4 Relative risk of lung cancer for nonsmokers according to smoking habits of spouses in epidemiological studies from Japan (bars indicate 95% confidence intervals).

men with occupational exposure to ETS (43,49); however, for women the findings appear less consistent (46,47,49,56,59,61). In general, the results using measures of ETS exposure in adulthood other than smoking habits of spouses gave a less coherent picture. This also holds true for studies trying to assess the total ETS exposure from different sources.

Some of the studies on passive smoking and lung cancer included information on ETS exposure in childhood. The results of these investigations are summarized in Table 4. Only the study by Janerich et al. (58) provided clear evidence of an increased lung cancer risk related to ETS exposure in childhood or adolescence. No consistent association was evident from the other studies, although two of three studies suggested an increased lung cancer risk if the mother smoked. It should be noted that parental smoking does not necessarily imply ETS exposure during childhood, e.g., if the parents took up smoking late in life.

In view of the substantial differences in risk associated with smoking for different histological types of lung cancer, it is of interest to assess such evidence also for ETS exposure. However, only a few of the studies on ETS and lung cancer included information on histological type. Some of these studies suggested higher relative risks for squamous/small-cell carcinomas than for other types (33,45,

Table 4 Summary of Findings on ETS Exposure in Childhood and Lung Cancer in Nonsmokers

Measure of exposure	Results (relative risk and 95% confidence interval)		Ref.
Maternal or paternal smoking	"No significant increase in risk"		39
Exposure in childhood	0.91	(0.74–1.12)	46
Parental smoking	0.6	(0.2–1.7)	47
Household exposure to cigarette smoke during childhood	0.7	(0.2–2.3)[a]	45
At least one smoking parent	1.0	(0.4–2.3)	33
Father smoker	0.9	(0.4–2.3)	57
Mother smoker	0.3	(0.5–18.8)	
ETS exposure during childhood or adolescence:			58
1–24 smoker-years	1.09	(0.68–1.73)	
>25 smoker-years	2.07	(1.16–3.68)	
Smoking by father	0.60	(0.40–0.91)	
Smoking by mother	1.71	(0.95–3.10)	60
Smoking by other family members during childhood	1.13	(0.69–1.87)	
Mother smoker	0.9	(0.6–1.1)[b]	61
Father smoker	1.1	(0.8–1.4)	
25 or more years of exposure to parental smoking	1.7	(0.8–3.6)	62

[a]Estimation based on children with exposure in childhood only and both childhood and adulthood.
[b]Confidence interval estimated from published data.

46,48). Most of the studies in which histopathological information was provided included predominantly adenocarcinomas; however, the investigations by Trichopoulos et al. (36,37) excluded this type.

V. Sources of Bias in the Epidemiological Studies

It is necessary to consider various sources of bias and their implications in the assessment of the epidemiological evidence on passive smoking and lung cancer. This is particularly relevant in view of the weak associations observed, i.e., relative risks mostly ranging between 0.5 and 2. The assessment of bias should preferentially involve also its quantitative implications for the estimated associations.

Bias in epidemiologic studies can be classified into three categories: selection bias, information bias (misclassification), and confounding (Rothman 1986). Selection bias may be a problem particularly in case-control studies, which was the design used for all but three of the investigations on passive smoking and lung cancer (see Table 3). A minority of these studies were population based, with cases from cancer or mortality registers and controls from the general population (33, 47,48,51,52,54,58,61). The remaining case-control studies were hospital based, often with hospital controls, who may not be representative for the exposure distribution in the source population for the cases. A matching on vital status in the selection of controls was employed in some studies (33,40,48) to achieve comparability in the acquisition of exposure information between cases and controls. This will result in an underestimation of the relative risk for factors associated with premature death, such as smoking (69), but should be of lesser importance for passive smoking.

Information bias may affect both the determination of exposure and of health effects. Nondifferential misclassification of exposure resulting from crude exposure estimates occurs in most epidemiological studies. As a rule this will dilute any associations between exposure and effect. In the studies on ETS and lung cancer, the exposure data were obtained from interviews or questionnaires, and with few exceptions no validation of the information was attempted. The most common measure of exposure was smoking of spouses, and it has been shown that nonsmokers living with smokers, on an average, have a higher cotinine excretion than nonsmokers living with nonsmokers (21,70–72). Smoking by spouses may be a more accurate predictor of ETS exposure for women than for men, where other sources predominate (73,74). It is clear, however, that there are many sources of ETS exposure that should be considered if the total exposure is to be assessed and that this depends also on cultural factors (71,75,76). The failure in most studies to obtain clearer associations between ETS exposure and lung cancer risk using more complex exposure models than smoking of spouses may partly be explained by the fact that such exposures are reported less reliably (77).

Attempts have been made to quantitatively assess the influence of nondifferential misclassification of exposure on the risk estimates (78,79). Using data on nicotine exposure and biological markers, it is suggested that the relative risk comparing exposed with truly unexposed to ETS should be more in the order 1.5–1.6 if the observed relative risk comparing nonsmokers living with smokers and nonsmokers is 1.35. It should be emphasized that only recent exposure is included in these calculations and that the imprecision will be even greater if lifetime exposure is of importance.

Misclassification of exposure may also be differential between cases and controls. Some of the studies on ETS and lung cancer that included deceased subjects did not match on vital status in the selection of controls (33,39,46,50,52). As a rule this led to a higher percentage of surrogate respondents for the cases because of the high lethality of lung cancer (see Table 3). A difference in the quality of the information on ETS exposure between index and surrogate respondents would then lead to biased estimates of the relative risks; however, one study suggests that this would be unimportant (73).

Nondifferential misclassification of the health effects will also result in a dilution of the associations. Secondary lung tumors and carcinomas with unknown primary site appeared in about one-sixth of reported cases of lung cancer on death certificates in the United States (30) and in central health registers in Sweden (33) among female nonsmokers. In many of the studies on passive smoking and lung cancer, there is an inadequate description of the diagnostic criteria, and some misclassification of outcome cannot be excluded.

Probably the most important potential source of bias in the epidemiological studies on ETS and lung cancer is confounding by unreported active smoking. There is a tendency for smokers to marry smokers, and in conjunction with some misclassification of smokers as nonsmokers this would tend to produce a spurious association between spouse smoking and lung cancer. Unfortunately there is limited empirical information that can be used to estimate the extent of this bias, and differences in assumptions may lead to quite discrepant conclusions regarding its magnitude (78,80).

One crucial factor for estimation of this bias is the proportion of those classified as nonsmokers who actually have been smokers. Using biological markers of nicotine exposure it has been indicated that up to 3% of subjects classifying themselves as nonsmokers have levels consistent with regular smoking (70–72, 78). In populations with a widespread use of smokeless tobacco, it may be unfeasible to rely on biological markers of nicotine exposure for estimating the proportion of smoking deceivers (81). Studies involving multiple reports of smoking over several years as well as studies using surrogates suggest that in the order of about 5% of ever-smokers may deny smoking (80,82). Several investigations indicate that surrogates can provide valid information to separate smokers from nonsmokers (69,83–85), which makes this source of information useful for validation. Very limited and inconclusive data are available for smoking misclassification at interview with newly diagnosed lung cancer cases, which was the source of information in most epidemiological studies on ETS exposure and lung cancer.

A few attempts have been made to quantify the bias from confounding by smoking on the risk estimates for lung cancer in nonsmokers living with smokers (78,80,82). Based on some empirical information and with reasonable assumptions, it appears that in women, who constitute more than 90% of the subjects in the studies on ETS and lung cancer, the smoking confounding bias may explain about 10–30% of the excess risk. Correcting for this bias would reduce the overall relative risk in nonsmoking women living with smokers from 1.23 to about 1.15–1.20. In men the smoking confounding bias would be greater because of higher smoking rates in the population.

Other confounding factors may also affect the observed associations between passive smoking and lung cancer. In particular, it has been indicated that nonsmokers living with smokers have a lower intake of nutritional elements that may be protective for lung cancer, including beta-carotene (86,87). However, there was no confounding by dietary factors in two studies showing an increased risk of lung cancer in passive smokers (35,59). It seems unlikely that the effects of other confounding factors would exceed those of smoking.

VI. Magnitude of Effects

In assessing the evidence on ETS and lung cancer it is of interest to make a quantitative comparison with exposure–response relationships for smokers. Using a multistage model developed from the Doll and Peto data for British doctors, it has been estimated that a dose of 0.5 cigarette equivalent a day from birth to age 65 would result in a relative risk of 1.36 in comparison with a nonexposed nonsmoker (88). For exposure starting at age 20 the relative risk would be 1.22, and only 1.11 if exposure occurred from birth to age 20. Allowing for passive smoking at a rate of one cigarette a day in the British doctors cohort would increase these estimates to 1.49, 1.33, and 1.13, respectively.

Using the "uncorrected" relative risk estimates for lung cancer in nonsmokers living with smokers from the previous section and the percentage of smokers living with smokers in the population the etiological fraction (EF) may be estimated, i.e., the fraction of the total number of cases that may be attributable to the exposure. In women the EF is between 0.10 and 0.15 assuming a relative risk of 1.23 and that between 50 and 75% in different populations have been married to smokers. Based on data indicating that between 4 and 40% of the nonsmoking men had been married to smokers in the published studies and a pooled relative risk of 1.82, the EF would be 0.03–0.25.

As indicated in the previous section, nondifferential misclassification of ETS exposure and confounding by smoking would result in bias working in opposite directions. The quantitative estimates indicate that the net effect would be a relative risk associated with ETS exposure at least as great as the one calculated for nonsmokers living with smokers. There is inadequate evidence for a quantitative estimation of other sources of bias.

The evidence on ETS and lung cancer has been thoroughly reviewed by various groups (1,2,5). The conclusions reached are quite coherent in that environmental tobacco smoke can cause lung cancer. Subsequent evidence provides no reason to change the conclusions. For the quantitative assessment there is, however, a need for additional data on misreporting of smoking by lung cancer cases to enable a more detailed estimation of confounding and for more precise information on lifetime ETS exposure to reduce misclassification bias.

VII. Conclusions

Large segments of the population in many countries are exposed to ETS, which means that even small effects of this exposure may be of public health significance.

Using biological markers, it has been estimated that the daily exposure to nicotine in passive smokers may correspond to a dose received from 0.1–1 cigarette in a smoker. The relative exposure for passive smokers in comparison with smokers varies substantially for different components in the smoke.

More than 25 epidemiological studies have been published on passive smoking and lung cancer. The most common approach in the analysis has been to base the exposure classification on smoking habits of spouses. Taking the studies together there is statistically significant increase in the lung cancer risk of about 20–30% in nonsmokers married to smokers. Higher risks in those married to heavy smokers were often observed, supporting a causal association.

It is probable that a part of the increased risk related to smoking of spouses is explained by confounding by smoking. On the other hand, nondifferential misclassification of ETS exposure, resulting from crude exposure measures, will give rise to an underestimation of the true risks. The available empirical data suggest that bias cannot explain the observed association between ETS exposure and lung cancer. An overall assessment taking into consideration the presence of carcinogens in ETS, exposure estimates in passive smokers, exposure–response relationships in smokers, and the epidemiological evidence on lung cancer in passive smokers indicates that ETS is of carcinogenic importance.

Acknowledgment

I am grateful for the assistance from Peter Lee, James Repace, Jonathan Samet, and Judson Wells in providing material for this chapter.

References

1. NRC. (1986). Environmental tobacco smoke: Measuring exposures and assessing health effects. U. S. National Research Council. Washington. D. C., National Academy Press.
2. U. S. Surgeon General. (1986). The health consequences of involuntary smoking. Washington, D. C., United States Department of Health and Human Services.
3. Pershagen, G. (1989). Environmental tobacco smoke and cancer. In *Assessment of inhalation hazards*. Edited by U. Mohr. Berlin, Springer, pp. 275–284.
4. Samet, J. M. (1991). The health effects of environmental tobacco smoke. *Crit. Rev. Environ. Toxicol.* (in press).
5. IARC. (1986). Monographs on the evaluation of the carcinogenic risk of chemicals to humans: Tobacco smoking. Lyon. International Agency for Research on Cancer.
6. Spengler, J. D., Dockery, D. W., Turner, W. A., Wolfson, J. M., and Ferris, B. J. (1981). Long term measurements of respirable sulphates and particles inside and outside homes. *Atmos. Environ.* 15:23–30.
7. Brunekreef, B., and Boleij, J. S. M. (1982). Long-term average suspended particulate concentrations in smoker's homes. *Int. Arch. Occup. Environ. Health* 50:299–302.

8. Repace, J. L., and Lowrey, A. H. (1980). Indoor air pollution, tobacco smoke and public health. *Science* 208:464–472.
9. Husgafvel-Pursiainen, K., Sorsa, M., Moeller, M., and Benestad, C. (1986). Genotoxicity and polynuclear aromatic hydrocarbon analysis of environmental tobacco smoke samples from restaurants. *Mutagenesis* 1:287–292.
10. Löfroth, G., Ling, P. I., and Agurell, E. (1988). Public exposure to environmental tobacco smoke. *Mut. Res.* 202:103–110.
11. Bergman, H., Edling, C., and Axelson, O. (1986). Indoor radon daughter concentrations and passive smoking. *Environ. Int.* 12:17–19.
12. James, A. C. (1988). Lung dosimetry. In *Radon and Its Decay Products in Indoor Air*. Edited by W. W. Nazaroff and A. V. Nero. New York, Wiley, pp. 259–209.
13. Brunneman, K. D. and Hoffman, D. (1974). The pH of tobacco smoke. *Food Cosmet. Toxicol.* 12:115–124.
14. Badre, R., Guillerm, R., Abran, N., Bourdin, M., and Dumas, C. (1978). Atmospheric pollution by smoking. *Ann. Pharm. Fr.* 36:443–452.
15. Jarvis, M. J., Russell, M. A. H., Benowitz, N. L., and Feyerabend, C. (1988). Elimination of cotinine from body fluids: Implications for noninvasive measurement of tobacco smoke exposure. *Am. J. Public Health* 78:696–698.
16. Haley, N. J., Sepkovic, D. W., and Hoffman, D. (1989). Elimination of cotinine from body fluids: Disposition in smokers and nonsmokers. *Am. J. Public Health* 79:1046–1048.
17. Curvall, M., Elwin, C. E., Kazemi-Vala, E., Warholm, C., and Enzell, C. R. (1990). The pharmacokinetics of cotinine in plasma and saliva from nonsmoking healthy volunteers. *Eur. J. Clin. Pharmacol.* 38:281–287.
18. Kyerematen, G. A., Damiano, M. D., Dvorchik, B. H., and Vesell, E. S. (1982). Smoking-induced changes in nicotine disposition: Application of a new HPLC assay for nicotine and its metabolites. *Clin. Pharamacol. Ther.* 32:769–780.
19. Jarvis, M. J., Russell, M. A. H., and Feyerabend, C. (1983). Absorption of nicotine and carbon monoxide from passive smoking under natural conditions of exposure. *Thorax* 38:829–833.
20. Jarvis, M. J., and Russell, M. A. H. (1984). Measurement and estimation of smoke dosage to nonsmokers from environmental tobacco smoke. *Eur. J. Respir. Dis.* 65:68–75.
21. Wald, N. J., and Ritchie, C. (1984). Validation of studies on lung cancer in nonsmokers married to smokers. *Lancet* i:1067.
22. Husgafvel-Pursiainen, K., Sorsa, M., Engström, K., and Einistö, P. (1987). Passive smoking at work: Biochemical and biological measures of exposure to environmental tobacco smoke. *Int. Arch. Occup. Environ. Health* 59:337–345.
23. Wall, M. A., Johnson, J., Jacob, P., and Benowitz, N. L. (1988). Cotinine in serum, saliva, and urine of nonsmokers, passive smokers, and active smokers. *Am. J. Public Health* 78:699–701.
24. Greenberg, R. A., Haley, N. J., Etzel, R., and Loda, F. A. (1984). Measuring the exposure of infants to tobacco smoke. *N. Engl. J. Med.* 310:1075–1078.
25. Henderson, F. W., Reid, H. F., Morris, R., Wang, O. -L., Ping, C. H., Helms, R. W., Forehand, L., Mumford, J., Lewtas, J., Haley, N. J., and Hammond, S. K. (1989). Home air nicotine levels and urinary cotinine excretion in preschool children. *Am. Rev. Respir. Dis.* 140:197–201.

26. Rylander, E., Pershagen, G., Curvall, M., and Kazemi-Vala, E. (1989). Exposure to environmental tobacco smoke and urinary excretion of cotinine and nicotine in children. *Acta. Paediatr. Scand.* 78:449–450.
27. Idle, J. F. (1990). Titrating exposure to tobacco smoke using cotinine—a minefield of misunderstandings. *J. Clin. Epidemiol.* 43:313–317.
28. Coultas, D. B., Samet, J. M., McCarthy, J. F., and Spengler, J. D. (1990). Variability of measures of exposure to environmental tobacco smoke in the home. *Am. Rev. Resp. Dis.* 142:602–606.
29. Cederlöf, R. Friberg, L., Hrubec, Z., and Lorich, U. (1975). The relationship of smoking and some social covariables to mortality and cancer morbidity. Stockholm, Department of Environmental Hygiene, Karolinska Institute.
30. Garfinkel, L. (1981). Time trends in lung cancer mortality among nonsmokers and a note on passive smoking. *J. Natl. Cancer Inst.* 66:1061–1066.
31. Hirayama, T. (1981). Non smoking wives of heavy smokers have a higher risk of lung cancer: A study from Japan. *Br. Med. J.* 282:183–185.
32. Koo, L. C., Ho, J. H. C., and Lee, N. (1985). An analysis of some risk factors for lung cancer in Hong Kong. *Int. J. Cancer* 35:149–155.
33. Pershagen, G., Hrubec, Z., and Svensson, C. (1987). Passive smoking and lung cancer in Swedish women. *Am. J. Epidemiol.* 125:17–24.
34. Wald, N., Nanchahal, K., Cuckle, H., and Thompson, S. (1990). Lung cancer and passive smoking. *Br. J. Cancer* 61:337.
35. Hirayama, T. (1984). Lung cancer in Japan: Effects of nutrition and passive smoking. In *Lung Cancer: Causes and Prevention*. Edited by M. Mizell and P. Correa. New York, Chemie International, pp. 175–196.
36. Trichopoulos, D., Kalandidi, A., Sparros, L., and Mac Mahon, B. (1981). Lung cancer and passive smoking. *Int. J. Cancer* 27:1–4.
37. Trichopoulos, D., Kalandidi, A., and Sparros, L. (1983). Lung cancer and passive smoking: Conclusion of the Greek study. *Lancet* ii:677–678
38. Chan, W. C., and Fung, S. C. (1982). Lung cancer in nonsmokers in Hong Kong. In *Cancer campaign*. Vol. 6. *Cancer epidemiology*. Edited by E. Grundman. Stuttgart, Fischer, pp. 199–202.
39. Correa, P., Pickle, L. W., Fontham, E., Lin, Y., and Haenszel, W. (1983). Passive smoking and lung cancer. *Lancet* ii:595–597.
40. Buffler, P. A., Pickle, L. W., Mason, T. J., and Contant, C. (1984). The causes of lung cancer in Texas. In *Lung Cancer: Causes and Prevention*. Edited by M. Mizell and P. Correa. New York, Chemie International, pp. 83–99.
41. Gillis, C. R., Hole, D. J., Hawthorne, V. M., and Boyle, P. (1984). The effect of environmental tobacco smoke in two urban communities in the west of Scotland. *Eur. J. Respir. Dis.* 65:121–126.
42. Hole, D. J., Gillis, C. R., Chopra, C., and Hawthorne, V. M. (1989). Passive smoking and cardiorespiratory health in a general population in the west of Scotland. *Br. Med. J.* 299:423–427.
43. Kabat, G. C., and Wynder, E. L. (1984). Lung cancer in nonsmokers. *Cancer* 53: 1214–1221.
44. Koo, L. C., Ho, J. H. C., and Saw, D. (1984). Is passive smoking an added risk factor for lung cancer in Chinese women? *J. Exp. Clin. Cancer Res.* 3:277–283.

45. Koo, L. C., Ho, J. H. C., Saw, D., and Ho, C. (1987). Measurements of passive smoking and estimates of lung cancer risk among nonsmoking Chinese females. *Int. J. Cancer* 39:162–169.
46. Garfinkel, L., Auerbach, O., and Joubert, L. (1985). Involuntary smoking and lung cancer: A case control study. *J. Natl. Cancer Inst.* 75:463–469.
47. Wu, A. H., Henderson, B. E., Pike, M. C., and Yu, M. D. (1985). Smoking and other risk factors for lung cancer in women. *J. Natl. Cancer Inst.* 74:747–751.
48. Akiba, S., Kato, H., and Blot, W. J. (1986). Passive smoking and lung cancer among Japanese women. *Cancer Res.* 46:4804–4807.
49. Lee, P. N., Chamberlain, J., and Alderson, M. R. (1986). Relationship of passive smoking to risk of lung cancer and other smoking-associated diseases. *Br. J. Cancer* 54:97–105.
50. Brownson, R. C., Reif, J. S., Keefe, T. J., Ferguson, S. W., and Pritz, J. A. (1987). Risk factors for adenocarcinoma of the lung. *Am. J. Epidemiol.* 125:25–34.
51. Gao, Y. T., Blot, W. J., Zheng, W., Ershow, A. G., Hsu, C. W., Levin, L. I., Zhang, R., and Fraumeni, J. F. (1987). Lung cancer among Chinese women. *Int. J. Cancer* 40: 604–609.
52. Humble, C. G., Samet, J. M., and Pathak, D. R. (1987). Marriage to a smoker and lung cancer risk. *Am. J. Public Health* 77:598–602.
53. Lam, T. H., Kung, I. T. M., Wong, C. M., Lam, W. K., Kleevens, J. W. L., Saw, D., Hsu, C., Seneviratne, S., Lam, S. Y., Lo, K. K., and Chang, W. C. (1987). Smoking, passive smoking and histological types of lung cancer in Hong Kong Chinese women. *Br. J. Cancer* 56:673–678.
54. Geng, G. Y., Liang, Z. H., Zhang, A. Y., and Wu, G. L. (1988). On the relationship between smoking and female lung cancer. In *Smoking and Health*. Edited by M. Aoki, S. Hisamichi, and S. Tominaga. Amsterdam, Elsevier, pp. 483–490.
55. Inoue, R., and Hirayama, T. (1988). Passive smoking and lung cancer in women. In *Smoking and Health*. Edited by M. Aoki, S. Misamichi, and S. Tominaga. Amsterdam, Elsevier, pp. 283–285.
56. Shimizu, H. M., Morishita, K., Mizuno, K., Masuda, T., Ogura, Y., Santo, M., Nishimura, M., Kunishima, K., Karasawa, K., Nishiwaki, K., Yamamoto, M., Hisamichi, S., and Tominaga, S. (1988). A case-control study of lung cancer in nonsmoking women. *Tohoku J. Exp. Med.* 154:389–397.
57. Svensson, C., Pershagen, G., and Klominek, J. (1989). Smoking and passive smoking in relation to lung cancer in women. *Acta Oncol.* 28:623–629.
58. Janerich, D. T., Thompson, W. D., Varela, L. R., Greenwald, P., Chorost, S., Tucci, C., Zaman, M. B., Melamed, M. R., Kiely, M., and McKneally, M. F. (1990). Lung cancer and exposure to tobacco smoke in the household. *N. Engl. J. Med.* 323: 632–636.
59. Kalandidi, A., Katsouyanni, K., Voropoulou, N., Bastas, G., Saracci, R., and Trichopoulos, D. (1990). Passive smoking and diet in the etiology of lung cancer among nonsmokers. *Cancer Causes Control* 1:15–21.
60. Sobue, T., Suzuki, R., Nakayama, N., Inubuse, C., Matsuda, M., Doi, O., Mori, T., Furuse, K., Fukuoka, H., Yasumitsu, T., Kuwabara, O., Ichigaya, M., Kurata, M., Kuwabara, M., Nakahara, N., Endo, S., and Hattori, S. (1990). Passive smoking

among nonsmoking women and the relationship between indoor air pollution and lung cancer incidence—Results of a multicenter case-control study. *Gan to Rinsho* 36: 329–333.

61. Wu-Williams, A. H., Dai, X. D., Blot, W., Xu, Z. Y., Sun, X. W., Xiao, H. P., Stone, B. J., Yu, S. F., Feng, Y. P., Ershow, A. G., Sun, J., Fraumeni, J. F., Jr., and Henderson, B. E. (1990). Lung cancer among women in northeast China. *Br. J. Cancer* 52:982–987.
62. Stockwell, H. G., Candelora, E. C., Armstrong, A. W., and Pinkham, P. A. (1991). Environmental tobacco smoke and lung cancer in never smoking women. *Am. J. Epidemiol.* (in press).
63. Knoth, A., Bohn, H., and Schmidt, F. (1985). Passives Rauchen als Lungenkrebsursache bei Nichtraucherinnen. *Med. Klin.* 78:66–69.
64. Sandler, D. P., Everson, R. B., and Wilcox, A. J. (1985). Passive smoking in adulthood and cancer risk. *Am. J. Epidemiol.* 121:37–48.
65. Dalager, N. A., Pickle, L. W., Mason, T. J., Correa, P., Fontham, E., Stemhagen, A., Buffler, P. A., Ziegler, R. G., and Fraumeni, J. F., Jr. (1986). The relation of passive smoking to lung cancer. *Cancer Res.* 46:4808–4811.
66. Lloyd, O. L., Ireland, E., Tyrrell, H., and Williams, F. (1986). Respiratory cancer in a Scottish industrial community: A retrospective case-control study. *J. Soc. Occup. Med.* 35:2–8.
67. Axelson, O., Andersson, K., Desai, G., Fagerlund, I., Jansson, B., Karlsson, C., and Wingren, G. (1988). Indoor radon exposure and active and passive smoking in relation to the occurrence of lung cancer. *Scand. J. Work Environ. Health* 14:286–292.
68. Miettinen, O. (1976). Estimability and estimation in case referent studies. *Am. J. Epidemiol.* 103:226–235.
69. McLaughlin, J. K., Dietz, M. S., Mehl, E. S., and Blot, W. J (1985). Reliability of surrogate information on cigarette smoking by type of informant. *Am. J. Epidemiol.* 126:144–146.
70. Lee, P. N. (1987). Passive smoking and lung cancer association: A result of bias? *Hum. Toxicol.* 6:517–524.
71. Riboli, E., Preston-Martin, S., Saracci, R., Haley, N. J., Trichopoulos, D., Becher, H., Burch, J. D., Fontham, E. T. H., Gao, Y. -T., Jindal, S. K., Koo, L. C., LeMarchand, L., Segnan, N., Shimuzu, H., Stanta, G., Wu-Williams, A. H., and Zatonski, W. (1990). Exposure of nonsmoking women to environmental tobacco smoke: A ten-country collaborative study. *Cancer Causes Control* 1:243–252.
72. Thompson, S. G., Stone, R., Nanchahal, K., and Wald, N. J. (1990). Relation of urinary cotinine concentrations to cigarette smoking and to exposure to other people's smoke. *Thorax* 45:356–361.
73. Cummings, K. M., Markello, S. J., Mahoney, M. C., and Marshall, J. R. (1989). Measurement of lifetime exposure to passive smoke. *Am. J. Epidemiol.* 130: 122–132.
74. Sandler, D. P., Helsing, K. J., Comstock, G. W., and Shore, D. L. (1989). Factors associated with past household exposure to tobacco smoke. *Am. J. Epidemiol.* 129: 380–387.
75. Coughlin, J., Hammond, S. K., and Gann, P. H. (1989). Development of epidemi-

ologic tools for measuring environmental tobacco smoke exposure. *Am. J. Epidemiol.* 130:696–704.
76. Cummings, K. M., Markello, S. J., Mahoney, M., Bhargawa, A. K., Mc Elroy, P. D., and Marshall, J. R. (1990). Measurement of current exposure to environmental tobacco smoke. *Arch. Environ. Health* 45:74–78.
77. Pron, G. E., Burch, D. J., Howe, G. R., and Miller, A. B. (1988). The reliability of passive smoking histories reported in a case-control study of lung cancer. *Am. J. Epidemiol.* 127:267–273.
78. Wald, N. J., Nanchahal, K., Thompson, S. G., and Cuckle, H. S. (1986). Does breathing other people's tobacco smoke cause lung cancer? *Br. Med. J.* 293:1217–1222.
79. Gann, P., Coghlin-Strom, J., and Hammond, K. (1988). Measurement of bias due to misclassification in epidemiologic studies of passive smoking. *Am. J. Epidemiol.* 128:920.
80. Lee, P. N. (1988). *Misclassification of Smoking Habits and Passive Smoking*. Berlin, Springer.
81. Bauman, K. E., Koch, G. G., Bryan, E. S., Haley, N. J., Downtown, M. I., and Orlandi, M. A. (1989). On the measurement of tobacco use by adolescents. *Am. J. Epidemiol.* 130:327–337.
82. Wells, A. J. (1990). Smoker misclassification does not account for observed passive smoking risk for lung cancer. Submission to indoor air quality and total human exposure committee science advisory board. Washington, D. C., United States Environmental Protection Agency.
83. Pershagen, G. (1984). Validity of questionnaire data on smoking and other exposures, with special reference to environmental tobacco smoke. *Eur. J. Resp. Dis.* 65:76–80.
84. Metzner, H. L., Lamphiear, D. E., Thompson, F. E., Oh, M. S., and Hawthorne, V. M. (1989). Comparison of surrogate and subject reports of dietary practices, smoking habits and weight among married couples in the Tecumseh diet methodology study. *J. Clin. Epidemiol.* 42:367–375.
85. U. S. Surgeon General (1990). The health benefits of smoking cessation. Washington, D. C., United States Department of Health and Human Services.
86. Koo, L. C., Ho, J. H. C., and Rylander, R. (1988). Life-history correlates of environmental tobacco smoke: A study on nonsmoking Hong Kong Chinese wives with smoking versus nonsmoking husbands. *Soc. Sci. Med.* 26:751–760.
87. Sidney, S., Caan, B. J., and Friedman, G. D. (1989). Dietary intake of carotene in nonsmokers with and without passive smoking at home. *Am. J. Epidemiol.* 129:1305–1309.
88. Darby, S. C., and Pike, M. C. (1988). Lung cancer and passive smoking: Predicted effects from a mathematical model for cigarette smoking and lung cancer. *Br. J. Cancer* 58:825–831.

6

Air Pollution and Lung Cancer

FRANK E. SPEIZER

Brigham and Women's Hospital and Harvard Medical School
Boston, Massachusetts

JONATHAN M. SAMET

University of New Mexico School of Medicine
and the New Mexico Tumor Registry
Albuquerque, New Mexico

I. Introduction

In the 1940s and 1950s, as the epidemic occurrence of lung cancer in males of Europe and the United States was recognized, suspect causal agents included not only tobacco smoking but also pollution of outdoor air by industry, vehicles, power plants, and residential fires (1,2). In many industrialized cities, air pollution was dramatically visible and associated with acute increases in numbers of deaths during episodes of high pollution (3,4). By midcentury, chemical carcinogenesis was well documented in animal models and by clinical and epidemiological observations. As outdoor air pollution worsened and lung cancer rates increased, it was plausible to postulate a causal link. However, as evidence accumulated on cigarette smoking as the predominant risk factor for lung cancer, air pollution was judged to have a small effect at most (5).

In the 1990s, although cigarette smoking is now established as the principal cause of lung cancer, concern remains that outdoor air pollution also contributes to the population's burden of lung cancer. Outdoor air has been shown to be contaminated by carcinogens emitted by industries, power plants, motor vehicles, and burning of coal and wood for space heating. The presence of carcinogens in outdoor air and the involuntary nature of the exposure sustained by the general population have kept the contribution of outdoor air pollution to lung cancer as a public health concern. In fact, the extent of lung cancer attributable to air pollution has been a subject of persistent controversy.

Continued uncertainty concerning the importance of outdoor air pollution as a cause of lung cancer largely reflects limitations of available epidemiological methodology. In most countries, nearly all cases of lung cancer are attributable to active cigarette smoking, and other causes, such as air pollution, cannot be adequately assessed without addressing confounding or effect modification by active smoking. Even passive smoking, now recognized as a cause of lung cancer in never smokers, should be considered as a potential confounding factor in addressing air pollution in never smokers (6). Under conditions of exposure found in most environments, the effect of outdoor air pollution on lung cancer risk is likely to be small in relation to that of tobacco smoking. Thus, it is difficult to design and carry out analytic epidemiological investigations, i.e., case-control and cohort studies, to detect the effect of outdoor air pollution on lung cancer risk.

Estimates of air pollution exposure are of necessity based on surrogate indexes for the actual carcinogens. Exposure misclassification is inevitable and made worse by the changing nature of air pollution over time and across the diverse locations in which subjects may reside. Furthermore, outdoor air pollution is a complex mixture, variable over time and regions; biologically significant interactions among the mixtures' components may occur. The investigation of air pollution and lung cancer is further complicated by the complexity of considering relevant occupational and lifestyle factors and of accurately assessing lifetime cigarette smoking.

This chapter provides a perspective on the association of air pollution with lung cancer, emphasizing more recent epidemiological studies and risk assessments. A recent monograph provides a more complete review (7), and several symposia have addressed this subject (8,9). Past reviews more extensively cover the earlier literature on air pollution and lung cancer (10–12).

II. Biological Plausibility

A. Descriptive Observations

Descriptive data on lung cancer rates provided initial support for the hypothesis that urban air pollution increased lung cancer risk (13,10,14). The relevant findings included higher rates of lung cancer in urban areas than in rural areas and sustained higher lung cancer rates in migrants from countries with higher pollution exposures and higher lung cancer risks to countries with lower pollution exposures and lower lung cancer risks.

Urban–rural gradients in lung cancer mortality rates were evident in data for the 1950s and 1960s from England and Wales, Scandinavian countries, and the

United States (10,14). The urban–rural gradients were as large as twofold but potentially attributable not only to an effect of air pollution but also to differences in cigarette smoking patterns of urban and rural dwellers. In several studies, the urban–rural gradients were found to persist even after stratification by intensity of cigarette smoking. For example, Stocks and Campbell (13) calculated smoking-specific lung cancer rates for rural areas near Liverpool and for Liverpool itself (Table 1). The rates were consistently higher in Liverpool in comparison with the rural areas within the smoking strata. These early studies comparing urban to rural gradients were likely to have been flawed, however, by not fully taking into account differences in the smoking patterns of urban and rural dwellers. Earlier in the century, urban dwellers probably started smoking at a younger age and smoked more cigarettes than rural dwellers (15). Doll and Peto (15) demonstrated that variation in age of starting to smoke has a major impact on lung cancer rates. Additionally, passive smoking, which was identified as a risk factor for lung cancer in the 1980s (6), was not considered in any of these analyses. Thus, urban–rural gradients in lung cancer cannot be attributed with certainty to air pollution exposure alone. A recent summary from several regions in Europe, Japan, and Australia (7), comparing lung cancer risks in urban and rural regions, showed urban–rural ratios above unity ranging up to 1.6 in men and to 1.9 in women (Table 2). Although smoking habits and occupational exposures were not taken into account in this summary, these 1980s data appear consistent and suggest that air pollution still warrants consideration as a lung cancer risk factor.

Support for a role of ambient air pollution as a risk factor for lung cancer was found in data from rural England in the demonstration of associations between surrogate measures of pollution exposure and lung cancer rates. For example, Curwen and colleagues (2) analyzed data from the 1940s for rural England and found that risk of lung cancer increased monotonically with increasing number of

Table 1 Lung Cancer Death Rates (per 100,000) for Men in Rural Areas and Liverpool, 1952–1954, by Age, Smoking, and Residence Location

	Age 45–54		Age 55–64		Age 65–74	
Smoking status	Rural	Liverpool	Rural	Liverpool	Rural	Liverpool
Nonsmokers	0	31	0	147	70	336
Pipe smokers	0	104	34	143	145	232
Cigarette smokers						
Light	69	112	70	378	154	592
Moderate	90	138	205	386	362	473
Heavy	117	205	626	543	506	588

Source: Ref. 13.

Table 2 Age-Standardized Rates per 100,000 Population for Mortality from Carcinoma of the Bronchus and Trachea in Urban and Rural Areas

	Males			Females		
Registry	Urban	Rural	Ratio	Urban	Rural	Ratio
Japan, Miyagi	30.9	28.4	1.1	9.2	8.1	1.1
Czechoslovakia, Slovakia	68.2	70.5	1.0	9.4	6.5	1.4
FRG, Saarland	77.7	63.0	1.2	7.7	6.0	1.3
France, Calvados	46.1	39.6	1.2	3.4	2.9	1.2
France, Doubs	56.9	40.1	1.4	3.3	2.0	1.7
Hungary, Szabolcs	61.8	50.9	1.2	10.3	6.2	1.7
Norway	39.4	24.5	1.6	9.6	5.2	1.9
Romania, Cluj County	35.2	35.3	1.0	6.7	4.7	1.4
Switzerland, Vaud	63.8	56.6	1.1	8.7	5.6	1.6
U.K., England and Wales	74.8	56.2	1.3	19.7	15.1	1.3
Australia, New South Wales	55.5	46.8	1.2	12.2	8.3	1.5

Source: Refs. 7, 16.

persons per acre, a surrogate for ambient smoke exposure (Fig. 1). Stocks (17) cited correlations of lung cancer rates with air pollution indices and with measures of fuel consumption. These associations also may have been confounded by cigarette smoking, however. Others have explained urban–rural gradients on the basis of smoking and occupational differences (18) or have been unable to find such differences (19).

Studies of population migration from high-exposure, high-risk countries to lower-exposure countries have been used to suggest a gradient of risk related to general environmental conditions including air pollutants (10,12). One early study, by Reid and colleagues (20), compared Norwegian and British migrants to the United States in the early 1960s with native-born U.S. residents and residents who did not migrate. Migrants were found to have lung cancer rates between the rates of the country of origin and those of native-born U.S. residents, whether the rates were higher (England and Wales) or lower (Norway) than the U.S. rates (Fig. 2). In these studies, potential confounding by cigarette smoking and occupational exposures could not be fully controlled; however, the hypothesis that migrants have lasting risk related to their country of origin, which reflects exposure to ambient air pollutants, was considered tenable in an earlier review of these data (21).

Additional evidence in support of an association of air pollution with lung cancer is provided by several occupational studies of workers exposed to combustion products from fossil fuels. Doll and colleagues (22) followed 3028 workers for 12 years and found that those exposed to emissions from retort coal gas plants

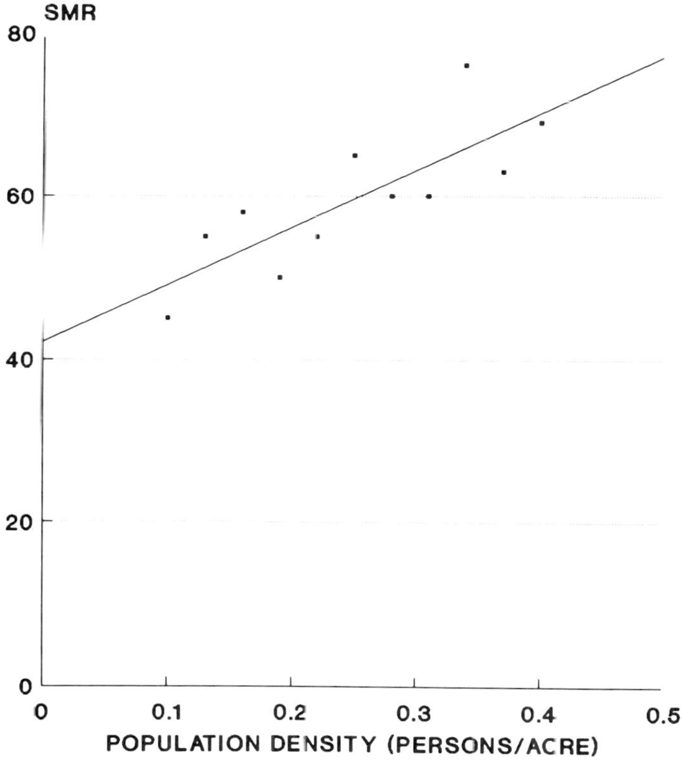

Figure 1 Cancer of the lung in males: Relation of the standard mortality ratio to population density in rural districts of England and Wales. (From Ref. 2, reprinted with permission.)

had a risk of lung cancer approximately twofold higher than in unexposed workers with similar smoking habits. Studies of coke oven workers in the steel industry of the United States workers showed a 2.5- to 10-fold higher risk among the most heavily exposed workers in comparison with unexposed workers (23). At lower levels of occupational exposure, excess lung cancer risk has not been so readily demonstrated. For example, roofers exposed to coal tar fumes while working primarily outdoors had an approximately 50% increase in lung cancer risk after 20 years of exposure and a 150% increase after 40 years (24).

B. Exposure Assessment

Combustion products, principally polycyclic hydrocarbons, have long been considered as the agents responsible for the carcinogenic potential of outdoor air pollution. Animal studies have documented the mutagenic or carcinogenic activ-

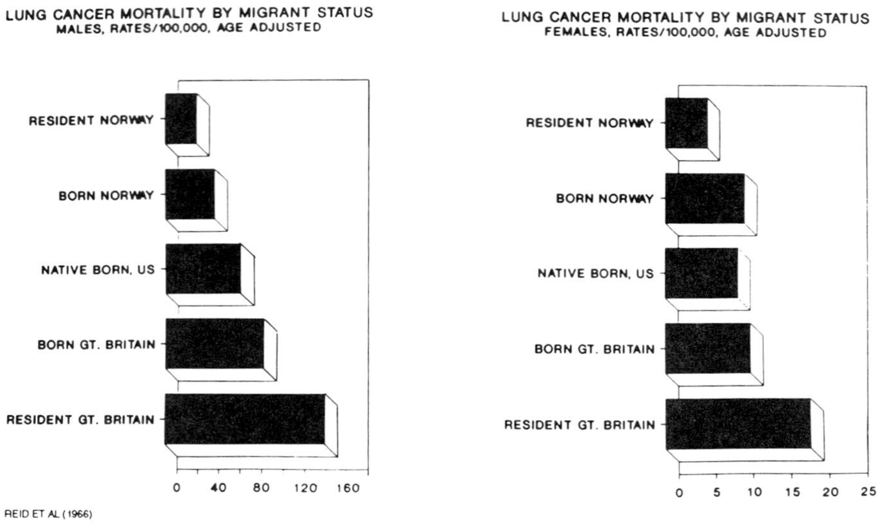

Figure 2 Lung cancer mortality rates, age-adjusted per 100,000, by migrant status. (From Table 13, Ref. 20.)

ity of many of the gases and the particles emitted by combustion processes (25). Known carcinogens can be found in the particles and gases emitted during the burning of fossil fuels. Benzo[*a*]pyrene, a carcinogenic polycyclic aromatic hydrocarbon, is often used as an index of carcinogenic activity produced by fossil fuel combustion. However, ambient air may be contaminated by elements and compounds considered to be carcinogens but not derived from the burning of fossil fuels (Table 3). Thus, three broad classes of putative carcinogenic agents present in ambient air as a result of either fossil fuel combustion or natural processes can be identified. The classes include specific inorganic elements resulting from the burning of coal or oil; radionuclides occurring naturally, from mining operations, or from combustion; and organic combustion products. Unfortunately, there are essentially no data from long-term ambient monitoring systems with which to document exposure to combustion products.

As indicated above, surrogate measures have been used, including estimates of population density and, where available, such measures as coal consumption, total particulate concentrations, measures of SO_2, and measures of vehicle density, which have been used to estimate exposure. In many regions, vehicle exhaust is a predominant source of ambient air pollution. Robertson (27) used motor vehicle registrations per square mile as a surrogate for city-to-city variation in air pollution exposure. In an analysis that used this exposure measure with

Table 3 Concentration of Selected Known Carcinogens in Urban and Rural Air

Substance	Range of concentration	
	Urban air	Rural air
Inorganic particles (ng/m³)		
Arsenic	2–130	<0.5–5
Asbestos	10–100	—
Beryllium	<0.2–8	—
Cadmium	4–250	—
Chromium	5–120	<1–10
Nickel	10–1000	<10
Uranium	0.01–2	—
Radionuclides (Ci/m³)		
^{210}Pb	$(1–30) \times 10^{-15}$	$(5.5–10) \times 10^{-15}$
^{212}Pb	$(0.1–4) \times 10^{-15}$	$(0.03–0.06) \times 10^{-15}$
^{226}Ra	$(50–100) \times 10^{-18}$	—
^{222}Rn	$(20–1000) \times 10^{-12}$	$(0.1–20) \times 10^{-12}$
^{228}Th	$(10–50) \times 10^{-18}$	—
^{230}Th	$(20–70) \times 10^{-18}$	—
^{232}Th	$(10–50) \times 10^{-18}$	—
^{234}U + ^{238}U	$(10–40) \times 10^{-17}$	—
Gaseous and particulate organic species (ng/m³)		
Dimethylnitrosamine	20–100	—
Benzene	5–90	—
Benzo[*a*]pyrene	1–50	—
1,2-Benzanthracene	1–70	—
Benzene-soluble organics	1000–20,000	200–300

Source: Ref. 26.

an 8- to 16-year lag and adjusted for other factors, Robertson found that the number of motor vehicles registered was a strong predictor of total age-adjusted cancer rates. Data on respiratory cancer were not reported separately.

For the volatile organic compounds, the Total Exposure Assessment Methodology (TEAM) Study conducted by the U. S. Environmental Protection Agency showed that emissions and personal exposure are not closely linked for many volatile organic compounds (28). For example, measurements of benzene exposure were made outdoors, indoors, and in the breathing zones of the subjects. For benzene, 83% of the emissions were estimated to come from motor vehicles, 14% from industrial activity, and only 3% from personal activities in the home including 0.1% from cigarettes. By contrast, estimates of exposures showed 51% from active smoking and another 5% from passive smoking. Exposures to motor accounted for approximately 20% of total exposure, personal home activities another 20%, and outdoor exposures from industrial sources accounted for only 3%. This analysis for benzene illustrates the potential for misclassification of exposure if there are significant sources of exposure to the air pollutant of concern other than outdoor air.

Other pollutants of concern for lung cancer originate from industrial sources, either as emissions from the factories or from user end products. Agents of concern include metals (e.g., arsenic, cadmium, and nickel), fibers (e.g., asbestos), and chemicals (e.g., bis-(chloromethyl) ether and formaldehyde). With the exception of formaldehyde, which can be found as a ubiquitous consequence of off-gassing from many consumer materials, and nickel, which is released in small quantities from fossil fuel combustion in stationary sources, these agents occur primarily in and around occupational settings. The work to date suggests that the bulk of the lung cancer risk from these agents (which is difficult to measure) is borne by workers in industries handling these materials and not by the populations in the surrounding communities.

C. Summary

Support for considering outdoor air pollution as a cause of lung cancer was originally derived from multiple lines of evidence. While both toxicological considerations and descriptive data on patterns of lung cancer occurrence support the hypothesis that outdoor air pollution causes lung cancer, numerous epidemiological studies conducted since the 1950s have established cigarette smoking as the cause of most cases and point to the need for consideration of cigarette smoking in assessing air pollution as a risk factor. Newer studies, designed with an understanding of the role of cigarette smoking, have more rigorously evaluated air pollution as a risk factor for lung cancer.

III. Recent Epidemiological Evidence

In this section, we review key epidemiological studies that have been performed on air pollution and lung cancer since the recognition that cigarette smoking causes most cases of lung cancer. Emphasis is placed on the more recent cohort and case-control studies that have collected information on cigarette smoking. We review the results of these studies on general outdoor air pollution, the epidemiological and toxicological evidence on diesel exhaust which emerged as a major concern during the 1970s, and the findings of studies on point sources of pollution within communities. Data on trends of lung cancer also have been considered; however, the difficulty of separating temporal effects of pollution from those of smoking render these data uninformative.

A. Cohort and Case-Control Studies

In cohort and case-control studies, information can be collected on cigarette smoking so that confounding by smoking or modification by smoking of the effect of air pollution on lung cancer risk can be addressed. In the studies reported to date, however, exposure has been estimated by surrogate indexes, supplemented in a few studies by some measurements of total particulate matter or concentrations of a carcinogenic component of the air pollution mixture.

Table 4 summarizes several cohort studies implemented during the 1950s and 1960s (15,29–34). The subjects were recruited as volunteers from special

Table 4 Cohort Studies of General Populations

Population/Dates	No. of lung cancers	Relative risk/comments	Ref.
187,783 white men from nine U.S. states, 1952–1955	448	RR = 1.3 for urban vs. rural, adjusted for age and smoking. Increases seen in both smokers and non smokers. Age started smoking not considered.	29
69,868 men in California, 1957–1962	304	RR = 1.3 for urban vs. rural counties, adjusted for smoking. Additive effect of smoking in urban area suggested	30
One million men and women in 25 U.S. states, 1959–1965	1510 (in men)	RR = 1.26 with exposure to dust and fumes and RR = 1.07 without for urban vs. rural, adjusted for age and smoking. No specific data for smoking groups.	31
25,444 men in Sweden with smoking habits known, 1963–1979	116 (to 1972)	Among smokers RR = 1.4 for urban vs. rural; RR = 1.1 for towns vs. rural. Two few cases among nonsmokers.	32,33
34,400 British male doctors, 1951–71	401	RR = 1.03 urban vs. rural, age and smoking adjusted. Lung cancers ratio urban vs. rural = 1.03. Smoking habits assessed in 1951. Smoking determined while in school; thus all urban, even though subsequently residing throughout country.	15
4,475 Finnish men, 1964–79	233	RR = 1.05 urban/urbanized vs. rural among smokers for lung and larynx. Non- and past smokers RR = 1.86 (NS).	34

groups or from the general population. Residence location at the time of recruitment was used as the index of pollution exposure in these studies, and smoking was controlled in estimating the effect of residence location. However, detailed smoking variables were not used, and age at start of smoking was not considered in any of the studies.

Case-control studies incorporating estimates of exposure based on measures of particulates, sulfur oxides, or benzo[*a*]pyrene and cigarette smoking provide inconsistent findings, with urban–rural differences affected by smoking status (13,18,35–41). Generally, the effects in nonsmokers give relative risks for urban compared with rural of 1.1–1.4, which in most studies were not significantly different from 1.0 (Table 5). In contrast, in smokers the urban effect appears to be more than additive. The relative risks, however, are below 1.8 (except for a recent study from China—see Table 5).

Diesel exhaust is a complex mixture that comprises particles in the respirable size range with various organic constituents having carcinogenic activity. Interest in diesel exhaust as a risk factor for lung cancer developed in part because of widespread use of diesel engines in automobiles during the 1980s. Data are available on lung cancer and diesel exhaust from both case-control (42–49) and cohort studies (50–60) of worker groups in the general population (Tables 6 and 7). Many of the studies are flawed by lack of specific exposure measures or data on smoking habits; however, the preponderance of the evidence was considered sufficient for the World Health Organization International Agency for Research on Cancer (IARC) to declare diesel engine exhaust a "probable carcinogen" (61). In most of the studies reviewed, occupational cohorts were assessed to make estimates that might be applicable to general populations. For example, Garshick and colleagues showed a modest 40% increase in lung cancer risk in railroad workers exposed to diesel exhaust. The excess was found both in a retrospective cohort of 55,000 workers traced between 1959 and 1980 (52) and in a case-control study of deaths occurring during 1981–82 (47). In the case-control study, smoking was controlled using next-of-kin reports of smoking habits.

The importance of this study was increased by the use of direct measures to estimate the diesel exhaust exposure that might have occurred during the working lives of the railroad workers. For workers aged less than 65 years, this estimation was possible because the conversion to diesel of the U.S. railroad industry only started in the early 1950s and was essentially completed by 1959. Thus, environmental and personal exposure measurements made in selected job categories in railroad yards that had not changed significantly in the last 30 years reflected the kinds of exposure these men had sustained over most of their working lives (62,63). Although absolute values of exposure have not been used in the analyses of lung cancer risks presented to date, the measured industrial hygiene data from selected worksites indicate a gradient of exposure that suggests the job categories used to characterize exposure groups were reasonable. Those workers, such as

Table 5 Case-Control Studies in General Population

Cases/Dates	Estimate of exposure	Relative risk	Comment	Ref.
725 male cases northern Wales and Liverpool, England. 12,000 hospital controls, 1952–1954	4–7-fold higher particulate and benz(*a*)pyrene urban vs. rural	RR = 1.1–3.4 in different smoking groups	Additive effect of smoking and urbanization association suggested	13
780–2873 men and 138–199 women northeastern England and northern Ireland, 1972	Urban areas defined as "high" some monthly averages of TSP exceeded 100 μg/m^3	RR, age and smoking adjusted—1.1–1.5 compared to living controls, urban vs. rural	Combined effect of urban and smoking more than additive	35,36
1425 males and 576 females in Los Angeles County, 1972–75	Benz(*a*)pyrene measured at 3 ng/m^3 higher (10–20 fold higher in past)	"High" RR fully explained by occupational exposures	No association with duration of residence in area	18
417 white male, hospital cases, Buffalo, NY, 1957–65	Two-year average TSP 200 μg/m^3 in heavily exposed area	RR in nonsmokers = 1.1; in smokers = 1.4 with more than 50 years in high area	Combined effect of smoking and exposure greater than additive	37
283 male, 139 female New Mexico cases, 1980–82	Urbanization defined as years in counties with >50,000 people	No consistent association with degree or duration of urbanization	Documents higher smoking amounts and rates in residents from urban areas	38
180 male, 79 female cases, Osaka, Japan, 1960–66	Two-fold higher particulate and 3-fold higher benz(*a*)pyrene in high vs. low regions	RR = 1.8 for men, 1.2 for women, adjusted for age and smoking; urban vs. rural	Increased risk seen primarily in smokers	39
910 male, 198 female Cracow, Poland, 1980–85	TSP and SO_2 both above 150 μg/m^3 compared to both below 104 μg/m^3	RR = 1.46 in men, 1.17 in women, adjusted for age, smoking and occupation. High vs. low regions. Significant in men only.	Effect more than additive to smoking and occupation	40
729 male, 520 female Shenyang, China, 1985–87	Reported "smokey" environments, coal burning stoves	RR = 2.3, adjusted for age, education and smoking. Highest vs. lowest exposure	Effect of indoor exposure higher in females (2.0) than males (1.3)	41

Table 6 Case-Control Studies Associating Lung Cancer and Potential Diesel Exhaust Exposure

Population/Dates	Exposure estimate	Risks	Comment	Ref.
10% random sample of U.S. cases 7,518 cases	Personal interviews	RR = lung Ca = 1.5 (not significant) in truck drivers	Adjusted for smoking. Relatively low compliance.	42
England ages <40, 598 cases and matched controls, 1975–79	Death certificate	RR* = 1.3 for all occupations with potential for diesel exposure	Short latency. No smoking data.	43
502 histologically confirmed cases and matched controls, U.S. hospitals, 1980–82	Personal interviews	RR, smoking adjusted 1.4 (not significant)	Smoking related cancers excluded from control group.	44
376 histologically confirmed cases and matched controls, Florence, Italy hospitals, 1981–83	Structural questionnaire	RR, smoking and age adjusted = 1.8	Ever vs. never in job with potential exposure.	45
604 cases from Swedish cancer registry died before 1979. Controls matched from death register plus matched living controls	Mailed questionnaire to surviving relatives and/or living controls	RR, smoking adjusted = 1.2 (not significant)	Results similar for dead or living controls	46
1256 cases in railroad workers and matched controls. Died 1981–82	Mailed questionnaire to surviving relatives	RR for 20 years exposure adjusted for smoking 1.4 in workers <65, 0.9 in older workers	Exposure determined by job codes. Older workers less exposed to diesel.	47
506 cases ages 25–84, New Mexico, and matched controls, 1980–82	Personal and next-of-kin interviews	RR = 0.6 (CI 0.2–1.6) adjusted for smoking, age and ethnic group	Less than 65, random telephone directory; over age 65, insurance claims.	48
1625 histologically confirmed cases and matched controls in men, France, 1976–80	Interviewing, questionnaire and hospital records	RR, adjusted for smoking, miners = 2.1; transport equipment operators = 1.4; motor vehicle operators = 1.4	No relationship to increased durations of exposure.	49

*Where no statement or confidence limit is given RR significantly different from 1.0.

Table 7 Cohort Studies of Diesel Exhaust Exposure and Lung Cancer

Population/Dates	No. of lung cancers	Relative risk/comments	Ref.
~38,000 railroad workers, 1953–58	154	No excess compared to national rates, little exposure to diesel. Smoking habits not considered	50
43,826 retired railroad workers, 1965–77	897	RR (compared to unexposed) for possible exp. = 1.2, probable exp. = 1.4. Controlled for asbestos and coal dust exposure, no information on smoking.	51
55,407 railroad workers age 40–64 in 1959 with 10+ years of service, 1959–80	1694	RR = 1.3–1.5 in age groups with longest exposure to diesel after 1959. Controlled for asbestos and welding. Smoking indirectly assessed.	52
~20,000 London transportation workers age 45–64, 1950–54	77	Overall no effect compared to SMR for England and Wales; no data on smoking.	53
~20,000 London transportation workers age 45–64 in 1949, 1949–74	667	Overall no excess when compared to general population; within five job categories highest SMR in highest exposure group.	54
8684 bus garage maintenance workers, 1967–75	205	SMR = 101 for lung cancer, 151 for leukemia, 121 for brain cancer, and 84 for all causes; none significant but follow-up time short.	55
694 bus company employees, 1951–83	195	SMR = 80 for all causes and 70 for cancer. No smoking history.	56
35,892 professional drivers, 1961–73	1143	RR lung cancers = 1.3. Smoking habits comparable to total population.	57
34,156 heavy construction vehicle operators, 1964–78	3345	SMR lung cancer = 99. Significant upward trend for lung cancers by duration in union.	58
6071 shipyard dockers, 1961–80	86	SMR = 89 for all causes and 132 for lung cancer. No smoking data.	59
3886 potash miners and millers (underground mines), 1940–67	433	No excess in mines using diesel.	60

*Total deaths.

engineers and brakemen, considered more likely to have higher exposures to diesel exhaust compared to clerks and conductors, did indeed have higher levels when personal and worksite monitoring was considered.

The epidemiological findings are supported by animal studies involving repeated long-term exposures to diesel exhaust; the studies demonstrate, in two different strains of rats, an increased incidence of both benign and malignant lung tumors that is related to dose. Similar studies in mice and hamsters have not shown such consistent results; some studies found excess adenocarcinomas and others showed no excess tumors beyond expectation from historical controls (61).

To summarize and evaluate evidence for carcinogenicity of air pollutants, Lewtas (64) used information compiled between 1987 and 1989 by the WHO IARC Working Groups. She points out that of the some 3000 chemicals identified in ambient air, only approximately 10% have been studied by experimental carcinogenic procedures. Many of the agents identified have been found to be carcinogenic in animals; however, for most of the chemicals and mixtures the data are inadequate in terms of both biochemical and animal studies. Furthermore, few of the identified agents have been studied in human populations, and a determination of human risk cannot be made. In addition, the fact that each agent is classified independently and most of these agents occur as complex mixtures, as well as the complex nature of the environments in which populations exist, make correct calculations of attribute risks to these complex mixtures almost impossible.

B. Use of Point Source Exposures or Clusters of Disease

Studies of populations living in the vicinity of point sources of industrial pollution emissions have been used to suggest the possibility of an association between ambient levels of these emissions and risk of lung cancer. Specific localized sources within communities frequently have been of concern. Such point sources are likely to be effluents from power plants or heavy industries. Examples include locations such as regions in the neighborhoods of petrochemical plants (65), arsenic-producing industries (66,67), and iron foundries (68). In addition, waste incinerators are likely to become increasingly prominent as community sources of airborne carcinogens (69,70). Emissions from many point sources are often known to contain carcinogens. Researchers may be challenged to quantitate the lung cancer risk associated with the point source or to assess clusters of lung cancer attributed to the point source (71).

Elliott and colleagues (70) describe an investigation of larynx and lung cancer near incinerators of waste solvents and oils in Great Britain. The investigation was initiated because of reports of a possible cluster of cases of laryngeal cancer near an incinerator. The investigators examined the relationship between proximity to the source and cancer incidence for the putative index incinerator and nine other incinerators. In an analysis based upon the Poisson distribution, the investigators found that the risk did not decrease with distance from the source for either cancer.

This investigation exemplifies the persistent problem of point sources of carcinogens in communities. Public concern is appropriate, but epidemiological methods may not be sufficiently sensitive to detect a potential important increased risk. Unless the exposed population is quite large, only unexpectedly high and possibly implausible increments in risk will be detectable. Clusters, apparently excess cases in a particular geographical region over a particular time interval, represent similarly difficult problems for epidemiologists. While often dramatically publicized concerns are raised by the media, clusters are infrequently linked to causal agents by simple (and often poorly conceived) retrospective epidemiological investigations.

Investigations around point sources are made difficult by population mobility and other problems in assigning exposure, by potential confounding, and by the possibility of selection bias. Population-exposure estimates based on residence location suffer from significant measurement error because mobility as persons move freely within and between communities may reduce presumed gradients of exposure. Selection bias would occur if mobility varied with susceptibility to the emitted pollutants; such a bias seems unlikely for lung cancer, a disease typically requiring lengthy exposure and lacking clear indicators of susceptibility. In addition to population mobility, exposure misclassification can be anticipated from the crudeness of exposure measures such as proximity to the point source, limited air monitoring data, and lack of insightful information on local micrometeorology. Confounding may arise from smoking or occupational factors, possible employment in the workforce at the point source, or other unmeasured factors that bring selected population groups into proximity to point sources.

Investigations of lung cancer around arsenic-emitting industries are illustrative. Arsenic, an established respiratory carcinogen, is emitted in the smelting of copper, lead, and zinc ores. Ecological studies have suggested increased lung cancer rates in areas around nonferrous smelters (66,72). However, these studies have been flawed by limited power and have proved uninformative when pooled.

Because of limitations of population exposure estimates, and other factors mentioned above, epidemiological methods may not be useful to quantitate the risks of point sources with sufficient certainty to exclude effects which may be of a magnitude that they have significant public health relevance.

IV. Quantitative Risk Assessment

For many of the reasons suggested above to be able to guide public health and regulatory policy, estimates have been made of the numbers of lung cancer cases attributable to outdoor air pollution. Such estimates can be made using a formal risk assessment approach, using a mathematical model to combine the distribution of exposures in the population of interest with a potency factor that describes the increase in risk with an increase in exposure. Estimates also have been based on critical, although less formal, analysis of the literature. These estimates of attributable risk from air pollution have varied widely, with earlier estimates in the 1950s suggesting upwards of 10% of all lung cancers to the most recent estimate by the U.S. Environmental Protection Agency (73) of less than 1% of all cancers (albeit most of these would be expected to be lung cancers).

However, all estimates in this field have been limited by a lack of population-based information on exposures and failure to control fully for possible important confounding from cigarette smoking and occupational exposures. It is unlikely that these limitations of epidemiological studies of outdoor air pollutants and lung cancer will ever be addressed to the satisfaction of all potential critics.

In summary, full understanding of the role of air pollution in the causal pathway of lung cancer cannot possibly come from analytic epidemiological studies alone. Most of the previous work can be considered as supporting or being consistent with a role for air pollution in the sense that these studies indicate a small but distinctly positive effect of general environmental exposures on lung cancer risk. The plausibility of this link is supported by mutagenic and carcinogenic testing in multiple species of specific compounds found in ambient environments, albeit at considerably higher doses. However, until biological markers of cumulative exposure to suspect environmental carcinogen are found, it appears to be futile to try further to quantitate the risk of lung cancer from ambient environmental agents through epidemiological studies alone. We do not conclude that epidemiological studies should not be done. However, the specific design of such studies should take into account the possible magnitude of the effect being sought and, when appropriate, should be planned to take advantage of possible higher exposures in subgroups. Methods for extrapolating from higher exposure to lower exposure may need further development. Further work also will be needed to develop more formal methods for combining data from toxicology, molecular biology, and other disciplines.

References

1. Doll, R., and Hill, A. B. (1950). Smoking and carcinoma of the lung: Preliminary report. *Br. Med. J.* 2:739–748.
2. Curwen, M. P., Kennaway, E. L., and Kennaway, N. M. (1954). The incidence of cancer of the lung and larynx in urban and rural districts. *Br. J. Cancer* 8:181–198.
3. Shy, C. M., Goldsmith, J. R., Hackney, J. D., Lebowitz, M. D., and Manzel, D. B. (1978). Health effects of air pollution. *Am. Thoracic Soc. News* 4:22–63.
4. Brimblecombe, P. (1987). *The Big Smoke: A History of Air Pollution in London Since Medieval Times*. London, Methuen & Co.

5. U.S. Department of Health, Education and Welfare. (1964). *Smoking and Health*: Report of the Advisory Committee to the Surgeon General of the Public Health Service. Washington, D.C., U.S. Government Printing Office.
6. U.S. Department of Health and Human Services. (1986). *The Health Consequences of Involuntary Smoking*: A Report of the Surgeon General. Washington, D.C., U.S. Government Printing Office.
7. Tomatis, L. (ed.) (1990). *Cancer: Causes, Occurrence and Control*. Lyon, WHO IARC Scientific Publication No. 100, p. 231.
8. Task Group (1978). Air pollution and cancer: Risk assessment methodology and epidemiological evidence. *Environ. Health Perspect.* 22:1–12.
9. Holmberg, B., and Ahlborg, U. (1983). Consensus report: Mutagenicity and carcinogenicity of car exhausts and coal combustion emissions. *Environ. Health Perspect.* 47:1–30.
10. Shy, C. (1976). Lung cancer and the urban environment; a review. In *Clinical Implications of Air Pollution Research*. Edited by A. J. Finkel and W. C. Duel. Acton, MA, Publishing Science Group, Inc., pp. 3–38.
11. Friberg, L., and Cederlof, R. (1978). Late effects of air pollution with special reference to lung cancer. *Environ. Health Perspect.* 22:45–66.
12. Winkelstein, W., Jr., and Levin, L. I. (1983). Air pollution and cancer. In *Reviews of Cancer Epidemiology*. Edited by A. M. Lilienfeld, New York, Elsevier, pp. 211–239.
13. Stocks, P., and Campbell, J. (1955). Lung cancer death rates among non smokers and pipe and cigarette smokers. *Br. Med. J.* 2:923–929.
14. Doll, R. (1978). Atmospheric pollution and lung cancer. *Environ. Health Perspect.* 22:23–31.
15. Doll, R., and Peto, R. (1981). The causes of cancer: Quantitative estimates of avoidable risks of cancer in the United States today. *JNCI* 66:1191–1308.
16. Muir, C., Waterhouse, J., Mack, T., Powell, J., and Whelan, S (eds.) (1987). *Cancer Incidence in Five Continents*, Vol. V. IARC Scientific Publication No. 88, Lyon, IARC.
17. Stocks, P. (1966). Recent epidemiological studies of lung cancers mortality in cigarette smoking and air pollution, with discussion of a new hypothesis of causation. *Br. J. Cancer* 20:595–623.
18. Pike, M. C., Jing, J. S., Rosario, I. P., Henderson, B. E., and Menck, H. R. (1979). Occupation: "Explanation" of an apparent air pollution related localized excess of lung cancer in Los Angeles County. In *Energy and Health*. Edited by N. Breslow and A. Whitemore. Philadelphia, SIAM, pp. 3–16.
19. Trichopoulos, D., Hatzakis, A., Wynder, E., Katsouyanni, K., and Kalandidi, A. (1987). Time trends of tobacco smoking, air pollution, and lung cancer in Athens. *Environ. Res.* 44:169–178.
20. Reid, D. D., Cornfield, J., Markush, R. E., Siegel, D., Pederson, E., and Haenszel, W. (1966). Studies of disease among migrants and native populations in Great Britain, Norway and the United States. III Prevalence of cardiorespiratory symptoms among migrants and native born in the United States. In *Epidemiological Study of Cancer and Other Chronic Diseases*. Edited by W. Haenszel. National Cancer Institute, Monograph 19, Bethesda, MD, National Cancer Institute, pp. 321–346.

21. Speizer, F. E. (1986). Overview of the risk of respiratory cancer from airborne contaminants. *Environ. Health Perspect.* 70:9–15.
22. Doll, R., Vessey, M. B., Beasley, R. W. R., Buckley, A. R., Fear, C. C., Fisher, R. E. W., Gammon, E. J., Gunn, W., Hughes, G. O., Lee, K., and Norman-Smith, B. (1972). Mortality of gas workers—final report of a prospective study. *Br. J. Ind. Med.* 29:394–406.
23. Redmond, C., Stobino, B. R., and Cypress, E. H. (1976). Cancer experience among coke byproducts workers. *Ann. N.Y. Acad. Sci.* 271:102–115.
24. Hammond, E. C., Selikoff, I. J., Lawther, P. L., and Seidman, H. (1976). Inhalation of benzpyrene and cancer in man. *Ann. N.Y. Acad. Sci.* 271:116–124.
25. Nesnow, S., and Lewtas, J. (1981). Mutagenic and carcinogenic potency of extracts of diesel and related environmental emissions: Summary and discussion of results. *Environ. Int.* 5:393–401.
26. Natusch, D. F. S. (1978). Potentially carcinogenic species emitted to the atmosphere by fossil-fueled power plants. *Environ. Health Perspect.* 22:79–90.
27. Robertson, L. S. (1980). Environmental correlates of intercity variation in age-adjusted cancer mortality rates. *Environ. Health Perspect.* 36:197–203.
28. Wallace, L. A. (1989). Major sources of benzene exposure. *Environ. Health Perspect.* 82:165–169.
29. Hammond, E. C., and Horn, D. (1958). Smoking and death rates—report on forty-four months of follow-up of 187,783 men. *JAMA* 166:1294–1308.
30. Buell, P., Dunn, J. E., and Breslow, L. (1967). Cancer of the lung and Los Angeles type air pollution. *Cancer* 20:2139–2147.
31. Hammond, E. C. (1972). Smoking habits and air pollution in relation to lung cancer. *Environmental Factors in Respiratory Disease*. Edited by D. H. K. Lee. New York, Academic Press, pp. 177–198.
32. Cederlof, R., Friberg, L., Hrubec, Z., and Lorich, U. (1975). The relationship of smoking and some social covariables to mortality and cancer morbidity. Stockholm, Karolinska Institutet.
33. Pershagen, G., and Simanato, L. (1991). Epidemiological evidence on air pollution and cancer. In *Air Pollution and Human Cancer*. Edited by L. Tomatis. pp. 63–74.
34. Tenkanen, L., and Teppo, L. (1987). Migration, marital status and smoking as risk determinants of cancer. *Scand. J. Soc. Med.* 15:67–72.
35. Dean, G. (1966). Lung cancer and bronchitis in Northern Ireland. *Br. Med. J.* 1: 1506–1514.
36. Dean, G., Lee, P. N., Todd, G. F., and Wicken, A. J. (1977,78). Report on a second retrospective mortality study in North-East England. Parts 1 and 2. London, Tobacco Research Council.
37. Vena, J. E. (1982). Air pollution as a risk factor in lung cancer. *Am. J. Epidemiol.* 116:42–56.
38. Samet, J. M., Humble, C. G., Skipper, B. E., and Pathak, D. R. (1987). History of residence and lung cancer risk in New Mexico. *Am. J. Epidemiol.* 125:800–811.
39. Hitosugi, M. (1968). Epidemiological study of lung cancer with special reference to the effect of air pollution and smoking habit. *Bull. Inst. Publ. Health* 17:236–255.
40. Jedrychowski, W., Becher, H., Wahrendorf, J., and Basa-Cierpialek, Z. (1990). A

case-control study of lung cancer with special reference to the effect of air pollution in Poland. *J. Epidemiol. Community Health* 44:114–120.
41. Xu, Z. Y., Blot, W. J., Xiao, H. P., Wu, A., Feng, Y. P., Stone, B. J., Sun, J., Ershow, A. G., Henderson, B. E., and Fraumeni, J. F. (1989). Smoking, air pollution, and the high rates of lung cancer in Shenyang, China. *JNCI* 81:1800–1806.
42. Williams, R. R., Stegens, N. L., and Goldsmith, J. R. (1977). Associations of cancer site and type with occupation and industry from the Third National Cancer Survey interview. *JNCI* 59:1147–1185.
43. Coggon, D., Pannett, B., and Acheson, E. D. (1984). Use of job-exposure matrix in an occupational analysis of lung and bladder cancers on the basis of death certificates. *JNCI* 72:61–65.
44. Hall, N. E. L., and Wynder, E. L. (1984). Diesel exhaust exposure and lung cancer: A case-control study. *Environ. Res.* 34:77–86.
45. Buitti, E., Kriebel, D., Geddes, M., Santucci, M., and Pucci, N. (1985). A case-control study of lung cancer in Florence, Italy. I. Occupational risk factors. *J. Epidemiol. Community Health* 39:244–250.
46. Damber, L. A., and Larsson, L. G. (1987). Occupation and male lung cancer: A case-control study in northern Sweden. *Br. J. Ind. Med.* 44:446–453.
47. Garshick, E., Schenker, M. B., Munoz, A., Segal, M., Smith, T. J., Woskie, S. R., Hammond, S. K., and Speizer, F. E. (1987). A case-control study of lung cancer and diesel exhaust exposure in railroad workers. *Am. Rev. Respir. Dis.* 135:1242–1248.
48. Lerchen, M. L., Wiggins, C. L., and Samet, J. M. (1987). Lung cancer and occupation in New Mexico. *JNCI* 79:639–645.
49. Benhamou, S., Benhamou, E., and Flamant, R. (1988). Occupational risk factors of lung cancer in a French case-control study. *Br. J. Ind. Med.* 45:231–233.
50. Kaplan, I. (1959). Relationship of noxious gases to carcinoma of the lung in railroad workers. *J. Am. Med. Assoc.* 171:97–101.
51. Howe, G. R., Fraser, D., Lindsay, J., Presnal, B., and Yu, S. Z. (1983). Cancer mortality (1965–77) in relation to diesel fume and coal exposure in a cohort of retired railway workers. *JNCI* 70:1015–1019.
52. Garshick, E., Schenker, M. B., Munoz, A., Segal, M., Smith, T. J., Woskie, S. R., Hammond, S. K., and Speizer, F. E. (1988). A retrospective cohort study of lung cancer and diesel exhaust exposure in railroad workers. *Am Rev. Respir. Dis.* 137: 820–825.
53. Raffle, P. A. B. (1957). The health of the worker. *Br. J. Ind. Med.* 14:73–80.
54. Waller, R. E. (1981). Trends in lung cancer in London in relation to exposure to diesel fumes. *Environ. Int.* 5:479–483.
55. Rushton, L., Alderson, M. R., and Nagarajah, C. R. (1983). Epidemiological survey of maintenance workers in London Transport executive bus garages and Chiswick works. *Br. J. Ind. Med.* 40:340–345.
56. Edling, C., Anjou, C. G., Axelson, O., and Kling, H. (1987). Mortality among personnel exposed to diesel exhaust. *Int. Arch. Occup. Environ. Health* 59:559–565.
57. Ahlberg, J., Ahlbom, A., Lipping, H., Norell, S., and Osterblom, L. (1981). Cancer among professional drivers—a problem-oriented register-based study (Swed.) *Lakartidningen* 78:1545–1546.

58. Wong, O., Morgan, R. W., Kheifets, L., Larson, S. R., and Whorton, M. D. (1985). Mortality among members of a heavy construction equipment operators union with potential exposure to diesel exhaust emissions. *Br. J. Ind. Med.* 42:435–448.
59. Gustafsson, L., Wall, S., Larsson, L. G., and Skog, B. (1986). Mortality and cancer incidence among Swedish dock workers—a retrospective cohort study. *Scand. J. Work Environ. Health* 12:22–26.
60. Waxweiler, R. J., Wagoner, J. K., and Archer, V. E. (1973). Mortality of potash workers. *J. Occup. Med.* 15:486–489.
61. WHO. (1989). Diesel and gasoline engine exhaust and some nitroarenes. IARC Monographs on the evaluation of carcinogenic risks to humans. Vol. 46, p. 143.
62. Woskie, S. R., Smith, T. J., Hammond, S. K., Schenker, M. B., Garshick, E., and Speizer, F. E. (1988). Estimation of the diesel exhaust exposures of railroad workers: II. National and historic exposures. *Am. J. Ind. Med.* 13:395–404.
63. Woskie, S. R., Smith, T. J., Hammond, S. K., Schenker, M. B., Garshick, E., and Speizer, F. E. (1988). Estimation of the diesel exhaust exposures of railroad workers: I. Current exposures. *Am. J. Ind. Med.* 13:381–394.
64. Lewtas, J. (1991). Experimental evidence for the carcinogenicity of air pollutants. In *Air Pollution and Human Cancer*. Edited by L. Tomatis. pp. 49–62.
65. Kaldor, M. S., Harris, J. A., Glazer, E., Glaser, S., Neutra, R., Mayberry, R., Nelson, V., Robinson, L., and Reeds, D. (1984). Statistical association between cancer incidence and major-cause mortality, and estimated residential exposure to air emissions from petroleum and chemical plants. *Environ. Health Perspect.* 54:319–332.
66. Blot, W. J., and Fraumeni, J. F. (1975). Arsenical air pollution and lung cancer. *Lancet* 2:142–144.
67. Hughes, J. P., Polissar, L., and VanBelle, G. (1988). Evaluation and synthesis of health effects studies of communities surrounding arsenic producing industries. 17: 407–413.
68. Smith, G. H., Williams. F. L. R., and Lloyd, O. L. (1987). Respiratory cancer and air pollution from iron foundries in a Scottish town: One epidemiological and environmental study. *Br. J. Ind. Med.* 44:795–802.
69. National Research Council (1991). *Environmental Epidemiology: Public Health and Hazardous Waste* Vol. 1. Washington, D.C., National Academy Press.
70. Elliott, P., Hill, M., Beresford, J., Kleinschmidt, I., Jolley, D., Pattenden, S., Rodrigues, L., Westlake, A., and Rose, G. (1992). Incidence of cancer of the larynx and lung near incinerators of waste solvents and oils in Great Britain. *Lancet* 339: 854–858.
71. Rothman, K. J., (1990). A sobering start for the cluster busters' conference. *Am. J. Epidemiol.* 132(Suppl. No. 1):5–13.
72. Pershagen, G. (1990). Air pollution and cancer. In *Complex Mixtures and Cancer Risk*, Edited by H. Vainio, M. Sorsa, and A. J. McMichael. Lyon, IARC, pp. 240–251.
73. U.S. EPA. (1990). Cancer risk from outdoor exposure to air toxics, Vol. 1, Final Report. Research Triangle Park, EPA-450/1-90-004a, pp. 1.1–1.6.

7

Indoor Air Pollution in Developing Countries

KIRK R. SMITH
East-West Center
Honolulu, Hawaii

YOUCHENG LIU
Harvard School of Public Health
Boston, Massachusetts

Air pollution in general and indoor air pollution in particular have long been considered to be associated with industrialization and urbanization and, thus, with the large cities of developed countries where most monitoring and control measures have focused. In recent years, however, the Global Environment Monitoring System program has demonstrated quite convincingly that the worst reported ambient conditions actually lie in the cities of developing countries (1). Similarly, although most studies of indoor air quality have been done in developed-country buildings, for many important pollutants the largest indoor pollutant concentrations and exposures again can be found in the developing countries in both rural and urban households (2).

Worldwide, there are four principal classes of indoor pollutants, derived from:

1. Combustion, e.g., carbon monoxide, aerosols, volatile organics, and sulfur and nitrogen oxides from cooking stoves, space heaters, and tobacco (environmental tobacco smoke [ETS]).
2. Building materials, furnishings, and chemical products, e.g., pesticides, volatile organic compounds, formaldehyde, asbestos.
3. Soil gas from ground under a building—radon.
4. Biological processes, e.g., mold, mildew, mites.

The first three of these classes contain known carcinogens that have been associated with human lung cancer (see Ref. 3).

As with outdoor emissions, the impact of indoor emissions on actual concentrations depends directly on mixing volume, i.e., the amount of air into which the pollution is mixed, and ventilation, the flow of air into and out of this volume. In general, most housing in developed countries lies in temperate latitudes and thus has relatively low air exchange rates, i.e., typically one air change per hour or less. Under these conditions, even rather low emission rates can result in indoor concentrations that exceed those outdoors, considering also that indoor air quality is affected by outdoor levels. Since people spend a great proportion of time indoors, typically 90% or more, indoor pollution often dominates total exposure to such pollutants as particulates and nitrogen dioxide.

Much housing in the developing world, however, lies in tropical and subtropical regions and typically has much more ventilation. In these circumstances, it takes fairly high emission rates to produce significant indoor pollutant levels. Unfortunately, there seem to be many situations in which such strong indoor sources exist. In addition, although a minority, there are still hundreds of millions of people in developing countries, the majority in China, who use solid fuels for space heating for a significant part of the year and, thus, share with developed countries the difficulty of making trade-offs among space-heating costs, fuel quality and efficiency, ventilation, and indoor air quality.

I. Indoor Sources

This chapter primarily focuses on the largest indoor sources of pollution in most developing countries—cooking and heating stoves—leaving aside ETS, asbestos, and radon, which are covered in other chapters, and such minor combustion sources as incense and mosquito coils.

After tobacco, the most common indoor pollution source of concern in developed-country studies has been gas cookstoves. In the global context, however, gas stoves are near the upper end of a historic evolution in the quality of household fuels, sometimes called the energy ladder (4). As illustrated in Figure 1, on the lowest rungs are those households that rely on dried animal dung and scavenged twigs and grass for cooking. The next step might be crop residues, followed by wood, and then charcoal. The first nonbiomass fuel on the ladder might be kerosene, as in India, or coal, as in China. Highest on the ladder lie bottled and piped gases and, for some rich communities, electricity. In general, each step involves increases in the cooking system's technology, cleanliness, efficiency, and up-front cost.

When learning to control fire, essentially all of humanity entered this ladder in the middle, with wood fuel. Now, many millennia later, fully half have moved

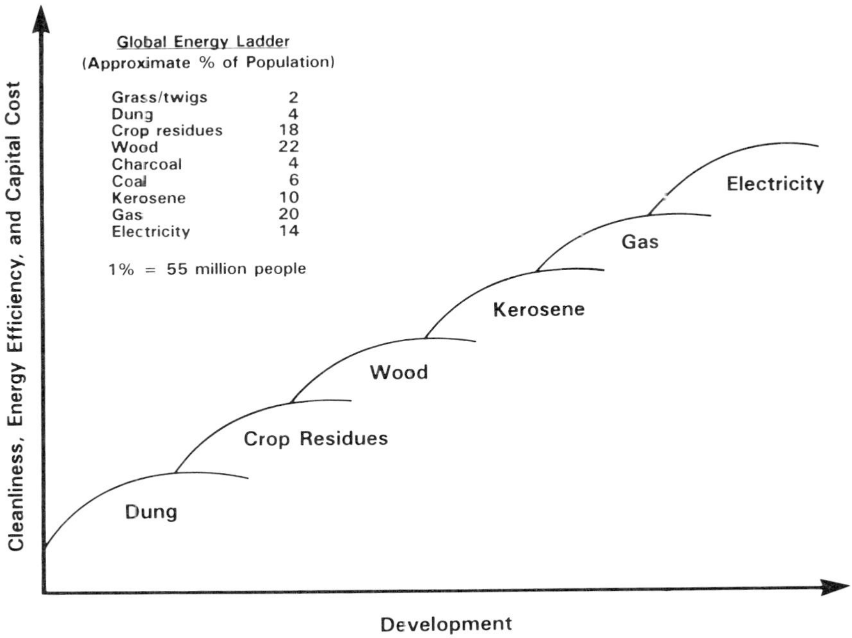

Figure 1 Shown here is a typical household energy ladder for South Asia. In other places, there may be variations, i.e., certain rungs shown here may be skipped and others added. For example, in Africa, charcoal use is significant, as is coal in China, where, by contrast, little kerosene is used. Listed are rough estimates by the authors of the percentage of the world's population at each major rung, including rungs not important in South Asia. Note that about half the population of the world uses unprocessed solid fuels, mostly biomass.

up the ladder to the modern fuels. The remainder, however, either still use wood or, for a significant fraction of humanity, have slipped down the ladder to the poorer-quality biomass fuels.

On a global scale, thus, somewhat more than half of the world's households cook daily with unprocessed solid fuels, i.e., biomass or coal. An unknown, but significant, proportion of this cooking is done under conditions releasing effluents into the living area. Although ventilation rates are often relatively high in the homes of developing countries, the pollutant emission factors for such fuels are so great that indoor concentrations and exposures can be quite substantial. Compared with gas stoves, for example, even stoves using one of the cleaner biofuels, wood, typically release 50 times more pollution during the cooking of a similar meal (5).

Although less prevalent, space heating with unprocessed solid fuels can also lead to high indoor air pollution levels. For part of the year in much of South Asia, for example, as well as in high-latitude or high-elevation parts of developing countries in all four major regions (Asia, Africa, Latin America, and Oceania), unvented space heating with biomass fuels is common. In addition, with or without venting, in much of temperate China, significant indoor concentrations result because of the high emission rates of coal fuels in simple cooking and heating stoves. Household coal use is increasing in other developing countries as well, particularly in Africa.

II. Pollutants

In spite of the long history of fascination with fire and hundreds of years of scientific investigations, we remain unable to predict the detailed behavior of combustion in any but the simplest configurations of fuel and air. Nevertheless, empirical evidence has shown that unprocessed solid fuels produce hundreds of chemical compounds because of the incomplete combustion that occurs under the operating conditions of simple stoves, which are often little more than a pit, three rocks, or a small open-ended box of clay. Both coal and biomass stoves pollute under these conditions, although the mix of compounds from each is significantly different. Unlike coal, biomass generally contains few inorganic contaminants, such as sulfur, trace metals, and ash, and, thus, can, under proper conditions, be burned with no releases other than the products of complete combustion, i.e., carbon dioxide and water. Unfortunately, it has turned out to be difficult to reliably create these needed combustion conditions in modestly priced household devices.

As with tobacco smoke, which is also the result of open biomass combustion, the smoke (here defined as total airborne effluent) from solid fuel combustion is a complicated and unstable mixture of aerosol (droplets and solid particles) and gases. Biomass smoke contains significant amounts of several of the health-relevant pollutants for which most countries have set standards: carbon monoxide, particulates, hydrocarbons, and, to a lesser extent, nitrogen oxides. More importantly, perhaps, the aerosol contains many organic compounds that are considered toxic, carcinogenic, or mutagenic, including formaldehyde, benzene, and polyaromatic hydrocarbons. Coal smoke contains all these and other pollutants because of fuel contaminants, e.g., sulfur oxides, inorganic ash particles, and toxic elements such as lead and fluorine. Table 1 lists some toxic organics typically found in wood smokes; however, it is difficult to make generalizations about the relative amounts of each pollutant because emissions can vary with small changes in fuel quality and configuration and other combustion characteristics (6). Comparatively little detailed research has focused on such variation.

The toxicologic characteristics of these emissions suggest potential links to four important categories of ill health: acute respiratory infections in children, adverse pregnancy outcomes, chronic lung diseases, and lung cancer (7–10). This chapter focuses only on the last of these.

Table 1 Toxic Organic Air Pollutants in Smoke from Wood Combustion

Pollutant	Category	Carcinogenic activity	Emission factor (mg/kg)	
			1 Stove	2 Fireplace
Acenaphthylene	1		64.0	10.2
Fluorine	1		20.0	4.7
Anthracene/phenanthrene	1		96.0	8.8
Phenol	1,3,4		100.0	20.0
Fluoranthene	1,4		22.0	1.6
Pyrene	1,4		19.0	1.6
Benz[*a*]anthracene	1,2	±	17.7	1.9
Chrysene	1,2	+	0.5	0.6
Benzofluoranthenes	1,2		13.5	1.9
Benzo[*b*]fluoranthene		++		
Benzo[*j*]fluoranthene		++		
Benzopyrenes	2		9.0	1.5
Benzo[*a*]pyrene (BaP)	1,2	+++	2.5	0.73
Indeno [1,2,3-*ed*]pyrene	1,2	+	2.0	
Benzo[*ghi*]perylene	1		5.9	1.4
Dibenzanthracene	1,2		1.0	0.18
Dibenz[*a,h*]anthracene	1,2	+++		
Dibenz[*a,c*]anthracene	2			
Ancenaphthene	1		6.4	0.12
Ethyl benzene	1		41.0	9.1
Phenanthrene	1		8.4	0.8
Dimethylbenzanthracene	2		2.5	
Benzo[*c*]phenanthrene	2	+++	2.5	8.0
Methylcholanthene	2			
3-Methylcholanthene	2	++++	0.5	
Dibenzopyrenes	2		0.7	0.4
Dibenzo[*a,l*]pyrene	2	high		
Dibenzo[*a,h*]pyrene	2	+++		
Dibenzo[*a,e*]pyrene	2	+++		
Dibenzocarbazoles	2			
Dibenzo[*a,g*]carbazole	2	±		
Dibenzo[*c,g*]carbazole	2	+++		
Dibenzo[*a,i*]carbazole	2	+		
Formaldehyde (HCHO)	3.2(?)	±	200.0	400.0
Propionaldehyde	3		200.0	
Acetaldehyde	3		100.0	
Isobutraldehyde	3		300.0	500.0
Cresols	3		200.0	60.0
Catechol	4		10.0	14.0

1 = Toxic chemicals categorized by USEPA as "priority pollutants."
2 = Carcinogenic compounds.
3 = Cilia-toxic and mucus-coagulating agents.
4 = Cancer-initiating, cancer-promoting, or co-carcinogenic compounds.
Source: Refs. 5,6.

III. Exposures

Although large-scale systematic measurement surveys have not yet been conducted, the results of a number of studies from different parts of the world provide some insight into typical indoor concentrations of the major pollutants produced by solid-fueled household stoves in developing countries. For illustration, Table 2 (biomass) and Tables 3 and 4 (coal) list the findings of studies of particle concentrations, either total or those in the size range that penetrate to the deep lung, the respirable fraction (11–15). Compared to national standards, World Health Organization (WHO) recommendations, or concentrations typical in even the dirtiest of cities, these indoor levels are dramatically elevated.

At this time, an accurate estimate of the total developing-country population exposed to "excessive" indoor concentrations cannot be made. We lack both internationally recognized standards for household concentrations as well as sufficient measurements. Assuming that such standards would be at least as stringent as outdoor standards, the total number of people exposed excessively indoors clearly rivals or exceeds that exposed to excessive ambient concentrations in all the world's cities (1), i.e., 0.5–1.5 billion. Given the greater time spent indoors and the known magnitude of concentrations in many situations, however, the contribution to the total global dose-equivalent (amount actually inhaled) from indoor combustion in developing countries is probably higher for some pollutants, e.g., particulates, than from any other source (2). Pinpointing the actual sources of exposure is further complicated in many urban and even some rural areas, by the contribution of outdoor sources to indoor levels.

Although an imperfect marker (16), the most common indicator for estimating the lung cancer risk of combustion-derived particles has been their content of one particular carcinogenic polyaromatic hydrocarbon (PAH), benzo[*a*]pyrene (BaP) (17). To convert the particulate concentrations in Tables 2–4 to equivalent BaP levels, the BaP/TSP ratio that has been measured in several developing-country situations for wood and coal can be applied to the total suspended particulate (TSP) concentrations (18–31). As shown in Table 5, typical BaP/particulate ratios for biomass smoke seem to be approximately 60–200 $\mu g/g$. For Chinese coal used in urban areas, BaP/particulate ratios measured in China range from 100 to 300 $\mu g/g$. With the particularly smoky coal used in some rural areas of China, to be further discussed below, the ratio may be about twice as large.

Homes where biomass is burned tend to have higher TSP levels than urban Chinese households using coal. These particles, however, tend to have a lower BaP content per unit mass than those from coal burning, leading to indoor BaP concentrations similar to those found in most coal-burning homes of China, i.e., concentrations from one to a few hundred ng/m^3. In the Chinese rural county, Xuan Wei, however, mean indoor BaP concentrations of 15,000 ng/m^3 were found in a small study of four homes using a particularly smoky coal for cooking on open pits (32). In urban China, in contrast, typical indoor BaP concentrations are 20–200 ng/m^3 (15). Levels are 50–100 times less in developed-country homes heated

Table 2 Indoor Air Pollution from Biofuel Combustion in Developing Countries

Location	Year	Description		n	Particulate concentration ($\mu g/m^3$)
A. KITCHEN AREA CONCENTRATION					
Papua New Guinea	1968	Overnight at floor level		9	200–4900
	1974	Overnight at sitting level		6	200–4900
Kenya	1971/2	Overnight	highlands	5	2700–7900
			lowlands	3	300–1500
	1988	24 h		64	1200–1900 (RSP)
India	1982	15 min cooking	wood	22	15,800
			dung	32	18,300
			charcoal	10	5500
	1988	Cooking (0.7 m to ceiling)		390	4000–21,000
Nepal	1986	Cooking—wood (geometric mean)		17	4700
China	1987	All day—wood		?	2600 (RSP)
The Gambia	1988	24 h		36	1000–2500 (RSP)
Zimbabwe	1990	2 h, during cooking[a]		40	1300 (RSP)
B. EXPOSURES DURING COOKING					
India	1983	4 villages		65	6800
	1987	8 villages[b]		165	3700
	1987	2 villages[b]		44	3600
	1988	5 villages		129	4700
	1991	3 villages	winter	95	6800
			summer		5400
			monsoon		4800
Nepal	1986	2 villages[b]		49	2000
	1990	1 village	before[c]	20	8200 (RSP)
			after	20	3000 (RSP)

RSP, respirable particulate fraction.

[a]Households with children having lower respiratory disease had 3.1 times higher concentration than those children having upper respiratory disease. Thirty-three of these households burned wood.

[b]Approximately half "improved cookstoves."

[c]Cooks' exposures measured before and after introduction of improved stoves.

Shown are the range of measurements for particulates in micrograms per cubic meter, the number of measurements (n), the country where the study took place, the year of publication, and a brief description. The studies are not completely comparable because of different measurement protocols and equipment but, nevertheless, are fairly consistent. Area concentrations are measured with stationary instruments placed indoors at breathing height. Exposure rates were measured with instruments worn by cooks during food preparation. For comparisons, the U.S. 24-h standard, not to be exceeded more than once per year, has been 260 $\mu g/m^3$ and the Japanese 1-h standard is 200 $\mu g/m^3$. Some of the studies listed here also measured other pollutants, including carbon monoxide and benzo[*a*]pyrene, which were sometimes found in concentrations well above those found in public settings in developed countries, as well as nitrogen and sulfur oxides and formaldehyde, which were found in concentrations roughly equal to the high end of those measured in indoor developed-country conditions.

Source: Refs. 11–14.

Table 3 Representative Indoor Concentrations of Particulates in Rural Chinese Households Using Coal

Location and publication year	Description	n	N#	Concentration (μg/m^3)
Huangxian				
Shandong	Brick bed (*kang*) used	—	—	618–948
(Suburb)	Arithmetic mean	—	—	490
Shanghai	CO, SO, NO also measured			
Xuan Wei	4 h/day, 2 days, 1.5 m		4	
Yunnan	from fire			
1987	High-vol sampler			24,400
	Med-vol sampler			25,800
Xinli Village				
Jilin	24 h, 5 months	38	20	1210–1650 (TSP)
1987	New and old houses			1040–1240 (PM10)
	Korean nationality			
Gansu				
1989	2 times/day, 3 days	—	4	1876–5117
	Room center, breathing zone (1.5 m)			
	Herders' houses			
	Animal dung also used in same village			
Inner Mongolia				
1990	2 times/day	—	12	500–1743 (TSP)
	Summer/winter			393–1559 (PM10)
Xiangshan				
Henan	3 times/day	—	40	340–1860
1990	1.5 h average			
	Unvented			
	Bedroom/kitchen connected			100–128

Values reproduced from original papers. In many cases, however, the degree of precision is substantially less than implied.
n, Number of data points; N#, number of households; PM10, particulate fraction under 10 μm in diameter.
Source: Ref. 15.

with solid fuels, and concentrations in ambient air are typically less than 1 ng/m^3 (33). For comparison, the annual ambient guideline in China and the former Soviet Union is 1 ng/m^3 (28).

Exposure to combustion-derived particulates can also be expressed as "cigarette equivalents," based on the relative amount of BaP inhaled (20 ng/cigarette) (34). At 300 ng/m^3, 3 h of cooking per day would produce BaP

Table 4 Representative Indoor Concentrations of Particulates Resulting in Urban Chinese Households Using Coal

Location and publication year	Description	*n*	N#	Concentration (μg/m³)
Hebei 1982	4 times/day, 1 day in summer 3 days in winter Stoves with/without flue and *kang* compared Housing type compared	—	00	501.1–1816
Hefei Anhui 1986	Standard sampling 2 months Kitchen/bedroom compared	29	5	480–550
Harbin Heilongjiang 1989	3 days continuous sampling 72 h average PM10	—	34	390–1030
Shanghai	1 time/day, 7 am–7 pm 3 cooking periods included 1 m from stove in kitchen No smoking when sampling Different ventilation compared	—	—	386–2831 (TSP) 337–2720 (PM10)
Anhui 1990	Stoves with flue compared with those without flue/bad ventilation Housing type considered 5 months	270	—	690–880
Shanghai, Wuhan Chengde, Shengyang	24 h, 2 days each home Dupont P-2500 sampler Summer/winter average No smoking during sampling	—	60	270 (bedroom) 1546 (classroom)
Lanzou Gansu 1991	Summer/winter 3 times/day, 5 days Average of 3 housing types	—	18	700–900

Values reproduced from original papers. In many cases, however, the degree of precision is substantially less than implied.

n, Number of data points; N#, number of households; PM10, particulate fraction under 10 μm in diameter.

Source: Ref. 15.

Table 5 Measured BaP/Particulate Ratios in Developing-Country Cookstove Emissions

Location	Sample no.—type	BaP/TSP ratio (μg/g) Mean of ratios (CV) or [ratio of means]	Ref.
BIOMASS			
Kenya	7—?	12 (1.2)	18
Gujarat, India	65—cooking (personal)	510–1000 (1.4)	19
Xuan Wei, China	?—breathing ht. (0.52–2 h)	[140, 225, 550]	20,21
Bhopal, India	70—ceiling	120 (0.81)	22
	58—breathing ht.	67 (1.5)	
	76—personal	39 (0.92)	
	(all cooking periods)		
Basse, The Gambia	32—breathing ht. (24 h)	120 (0.40)—BaP/IP	23
Maragua, Kenya	20—breathing ht. (24 h)	60 (0.83)—BaP/RSP	24,25
COAL			
Taiyuan, China	?—winter (kitchen)	[110]	26
	(bedroom)	[250]	
Jilin, China	4—old houses	[230]	27
	4—new houses	[280]	
Shanghai, China	24—winter	[27]	28
Guangzhou, China	21—5 days each season	[350]	29
Xuan Wei, China	?—?: Smoky coal	[450–510]	30
	Smokeless coal	[55–130]	
Xuan Wei, China	4—? Smoky coal	[600]	31
	Smokeless coal	[300]	

RSP, respirable suspended particulates; IP, inspired particulates.

exposures to the cooks equivalent to smoking about two (20-cigarette) packs per day. The 24-h indoor measurements in the two African studies listed in Table 2 imply that, on average, for every 3 h in the house, a person would be exposed to the BaP equivalent of one pack of cigarettes. A woman cooking and otherwise staying half the day in the house, therefore, might have a total daily BaP exposure roughly equivalent to five packs.

Caution is required, however, in interpreting this cigarette analogy. In particular, the comparison refers only to BaP, which is relatively more concentrated in wood smoke and coal smoke than in tobacco smoke—1.5 μg/g of particulates for ETS, according to the U.S. Surgeon General (34). If estimated by particulates alone, the cook experiences an exposure equivalent to only a few cigarettes per day (5), much lower than that of typical active smokers, but well above typical ETS exposures (35).

IV. Calculated Risks

Dose-response modeling can be used to estimate the potential lung cancer risks of indoor exposure to combustion emissions. The World Health Organization (17) has estimated the lifetime lung cancer risk of breathing 1.0 ng/m^3 BaP to be 9×10^{-5}. Using a linear dose-response assumption, adult women breathing at 350 ng/m^3 during 4 h of cooking with wood and 150 ng/m^3 for another 8 h per day have an equivalent annual exposure rate of 110 ng/m^3. This dose corresponds to a lifetime additional lung cancer risk of 1% or, by simply dividing by a 70-year lifetime, a gross annual mortality of 15/100,000. This estimate is substantially greater than observed lung cancer mortality for women in most rural areas of developing countries (36).

For women cooking with smoky coal in Xuan Wei, the exposure rate might be as much as 10 times greater (1100 ng/m^3) (see Table 7). The associated estimate of additional lifetime lung cancer risk is seemingly unrealistically high, i.e., 10%. Simply dividing by a 70-year life span, however, implies an annual mortality rate of about 150/100,000, a rate that has been observed in some areas of Xuan Wei.

Of course, comprehensive risk assessments require detailed understanding of exposures, which does not exist at present. Information is needed not only on indoor concentrations, but also on the activity patterns of householders, including time spent indoors and time spent cooking. Such data are scarce, but the additional research to gather them would benefit both developed and developing countries through better risk assessment capability.

V. Epidemiology

Although, by comparison to developed countries, the exposures received in many developing-country households are remarkably high, environmental epidemiological studies have been difficult because of the long latencies between dose and effect relevant to cancer, the complexity of the pollutant mixtures, the impossibility of estimating lifetime exposures, the apparent homogeneity of exposures in some areas, and the potential confounding by other risk factors, such as active and passive smoking and chronic and acute lung diseases. In addition, those regions with households lowest on the energy ladder tend not to have extensive medical and public health infrastructures, and thus the population's health is represented poorly in health records. Thus, few studies have been done in areas with biomass-using populations.

In China, however, where solid fuels are extensively used, medical records have been relatively well maintained for several decades, a combination leading to important research opportunities (37). In addition, a major effort was made in the

1970s to gather the data needed to produce the detailed Cancer Atlas of China (38). In recent years, therefore, there have been a number of studies of lung cancer directly focusing on Chinese coal-burning households. Even in China, however, relatively little effort has been directed toward biomass-using households, which still comprise the majority nationwide.

A. Cancer from Biomass Smoke

As indicated in Table 1, biomass smoke contains many chemicals known to cause cancer in laboratory animals and found in mixtures known to cause cancer in humans. In the early 1970s, based on a small study in Kenya (seven measurements of particulate and PAH levels in households of different elevations), it was proposed that nasopharyngeal cancer might be associated with biomass smoke (16,39). Kodama and Dollar (40) proposed a mechanism involving rapid dissolution of hygroscopic aerosols, including the nonrespirable fraction, in the upper respiratory tract. Later studies in Chinese populations of Malaysia (41) and Hong Kong (42), however, failed to confirm this association. Any effect of biomass smoke is now generally thought to be small compared to the effects of other factors such as diet.

Lung cancer, which, based on risk extrapolations from animal studies, might be expected to be prevalent in biomass-using areas, is relatively rare (43). Indeed, some of the lowest lung cancer rates in the world are found in rural nonsmoking women in developing countries. Not only are crude rates low, but so are age-adjusted rates, which control for the disparate age distribution of different countries. On the other hand, in many developing countries, the ratio of nonsmoking to smoking women among lung cancer cases is higher than for men (36), implying that smoking is a relatively less important risk factor for women.

A hospital-based case-control study in Osaka, Japan (44) compared 144 women lung-cancer patients (mean age of 60) with an unmatched group of 713 controls, both groups being nonsmokers, as shown in Table 6 (29,44–53). Logistic regression analysis was conducted to adjust for the differences in age distribution and education observed in the two groups. Although none of the patients or controls were still using biomass, those women who reported cooking with straw or wood fuel when they were 30 years old had an 80% increased chance of having lung cancer (odds ratio (OR) = 1.8{95% confidence interval: 1.1–2.9}). The increased risk based on cooking at age 15 was not significant, nor were the effects for use of different heating fuels, ETS during childhood, or presence of a smoking husband. An increase was noted, however, for presence of a nonhusband smoking householder (usually son or father).

The authors point out that it is important to allow for the long latency period of cancer in such studies. By classifying according to cooking fuel at a particular age (in this case, 30), they believe that an association was found that would have been obscured if classification had been based on "never-used" versus "ever-used."

In Harbin, China, where lung cancer rates were found to be rising (54), 55 women patients with adenocarcinoma of the lung were matched by age with 55 controls (51). Screening analysis found that cooking with biomass (wood, crop residues, and bark) was associated with an odds ratio of 2.4 compared to using gas. This risk, however, was not significant after using logistic regression to adjust for occupation, history of respiratory disease, and house characteristics. (As discussed below, coal use was associated with substantially higher risks.)

As shown in Table 6, no significant association was found between lung cancer and exposure to cooking fuel (kerosene, gas) smoke (43,55) in a Hong Kong case-control study of nonsmoking women. Similar negative results were reported by the same authors for ETS exposure (56) and incense burning (57). These authors have suggested that dietary differences may explain the observed variation in lung cancer rates among nonsmoking Chinese women of different ethnic groups (58).

A case-control study in Singapore found no association of lung cancer with various indicators of cooking exposure (including use of the fuels, wood, charcoal, gas, and kerosene), although the authors state that such an effect cannot be excluded because of the universal changes in cooking practices among cases and controls (59). Significant elevated risks for women were found for presence of a religious altar where incense was burned (OR = 1.5) and for burning of incense during sleep (OR = 4.1).

B. Coal Smoke and Lung Cancer

In contrast to biomass, there are a number of epidemiological investigations of the health impacts of cooking with coal in open stoves, all conducted in China and some published only in China, where coal use for cooking is common (60). A range of adverse effects have been found, including stroke, lowered lung function, fluorosis, and strong associations with lung cancer.

Ecologic Studies. A number of investigators have noted ecological associations between lung cancer rates and indicators of indoor coal smoke exposures in regions and cities of China. Xiao and Xu (61) analyzed women's lung cancer rates in 16 Chinese metropolitan cities with populations over 1 million in which the age-adjusted rate varied from 4.7–12.5 per 100,000 (national average was 3.2) and latitudes from 28.1–45.8, but with similar rates of smoking. The correlation coefficient ($r = 0.69$) between lung cancer mortality and latitude was statistically significant, with the positive correlation implying that higher latitudes were associated with higher cancer rates. For men, the correlation was smaller ($r = 0.17$) and not statistically significant. Neither gender showed a trend with latitude for bladder cancer. In addition, the men/women ratio declines with

Table 6 Summary of Epidemiological Studies of Lung Cancer from Indoor Air Pollution Due to Fuel Combustion

Study	Design	Exposure	Population
DEVELOPED COUNTRIES–CASE CONTROL			
Los Angeles, 1981–2; Wu et al., 1985 (45)	Case-control 149 adenocarcinomas Neighborhood controls Age-matched	Telephone interview about heating and cooking fuels ever used and childhood pneumonia	White women <76 born in N. America or Europe
Osaka, Japan, 1986–8; Sobue et al., 1990 (44)	Case-control $n = 144 + 713$ Nonsmokers Hospitalized controls	Reported cooking with biofuels at age 30	Adult women mean = 60 + 56
CHINA–ECOLOGIC			
Wuhan, 1983–4; Yang and Li, 1990 (46)	Cancer mortality in 170,000 people of 2 districts	One district—69% coal use; other—42%. Rest is gas SO_2, NO_x, CO	All deaths 1978–82
Guangzhou, 1976, 1989; Cai, 1990 (47)	Correlation Adjusted mortality of lung cancer/malignant carcinoma	SO_2, NO_x, CO, dust measured 4 districts	Residents
Benxi, 1988; Qu et al., 1990 (48)	Retrospective Follow-up $n = 101$ deaths in 100,000 people	Living in areas heavy polluted (coal); slightly polluted (gas); control (village-biomass) PAH, SO_2, CO, NO_x Indoor/outdoor	All deaths 1977–81
CHINA–CASE CONTROL			
Shanghai, 1984–6; Gao et al., 1987 (49)	Case-control $n = 672 + 735$ Matching by age across city	Current cook fuel use Frequency of rapeseed oil use	Adult women

Outcome	OR (95% confidence interval)	Remarks
Diagnosis microscopically (incidence)	[a]Childhood coal burning 2.3 (1.0–5.5) Childhood pneumonia 2.7 (1.1–6.7)	Adjusted for smoking. Multiple regression analysis did not change results much. PAR of childhood lung disease and coal smoke: 22%. Squamous cell carcinoma explained by smoking.
Hospitalized confirmed by biopsy (incidence)	1.8 (1.1–2.9)	Adjusted for age and education. Logistic regression with ETS. No effect at age 15.
National disease surveillance (deaths)	26—high coal use; 12—low coal use (per 100,000)	80 homes chosen randomly for monitoring, 2 seasons, indoor/outdoor, coal/gas.
Respiratory immunological (deaths)	MC/SO_2:r = 0.88+ MC/NO_x:r = 0.31 MC/CO:r = 0.34 MC/TSP:r = 0.56 LC/SO_2:r = 0.77 LC/NO_x:r = 0.34 LC/CO:r = 0.10 LC/TSP:r = 0.39	MC: malignant carcinoma LC: lung cancer Mortality data from 1976 Pollution data from 1989 "+" = significant
90% diagnosed by pathology and x-ray. No diagnosis after death (deaths)	SMR: 9.5,5.6—heavy 6.4, 3.9—slight 2.7, 1.6—control (adjusted to national, provincial age distributions)	5 day indoor/outdoor monitoring in 3 seasons. BaP ng/m^3 heavy: 114/173; slight: 43/33; control: 33/9.3
Hospitalized w/ biopsy and x-ray (incidence)	[a]Coal—0.9 Wood—1.0 Rapeseed—1.4 (1.1–1.8)	Adjusted for age, education, and smoking. No trend with years of coal use. Significant OR[a] with reported smokiness (1.6 {1–2.5}) and eye irritation (1.6 {1.2–2.1}).

Table 6 Continued

Study	Design	Exposure	Population
Shenyang, 1985–7; Xu et al., 1989 (50)	Case-control $n = 1249 + 1345$ Age and gender matched controls across city	Years of *kang* use Years w/*kang*, place of cookstove indoor pollution index (IAPI), smokiness	Adults Men median—59 Women—56
Harbin, 1985–9; Wang et al., 1989 (51)	Case-control $n = 55 + 55$ Matched by age and gender	Coal, biofuels Winter indoor smoke pollution (WISP) 10 y of residence Coal consumption index (CCI) TSP, BaP, IP Indoor cooking	Adult women
Shenyang and Harbin, 1985–7; Wu-Williams et al., 1990 (52)	Case-control $n = 965 + 959$ Matching by age across cities	Years of *kang* use; coal heated wall/floor; frequency deep frying; eye irritation	Adult women, includes group in Xu et al., 1989 (50)
Guangzhou, 1985; Du and Ou, 1990 (29)	Case-control $n = 662 + 662$ Matched by age, gender, and street	Coal briquette or gas in cookstove BaP in urine TSP, BaP, SO_2, NO_x, radon, thoron	Deaths
Xuan Wei, 1985–6; Liu et al., 1991 (53)	Case-control $n = 110 + 426$ Matched by age, gender, and village Controls effectively matched by fuel and house type	Years of cooking For men, frequency of cooking. For both, chronic bronchitis (CB).	Adults Mean: 50 y
Shunyi County, 1989; Liu and Hu, 1991 (unpublished)	Case-control $n = 220 + 440$ Controls matched by age, gender, and village	Use of coal cakes for cooking and heating—no flues.	Farmer deaths 1981–86

Outcome	OR (95% confidence interval)	Remarks
Hospitalized confirmed by biopsy (incidence)	[a]20+ years *kang* use—2.1–2.2; 50+ years *kang*—3.4, women; 30+ years bedroom—2.1–7.8 (men-women); IAPI and reported smokiness significant	Adjusted for smoking, age, education, indoor pollution index, etc. PAR of IAQ—men, 13%; women, 17%. Smoking—55% + 37%.
Hospitalized adenocarcinoma (incidence)	CCI: 6.2 (2.1–18) WISP: 3.4 (1.2–12) Low ceilings: 4.3 (1.0–18)	Mantel-Haenzel used for screening Logistic regression Biofuel: 2.4 (0.9–6.4) Smoking: no significance TSP: 0.57 mg/m^3 BaP:27 ng/m^3
Hospitalized confirmed by biopsy (incidence)	[a]21+ y *kang* use—1.5 (1.1–2.0) 1–20 y coal heat—1.5 (1.1–2.1) 21+ y coal heat—1.4 (1.1–1.9) Deep fry—2.0 (1.4–2.8) Eye irritation—1.7 (1.2–2.6)	Adjusted for age, smoking, and education. Increasing trend with frequency of deep frying.
Hospital records (deaths)	5.8 for women smokers 3.1 for nonsmokers with n = 21	Mantel-Haenzel test used. No adjustment information given BaP ng/m^3 coal: 120; LPG: 22.
17% diagnosed by pathology; 83% by x-ray. Follow-up done (incidence)	Women: CB: 7.4 (2.4–22.4) Year 31–44: 9.2 (1.8–47) 45 + 4.7 (1.6–134) Men: CB: 7.3 (2.7–20) Freq: 3.4 (1.3–8.9)	Mantel-Haenzel analysis followed by logistic regression. Smoking risks unusually low.
Reconfirm diagnosis (deaths)	2.0 (1.2–3.4)	Men/women lung cancer rate—1.65; PAR smoking = men, 99.6%; women, 39%. Analysis adjusted for smoking. Logistic regression employed.

OR, odds ratio.

[a]These were reported as "Relative Risks" by the original authors.

latitude, reaching levels as low as anywhere else in the world—1.5 or less. (They found similar relationships, e.g., $r = 0.75$ for women's lung cancer, for another group of 10 cities of populations between 500,000 and 1 million.) Overall, women had a much higher proportion of adenocarcinoma than men.

There were no significant relationships, however, between several measures of ambient air pollution and total age-adjusted lung cancer rates among these cities, although within the city of Shenyang there was a significant relationship ($r = 0.79$) among age-adjusted 1976–78 lung cancer rates and 1972–73 ambient particulate concentrations in seven communes (sections of the city). A similar relationship ($r = 0.81$) was also found between these cancer rates and 1955–57 dustfalls measured in 12 Shenyang communes.

Among other possibilities (smoking, diet, respiratory infections, outdoor air pollution), the authors point out that the latitudinal, gender, and cancer-site patterns in China are most consistent with indoor air pollution from coal heating as a risk factor (62). Yang and colleagues compared various factors in the high and low lung cancer mortality regions (26 vs. 12 per 100,000) in Wuhan city to find that there were significant differences in stove types (coal vs. gas fuel), house density, and indoor sulfur dioxide and nitrogen oxides, but not for carbon monoxide (46,63).

Measured indoor and outdoor CO, SO_2, TSP, and NO_x levels in four homes in each of four districts in Guangzhou in 1989 were compared with 1976 cancer mortality rates (47). As shown in Table 6, a significant correlation was found only with total cancer and SO_2. No significant correlations were found for lung cancer mortality alone. Compared with those using coal, homes with gas stoves had significantly lower concentrations of all pollutants except NO_x.

In the northeastern city Benxi, Qu et al. (48) monitored indoor and outdoor pollution in three seasons in three residential districts: heavily polluted where coal was the principal household fuel, lightly polluted where gas was used, and a "control" district outside the city where biomass was used. They found significant differences in the levels of various polyaromatic hydrocarbons, such as particulate BaP, generally in the pattern coal > biomass > gas. A similar pattern was found for indoor levels of CO, but not for NO_x, or, consistently, with SO_2. Based on standardized mortality ratios (SMRs) adjusted either for the national or provincial age distributions, however, lung cancer mortality was found to vary in the pattern coal > gas > biomass (see Table 6). This would seem to show that simple (unadjusted for time and activity) BaP concentration is not a good indicator for lung cancer. Unfortunately, particulate concentrations themselves were not given.

In Xuan Wei, the rural county in Yunnan Province (southern China) mentioned above, the annual age-adjusted (China's 1964 age distribution) lung cancer mortality rate in 1973–1979 was 28/100,000 for men and 25/100,000 for women, about three and eight times higher, respectively, than the China averages (64). Lung cancer mortality rates were much greater in some districts (communes) of the county, however, the highest being more than 150/100,000, while the lowest was less than 1, a difference of about a factor of 200. Until the 1980s, high-tar bituminous coal burned in open pits was the main cooking and heating arrangement in the high-mortality districts, while "smokeless" coal, usually with a clay binder, and wood were used in low-mortality regions (65).*

The rate of lung cancer mortality in farmers was higher than those in other occupations, and there was little difference between sexes. Indeed, in at least one district, women had a higher rate of lung cancer than men, in spite of sharing in the overall low smoking rate for women in rural China. This pattern suggests a strong nonoccupational carcinogenic factor affecting women (66). Ongoing research involving indoor air monitoring, epidemiological studies, and animal exposure tests on- and off-site is being conducted by the Chinese Academy of Preventive Medical Sciences and local public health and antiepidemic stations with assistance from the U.S. Environmental Protection Agency (20,64,67).

A pilot measurement program revealed extremely high pollution concentrations in Xuan Wei homes using either coal or biomass, although coal particulate levels were generally higher (see Tables 2–4). The data indicate a strong correlation of fuel type used in the past with lung cancer mortality rates in the 1970s, e.g., $r = 0.82$ for gross rates and the percent of households using smoky coal. This implies that risk may be adequately indicated by such relatively gross measures as particulate concentration. The plausibility of this association is supported by laboratory data showing mutagenicity per gram of particulates to be similar for emissions from the three major fuels—smoky coal, wood, smokeless coal (68).

In contrast, mouse skin tumorigenicity seems to be much stronger in extracts from the coal smoke (31). Another characteristic of the Xuan Wei studies, however, is the difficulty of comparing the results of one paper with another because denominators were not used consistently. In Mumford et al. (31), for example, PAH yields are reported in terms of extracted organics from particulates and in terms of air volume, but not in terms of suspended particulate mass, which is the usual air pollution measure. Not given also are the percentages of particulate mass that have been extracted so that the reader can do the conversion.†

Where differences in air concentrations and mutagenic character do not

---

*The available English literature about Xuan Wei is also not clear about the history of fuels used in the households, e.g., the extent, timing, and effectiveness of interventions taken to reduce excessive exposures.

†In other papers (e.g., Ref. 21) there are values for particulate mass, but it is unclear if the same data set is being used. It is often also unclear how the houses used for pollution monitoring were chosen and thus how well they represent the conditions under which the population was exposed. There is also some confusion because some of the Xuan Wei papers use gross and others use age-adjusted cancer rates. In addition, some apply linear and some apply log-linear regression. (Changes in approach are inevitable in an ongoing research program, of course, but it would be useful to the reader if there were clearer connections made between the results published in different papers.)

seem to explain observed lung cancer rates, the investigators reason that the differences observed are due to different size distributions of the particles from coal and wood burning. They argue that those from wood combustion are significantly larger and thus do not deposit as much in the deep lung (21). This hypothesis seems to be based on only a few electron microscope photos, however (64), and is quite at variance with the existing literature on wood smoke particle size distributions (see Refs. 69,70). The physiological justification for this explanation is also questionable, since most lung cancers start in the proximal airways.

Analysis at the district level shows a strong correlation ($r = 0.78, p < 0.01$) between indoor particulate BaP concentrations due to each fuel as measured today (400–2500 ng/m^3)—weighted by the estimated fraction of homes using each fuel before 1958—and compared to the 1973–79 district-specific mortality rates for lung cancer (71). These data are summarized in Table 7.

There are anomalies, however, that have not yet been explained, but that may be associated with differences in coal quality coming from the small local mines (67). In Bao Shan District, for example, high indoor concentrations must have existed in the past as they did in other districts using predominantly smoky coal (see Table 7). Nevertheless, this area has a low lung cancer mortality, 9.2/100,000, compared to more than 100/100,000 in some other smoky coal districts (68). To

Table 7 Percentage of Households Burning Fuel Before 1958, BaP Concentration in Indoor Air, and 1973–1979 Age-Adjusted Lung Cancer Mortality per 100,000 in 11 Xuan Wei Communes

Commune	Smoky coal (%)	Wood (%)	Smokeless coal (%)	BaP (ng/m^3)	Mortality rate
Chengguan	100.0	0.0	0.0	1090	174
Laibin	89.7	8.7	1.6	680	128
Roncheng	81.9	18.1	0.0	2490	104
Longtan	78.0	22.0	0.0	560	23.0
Longchang	76.1	17.9	6.0	1080	39.4
Banqiao	34.0	16.4	49.6	400	19.0
Baoshan	87.1	12.9	0.0	464	9.18
Haidai	49.7	22.5	27.8	539	13.4
Puli	35.2	52.0	12.8	286	7.49
Luoshui	2.7	39.0	58.3	438	9.55
Reshui	0.0	66.6	33.4	356	2.08

Particulate BaP concentration based on recent indoor measurements during burning, weighted by the duration of burning at each time of day for each fuel, and then weighted by the estimated percentage of households using each fuel before 1958. No modification for seasonal variation or time-activity patterns of the householders.
Source: Ref. 71.

date, the investigators have not been able to definitively identify any chemical or physical features of the several different kinds of local smoky coals that would help explain this discrepancy.

One possibility currently under investigation is that the emissions may be less carcinogenic if the coal is mixed with binder, as may have been more common in the past in Bao Shan (72). Another possibility is proffered by Zhou et al. (73), who provide evidence that the carcinogenic effect of the coal smoke may be more closely related to the number of free radicals than to the total PAH or BaP. Still another is an association of higher risk with the amount of three- to four-ring alkylated PAH (74).

Case-Control Studies. As shown in Table 6, there have been several hospital-based case-control studies of lung cancer and indoor coal smoke in China. A study of 672 women lung cancer patients and 735 population-based controls in Shanghai confirmed smoking to be an important risk factor, but much less so for adenocarcinoma (75). At 20 per 100,000, the age-adjusted women's lung cancer incidence rate is one of the highest in the world, but only 6% (population attributable risk {95% confidence interval: 0–12%}) of the adenocarcinoma, which accounted for 61% of the cases, could be attributed to smoking. Adjusted for smoking, age, and education, Gao et al. (49) also found a significant odds ratio (1.4 {1.1–1.8}) according to the frequency of using rapeseed oil in cooking. Independent association was also found for reported eye irritation during cooking, reported smoky conditions, and for the number of dishes prepared per week. No significant odds ratios were associated with type of cooking fuel, although the extent of information obtained on cooking histories is unclear. No differences were found in these factors based on type of carcinoma. The possibility that cooking with rapeseed oil is a cause of lung cancer is supported by studies that show mutagenicity of the condensed volatiles resulting from heating of rapeseed but not soybean oil (76).

Xu et al. (50) interviewed 1249 lung cancer patients and 1345 population-based controls in Shenyang. Smoking was found to account for about 55% of lung cancer in men, but only 37% in women. Calculated odds ratios, as shown in Table 8, were adjusted for age, education, and smoking. Significantly elevated risks in men and women were found according to the number of years people had lived in the presence of and had used the coal *kang* (heated bed) and, for women, whether they had lived for more than 30 years in homes where the cookstove was in the bedroom. An elevated risk was also found for men living more than 20 years in a household having a coal-fired radiator/heating system extending to more than one room. Risks decreased, but not significantly, as use of gas for cooking or heating increased. The simple presence of a standing coal stove was not associated with changes in risk.

The authors propose an "overall indoor air pollution index," based on three indicators: coal central heating, coal cooking fuel, and location of cookstove. As

Table 8 Odds Ratios of Lung Cancer According to Home Heating and Cooking Characteristics in Shenyang, Adjusted for Age, Education, and Smoking

		Odds ratio	
	Years of use	Men	Women
Heating method			
Kang (coal)	0	1.0	1.0
	1–39	0.8	2.4
	40–49	0.9	1.9
	50+	1.0	3.4*
Burning *kang*	0	1.0	1.0
	1–19	1.7*	1.3
	20+	2.1	2.3*
Single standing coal stove	0	1.0	1.0
	1–39	0.8	0.9
	40–49	1.0	0.9
	50+	1.0	1.2
Coal stove with pipes extending to other rooms	0	1.0	1.0
	1–19	1.1	1.4
	20+	2.3*	1.5
Central heating (gas)	0	1.0	1.0
	1–9	1.1	0.8
	10–29	0.7	0.7
	30+	0.8	0.8
Cooking method and location			
Gas fuel	0	1.0	1.0
	1–9	1.2	0.9
	10+	2.1*	0.8
Cooking place in bedroom	0	1.0	1.0
	1–29	1.2	1.5
	30+	2.1*	1.8*

*$p < 0.05$.
Source: Ref. 50.

shown in Table 9, increasing odds ratios were associated with nearly every increase in the index for both men and women, particularly for squamous cell carcinoma. Overall, the indoor air pollution index accounted for 13% and 17% of the lung cancer in men and women, respectively. Like smoking, indoor air pollution seemed to account for less adenocarcinoma than squamous cell carcinoma: the population attributable risk was 16% compared to 12% for women; 18% compared to 7% for men (neither significant). Unfortunately, the index did not take

Table 9 Odds Ratio (OR) and Confidence Interval (CI) for Lung Cancer According to Index of Indoor Air Pollution Exposure in Shenyang, Adjusted by Age, Education, and Smoking

Air pollution index[a]	All cell types		Squamous cell/ Oat cell carcinoma	
	OR	95% CI	OR	95% CI
		Men		
0–0.9	1.0	—	1.0	—
1.0–1.4	1.1	0.8–1.4	1.3	0.9–1.7
1.5–1.9	1.2	0.9–1.6	1.5	1.0–2.0
2.0+	1.6	1.1–2.3	1.9	1.0–2.6
		Women		
0–0.9	1.0	—	1.0	—
1.0–1.4	1.2	0.9–1.6	1.1	0.7–1.7
1.5–1.9	1.3	0.9–1.9	1.2	0.7–2.0
2.0+	1.5	1.0–2.4	2.0	1.1–3.6

[a]Air pollution index based on the sum of three factors: existence of coal-based room or central (noncoal) heating (1 or 0); cooking fuel is gas (0), only summer is gas (0.5), coal (1); cooking place is kitchen (0), in bedroom during winter (0.5), or in bedroom all year (1). This was weighted by percentage of time the person lived in such conditions, but by total time and thus could range from 0 to 3. None of the ORs for adenocarcinoma were significant at 95%.
Source: Ref. 53.

into account the number of years of exposure, but only the percent of total time in each situation, e.g., whether 1 year or 50 years.

Combining the women's data from this Shenyang study with those from a similar study in nearby Harbin, Wu-Williams et al. (52) analyzed questionnaires from 965 lung cancer patients and 959 controls. Logistic regression included variables for age, smoking, and education. Significantly higher risks were found for presence and use of *kang*, as in the Shenyang study alone. In addition, however, significant risks were also noted by number of years living in the presence of a coal stove, heated brick walls/floors, and coal burners, as well as reported current eye irritation and current amount of deep-frying. No significant differences were found between the two major types of carcinoma. In a multivariate analysis, current deep-frying and years of *kang* use and heated brick wall/floor remained significant, along with several factors not related to indoor air.

The same Harbin case-control study listed above under biomass showed that, after logistic regression, a high coal consumption per square meter of living area (OR = 6.2) indoor pollution in winter (OR = 3.4), and low ceiling height in the living room (OR = 4.3) were the main risk factors for women's lung adenocarcinoma (51). (The cutpoints between "high" and "low" for these parameters were not given.) Monitoring showed that the average air concentrations of TSP and BaP in bedrooms in winter were 4.4 and 27 times higher than the maximum allowable air concentrations in China, which are 150 $\mu g/m^3$ and 1 ng/m^3, respectively. No significant association between women's lung adenocarcinoma and active cigarette smoking or passive smoking was found (77). Indeed, a combined analysis of eight studies in China found the odds ratio for smoking to be just 3.1 for men and 2.3 for women, substantially less than found in developed nations.

In Guangzhou, the highest age-adjusted mortality rates of lung cancer for those women in one job category for more than 10 years were found among homemakers (29). In addition, the lung cancer mortality rates of Guangzhou women have been increasing dramatically, from 18 (1976) to 25 (1985) per 100,000, even though their smoking rate is less than 5%. These findings are quite distinct from the Shanghai data of Gao et al. (49), where no significant elevated risk was found for those women who had never worked outside the home.

Also in Guangzhou, there were 349 homemakers among 1243 female lung cancer deaths recorded during the period of one study (78). These women had no previous occupational exposure, 40% were nonsmokers, and none seemed to be exposed to significant outdoor air pollution. The epidemiological survey showed that female lung cancer mortality was related to exposure to coal combustion and cooking (32). The investigators monitored kitchens for suspended particulates, deposited dust, and BaP in deposited dust. They found (as expected) that concentrations were much higher in kitchens using coal compared to those using liquefied petroleum gas (LPG) for cooking.

Another Guangzhou study compared 662 lung cancer deaths and 662 controls living on the same street and matched by age and gender in Guangzhou (29). Indoor pollutant concentrations were high, with particle BaP concentrations averaging 120 ng/m^3 in a subsample of 21 coal-using kitchens, based on 5 days of monitoring each season. Comparable kitchens with gas stoves averaged 22 ng/m^3. Women who cooked in the coal stove homes also had significantly higher ($1.4\times$) levels of urinary BaP than those cooking with gas. The ratio of risks for lung cancer associated with coal stove smoke was about 6 for smoking women (3.1 for nonsmokers), but was not significantly increased for men. Men had a higher odds ratio (3.3 vs. 1.8) for smoking, however.

An unpublished case-control study in Shunyi County, near Beijing, reconfirmed 220 deaths from lung cancer over 6 years in a population of about 500,000 and found 440 controls matched by neighborhood, age, and gender (J. Liu and H. Hu, unpublished). Age-adjusted lung cancer mortality was 7.3/100,000 for men and 4.7/100,000 for women, resulting in a low gender ratio (1.6 compared to the world average of more than 5). Following univariate analysis, logistic regression was performed, identifying burning of coal without flue (OR = 2 {1.2–3.4}) and past chronic respiratory disease (OR = 2.2 {1.4–3.7}) as significant risks, along with smoking and past severe psychiatric attack. The authors point out that coal use can be significantly associated with lung cancer risk even in rural areas where overall lung cancer rates remain low.

A case-control study in Xuan Wei county matched 110 lung cancer patients with 426 controls by age, gender, occupation, and village, the latter effectively matching them also by cooking fuel and house type (71). As shown in Table 10, for women, years of cooking, but not the age of starting to cook, were associated with increased risk. For men, frequent cooking was associated with an increased risk. A strong association was found between lung cancer and a history of chronic bronchitis (see Table 6). The extremely heavy indoor air pollution levels from coal cookfires in this area were suggested as a reason that the risks found for active and

Table 10 Odds Ratio (OR) and Confidence Interval (CI) for Lung Cancer According to Cooking History and Passive Smoking in Xuan Wei

	OR	95% CI
Women		
Age of starting to cook		
>14.7	1.0	
11–14.7	2.4	1.1–5.2
<10	1.3	0.45–3.5
Trend (*p*-value)	>0.05	
Years of cooking		
<30	1.0	
31–44	9.2	1.8–47
>45	15	1.6–130
Trend (*p*-value)	>0.05	
Passive smoking		
No	1.0	
Yes	0.77	0.30–2.0
Men		
Often cooks food		
No	1.0	
Yes	3.4	1.3–8.9

ORs have been rounded to two places of precision.
Source: Ref. 53.

passive smoking were less than observed elsewhere in China. Another case-control study (not listed in Table 6) has been underway in Xuan Wei in which cases and controls are not matched for fuel type, potentially allowing simultaneous assessment of the effect of fuel in relation to other risk factors (21). Preliminary results, however, indicate fairly modest odds ratios (1.3–4) for past use of smoky coal and a surprising similarity of these risks for men and women (68).

Although the environmental, toxicological, and epidemiological studies published to date on Xuan Wei have done an excellent job of outlining what, short of smoking, would appear to be one of the most striking patterns in history of cancer risk from air pollution, there clearly is much more to learn.

Developed-Country Studies. A case-control study among 149 lung cancer cases and 149 controls consisting of white women in Los Angeles found that reported exposure to coal burning in stoves or fireplaces during the majority of childhood and teenage years was a significant risk factor (2.3) for adenocarcinoma (45). Also significant was childhood pneumonia (2.7), which may also have indoor air pollution as a risk factor (79). Together, childhood coal smoke exposures and pneumonia accounted for 22% of the adenocarcinoma. Squamous cell carcinoma, which was also studied, was not significantly associated with these risk factors and could be almost entirely explained by smoking, a finding different from most of the Chinese studies, which found little difference (none significant) between the two types.

A case-control study was described by Hodgson and Kuller (80) in which all lung cancer deaths for 1 year in two Pennsylvania counties were considered cases. Interviews were conducted with two sets of controls: one chosen among heart-disease patients matched by age, gender, race, and urban status, the other from the same neighborhood. One question related to fuel source for heating—gas, coal, or oil. Surprisingly, they found significant risks compared to electric heating only for gas heating among the neighborhood control series (3.3 {1–12} 5 years; 2.7 {1–7.2} 10 years). Collinearity between pack-years of smoking and gas heating was examined and rejected as a possible explanation. The authors take the reasonable position that the inconsistency of the results put them in considerable doubt.

A small case-control study in Germany involving 80 lung cancer cases and 160 controls did not identify significant lung cancer risks for indoor or outdoor air pollution (81). The investigators had difficulty reconstructing exposure histories, partly because of the high rate of mobility in the population, an average of five residences per person.

Using the U.S. National Household Interview Survey, Sterling et al. (82) compared the standardized morbidity and mortality ratios (SmR and SMR) between working women and homemakers and found a significant excess risk (ratio of SmRs = 1.6 {1.0–2.4}) for the incidence of all cancers among white but not black homemakers. Adjustments were made for age and to account for the overall differences in chronic disease rates, because women with chronic diseases may be less likely to work outside the home. The authors attributed the remaining cancer risk to the common household exposures to a wide range of chemicals.

VI. Feasible Interventions

The only fully effective long-term solution to the high household pollutant concentrations that lead to significant risks of lung cancer and other forms of ill-health would seem to be cleaner fuels, i.e., progress up the energy ladder in Figure 1. Unfortunately, there are hundreds of millions of households worldwide that will not be able to move up for many decades, because of the relative costs and availabilities of the fossil fuels required. For many of these households, however, there are promising interim measures involving improved stoves and better ventilation that can have some effect.

In the 1980s, for example, principally in response to energy shortages but partly to reduce indoor air pollution exposures, a large number of programs to improve stoves were started in developing countries across the world (83). To design, build, and disseminate a low-cost stove that was acceptable and reliable turned out to be a much more challenging task than first envisioned, however. Consequently, there have been many false starts and disappointments. Nevertheless, by the end of the 1980s, there had also been a number of successes. Principal among these was the Chinese National Improved Biomass Stove Program, which installed 120 million improved biomass stoves during the decade, more than 10 times the total in all the rest of the world, although there has been less effort devoted to improved coal stoves (84). Kenya and Sri Lanka also had notable successes (85).

Needed, however, is a more concerted effort to achieve and verify exposure reductions along with improved fuel efficiency, which has been the chief aim of most programs. Significant benefit may accrue from such programs, not only with regard to lowering of lung cancer risk, but also from reduction of other health impacts of greater current importance in developing countries, such as childhood pneumonia (79).

VII. Summary

The easiest criticism to levy against most of the lung cancer epidemiological studies discussed above is that they do not have precise measures of exposure. On the other hand, how can they, given the long, but uncertain, latency period for lung cancer and the physical impossibility of reconstructing exposure histories over decades past? As these studies mature, however, it may be possible to reduce the uncertainty of long-latency exposure estimates. For example, some of the Xuan Wei studies have had to combine data from questionnaires about pre-1958 conditions, measured air pollution levels in the 1980s, and cancer rates in the 1970s. Now that the general outlines of the health impact have been identified, it may be worth the extra work needed to develop more complete exposure histories by investigating changes in behavior, food, fuel, cooking, housing, and other factors that may influence exposure.*

Another example is the Shanghai study where cooking with rapeseed oil was identified as a major risk factor. This factor, however, was apparently not examined in historical context. Indeed, this and several other studies used questions related to present cooking patterns (e.g., "perceived smokiness," "frequency of eye irritation") as exposure indicators. Without evidence that cooking behavior has remained constant for many decades, it is difficult to interpret these indicators.

A confounding factor that does not seem to have been examined in detail in any of the present studies is previous history of chronic or acute respiratory disease (e.g., chronic bronchitis and childhood pneumonia) (86). Several of the studies above found these to be risk factors for lung cancer. These are also known to have indoor air pollution as a risk factor, however. It might thus be fruitful to attempt to distinguish the degree to which indoor pollution acts to enhance lung cancer risk through its impact on these other respiratory diseases compared to its more direct impact.

There would also seem to be discrepancies with regard to the differential impact of indoor pollution exposures on two major types of lung carcinoma. As pointed out above, the Chinese studies that examined cell type either find no difference (49,52) or a slightly increased risk for squamous cell carcinoma compared to adenocarcinoma (50). The Los Angeles study (45), however, determined that squamous cell carcinoma could be explained nearly entirely by smoking and that exposure to coal stoves was more closely related to adenocarcinoma, a finding more consistent with accepted concepts. It is possible that these differences are due to sample size and chance or to problems related to consistent diagnosis. It is intriguing to speculate, however, that there may be a set of carcinogens specific to each cell type that is found in a different balance in smokes from different fuels, i.e., that some stove smokes act more like tobacco smoke than others. This may also help explain some of the anomalous results that have come from the Xuan Wei coal smoke studies and the marked difference in the attributable risk of smoking in China (77).

In spite of these difficulties, the evidence from China seems fairly convincing that household coal smoke exposures enhance lung cancer risk. As listed in Table 6, the odds ratios of various indicators of coal smoke ranges from 2 to 6 for

---

*The ongoing Xuan Wei case-control study should reduce some of this uncertainty, along with avoiding any misclassification that may result from the necessity to rely on lung cancer diagnoses done in the 1970s.

most studies, with one study finding no significant risk (49) and one, Xuan Wei (53), finding odds ratios up to 9, a result consistent with the higher exposures experienced there compared to the other study households.

As a result, the governments of China and other developing countries considering expanded use of unvented and/or smoky coal for household applications would do well to reconsider. The health benefits from cleaning the coal and/or substituting cleaner fuels are probably substantial, and such interventions deserve a high priority, even in comparison to efforts to address the more obvious deterioration of urban ambient air quality.

The available evidence does not reveal much about biomass smoke, however, to which much larger populations are exposed worldwide. This is partly due to the relative absence of evidence (which, by itself, is not evidence of absence). Few studies have been done. Another reason probably is that biomass particulates do not seem to contain as much BaP and other carcinogenic PAH as coal. These reasons do not seem sufficient, however. In addition, there may also be other differences between the two mixtures that allow lung cancer rates to remain low in regions with long-term high biomass smoke exposures (87).* Thus, although other health endpoints (childhood pneumonia, adverse pregnancy outcomes, and chronic obstructive lung disease) appear to be of more current concern in groups heavily exposed to biomass smoke, the large populations and the high exposures involved warrant careful attention by the lung cancer research community as well.

Acknowledgments

We appreciate comments and suggestions by R. S Chapman, M. R. Dove, H. S. Hu, L. C. Koo, and H. F. Takeuchi.

References

1. Global Environment Monitoring System. (1988). *Assessment of Urban Air Quality*. Geneva, United Nations Environmental Program/World Health Organization.
2. Smith, K. R. (1988). Total exposure assessment: Implications for developing countries. *Environment* 30(10):16–20.
3. Samet, J. M., and Spengler, J. D. (eds.). (1991). *Indoor Air Pollution: A Health Perspective*. Baltimore, Johns Hopkins University Press.
4. Smith, K. R. (1990). Indoor air pollution and the pollution transition. In *Indoor Air Quality*. Edited by M. Kasuga. Berlin, Springer-Verlag, pp. 448–456.

---

*It is conceivable that there may even be support for the hypothesis that low exposures to some carcinogens are protective.

5. Smith, K. R. (1987). *Biofuels, Air Pollution, and Health: A Global Review*. New York, Plenum Press.
6. Cooper, J. A. (1980). Environmental impact of residential wood combustion emissions and its implications. *J. Air Pollut. Control Assoc.* 30:855–861.
7. WHO Consultative Group. (1992). *Epidemiological, Social, and Technical Aspects of Indoor Air Pollution from Biomass Fuels*. WHO/PEP/92.3A, Geneva, World Health Organization.
8. Chen, B. H., Hong, C. J., Pandey, M. R., and Smith, K. R. (1990). Indoor air pollution in developing countries. *WHO Stat. Q.* 43(3):127–138.
9. De Koning, H. W., Smith, K. R., and Last, J. M. (1985). Biomass fuel combustion and health. *Bull. WHO* 63(1):11–26.
10. Smith, K. R. (1990). Health effects in developing countries. In *Bioenergy and the Environment*. Edited by J. Pasztor and L. A. Kristoferson. Boulder, CO, Westview, pp. 301–322.
11. Pandey, M. R., Boleij, J. S. M., Smith, K. R., and Wafula, E. M. (1989). Indoor air pollution in developing countries and acute respiratory infection in children. *Lancet* 25:427–428.
12. Collings, D. A., Sithole, S. D., and Martin, K. S. (1990). Indoor woodsmoke pollution causing lower respiratory disease in children. *Trop. Doctor* 20:151–155.
13. Saksena, S., Prasad, R., Pal, R. C., and Joshi, V. (1992). Patterns of daily exposure to TSP and CO in the Garwal Himalaya. *Atmos. Environ.* 26A(11):2125–2134.
14. Pandey, M. R., Neupane, R. P., Gautam, A., and Shrestha, I. B. (1990). The effectiveness of smokeless stoves in reducing indoor air pollution in a rural hill region of Nepal. *Mountain Res. Dev.* 10(4):313–320.
15. Hu, H., Liu, Y., Smith, K. R., and Sinton, J. (1992). Indoor air pollution in China: Bibliography and database. Honolulu, Environment and Policy Institute, East-West Center.
16. Morris, S. C., and Grimshaw, C. A. (1990). Health effects in developed countries. In *Bioenergy and the Environment*. Edited by J. Pasztor and L. A. Kristoferson. Boulder, CO, Westview, pp. 323–348.
17. WHO. (1987). *Air Quality Guidelines for Europe*. Regional Publications, European Series No. 23. Copenhagen, WHO.
18. Clifford, P. (1972). Carcinogens in the nose and throat. *Proc. R. Soc. Med.* 65: 682–686.
19. Smith, K. R., Aggarwal, A. L., and Dave, R. M. (1983). Air pollution and rural biomass fuels in developing countries: A pilot village study in India and implications for research and policy. *Atmos. Environ.* 17:2343–2362.
20. He, X., et al. (1986). Lung cancer and indoor air pollution in China. In *Medicine in China: Cancer, Early Diagnosis and Control*. Edited by H. Huang. Hong Kong, University of Hong Kong (in Chinese).
21. Mumford, J. A., He, X. Z., and Chapman, R. S. (1990). Human lung cancer risks due to complex organic mixtures of combustion emissions. In *Occupational Cancer Epidemiology, Recent Results in Cancer Research*, #120. Berlin, Springer-Verlag, pp. 106–121.
22. Menon, P. (1988). Indoor spatial monitoring of combustion generated pollutants (TSP,

CO and BaP) by Indian cookstoves. Honolulu, Department of Meteorology, University of Hawaii (UHMET 88-01).

23. WHO. (1988). *Indoor Air Quality in the Base Area, The Gambia*. WHO/PEP/88.3, HEAL Project, World Health Observation. Geneva, WHO.
24. Boleij, J., Campbell, H., Wafula, E., et al. (1988). Biomass fuel combustion and indoor air quality in developing countries. In *Proceedings of the Indoor and Ambient Air Quality Symposium*. Edited by R. Perry and P. W. Kirk. London, Selper, pp. 24–29.
25. Wafula, E. M., Onyango, F. E., Thairu, H., et al. (1990). Indoor air pollution in a Kenyan village. *East Afr. Med. J.* 67(1):24–32.
26. Guo, L., et al. (1986). The improvement of indoor air pollution after using gas for cooking in Tai Yuan city. *Chin. J. Environ. Health* 2(4):32–33 (in Chinese).
27. Li, M., et al. (1990). Indoor air pollution and human health among ethnic Koreans. *Proc. of 3rd National Conference on Environmental Health*, Shenyang (in Chinese).
28. Yu, S-Z., Zhang, Z-F., and Ling, F. (1990). Indoor air pollution of coal fumes as a risk factor of stroke, Shanghai. In *Indoor Air '90*. Edited by D. S. Walkinshow. Proceedings of the Fifth International Conference on Indoor Air Quality and Climate. Toronto, Vol. 1, pp. 89–94.
29. Du, Y. X., and Ou, X. (1990). Indoor air pollution and woman lung cancer. In *Indoor Air '90*. Edited by D. S. Walkinshow. Proceedings of the Fifth International Conference on Indoor Air Quality and Climate. Toronto, Vol. 1, pp. 59–64.
30. Yang, R. D. (1988). Characteristics of indoor air pollution in medium-prevalence areas in Xuanwei County. *Chin. J. Environ. Health* 5(6):16–18 (in Chinese).
31. Mumford, J. L., Helmes, C. T., Lee, X., et al. (1990). Mouse skin tumorigenicity studies of indoor coal and wood combustion emissions from homes of residents in Xuan Wei, China with high lung cancer mortality. *Carcinogenesis* 11(3):397–403.
32. Ou, X. L., et al. (1989). Relationship between housewife lung cancer and domestic coal use. *Chin. J. Environ. Health* 5(1):4 (in Chinese).
33. Sloof, W., Janus, J. A., Matthijsen, A. J. C. M., et al. (eds.). (1989). *Integrated Criteria Document PAHs*. Report #758474011. Bilthoven, The Netherlands, National Institute of Public Health and Environmental Protection.
34. U.S. Surgeon General. (1982). The health consequences of smoking—cancer. *A Report of the Surgeon General*. Rockville, MD, U.S. Dept. of Health and Human Services.
35. USNRC. (1986). U.S. National Research Council, Committee on Passive Smoking. *Environmental Tobacco Smoke: Measuring Exposures and Assessing Health Effects*. Washington, D.C., National Academy Press.
36. Koo, L. C., and Ho, J. H. C. (1990). Worldwide epidemiological patterns of lung cancer in nonsmokers. *Int. J. Epidemiol.* 19(3 Suppl. 1):S14–S23.
37. Fraumeni, J. F. (1985). Opportunities for United States-People's Republic of China collaboration in cancer epidemiology. *Natl. Cancer Inst. Monograph*. 69:59–62.
38. Li, J., Liu, B., Li, G. Y., et al. (1979). *Atlas of Cancer Mortality in the People's Republic of China*. Shanghai, China, China Map Press.
39. Hoffman, D., and Wynder, E. L. (1971). Respiratory carcinogens: Their nature and precursors. In *International Symposium of Identification and Measurement of Environmental Pollutants*. Ottawa, National Research Council of Canada, pp. 9–16.

40. Kodama, A. M., and Dollar, A. M. (1983). Indoor fires and a possible cause of cancers of the upper respiratory and digestive systems in certain underdeveloped countries. *J. Environ. Health* 46(2):88–90.
41. Armstrong, R. W., Kutty, R. W., and Armstrong, M. J. (1978). Self-specific environments associated with nasopharyngeal carcinoma in Selangor, Malaysia. *Soc. Sci. Med.* 12D:149–156.
42. Yu, M. C., Ho, J. H. C., Henderson, B. E., et al. (1985). Epidemiology of nasopharyngeal carcinoma in Malaysia and Hong Kong. *Nat. Cancer Inst. Monogr.* 69: 203–207.
43. Koo, L. C. (1989). Environmental tobacco smoke and lung cancer: Is it smoke or the diet? In *Present and Future of Indoor Air Quality*. Edited by J. Bieva, et al. Amsterdam, Elsevier Science.
44. Sobue, T. (1990). Association of indoor air pollution and lifestyle with lung cancer in Osaka, Japan. *Int. J. Epidemiol.* 19(3 Suppl. 1):S62–S66.
45. Wu, A. H., Henderson, B. E., Pike, M. C., and Yu, M. C. (1985). Smoking and other risk factors for lung cancer in women. *JNCI* 74(4):747–751.
46. Yang, X., and Li, Y. B. (1990). A preliminary study of the impact of indoor air pollution on the health of the dwellers in Wuhan City. In *Indoor Air '90*. Edited by D. W. Walkinshow. Proceedings of the Fifth International Conference on Indoor Air Quality and Climate. Toronto, Vol. 1, pp. 83–88.
47. Cai, W. C. (1990). Indoor air pollution and human health in Guangzhou. *Proc. of 3rd National Conference on Environmental Health*. Shenyang, Nov. (in Chinese).
48. Qu, Z., Hao, R., and Ma, H. (1990). A survey on the relation between the pollution level of airborne polycyclic aromatic hydrocarbons in atmosphere and indoor air and the incidence of lung cancer in Benxi City. In *Indoor Air '90*. Edited by D. W. Walkinshow. Proceedings of the Fifth International Conference on Indoor Air Quality and Climate. Toronto, Vol. 1, pp. 119–124.
49. Gao, Y. T., Blot, W. J., Zheng, W., et al. (1987). Lung cancer among Chinese women. *Int. J. Cancer* 40:604–609.
50. Xu, Z. Y., Blot, W. J., Xiao, H. P., et al. (1989). Smoking, air pollution, and high rates of lung cancer in Shenyang, China. *JNCI* 81(23):1800–1806.
51. Wang, F. L., et al. (1989). Analysis of risk factors for female lung adenocarcinoma in Harbin indoor air pollution. *Chin. J. Prev. Med.* 23(5):270 (in Chinese).
52. Wu-Williams, A. H., Dai, X. D., Blot, W., et al. (1990). Lung cancer among women in north-east China. *Br. J. Cancer* 62:982–987.
53. Liu, Z. Y., He, X. Z., and Chapman, R. S. (1991). Smoking and other risk factors for lung cancer in Xuan Wei, China. *Int. J. Epidemiol.* 20(1):26–31.
54. Wang, X. Z. (1984). Indoor/outdoor air pollution and lung cancer. *Chin. J. Environ. Health* 2(5):7–12 (in Chinese).
55. Koo, L. C., Lee, N., and Ho, J. H. C. (1983). Do cooking fuels pose a risk for lung cancer? A case control study of women in Hong Kong. *Ecology Dis.* 2(4):255–265.
56. Koo, L. C., Ho, J. H., Saw, D., and Ho, C. Y. (1987). Measurements of passive smoking and estimates of risk for lung cancer among non-smoking Chinese females. *Int. J. Cancer* 39:162–169.
57. Koo, L. C., and Ho, J. H. C. (1991). Is incense hazardous to health? *International*

Symposium on Indoor Air Quality in Asia. Hong Kong, Cancer Research Laboratory, H. K. Anti-Cancer Society, Nam Long Hospital.

58. Koo, L. C., and Ho, J. H. C. (1990). Chronic bronchitis, lung cancer, nasopharyngeal cancer in Hong Kong. In *Epidemiology and Prevention of Cancer*. Edited by R. Sasaki and K. Aoki. University of Nagoya Press, Japan, pp. 131–134.
59. MacLennan, R., Da Costa, J., Day, N. E., et al. (1977). Risk factors for lung cancer in Singapore Chinese, a population with high female incidence rates. *Int. J. Cancer* 20: 854–860.
60. Hong, C. J. (1992). Health aspects of domestic use of biomass fuels and coal in China. In *Indoor Air Pollution from Biomass Fuel*. Working Papers from a WHO Consultation, WHO/PEP/92.3B. Geneva, World Health Organization, pp. 43–77.
61. Xiao, H., and Xu, Z. (1985). Air pollution and lung cancer in Liaoning Province: PRC. *Natl. Cancer Inst. Monogr.* 69:53–58.
62. Xu, Z. Y., Blot, W. J., and Fraumeni, J. F. (1986). Geographic variation of female lung cancer in China. *Am. J. Public Health* 76:1249–1250
63. Yang, X., et al. (1983). The relation of indoor air pollution and human health—a primary study. Workshop on Chinese Environmental Health (in Chinese), Beijing.
64. Mumford, J. L., He, X. Z., Chapman, R. S., et al. (1987). Lung cancer and indoor pollution in Xuan Wei, China. *Science* 235:217–235.
65. Yunnan Provincial Public Health and Anti-epidemic Station. (1987). Measures to prevent lung cancer in Xuanwei County. *Chin. J. Environ. Health* 4(3):2–4 (in Chinese).
66. Yunnan Provincial Public Health and Anti-Epidemic Station. (1984). Indoor air pollution monitoring in high and low lung-cancer prevalence regions in Xuanwei County. *Chin. J. Environ. Health* 1(5):14 (in Chinese).
67. Chapman, R. S., Mumford, J. L., Harris, D. B., et al. (1988). The epidemiology of lung cancer in Xuan Wei, China: Current progress, issues, and research strategies. *Arch. Environ. Health* 43(2):180–185.
68. Chapman, R. S., Mumford, J. L., He, X. Z., et al. (1989). Assessing indoor air pollution exposure and lung cancer risk in Xuan Wei, China. *J. Am. Coll. Toxicol.* 8(5):941–948.
69. Dasch, J. M. (1982). Particulate and gaseous emissions from wood-burning fireplaces. *Environ. Sci. Technol.* 16:635–645.
70. Kamens, R. M., Rives, G. D., Perry, J. M., et al. (1984). Mutagenic changes in dilute wood smoke as it ages and reacts with ozone and nitrogen dioxide: An outdoor chamber study. *Environ. Sci. Technol.* 18(7):523–530.
71. He, X., Chen, W., Liu, Z., and Chapman, R. S. (1991). An epidemiological study of lung cancer in Xuan Wei County, China: Current progress. Case-control study on lung cancer and cooking fuel. *Environ. Health Perspect.* 94:9–13.
72. Ren, W. S. (1984). Emission of BaP from combustion of four different fuels. *Chin. J. Environ. Health* 1(1):35–36 (in Chinese).
73. Zhou, S. W., Wei, Y. X., and Li, S. M. (1990). Free radicals and indoor air pollution in a high mortality area of lung cancer—Xuan Wei County, China. In *Indoor Air '90*. Edited by D. W. Walkinshow. Proceedings of the Fifth International Conference on Indoor Air Quality and Climate. Toronto, Vol. 1, pp. 137–142.

74. Chuang, J. C., Wise, S. A., Cao, S., and Mumford, J. L. (1992). Chemical characterization of mutagenic fractions of particles from indoor coal combustion: A study of lung cancer in Xuan Wei, China. *Environ. Sci. Technol.* 26:999–1004.
75. Gao, Y. T., Blot, W. J., Zheng, W., et al. (1988). Lung cancer and smoking in Shanghai. *Int. J. Epidemiol.* 17(2):277–280.
76. Liu, Z. Q., et al. (1987). Mutagenicity of condensate from frying process in kitchens. *Chin. J. Environ. Health* 4(6):10–11 (in Chinese).
77. Liu, Z. (1992). Smoking and lung cancer in China: Combined analysis of eight case-control studies. *Int. J. Epidemiol.* 21(2):197–201.
78. Du, Y. S., et al. (1984). A preliminary analysis of trends of lung cancer mortality in Guangzhou, China. *Acta Acad. Med. Guangzhou* 12(1):1–22 (in Chinese).
79. Smith, K. R., and Rogers, S. (in press). Reducing exposure to household biomass smoke. In *Interventions to Reduce Mortality from Pneumonia in Children*. Edited by S. Rogers. London, School of Hygiene and Tropical Medicine.
80. Hodgson, M. J., and Kuller, L. H. (1990). A population-based case-control study of lung cancer: Smoking, home-heating fuel, and occupation as risk factors. In *Indoor Air '90*. Edited by D. W. Walkinshow. Proceedings of the Fifth International Conference on Indoor Air Quality and Climate. Toronto, Vol. 1, pp. 429–433.
81. Molik, B., Jockel, K. H., Schoneberg, G., and Wichmann, H. E. (1990). Indoor and outdoor air pollution and lung cancer. In *Indoor Air '90*. Edited by D. W. Walkinshow. Proceedings of the Fifth International Conference on Indoor Air Quality and Climate. Toronto, Vol. 1, pp. 441–445.
82. Sterling, T., Weinkam, J., and Sterling, D. (1990). Exposure of homemakers to toxic contaminants: I. Differences in chronic conditions between homemakers and employed persons. In *Indoor Air '90*. Edited by D. W. Walkinshow. Proceedings of the Fifth International Conference on Indoor Air Quality and Climate. Toronto, Vol. 1, pp. 471–476.
83. Smith, K. R., ed. (1991). Project Reports. *Global Review of Improved Cookstove Programs*. Honolulu, Environment and Policy Institute, East-West Center.
84. Gu, S., Huang, K., Qiu, D., and Smith, K. R. (1991). 100-Million improved cookstoves in China: How was it done? Country Study #1. *Global Review of Improved Cookstove Programs*. Honolulu, Environment and Policy Institute, East-West Center.
85. Barnes, D., Openshaw, K., Smith, K. R., and Van der Plas, R. (1992). *An Evaluation of Improved Cookstove Programs: Prospects for Success or Failure*. Washington, D.C., ESMAP, World Bank.
86. Lu, B. Y., et al. (1984). Research on human airway resistance in high and low lung cancer prevalence regions in Xuan Wei County. *Chin. J. Environ. Health* 1(4):12–13 (in Chinese).
87. Rylander, R. (1990). Environmental exposures with increased risks for lung cancer? *Int. J. Epidemiol.* 19(3 Suppl. 1):S67–S72.

8

Asbestos and Man-Made Fibers

JANET M. HUGHES

Tulane University School of Public Health
and Tropical Medicine
New Orleans, Louisiana

HANS WEILL

Tulane University Medical Center
New Orleans, Louisiana

I. Introduction

Asbestos and man-made mineral fibers (MMMF) are two classes of fibrous minerals with worldwide economic and societal importance. They have been used in a broad range of products because of various desirable properties; many insulation materials use them for fire retardation, and their strength and surface properties make them useful for numerous other products, including construction materials and water pipes. While some of these items can be made with other materials, in some cases these are considerably more expensive.

Asbestos was first used commercially in the late 1800s. While concerns about possible lung cancer risk to workers began to appear in the 1930s, these were limited to anecdotal and case reports, and production continued to expand exponentially. A recent review of early asbestos work notes that asbestos was recognized as a lung carcinogen in Germany by 1943, but most of the basis for this was published in German and was not well recognized outside that country (1). Beginning in 1949, several reports of increased lung cancer risk among British workers appeared (2–4); by the mid-1960s the existence of a substantial lung cancer risk to past asbestos workers was well established. Though much was not understood about asbestos health risks, and exposure-response data for the malignant and nonmalignant effects did not become available until considerably later (the 1980s), concerns regarding asbestos-related risks caused commercial asbestos production to peak in the early 1970s and to decrease dramatically since that time (Fig. 1).

The primary continuing use of asbestos today is for asbestos cement products (75% of total consumption) and friction materials (15%), with the majority of the use by third world countries, where its continuing availability is considered of great economic importance. Because of this ongoing use and the fact that asbestos products are already in place throughout industrialized countries, concern for the potential health risks related to asbestos exposure continues. A recent proposed Environmental Protection Agency (EPA) ban (7) and phase-out of asbestos products in the United States has been overturned by a federal appellate court (8) on the basis that the agency had failed to explore less burdensome alternatives, with appropriate cost-benefit analyses, and that they failed "to evaluate the harm which will result from increased use of substitute products." The latter, referred to as "fibrous substitutes" by EPA, were designated by the court as "known carcinogens." (Man-made mineral fibers have actually been categorized by the International Agency for Research on Cancer [IARC] as 2B, *possibly carcinogenic to man*.) Notwithstanding the debate regarding the relative risks associated with asbestos and man-made mineral fiber exposures, the trends in use of each type of fiber in the United States amply illustrate increasingly

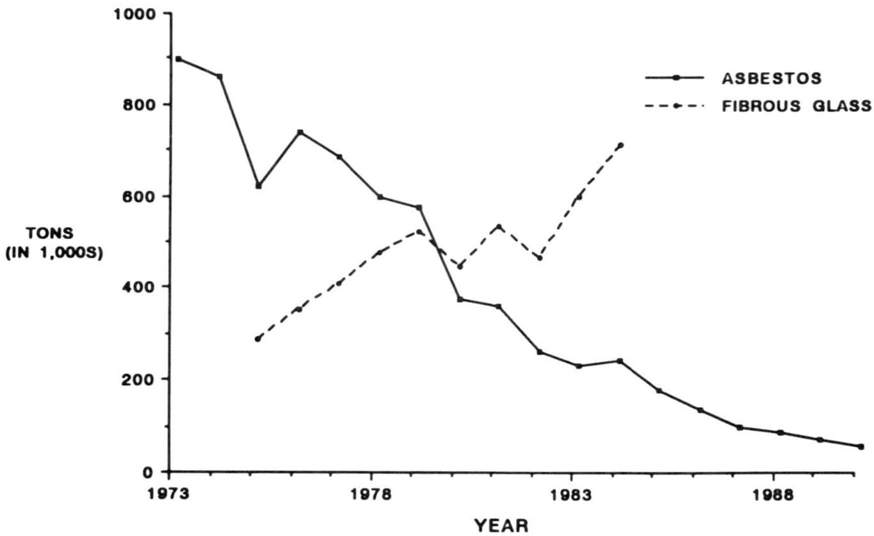

Figure 1 U.S. asbestos and fibrous glass use, 1973–1990. (From Refs. 5,6.)

stringent regulation of asbestos and the corresponding increase in use of MMMF (Fig. 1).

Because of the increased use of these substitutes and because of a number of similarities between these fibers and asbestos, concerns have been raised about the potential health risks from these materials. Although man-made mineral fibers (MMMF) have been the subject of considerable research over the past 15 years, information concerning potential MMMF risks is far more limited than that concerning asbestos.

II. Asbestos

A. Background

Asbestos is a class of naturally occurring, fibrous minerals, consisting primarily of two subgroups: serpentine, which includes chrysotile asbestos, and the amphiboles, of which amosite, crocidolite, and tremolite are important members. These classes differ both geometrically and chemically. Regarding structure, chrysotile fibers are generally curled while amphibole fibers are straight, and while there is considerable overlap in their distributions by length and diameter, chrysotile fibers tend to be shorter and thicker than those of amphiboles.

Chrysotile was the primary type of asbestos used in most products, accounting for over 95% of the asbestos used in U.S. buildings (9); most was imported from Canada, with only a relatively small amount mined in the United States. Though used in far less quantity than chrysotile, crocidolite and amosite were used widely, especially for certain products, and are particularly important regarding potential health risks; most of the amphibole fiber used in the United States was imported from South Africa. The use of asbestos in acoustical and thermal insulation products was discontinued in the mid-1970s, primarily because of the potential release of fiber from these products which may become friable. Remaining use is in products where asbestos is encapsulated in a cement or resin matrix, with less potential for fiber release, such as asbestos-cement sheets and pipe, brake linings, gaskets, packings, roof coatings, and floor tiles (Asbestos Institute, Montreal, personal communication).

Essentially all residents of industrialized countries have accumulated a substantial number of asbestos fibers in their lungs; the average number for adults is likely to be in the millions (10). The concentration of asbestos fibers in buildings and the outdoor air of communities varies, but in an EPA survey of 48 buildings (11), a mean of approximately 0.00007 fibers per milliliter of air (f/ml) was found using transmission electron microscopy (for fibers longer than 5μm in length). A recent comprehensive review of the concentration data available for estimating indoor airborne exposure levels, which summarized results from over 200 buildings, support this value of 0.00007 f/ml as an estimate of the mean level in asbestos-containing buildings (12). By contrast, the current allowable U.S. occupational exposure level is 0.2 f/ml by phase contrast microscopy, more than 2000 times higher; workers in the cohorts upon which the health risk data are based were primarily exposed, on average, to concentrations of 5–10 f/ml or more, with some considerably higher.

B. Overall Lung Cancer Risk; Fiber Type Differences

The early reports demonstrating increased lung cancer risk among British workers (2–4) linked this risk to workers with asbestosis. Since these reports, numerous studies have demonstrated increased lung cancer risk among past asbestos workers. This risk has been demonstrated by comparing the observed lung cancer mortality (O) to that expected (E), based usually on regional or national cancer rates. Increased risk among workers is not generally observed until 20 (possibly 15) years following initial exposure, a pattern consistent with a necessary "latency" period for an asbestos-induced cancer to develop. The relatively few studies with follow-up of workers for 35 or more years suggest that relative risks may be elevated during the period 20–35 years after initial exposure but may decrease after this period (see Ref. 13).

The overall results from 28 of these studies are summarized in Table 1. Primarily these are for men, and most include only observations 20 or more years after hire. Studies of shipyard workers were not included because of the possibility of multiple other exposures in this industry that might have affected lung cancer risk.

For workers in the 11 cohorts exposed almost exclusively to chrysotile asbestos, the overall lung cancer risk was elevated 23% (a total of 517 cases, compared with 420.8 expected). Of these, the greatest risk (a 69% increase) was for chrysotile textile workers. If these are excluded, the pooled risk was 16% higher than expected for the other chrysotile workers combined. By contrast, workers in the 17 cohorts exposed either to amphiboles alone or to mixtures of chrysotile and amphiboles experienced more than double the expected risk (1381 cases, 635.0 expected).

With the exception of textile manufacturing, for each industry segment risk to workers exposed to amphiboles was considerably higher than those exposed only to chrysotile.

One limitation of across-study comparisons such as in Table 1 is that exposures (in duration and/or concentration) of the populations may not be strictly comparable. An alternative comparison is possible using the available exposure-response data for some of these industries.

C. Exposure-Response Information

Quantitative exposure-response relationships have been developed primarily to enable a rational approach to setting workplace standards for allowable worker

Table 1 Lung Cancer Risk[a] in Combined Studies, by Industry Segment and Fiber Type

	Fibers					
	Chrysotile[b]			Amphiboles or mixed		
Industry	O	E	O/E	O	E	O/E
Mining/Milling	249	201.3	1.24	91	34.5	2.64
	(14,15)[c]			(16)		
Gas masks	6	4.8	1.25	33	15.8	2.09
	(17)			(17–19)		
Friction products	55[d]	23.9	1.65			
	106[e]	98.5	1.08			
	(20,21)					
Insulation				481	111.2	4.33
				(13,22,23)		
Assorted MFG	4	4.3	0.93	77	28.4	2.71
	(24)			(25)		
Asbestos Cement	58	56.3	1.03	395	266.9	1.48
	(26–29)			(29–35)		
Subtotal	423	365.2	1.16	1,077	456.8	2.36
Textiles	94	55.6	1.69	304	178.2	1.71
	(36,37)			(38–40)[f]		
Total	517	420.8	1.23	1,381	635.0	2.17

[a]O/E = observed/expected; for most studies, results are for at least 20 years after hire.
[b]Exclusively or very predominantly chrysotile.
[c]References to studies included in category.
[d]Men in lowest cumulative exposure category for Ref. 20.
[e]Other men in Ref. 20, those in Ref. 21.
[f]Textiles and other asbestos products from Ref. 40; laggers excluded.

exposure levels. However, in addition to their use in projecting lifetime cancer risk to workers, they have been used extensively for estimating potential risk for persons environmentally exposed and provide an assessment of lung cancer risk by fiber type while taking into account amount of exposure.

While there has been a relatively large number of reports demonstrating an increasing lung cancer risk to past workers with increasing years of exposure, most of these were unable to take into account the intensity (airborne fiber concentrations) of these workers' exposures. Only a relatively few studies quantitatively estimated exposure levels for individual workers, which, combined with time worked at each level, resulted in estimates of cumulative exposures. Several reviews of these relationships have been published (see Refs. 41,42), examining in detail the estimation of slopes from the available studies. There are several technical issues involved in deriving these slopes, including (1) the method for converting the unit used in the past for estimating exposure concentrations (millions of particles per cubic foot of air [mppcf]) to the current unit of f/ml; (2) statistical issues on how to fit the model to the available data (41); and (3) the possible flattening of exposure-response relationships due to errors in estimating exposures.

Only nine studies have been able to quantitatively assess the lung cancer exposure-response relationship and have observed a biologically sensible pattern of risk in relation to exposure, i.e., where there is excess risk, a general increase in this risk with increasing exposure, regardless of the shape of the relationship. (An additional study of textile workers (39) is excluded because of the very different and unexplained results for two subgroups of workers.)

In these studies, after allowing for an appropriate latency period, relative risk has generally been shown to be linearly related to cumulative exposure. This relationship can be expressed as:

$$O/E = 1 + b^{*}x \qquad (1)$$

where b is the slope of the line and x is cumulative exposure, usually expressed as f/ml-years (a past worker exposed to 10 f/ml for 10 years has a cumulative exposure of 100 f/ml-years). The slope of the line is the amount risk increases per unit increase in cumulative exposure. Since the data are based on workers, years here refers to work years, usually assumed to be approximately 40 h/week, 50 weeks/calendar year. For no exposure, the model assumes that risk is not elevated, i.e., the ratio O/E is 1.

By the equation, for a cumulative exposure of 100 f/ml-yrs, a relatively steep slope of 0.01 would correspond to a ratio of 2.0 (a 100% increase in lung cancer risk), whereas a shallow slope of 0.0005 would mean a ratio of 1.05 (a 5% increase in risk).

There is substantial variability in the slopes reported in these nine studies. In general, however, the slopes cluster into two groups: those with shallow slopes, approximately 0.0006 or less, and those with relatively steep slopes, approximately 0.01 (Fig. 2). The four studies with shallow slopes were all of workers exposed exclusively (or nearly so) to chrysotile asbestos; these include chrysotile miners (14), friction product manufacturing workers (20,21), and asbestos cement manufacturing workers (29). There were four cohorts with slopes of approximately 0.01 (ranging from approximately 0.0085 to 0.0107): mixed fiber textile manufacturing (38), chrysotile textile manufacturing (36), crocidolite mining (16), and mixed fiber cement manufacturing (29). Thus, of the four groups with steep slopes, three were exposed to amphibole fibers. A study of retirees from manufacturing of assorted products (25) reported an intermediate slope (approximately 0.002); these workers had been engaged in the manufacture of a broad range of materials, some using chrysotile alone and others using mixed fibers.

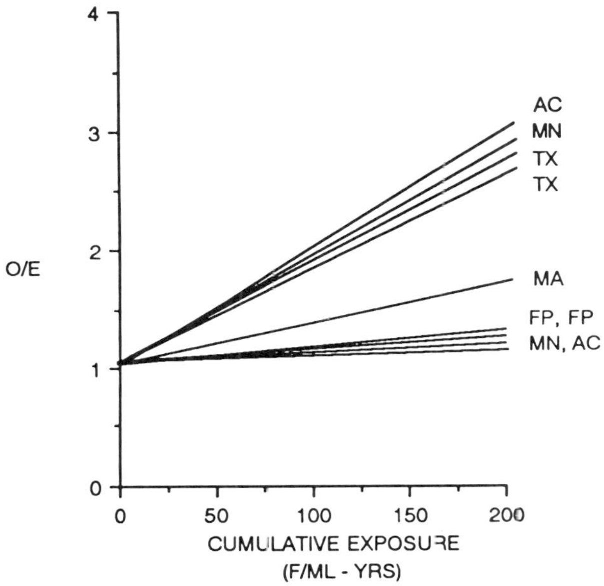

Figure 2 Lung cancer exposure-response relationships in nine studies of asbestos workers. AC = asbestos cement, MN = mining, TX = textile manufacturing, MA = assorted manufacturing, FP = friction product manufacturing.

These slopes can be compared within industry groupings. In mining, Quebec chrysotile miners (14) were observed to have a slope of 0.0005, while that for Australian crocidolite miners was approximately 0.01 (16). In asbestos cement product manufacturing, two plants in the same city, operating at approximately the same time and using predominantly chrysotile, had substantially different lung cancer experience (as well as mesothelioma); the plant with regular crocidolite use had a slope of approximately 0.01 while the slope for the other plant, with very restricted amosite use, was 0.0003 (29). In asbestos textile manufacturing, however, the slope for workers exposed only to chrysotile (36) was approximately the same as for those exposed to a mixture of fibers (38).

D. Other Factors

The reason for the increased risk in the asbestos textile industry, regardless of fiber type, has been the subject of much interest. The substantially elevated lung cancer risk (59/29.6 = 1.99) among the chrysotile textile workers in South Carolina (36) is particularly puzzling when compared with the risk (230/184.0 = 1.25) to workers at the Quebec chrysotile mine (14) which was the source of the asbestos used at the textile plant and where airborne exposure levels were apparently higher. Two possible explanations concerning risk to textile workers have been put forward. One is that carcinogenic mineral oils may have been used extensively in this industry (43); a case-control investigation failed to detect a role of mineral oil (44), but there is some question whether past records allow an accurate classification of workers according to mineral oil exposure.

Another possible explanation is that airborne fibers in textile plants, which are woven by machine into fabric, tend to be longer and thinner than in most other industrial settings, particularly mines. A comparison of the distributions of fibers by dimension in the lungs of Quebec mine and textile plant workers support this, with the percentage of fibers greater than 20 μm in length higher for plant workers than for miners (45).

Such a difference in fiber dimensions as a possible explanation of the differing lung cancer risk at these two locations is consistent with a large body of evidence from animal experiments, which demonstrates a gradient of risk with dimension—short, thick fibers being the least hazardous and long, thin fibers, the most (see, for example, Ref. 46).

E. Lung Fibrosis

The risk of asbestosis among past asbestos workers was recognized earlier than the risk of cancer. Beginning with the earliest reports of increased lung cancer risk among these workers, there has been interest in whether these are two separate, independent risks or if asbestos-induced lung cancer is a complication of the fibrosis. It has been suggested that asbestosis rather than asbestos *per se* accounts for the observed lung cancer risk in past workers (47,48). Of relevance is that increased lung cancer has been shown to be associated with other lung scarring such as that due to silicosis (49) and idiopathic pulmonary fibrosis or lung fibrosis associated with collagen vascular disorders (50). Findings from fundamental biological research are contributing to the credence of an association between asbestos-induced lung fibrosis and cancer. It has recently been suggested that the processes of inflammation, fibrosis and carcinogenesis are likely to be interrelated, with a central role hypothesized for the activated alveolar macrophage in fibrotic lungs (51).

There is an accumulating body of epidemiological evidence that elevated lung cancer risk among asbestos-exposed individuals may be restricted to those with fibrosis. Circumstantial evidence comes from two studies: of lung cancer cases among insulators, 82% had radiographic and 100% had histological evidence of asbestosis (52), while 90% of cases among London factory workers had histological evidence (40).

Two recent studies designed to address this issue, but with different methodologies, found strikingly similar results. An autopsy study of amphibole miners (53), using a standardized proportional mortality analysis, and a cohort study of asbestos cement workers (54), using standardized mortality ratios, observed no elevated risk among workers without asbestosis but substantially elevated risk for those with lung fibrosis (Table 2). In both studies, exposure estimates were available but could not account for these results.

Such an etiology for asbestos-induced lung cancer (asbestosis as a necessary precursor) would be important concerning potential lung cancer risk for current workers and for individuals environmentally exposed to asbestos. There is general agreement that environmental exposures do not result in lung fibrosis, and among current workers, asbestosis is decreasingly encountered and, when present, most often is of minimal severity.

F. Low Exposure Risk Estimation

In using Eq. (1) to estimate lifetime lung cancer risk in exposed populations, many risk assessments use a steep slope of 0.01 (55–57), even though for some applications, this is likely to result in a substantial overestimate. For many situations of interest, such as for building occupants, the exposure is only to chrysotile asbestos and there is a preponderance of short fibers; a considerably shallower slope may therefore be more appropriate.

The data upon which the model is based are for past, industrially exposed workers, whereas much of the current interest is in estimating potential risk for populations exposed to far lower, even environmental, exposure levels; use of the model for environmental and lower level occupational exposures therefore extrapolates far beyond the range of observations on workers, often by several orders of magnitude. The model assumes that risk is increased for any amount of expo-

Table 2 Lung Cancer Risk in Relation to Lung Fibrosis, Results of Two Studies

Autopsy Study (53)				Cohort Study (54)			
Histology (asbestosis category)	N	O/E	SPMR[a]	Radiography (abnormality category)	N	O/E	SMR[b]
None	302	8/12.4	65	None	420	10/9.5	105
				Pleural	62	2/1.5	133
Slight	69	11/3.6	306	0/1	83	4/2.3	178
Moderate	28	6/1.6	375	≥1/0	77	9/2.1	433

[a]Standardized proportional mortality ratio.
[b]Standardized mortality ratio.

sure, no matter how small, and is therefore referred to as a no-threshold model. It does not allow for the possibility of defense and repair mechanisms that may be capable of dealing with very small exposures and ignores the possibility that lung fibrosis may be a necessary precursor of increased lung cancer risk.

Assuming a slope of 0.01, in a working population exposed to indoor levels in buildings of 0.0001 f/ml for 20 years, the cumulative exposure is 0.002 f/ml-years, for a projected risk ratio of 1.00002, or an increase in relative risk of 0.002%. Thus, if the population consists of one million individuals with a background lifetime risk of 5% (50,000 individuals likely to die of lung cancer, a figure consistent for a mix of smokers and nonsmokers, men and women), then the asbestos exposure is estimated to increase this amount by 0.002%, or one case. Since approximately 50,000 would be expected to die of lung cancer anyway, the potential additional one case would be too small to be detectable.

Note that the estimated *number* of asbestos-attributable deaths depends on the background risk in the population. Therefore, if the current U.S. trend of reduced cigarette smoking among men continues and lung cancer mortality falls (as it already has for U.S. men younger than 45 years old), then the background risk (50,000 in the example above) will decline, resulting in a correspondingly lower number of projected additional cases.

III. Man-Made Mineral Fibers

A. Background

Although most commonly called man-made *mineral* fibers (MMMF), it has been pointed out that the technically correct term is *man-made vitreous fibers*, since minerals cannot be *man-made* (58). This point having been made, we will continue to refer to MMMF because of the prevalent use of this term.

The major categories of MMMF are fibrous glass (glass fibers, glass wool), rock wool, slag wool, and refractory ceramic fibers. In contrast to naturally occurring mineral fibers, MMMF are glassy and do not have a definite chemical composition or crystal structure. Asbestos can split longitudinally, whereas MMMF break predominantly across the fiber axis and do not form fibrils (as does chrysotile). Rock and slag wool are produced by blowing, centrifuging, or drawing molten rock or slag derived from metal smelting. The primary constituent of glass fibers is silica, usually in the form of finely powdered sand. Other ingredients include aluminum from kaolin clay or synthetic aluminum oxides, boric oxide, magnesium oxide, calcium oxide, fluoride, sodium sulfate, and iron oxide (6). Refractory ceramic fibers are made primarily by blowing and spinning and contain aluminum (or other oxides) and silica.

Although used in a wide range of products, many applications of specific MMMF are related to their thermal and acoustical insulation properties. Refractory ceramic fibers are primarily used for their resistance to very high temperatures (e.g., furnace insulation; aerospace applications). Glass fibers have also been used for air and liquid filtration and other special purposes. All MMMF can be in the respirable range in regard to physical dimension. These dimensions vary widely among fiber categories and products, and for some products many fibers are nonrespirable; for these reasons, actual counts of airborne fiber concentrations, taking into account fiber dimensions, are needed in order to quantify respirable fiber exposure levels. Such measured workplace concentrations of MMMF have been shown to be far lower (59) than those for asbestos known to have been present in past decades. In MMMF production and use, rock/slag wool and ceramic fibers have generally resulted in higher fiber concentrations than fibrous glass; an exception is special purpose fine-diameter glass fiber production, for which the concentrations have been shown to be higher than for the other fiber types. The question of durability of natural and man-made mineral fibers in the lungs is complex and depends upon, undoubtedly among other factors, dimension and chemical composition. What seems reasonably certain is that among asbestos fibers, chrysotile is far less durable than the amphiboles; for MMMF, ceramic fibers are more durable than glass and rock/slag wool fibers (60,61).

The likelihood of confounding carcinogenic exposures in this industry has been recognized (see Refs. 62,63) but incompletely identified and not quantified; these include asbestos, arsenic (from copper slag), polycyclic aromatic hydrocarbons, bitumen, and quartz. It is not likely that further detailed information in regard to these other exposures will be uncovered.

B. Epidemiological Studies

There have been two major studies of the mortality experience of MMMF workers, one of 16,661 male workers in 17 U.S. plants (64) and the other of 21,967 workers in 13 plants in seven European countries (65). The European study was conducted jointly by investigators from IARC and each of the seven countries. The U.S. study included exposure estimates for individual workers. The European study did not have quantitative information available concerning exposure levels, but considered employment during three "technological phases," for which the early and intermediate phases reportedly entailed considerably higher exposures than the late phase. Two smaller cohort studies of two Canadian plants have also been conducted (66,67), as well as two case-control investigations (68,69).

The lung cancer results (20 or more years from hire) for the U.S., European, and Canadian cohort studies appear in Table 3. Workers exposed exclusively to glass filament fibers are considered separately from other fibrous glass workers because of the higher nominal diameter of these fibers. Only a slightly elevated lung cancer risk was observed in two studies, neither of which was statistically significant.

Table 3 Lung Cancer Mortality[a] ≥20 Years from Hire, Results of Four Studies of MMMF Workers

Industry segment	U.S. study (64)	European study (65)	Canadian studies (66,67)[b]	Studies combined
FG[c] filament only	70/62.6	0/2.4	7/6.2	77/71.2
	111.9	0	114.0[f]	108.2
	[3][d]	[2][e]	[1]	[6]
FG (± filament)	280/246.6	46/41.3	12/6.2	338/294.1
	113.5*	111.4	194.2*	114.9**
	[8]	[5]	[1]	[14]
Rock/Slag wool	58/43.2	34/24.3	—	92/67.5
	134.2*	139.9*		136.2**
	[6]	[7]		[13]

[a]Observed number of lung cancer deaths/number expected based on regional rates; the U.S. study, respiratory cancer is reported.
[b]Reference 66 for FG, Ref. 67 for FG filament.
[c]FG = fibrous glass
[d]Number of plants.
[e]One plant produced FG during 1946–1960 and FG filament from 1961 on.
[f]15 or more years from hire.
*Observed significantly higher than expected, $p < 0.05$, Poisson distribution.
**Observed significantly higher than expected, $p < 0.01$, Poisson distribution.

For fibrous glass and rock/slag wool, the lung cancer results for the U.S. and European studies were remarkably similar. For fibrous glass, risk was elevated approximately 14% and 11%, respectively, an increase that was statistically significant in the larger U.S. study. Extensive analyses found no associations between risk and any exposure indices, including individual exposure estimates (U.S.), technological phase (Europe), or length of exposure. There was a relationship with time since hire in the European but not the U.S. study.

Lung cancer risk was higher in the smaller Canadian (66) study (20 or more years from hire, a standardized mortality ratio [SMR] of 194). However, risk was not related to exposure duration and was similarly elevated less than 10 (SMR = 244) and 10–20 years (SMR = 198) after hire. As stated by the authors, these observations are the opposite of what might be expected if the increase were caused by exposure.

In the U.S. study, four of the fibrous glass plants produced fine fibers, and it was possible to compare workers based on whether they were ever assigned to these areas of the plants. Contrary to earlier results (70), the later follow-up (64) observed no differences in lung cancer risk based on fine fiber exposure, even though exposure levels during fine fiber production were reportedly 10 times those during production of other glass fibers and similar to those for mineral wool (63).

Overall, risk for rock/slag wool workers was considerably higher than for fibrous glass workers and was significantly elevated in both studies. However, in the U.S. study, risk differed significantly among the six plants and was not related to any exposure indices or time since hire. In the European study, risk was not related to employment duration, but there were significant trends of risk with time since hire and technological phase (after accounting for time since hire).

The excess lung cancer risk among rock/slag wool workers in the European cohort was restricted to slag wool workers, who had an SMR (20 or more years after hire) of 188.5 (23/12.2) compared with 90.9 (11/12.1) for rock wool workers. A similar comparison is not possible in the U.S. study since all six rock/slag wool plants used slag either exclusively (four plants) or intermittently but with inadequate information for reliably categorizing workers by type of exposure.

The two case-control studies found no relationship between lung cancer and exposure. The first, an investigation of 73 lung cancers (and 536 controls) among employees of the English glass fiber plant in the European study, acquired more detailed exposure information than in the joint study; no relationship was observed between lung cancer and fine fiber exposure, duration of exposure or time since hire (68). A study of 55 lung cancers (and 98 controls) in nine U.S. slag wool plants, four of which had been included in the U.S. cohort study, had both smoking and exposure information available. Lung cancer risk was found to be associated with cigarette smoking but not to slag wool exposure indicators (69).

C. Interpreting the MMMF Information

Based on the accumulated data from two very large and two smaller studies, there is not conclusive evidence that lung cancer risk is elevated among fibrous glass workers. Risk was only slightly elevated, an increase potentially explained by unknown confounders such as cigarette smoking, a risk factor that could not be taken into account in these studies. Importantly, no relationship of risk with exposure has been demonstrated for this segment of the industry. It should be recognized, however, that airborne fiber levels were quite low, thereby limiting the power of these studies to detect such a relationship.

An elevated lung cancer risk has been demonstrated among rock/slag wool workers; however, these risks appear to be restricted to those exposed to slag wool. The strongest indication of an exposure-response relationship is the observation in the European study that risk was highest in the early and intermediate technological phases, when exposure levels were highest. The elevated risks in this segment of the industry are likely related to the workers' industrial exposures, but whether these risks can be attributed to the mineral fiber exposure is not clear.

In the U.S. study, there were significant differences in risk among rock/slag wool plants, differences that were not consistent with the estimated fiber exposures in these plants. There are possibly carcinogenic contaminants in this industry, especially in the slag wool segment, and there is evidence of past asbestos use in some of the rock/slag wool plants. However, in both the U.S. and European studies, risk in plants with known asbestos use does not appear to be substantially different from those without known use (63), but the limited availability of information on past asbestos use makes this observation inconclusive.

An earlier summary of the MMMF epidemiological evidence (57) noted that there was qualitative evidence of an exposure-response relationship because: (1) there was a similar hierarchy of fiber counts and lung cancer risks across the three sectors of the industry (rock/slag wool, glass wool, and glass filaments); and (2) glass wool workers exposed to small-diameter fibers had a higher risk than other such workers. However, results published since that review weakens this evidence. Risk (20 or more years from hire) for glass filament workers was similar to fibrous glass workers (see Table 3), even though fiber exposure levels were lower in the filament group. In the later U.S. follow-up, fine-fiber fibrous glass workers, whose fiber exposures were estimated to be 10 times higher than other fibrous glass workers and similar to workers in rock/slag wool production, were found to be at no higher risk than other fibrous glass workers.

While no mortality studies of ceramic fiber workers have been reported to date, the demonstrated greater tissue persistence of these fibers and animal inhalation studies indicating induction of tumors provide a strong basis for considerable concern in regard to potential carcinogenic risk to exposed humans.

In 1987, an IARC working group evaluated the epidemiological evidence concerning MMMF (6), concluding that there was: (1) inadequate evidence of carcinogenicity for glass wool and glass filament fibers; (2) limited evidence for rock/slag wool; and (3) no available data for ceramic fibers. When these conclusions were combined with an evaluation of the animal data, glass wool, rock/slag wool, and ceramic fibers were classified as Group 2B—possibly carcinogenic. Glass filament fibers were categorized as Group 3—not classifiable as to their carcinogenicity to humans. For rock/slag wool, the classification was based largely on the epidemiologic data. For glass and ceramic fibers, it was based largely on animal data, which were reasonably clear-cut for ceramic fibers but considerably less so for glass fibers.

IV. Discussion

Regarding lung cancer risk from asbestos exposure, with the exception of results for textile workers, lung cancer risk appears to be considerably higher for workers exposed to amphiboles than to chrysotile, controlling for amount of exposure. A possible explanation regarding a differing risk by fiber type is the differing durability of fibers in tissue; in vivo and in vitro experiments have demonstrated that chrysotile fibers are cleared by the lungs relatively rapidly, whereas amphibole fibers are durable, persisting in the lungs for long periods of time. While persistence per se of fibers in lung tissue has not been demonstrated to be related to increased risk (i.e., mineral-induced carcinogenesis may not require long-term residence in the target tissue), this determinant of pathogenic potency, which in turn is related to fiber type, is considered biologically plausible. The higher risk among textile workers, even those exposed only to chrysotile, compared with, for example, chrysotile miners with higher exposures, remains unexplained but may be related to the higher percentage of long fibers in textile manufacturing. This would be consistent with results from animal experiments, which have demonstrated that long, thin fibers are more pathogenic than short, coarse fibers (71,72).

The results noted here concerning factors affecting asbestos associated lung cancer risk have been summarized as indicating three overall influencing factors (inevitably labeled the "3 D's"): dose (both concentration and duration of exposure), durability, and dimension. The information concerning durability and dimension has been primarily a result of experimental work rather than epidemiological investigation.

Quantitative exposure-response relationships for humans have not, to date, taken durability and dimension of the fibers into account. Moreover, for most situations, risk assessments generally use the steep slope for the linear model, likely more appropriate for exposures involving amphiboles or asbestos textile exposures than for exposures such as to chrysotile-building products. This conservative approach, resulting in a likely substantial overestimate of risk, still produces risk estimates that indicate that lung cancer risk from general environmental asbestos exposures are extremely small, too low to be detected in an exposed population and smaller than many commonly accepted risks. Specifically, the earlier example of 20 years of exposure in a public building to 0.0001 f/ml of airborne asbestos corresponded to a projected risk of one lifetime lung cancer per million exposed, or approximately an annual rate of 0.02 cases (assuming a remaining lifetime of approximately 50 years). This risk is considerably lower than the annual death rates (per million) of approximately 60 for home accidents (ages 1–14), 18 for drowning, 16 for fires (ages 5–14), 14 for bicycling (ages 10–14), and 2 for floods (73,74).

For MMMF, epidemiological studies have demonstrated a clearly elevated lung cancer risk only for slag wool workers. Rock wool and fine glass fiber workers, whose fiber exposure levels were similar to those in slag wool production, were not found to be at elevated risk. Because of these observations and because the slag wool segment of the industry apparently has the greatest potential for contaminant carcinogenic exposures, it is not currently possible to determine how much of the risk in these workers can be ascribed to fiber and how much to such contaminant exposures.

In comparing epidemiological results of asbestos and MMMF workers, several important differences concerning these exposures are important to keep in mind. The first is the considerably lower airborne fiber exposure levels experienced by MMMF workers compared with past asbestos workers. For example, compared with 5–10 f/ml and higher airborne asbestos fiber concentrations for past asbestos workers, in the U.S. MMMF study, mean MMMF worker exposure levels were estimated as 0.35 f/ml for rock/slag wool, 0.04 f/ml for fibrous glass, 0.29 f/ml for fine diameter fibrous glass, and 0.01 f/ml for fibrous glass filament (63). This difference in exposure levels led to the observation that chrysotile asbestos exposure at 0.5 f/ml or lower for 20 years would be expected to result in only a small increase in lung cancer risk (57), approximately 10% or less [by Eq. (1), using a slope of 0.01].

Additionally, most industrial asbestos exposures were not contaminated with other possible carcinogens (with the possible exception of asbestos textile workers), whereas MMMF production includes numerous other exposures, including combustion by-products, contamination of the materials with other substances, and the possible past use of asbestos. And finally, asbestos fibers can have very much smaller diameters than MMMF, and most MMMF are cleared from the lungs far more rapidly than asbestos, particularly amphiboles.

V. Conclusions

It has now been firmly established by epidemiological studies that the risk of lung cancer in workers who have had occupational exposure to asbestos is dose-dependent. The observed risks in these studies have, however, been associated with far higher levels of asbestos exposure than those measured in the general indoor or outdoor environment, or indeed than current occupational exposures. Recent focus has therefore been on estimating risk at these lower exposure levels, assuming a linear, no-threshold model, making no adjustment for fiber type, and without taking into account the presence or absence of asbestosis. Resulting estimates have shown these risks to be low, particularly for environmental exposures. They may, however, be substantial *overestimates* (1) if lung fibrosis is a necessary condition for asbestos-related lung cancer risk and asbestosis is no longer a likely consequence of current exposures; (2) if fiber type is taken into account and exposures have been primarily to chrysotile; and (3) if smoking continues to decline in exposed populations—all factors likely to be operative in the future. Asbestosis as a necessary precursor for excess lung cancer risk would, in many circumstances, support a threshold model for risk estimation.

In contrast to asbestos-induced lung cancer risk, it has not been firmly established by human population-based studies that MMMF exposure increases the risk for lung cancer. Glass filament exposure surely does not constitute such a risk, glass fiber exposure is not likely to do so at manufacturing exposure levels, and while rock/slag wool production workers may have had an excess risk from past workplace exposures, dose-response relationships have not been demonstrated for the fiber component of their exposures. However, even absent epidemiological data, caution regarding refractory ceramic fiber exposure is justified on the basis of fiber characteristics in biological systems and the demonstrated carcinogenic effect of these fibers in animal models.

Finally, while recent evidence on fiber-induced lung cancer risk is encouraging from a public health standpoint, it continues to be prudent policy to control airborne concentrations of both asbestos and MMMF, with increased emphasis on occupational user exposures.

References

1. Enterline, P. E. (1991). Changing attitudes and opinions regarding asbestos and cancer, 1934–1965. *Am. J. Ind. Med.* 20:685–700.
2. Merewether, E. R. A. (1949). Annual report of the chief inspector of factories for the year 1947. London, HMSO.
3. Gloyne, S. R., and Leeds, M. D. (1951). Pneumoconiosis: A histological survey of necropsy material in 1,205 cases. *Lancet* 1:810–814.
4. Doll, R. (1955). Mortality from lung cancer in asbestos workers. *Br. J. Ind. Med.* 12: 81–86.
5. Virta, R. L. (1990). Asbestos. Annual Report. Washington, D.C., U.S. Department of the Interior, Bureau of Mines.
6. International Agency for Research on Cancer. (1988). *Man-Made Mineral Fibres and Radon*. IARC Monographs on the evaluation of carcinogenic risks to humans. Vol. 43. Lyon, IARC.
7. U.S. Environmental Protection Agency. (1989). EPA final rule on asbestos. *Fed. Reg.* 29:460.
8. U.S. Court of Appeals, Fifth Circuit. (1991). No. 89-4596. On petition for review of a rule of the Environmental Protection Agency, October 18.
9. Spengler, J. D. Özkaynak, H., McCarthy, J. F., and Lee, H. (1988). Summary of symposium on health aspects of exposure to asbestos in buildings. In *Proceedings of Symposium on Health Aspects of Exposure to Asbestos in Buildings, December 14–16, 1988*. Cambridge, MA, Harvard University, Energy and Environmental Policy Center, pp. 1–26.
10. Churg, A., and Wiggs, B. (1986) Fibre size and number in users of processed chrysotile ore, chrysotile miners, and members of the general population. *Am. J. Ind. Med.* 9:143–152.
11. Crump, K. S. (1990). *Science* 248:799.
12. Health Effects Institute—Asbestos Research, Asbestos Literature Review Panel. (1991). *Asbestos in Public and Commercial Buildings: A Literature Review and Synthesis of Current Knowledge*. Cambridge, MA, HEI-AR.

13. Selikoff, I. J., Hammond, E. C., and Seidman, H. (1979). Mortality experience of insulation workers in the United States and Canada, 1943–1976. *Ann. NY Acad. Sci.* 330:91–116.
14. McDonald, J. C., Liddell, F. D. K., Gibbs, G. W., Eyssen, G. E., and McDonald, A. D. (1980). Dust exposure and mortality in chrysotile mining, 1910–1975. *Br. J. Ind. Med.* 37:11–24.
15. Piolatto, G., Negri, E., La Vecchia, C., Pira, E., Decarli, A., and Peto, J. (1990). An update of cancer mortality among chrysotile asbestos miners in Balangero, northern Italy. *Br. J. Ind. Med.* 47:810–814.
16. Armstrong, B. K., De Klerk, N. H., Musk, A. W., and Hobbs, M. S. T. (1988). Mortality in miners and millers of crocidolite in Western Australia. *Br. J. Ind. Med.* 45:5–13.
17. Acheson, A. D., Gardner, M. J., Pippard, E. C., and Grime, L. P. (1982). The mortality of two groups of women who manufactured gas masks from chrysotile and crocidolite asbestos: a four-year follow-up. *Br. J. Ind. Med.* 39:344–348.
18. Jones, J. S. P., Smith, P. G., Pooley, F. D., Berry, G., Sawle, G. W., Wignall, B. K., Madeley, R. J., and Agarwal, A. (1980). The consequences of exposure to asbestos dust in a war-time gas mask factory. In *Biological Effects of Mineral Fibers*. Lyon, International Agency for Research on Cancer, pp. 637–653.
19. McDonald, J. C., and McDonald, A. D. (1981). Mesothelioma as an index of asbestos impact. In *Banbury Report No. 9, Quantification of Occupational Cancer*. Edited by Peto, R., and Schneiderman, M., Cold Spring Harbor, New York, Cold Spring Harbor Laboratory, pp. 73–85.
20. McDonald, A. D., Fry, J. S., Woolley, A. J., and McDonald J. C. (1984). Dust exposure and mortality in an American chrysotile asbestos friction products plant. *Br. J. Ind. Med.* 41:151–157.
21. Newhouse, M. L., and Sullivan, K. R. (1980). A mortality study of workers manufacturing friction materials: 1941–1986. *Br. J. Ind. Med.* 46:176.
22. Acheson, E. D., Gardner, M. J., Winter, P. D., and Bennett, C. (1984). Cancer in a factory using amosite asbestos. *Int. J. Epidemiol.* 13:3–10.
23. Seidman, H., Selikoff, I. J., and Gelb, S. K. (1986). Mortality experience of amosite asbestos factory workers: Dose-response relationships 5 to 40 years after onset of short-term work exposure. *Am. J. Ind. Med.* 10:479–514.
24. Weiss, W. (1977). Mortality of a cohort exposed to chrysotile asbestos. *J. Occup. Med.* 19:737–740.
25. Enterline, P. E., Hartley, J., and Henderson, V. (1987). Asbestos and cancer: A cohort followed up to death. *Br. J. Ind. Med.* 44:396–401.
26. Thomas, H. F., Benjamin, I. T., Elwood, P. C., and Sweetnam, P. M. (1982). Further follow-up study of workers from an asbestos cement factory. *Br. J. Ind. Med.* 39: 273–276.
27. Ohlson, C.-G., and Hogstedt, C. (1985). Lung cancer among asbestos cement workers. A Swedish cohort study and a review. *Br. J. Ind. Med.* 42:397–402.
28. Gardner, M. J., Winter, P. D., Pannett, B., and Powell, C. A. (1986). Follow-up study of workers manufacturing chrysotile asbestos cement products. *Br. J. Ind. Med.* 43: 726–732.

29. Hughes, J. M., Weill, H., and Hammad, Y. Y. (1987). Mortality of workers employed in two asbestos cement manufacturing plants. *Br. J. Ind. Med.* 44:161–174.
30. Albin, M., Jakobsson, K., Attewell, R., Johansson, L., and Welinder, H. (1990). Mortality and cancer morbidity in cohorts of asbestos cement workers and referents. *Br. J. Ind. Med.* 47:602–610.
31. Raffn, E., Lynge, E., Juel, K., and Korsgaard, B. (1989). Incidence of cancer and mortality among employees in the asbestos cement industry in Denmark. *Br. J. Ind. Med.* 46:90–96.
32. Finkelstein, M. M. (1984). Mortality among employees of an Ontario asbestos-cement factory. *Am. Rev. Respir. Dis.* 129:754–761.
33. Alies-Patin, A. M., and Velleron, A. J. (1985). Mortality of workers in a French asbestos cement factory, 1940–1982. *Br. J. Ind. Med.* 42:219–225.
34. Lacquet, L. M., and van der Linden, L. (1980). Roetgenographic lung changes, asbestosis and mortality in a Belgian asbestos-cement factory. In *Biological Effects of Mineral Fibers*. Edited by J. C. Wagner and W. Davis. Vol 2. IARC Scientific Publication No. 30. Lyon, International Agency for Research on Cancer, pp. 783–793.
35. Neuberger, M., and Kundi, M. (1990). Individual asbestos exposure: Smoking and mortality—a cohort study in the asbestos cement industry. *Br. J. Ind. Med.* 47: 615–620.
36. McDonald, A. D., Fry, J. S., Woolley, A. J., and McDonald, J. C. (1983). Dust exposure and mortality in an American chrysotile textile plant. *Br. J. Ind. Med.* 40: 361–367.
37. Robinson, C., Lemen, R., and Wagoner, J. K. (1979). Mortality patterns, 1940–1975, among workers employed in an asbestos textile friction and packing products manufacturing facility. In *Dusts and Disease*. Edited by R. Lemen and J. Dement. Park Forest, IL, Pathotex Publishers, pp. 131–144.
38. McDonald, A. D., Fry, J. S., Woolley, A. J., and McDonald, J. C. (1983). Dust exposure and mortality in an American factory using chrysotile, amosite and crocidolite in mainly textile manufacture. *Br. J. Ind. Med.* 40:368–374.
39. Peto, J., Doll, R., Hermon, C., Binns, W., Clayton, R., and Goffe, T. (1985). Relationship of mortality to measures of environmental asbestos pollution in an asbestos textile factory. *Ann. Occup. Hyg.* 29:305–355.
40. Newhouse, M. L., Berry, G., and Wagner, J. C. (1985). Mortality of factory workers in east London, 1933–1980. *Br. J. Ind. Med.* 42:4–11.
41. Liddell, F. D. K., and Hanley, J. A. (1985). Relations between asbestos exposure and lung cancer SMRs in occupational cohort studies. *Br. J. Ind. Med.* 42:389–396.
42. Gardner, M. J., (1989). A review of the available evidence for setting occupational exposure limits for asbestos, Annexe to report prepared by a World Health Organization Meeting, Oxford, April 10–11.
43. McDonald, J. C., and McDonald, A. D. (1986). Epidemiology of asbestos-related lung cancer. In *Asbestos-Related Malignancies*. Edited by A. Antman. Orlando, FL, Grune & Stratton, pp. 57–79.
44. Dement, J. M. (1991). Carcinogenicity of chrysotile asbestos: A case control study of textile workers. *Cell. Biol. Toxicol.* 7:59–65.

45. Sebastien, P., McDonald, J. C., McDonald, A. D., Case, B., and Harley, R. (1989). Respiratory cancer in chrysotile textile and mining industries: Exposure inferences from lung analysis. *Br. J. Ind. Med.* 46:180–187.
46. Davis, J. M. G. (1989). Mineral fibre carcinogenesis: Experimental data relating to the importance of fibre type, size, deposition, dissolution and migration. In *Non-Occupational Exposure to Mineral Fibres*. Edited by J. Bignon, J. Peto, and R. Saracci. Lyon, IARC Scientific Publications No. 90, pp. 33–45.
47. Browne, K. (1986). Is asbestos or asbestosis the cause of the increased risk of lung cancer in asbestos workers? *Br. J. Ind. Med.* 43:145–149.
48. Kuschner, M. (1987). The effects of MMMF on animal systems: Some reflections on their pathogenesis. *Ann. Occup. Hyg.* 31:791–797.
49. World Health Organization, International Agency for Research on Cancer. (1987). *Silica and some silicates, 1986*. Vol. 42. IARC monographs on the evaluation of the carcinogenic risk of chemicals to humans. Lyon, WHO.
50. Turner-Warwick, M., Lebowitz, M., Burrows, B., and Johnson, A. (1980). Cryptogenic fibrosing alveolitis and lung cancer. *Thorax* 35:496–499.
51. Rom, W. M., Travis, W. D., and Brody, A. R. (1991). Cellular and molecular basis of the asbestos-related diseases. *Am. Rev. Respir. Dis.* 143:408–422.
52. Kipen, H. M., Lilis, R., Suzuki, Y., Valciukas, J. A., and Selikoff, I. J. (1987). Pulmonary fibrosis in asbestos insulation workers with lung cancer: A radiological and histopathological evaluation. *Br. J. Ind. Med.* 44:96–100.
53. Sluis-Cremer, G. K., and Bezuidenhout, B. N. (1989). Relation between asbestosis and bronchial cancer in amphibole asbestos miners. *Br. J. Ind. Med.* 46:537–540.
54. Hughes, J., and Weill, H. (1991). Asbestosis as a necessary precursor of asbestos-related lung cancer: Results of a prospective mortality study in asbestos products manufacturing. *Br. J. Ind. Med.* 48:229–233.
55. Consumer Product Safety Commission. (1983). Report of the Chronic Hazard Advisory Panel on Asbestos, Washington, D.C.
56. Environmental Protection Agency. (1986). Airborne Asbestos Health Assessment Update. Washington, D.C.
57. Doll, R. (1987). Symposium on MMMF, Copenhagen, October, 1986: Overview and conclusions. *Ann. Occup. Hyg.* 31:805–819.
58. Nomenclature Committee of TIMA Inc. (1991). Nomenclature of man-made vitreous fibers. TIMA Inc.
59. Esmen, N., Corn, M., Hammad, Y., Whittier, D., and Kotsko, N. (1979). Summary of measurements of employee exposure to airborne dust and fiber in 16 facilities producing man-made mineral fibers. *Am. Ind. Hyg. Assoc.* 40:108–117.
60. Meek, M. E. (1991). Lung cancer and mesothelioma related to man-made mineral fibers: The toxicological evidence. In *Mineral Fibers and Health*. Edited by D. Liddell and C. Miller. Boca Raton, FL, CRC Press, pp. 265–282.
61. Davis, J. M. G. (1991). Information obtained from fiber-induced lesions in animals. In *Mineral Fibers and Health*. Edited by D. Liddell and C. Miller, Boca Raton, FL, CRC Press, pp. 249–263.
62. Öhberg, J. (1987). Technological development of the mineral wool industry in Europe. *Ann. Occup. Hyg.* 31(4B):529–545.

63. Enterline, P. E. (1991). Carcinogenic effects of man-made vitreous fibers. *Ann. Rev. Publ. Health* 12:459–480.
64. Marsh, G. M., Enterline, P. E., Stone, R. A., and Henderson, V. L. (1990). Morality among a cohort of U.S. man-made mineral fiber workers: 1985 follow-up. *J. Occup. Med.* 32:594–604.
65. Simonato, L., Fletcher, A. C., Cherrie, J., Andersen, A., Bertazzi, P., et al. (1987). European historical cohort study: Extension of the follow-up. *Ann. Occup. Hyg.* 31: 603–623.
66. Shannon, H. S., Jamieson, E., Julian, J. A., Muir, D. C. F., and Walsch, C. (1987). Mortality experience of glass fiber workers: extended follow-up. *Ann. Occup. Hyg.* 31:657–662.
67. Shannon, H. S., Jamieson, E., Julian, J. A., and Muir, D. C. F. (1990). Mortality of glass filament (textile) workers. *Br. J. Ind. Med.* 47:533–536.
68. Gardner, M. J., Magnani, C, Pannett, B., Fletcher, A. C., and Winter, P. D. (1988). Lung cancer among glass fibre production workers: A case-control study. *Br. J. Ind. Med.* 45:613–618.
69. Wong, O., and Foliart, D. A case-control study of lung cancer in a cohort of workers potentially exposed to slag wool fibers. *Br. J. Ind. Med.* (1991) 48:818–824.
70. Enterline, P. E., and Marsh, G. M. (1987). Mortality update of a cohort of US man-made mineral fiber workers. *Ann. Occup. Hyg.* 31:625–656.
71. Pott, F. (1978). Some aspects of dosimetry of the carcinogenic potency of asbestos and other fibrous dusts. *Staub-Reinhalt Luft* 38:486–490.
72. Stanton, M. F., Layard, M., Tegeris, A., et al. (1981). Relation of particle dimension to carcinogenicity in amphibole asbestos and other fibrous minerals. *JNCI* 67: 965–975.
73. Weill, H., and Hughes, J. M. (1986). Asbestos as a public health risk: Disease and policy. *Ann. Rev. Public Health* 7:171–192.
74. Commins, B. T. (1984). Estimates of risk from environmental asbestos in perspective. In *Non-occupational Exposure to Mineral Fibres*. Edited by J. Bignon, J. Peto, and R. Saracci. IARC Scientific Publication No. 90. Lyon, International Agency for Research on Cancer, pp. 476–485.

9

Arsenic and Lung Cancer

WILLIAM J. BLOT and JOSEPH F. FRAUMENI, JR.

National Cancer Institute
National Institutes of Health
Bethesda, Maryland

I. Introduction

Although arsenic has generally failed to induce cancer in experimental animals, epidemiological studies from around the world clearly indicate that inorganic arsenic is a pulmonary carcinogen in humans. The evidence derives primarily from observations of rising risk of lung cancer with increasing level of exposure to arsenic trioxide among copper smelter workers, although excesses of lung cancer have been documented among other population groups inhaling inorganic arsenic and possibly ingesting these compounds in drinking water or pharmaceuticals. This chapter summarizes results from these studies and examines the nature of the etiological association between arsenic exposure and lung cancer.

II. Occupational Exposures

In 1948, Hill and Faning (1) reported five deaths from lung cancer among workers manufacturing arsenic-containing pesticides used as sheep dip, whereas only one was expected based on the proportion of lung cancer deaths among other factory workers with little or no exposure to arsenic. Although there had been numerous reports of skin tumors following ingestion of arsenical compounds (2), this was the first suggestion that inorganic arsenic may increase the risk of lung cancer.

A. Smelters

The most extensive evidence implicating arsenic as a lung carcinogen has come from studies of nonferrous smelter workers, particularly copper smelters. Inorganic arsenic is a constituent of most copper ores and, to a lesser degree, of lead and zinc ores. Arsenic is removed during the smelting of these ores: some is recovered during the smelting process (most commercial arsenic trioxide is obtained from smelters), while the rest is emitted as an industrial air pollutant, which may be inhaled by workers and residents in adjacent neighborhoods. Elevated levels of arsenic have been detected in hair, urine, and lung tissue of exposed individuals (3–7).

In 1969, Lee and Fraumeni (8) reported a threefold increased standardized mortality ratio (SMR) from lung cancer among a cohort of approximately 8000 workers at a Montana copper smelter. This was the first large-scale epidemiological investigation of arsenic-exposed workers and the first to quantify risk according to estimated level of exposure of each worker. Earlier surveys of copper smelter workers had failed to detect an increased risk (9). Lee and Fraumeni showed that the SMRs for lung cancer rose in proportion to maximum arsenic exposure, with an eightfold excess among men who had worked in areas of the smelter, such as the arsenic roaster and Cottrell, where arsenic contamination was the most severe. Extended follow-up of this cohort confirmed that the excess lung cancer risk persisted through the 1970s and further clarified the level of risk according to

Table 1 SMRs for Lung Cancer According to Cumulative Exposure to Airborne Arsenic Among Montana Copper Smelter Workers

Cumulative arsenic exposure ($mg/m^3 \times$ years)	No. lung cancer deaths	SMR
<0.9	20	168
0.9–1.9	33	256
2.0–8.3	43	167
8.4–41.6	115	315
41.7–208.3	54	429
208.4–416.6	20	571
416.7+	17	680

Source: Adapted from Ref. 11.

intensity, duration, and timing of arsenic exposure (10–13). Table 1 shows that the SMRs for lung cancer tended to rise nearly linearly with estimated cumulative arsenic exposure. Risk also rose with alternative indices, including time-weighted average exposure and maximum level of exposure. Risk among these smelter workers and others did not consistently decline as years since cessation of exposure increased, but excess risk increased with age at first exposure (13,14).

Similar observations have come from follow-up of workers in copper smelters in Washington (15), Utah (16,17), and elsewhere in the United States (17), as well as in Japan (18), Sweden (19), and China (20). Table 2 lists results of evaluation of lung cancer mortality in these cohorts. Twofold or higher SMRs have been found in nearly all groups, with risk usually rising in proportion to arsenic exposure. In the United States, the highest arsenic levels (up to 3% arsenic) in the copper ores smelted were found at the Anaconda smelter in Montana, the Tacoma smelter in Washington, and the Garfield smelter in Utah (11,15,17). Lung cancer risks were elevated among workers at these smelters, but not at seven other American copper smelters where arsenic content of the feed ores was generally less than one-tenth as high (17).

Workers in the copper smelters were typically exposed to several pollutants in addition to arsenic trioxide. Prominent among these was sulfur dioxide (SO_2), since most ores were sulfide-based. Arsenic and SO_2 exposures tended to be highly correlated, but when the two factors were assessed jointly, the major effect on lung cancer was associated with arsenic and not SO_2 (10,17,19). The potentially interactive effects of arsenic and cigarette smoking have been evaluated in some of the smelter cohort studies. In Montana, most of the men had smoked, but risks of lung cancer increased with rising arsenic exposure among nonsmokers as well as smokers, and SMRs associated with high arsenic exposure were greater

Table 2 Cohort Studies of Lung Cancer Among Copper Smelter Workers

Study location	Size of cohort	No. of lung cancer deaths	SMR	Dose-response trends	Ref.
Montana	8047	302	286	+	11
Washington	2802	104	263	+	15
Utah	2288	48	211	+	17
Arizona, Nevada, Tennessee	3790	45	86		17
Japan	839	29	1189	+	18
Sweden	3916	103	372	+	19
China	NA	26	360		22

than SMRs associated with smoking (21). In combination, arsenic and smoking appeared to act in more of an additive than a multiplicative fashion in enhancing lung cancer risk. Similarly, among tin miners and smelter workers in southern China, heavy exposure to arsenic conveyed a higher risk than cigarette or water pipe smoking, and the effects appeared additive (22). In Sweden, although arsenic was found to be a strong risk factor among nonsmokers, smoking and cumulative arsenic exposure increased risk of lung cancer in a fashion between additive and multiplicative (23) (Table 3). In all studies, however, spareness of data has precluded clear-cut evaluations of the form of the interaction.

Only limited data are available on the histological types of lung cancer among arsenic-exposed workers. All cell types seem to be increased, although some studies suggest that lung adenocarcinoma may be disproportionately affected (24,25).

B. Miners

Workers mining copper and certain other ores with arsenic content are also exposed to airborne arsenical dusts. The numbers of studies have been smaller, but increased risks of lung cancer have been reported among Rhodesian gold miners (26), copper and other hard rock miners in the United States (27), and tin miners in China (22,28) and Great Britain (29). Although arsenic exposure was common to each of these groups, the underground miners often had concomitant exposure to radon, silica, or other potential carcinogens. Among one group of Chinese tin miners with little radon exposure, up to threefold excesses of lung cancer were associated with heavy exposure to arsenic dusts (25), and in another risks associated with heavy arsenic were of similar magnitude to those associated with heavy radon exposure (22).

Table 3 Odds Ratios for Lung Cancer According to Cumulative Arsenic Exposure and Smoking Status Among Swedish Copper Smelter Workers

Cumulative arsenic exposure ($mg/m^3 \times$ years)	Nonsmokers	Smokers
<0.25	1.0[a]	7.5
0.25–14.9	0.8	7.9
15–99.9	2.8	10.4
100+	7.1	29.6

[a]Reference category.
Source: Ref. 19.

C. Pesticide Manufacturers and Users

The major use of arsenic around the world has been in the making of insecticides, fungicides, and herbicides (30). As previously noted, the earliest report of arsenic-related lung cancer came from a study of workers making arsenic trioxide pesticides, which were used to control insects on sheep (1). The most common pesticides were calcium and lead arsenates, used in vineyards and orchards, but their production and application have declined substantially since peaking in the 1940s. Proportionate mortality surveys in the 1950s revealed that lung cancer was disproportionately represented among vineyard workers applying arsenicals in France and Germany (31,32). The workers were exposed not only through inhalation of airborne dusts, but also through ingestion of wine contaminated with arsenate residues. In Washington State, arsenical pesticides were extensively used in apple and pear orchards, but follow-up of orchardists has revealed little or no excess risk of lung cancer (33,34).

Increased risks of lung cancer have been documented among American workers involved in the production of arsenical pesticides. Among a cohort of men producing lead arsenate, calcium arsenate, sodium arsenite, and other pesticides in Baltimore, there was a 68% excess of lung cancer mortality overall, with the increase surpassing 10-fold for workers with high exposures for 15 or more years (36). In comparison, workers manufacturing nonarsenical pesticides at the plants showed no excess of lung cancer. Furthermore, there was an increased risk of lung cancer among 611 workers producing pesticides at a Michigan chemical plant, with SMRs rising with increasing cumulative arsenic exposure (37). Extended follow-up of this cohort into the 1980s revealed an overall twofold excess of respiratory cancer, with mild trends in risk associated with increasing duration of exposure and decreasing interval since cessation of employment (38).

Because of pesticide residues on tobacco, cigarette smokers may also inhale trace amounts of arsenic. Arsenic content of U.S. cigarettes rose to over 40 μg/cigarette in the 1950s before falling substantially by the 1960s (30).

D. Other Occupational Exposures

Industrial uses of arsenic extend to a variety of occupational groups. For example, high concentrations of urinary arsenic have been detected among workers handling wood treated with arsenic pentoxide preservatives, but cancer risk in this group has not been evaluated (39,40). Arsenic is also widely used in glass production. Although exposures to arsenic have not been quantified, increased risks of lung cancer have been reported among glass production workers (41). Further, arsenic is employed in the production of semiconductors, with documented airborne release of low levels during implantation of arsenic onto silicon wafers (42).

III. General Environmental Exposures

A. Arsenical Air Pollution

In 1975 an analysis of lung cancer mortality rates in U.S. counties where copper, lead, or zinc primary smelters were located revealed higher than expected rates among both males and females (43). Although data on smoking prevalences were unavailable and occupational exposures may have contributed to the pattern among men, the higher rates raised the possibility of a hazard from industrial emissions of inorganic arsenic. Such an effect seemed plausible because environmental studies in the vicinity of smelters revealed arsenical pollution, with elevated levels of urinary and hair arsenic in children living close to smelter stacks (3,4,6). Since publication of this correlational study, several investigations have characterized risk of lung cancer among residents near smelters according to indices of arsenical air pollution. Because pollutant levels fall sharply as distance of residence from the smelter increases, with most metallic fallout occurring within a few kilometers of the central stacks, and because most smelters are located in relatively remote areas, the populations studied have been small. Perhaps in part due to the small numbers, results have been mixed (44). Comparisons of residences of patients with lung cancer vs. breast and prostate cancers in 10 areas of the western United States where smelters were located found no significant differences, although only small percentages of the families lived within 2 km of the smelters (45,46). However, a review of lung cancer death certificates over a 35-year period among females living near the Tacoma copper smelter revealed a trend of rising risk with an index of arsenic exposure, with a 60% excess observed in the highest quintile of exposure (47). In Quebec, lung cancer rates were higher in a town where a copper smelter was located than in a neighboring community, with the excess not attributable to occupation or smoking (48).

Three case-control studies of lung cancer have found increased risks among residents exposed to smelter effluents after adjusting for smoking and occupation. In eastern Pennsylvania a 60% excess was found among residents living close to a zinc smelter and in areas where soil levels of arsenic were elevated (49). In northern Sweden a twofold excess was detected among men living near a copper smelter (50). A larger investigation was recently completed in Shenyang, China, where one of China's largest copper smelters is located in a highly populated urban area (20). After adjusting for smoking and work in the smelter, a threefold excess risk in the mid-1980s was found among men who lived within 1 km of the smelter, but not at greater distances. No concomitant excess risk was found among women.

Arsenical pollution has been reported also in the vicinity of a pesticide-manufacturing plant in Baltimore (51). Lung cancer mortality rates among men, but not women, in the affected census tracts were nearly twice as high as in matched control areas.

B. Arsenic-Contaminated Drinking Water

The strongest suggestion that ingested arsenic may result in an increased risk of lung cancer arises from recent observations among persons consuming arsenic-contaminated drinking water. In Taiwan, endemic arsenic poisoning has been linked to elevated mortality from several cancers (52,53). Most prominent are nonmelanoma skin cancers associated with chronic cutaneous arsenicism, along with cancers of the urinary tract (bladder and kidney). Lung cancer rates also varied with the extent of arsenic water concentrations, being more than twice as high among men and women in contaminated areas. In a case-control study that involved 76 cases in the endemic area and controlled for cigarette smoking, risk of lung cancer rose in proportion to duration of exposure to contaminated well water (54). The excess was threefold among those consuming arsenic-contaminated water for 40 or more years compared to nonusers. In Japan, an elevated proportion of lung cancer has been noted among villagers exposed to arsenic through industrial pollution (55). There also were chronic skin arsenicism and accompanying skin tumors, along with high arsenic water levels, suggesting that the excess lung cancer may be linked to arsenical water pollution as well as air pollution.

IV. Medical Exposures

Potassium arsenite (Fowler's solution) was prescribed as a treatment for several illnesses, especially of the skin, although its use was discontinued in the 1960s. In a recent followup of 478 patients treated with Fowler's solution for periods ranging from 2 weeks to 12 years during 1945–1969 in rural England, 14 respiratory cancer deaths were recorded, exactly equal to the 14.0 deaths expected based on English/Welsh national rates (56). There was a modest rise in risk with cumulative arsenic dose, but the trend was not significant. It is noteworthy that in a subset of the cohort given dermatological examinations, all of the cancer deaths occurred among the approximately 50% with skin keratoses and other signs of chronic arsenicism. In a small cohort of Danish skin disease patients treated with arsenical drugs, no significant excess of lung or other noncutaneous tumors was seen (57). Thus, there is no clear epidemiological support for the many clinical reports of lung cancer among persons with chronic arsenical dermatoses, including skin tumors induced by arsenic medications (58).

V. Mechanistic Pathways

The mechanisms by which the trivalent form of inorganic arsenic induce lung cancer are unknown. Few clues arise from carcinogenesis bioassays, because arsenic and its compounds have failed to either initiate or promote cancer in experimental animals (30). In addition, arsenic is considered at most a weak mutagen in *E. coli* and mammalian cells (30). Arsenic has long been known for its toxicity, however, and it can cause cell transformation, chromosomal aberrations, and sister chromatic exchanges, and it can inhibit DNA repair in animal systems (59–61). These effects are considerably greater for the trivalent (arsenite) than pentavalent (arsenate) forms of inorganic arsenic. Arsenic has recently been shown to induce amplification of oncogenes in culture, suggesting a role in the progression of initiated cells in the lung (61).

Epidemiological leads to causal mechanisms are also scarce, although mathematical modeling of risks is consistent with arsenic being more involved in late rather than early stages of carcinogenesis. Risk, however, does not decline substantially following cessation of exposure, as it does, for example, among cigarette smokers who quit smoking, as would be expected if arsenic acted at a penultimate stage of the lung cancer process. The available data indicate that lung cancer can be induced by arsenic alone, with exposures to smoking or other occupational agents (e.g., SO_2) not required for its carcinogenic effect.

VI. Conclusions

There is substantial epidemiological evidence that inhalation of inorganic arsenic in its trivalent forms is a cause of lung cancer in the workplace and in surrounding neighborhoods, although mechanisms of action are unclear. Recent data from Taiwan suggest that ingestion of arsenic in contaminated well water also may increase the risk of lung and other cancers, but further studies are needed to confirm this finding. Epidemiological and multidisciplinary research is also needed to determine whether pentavalent forms of inorganic arsenic increase the risk of lung cancer, to further evaluate interactions between arsenic and other environmental and susceptibility factors, and to apply laboratory probes that can elucidate carcinogenic processes at the molecular and cellular levels.

References

1. Hill, A. B., and Faning, E. L. (1948). Studies in the incidence of cancer in a factory handling inorganic compounds of arsenic. I. Mortality experience in the factory. *Br. J. Ind. Med.* 5:1–6.
2. Neubauer, O. (1947). Arsenical cancer: A review. *Br. J. Cancer* 1:192–251.
3. Milham, S., and Strong, T. (1974). Human arsenic exposure in relation to a copper smelter. *Environ. Res.* 7:176–182.
4. Baker, E. L., Hayes, C. G., Landrigan, P. J., Handke, J. L., Leger, F. I., Housworth, J., and Harrington, M. J. (1977). A nationwide survey of heavy metal absorption in

children living near primary copper, lead, and zinc smelters. *Am. J. Epidemiol.* 106: 261–273.

5. Webster, P. O., Brune, D., and Nordberg, G. (1981). Arsenic and selenium in lung, liver, and kidney tissue from dead smelter workers. *Br. J. Ind. Med.* 38:179–184.
6. Hartwell, T. D., Handy, R. W., Harris, B. J., Williams, S. R., and Gelbach, S. H. (1983). Heavy metal exposure in populations living around zinc and copper smelters. *Arch. Environ. Health* 38:284–295.
7. Blom, S., Lagerkvist, B., and Linderholm, H. (1985). Arsenic exposure to smelter workers. *Scand. J. Work. Environ. Health* 11:265–269.
8. Lee, A. M., and Fraumeni, J. F. (1969). Arsenic and respiratory cancer in man: An occupational study. *JNCI* 43:1045–1052.
9. Pinto, S. S., and Bennett, B. M. (1963). Effect of arsenic trioxide exposure on mortality. *Arch. Environ. Health* 7:583–591.
10. Lubin, J. H., Pottern, L. M., Blot, W. J., Tokudome, S., Stone, B. J., and Fraumeni, J. F. (1981). Respiratory cancer among copper smelter workers: Recent mortality statistics. *J. Occup. Med.* 23:779–784.
11. Lee-Feldstein, A. (1986). Cumulative exposure to arsenic and its relationship to respiratory cancer among copper smelter employees. *J. Occup. Med.* 28:296–302.
12. Lee-Feldstein, A. (1989). A comparison of several measures of exposure to arsenic; matched case-control study of copper smelter employees. *Am. J. Epidemiol.* 129: 112–124.
13. Brown, C. C., and Chu, K. C. (1983). Implications of the multistage theory of carcinogenesis applied to occupational arsenic exposure. *JNCI* 70:455–463.
14. Mazumder, S., Redmond, C. K., Enterline, P. E., Marsh, G. M., Costantino, J. P., Zhou, S. Y., and Patwardkan, R. N. (1989). Multistage modeling of lung cancer mortality among arsenic-exposed copper smelter workers. *Risk Anal.* 9:551–563.
15. Enterline, P. E., Henderson, V. L., and Marsh, G. M. (1987). Exposure to arsenic and respiratory cancer: A reanalysis. *Am. J. Epidemiol.* 125:929–938.
16. Rencher, A. C., Carter, M. W., and McKee, D. W. (1977). A retrospective epidemiologic study of mortality at a large western copper smelter. *J. Occup. Med.* 19: 754–758.
17. Enterline, P. E., Marsh, G. M., Esmen, N. A., Henderson, V. L., Callahan, C. M., and Paik, M. (1987). Some effects of cigarette smoking, arsenic and SO_2 on mortality among U.S. copper smelter workers. *J. Occup. Med.* 29:831–838.
18. Tokudome, S., and Kuratsune, M. (1976). A cohort study on mortality from cancer and other causes among workers at a metal refinery. *Int. J. Cancer* 17:310–317.
19. Jarup, L., and Pershagen, G. (1991). Arsenic exposure, smoking and lung cancer in smelter workers: A case-control study. *Am. J. Epidemiol.* 134:545–551.
20. Xu, Y. Z., Blot, W. J., Xiao, H. P., Wu, A., Feng, Y. P., Stone, B. J., Sun, J., Ershow, A., Henderson, B. E., and Fraumeni, J. F. (1989). Smoking, air pollution, and the high rates of lung cancer in Shenyang China. *JNCI* 81:1800–1806.
21. Welch, K., Higgins, I., Oh, M., and Burchfiel, C. (1982). Arsenic exposure, smoking, and respiratory cancer in copper smelter workers. *J. Occup. Med.* 37: 325–335.
22. Taylor, P. R., Qiao, Y. L., Schatzkin, A., Yao, S. X., Lubin, J., Mao, B. L., Rao, J. Y.,

McAdams, M., Xuan, X. Z., and Li, J. Y. (1959). Relation of arsenic exposure to lung cancer among tin miners in Yunnan Province China. *Br. J. Ind. Med.* 46:881–888.
23. Jarup, L., and Pershagen, G. (1991). Arsenic exposure, smoking and lung cancer in smelter workers: A case-control study. *Am. J. Epidemiol.* 134:545–551.
24. Wicks, M., Archer, V. E., Auerbach, O., and Kuschnver, M. (1981). Arsenic exposure in a copper smelter as related to histological types of lung cancer. *Am. J. Ind. Med.* 2:25–32.
25. Pershagen, G., Bergman, F., Klominek, J., Damber, L., and Wall, S. (1987). Histological types of lung cancer among smelter workers exposed to arsenic. *Br. J. Ind. Med.* 44:454–458.
26. Osburn, H. S. (1969). Lung cancer in a mining district in Rhodesia. *S. Afr. Med. J.* 43: 1307–1312.
27. Wagoner, J. K., Miller, R. W., Lundin, F. E., Fraumeni, J. F., and Haid, M. (1963). Unusual cancer mortality among a group of underground metal miners. *N. Engl. J. Med.* 269:284–289.
28. McLaughlin, J. K., Chen, J., Dosemeci, M., Chen, R., Rexing, S., Wu, Z., Hearl, F. B., McCawley, M. A., and Blot, W. J. (1992). A nested case-control study of lung cancer among silica-exposed workers in China. *Br. J. Ind. Med.* 49:167–171.
29. Hodgson, J. T., and Jones, R. D. (1990). Mortality of a cohort of tin miners 1941–86. *Br. J. Ind. Med.* 47:665–676.
30. International Agency for Research on Cancer. (1980). *Evaluation of the Carcinogenic Risk of Chemicals to Man*. Vol. 23, *Some Metals and Metallic Compounds*. Lyon, IARC.
31. Roth, F., (1957). The sequelae of chronic arsenic poisoning in Moselle vinters. *Germ. Med. Month.* 2:172–176.
32. Galy, P., Touraine, R., Brune, J., Boudier, P., and Gallois, P. (1963). Le cancer pulmonaire d'origine arsenicals des vignerons du Beaujolais. *J. Franc. Med. Chir. Thorac.* 17:303–311.
33. Nelson, W. E., Lykins, M. H., Mackey, J., Newill, V. A., Finklea, J. F., and Hammer, P. I. (1973). Mortality among orchard workers exposed to lead arsenate: A cohort study. *J. Chron. Dis.* 26:105–118.
34. Wicklund, K. G., Daling, J. R., Allard, J., and Weiss, N. S. (1988). Respiratory cancer among orchardists in Washington state, 1968 to 1980. *J. Occup. Med.* 30: 561–564.
36. Mabuchi, K., Lilienfeld, A., and Snell, L. M. (1979). Lung cancer among pesticide workers exposed to inorganic arsenicals. *Arch. Environ. Health* 34:312–320.
37. Ott, M. G., Holder, B. B., and Gordon, H. L. (1974). Respiratory cancer and occupational health. *Arch. Environ. Health* 29:250–255.
38. Sobel, W., Bond, G. G., Baldwin, C. L., and Ducommun, D. J. (1988). An update of respiratory cancer and occupational exposure to arsenicals. *Am. J. Ind. Med.* 13: 263–270.
39. Rosenberg, M. J., Landrigan, P. J., and Crowley, S. (1980). Low-level arsenic exposure in wood processing plants. *Am. J. Ind. Med.* 1:99–107.
40. Takahashi, W., Pfenninger, K., and Wong, L. (1983). Urinary arsenic, chromium, and copper levels in workers exposed to arsenic-based wood preservatives. *Arch. Environ. Health* 38:209–214.

41. Sankila, R., Karjalainen, S., Pukkalu, E., Oksanen, H., Hakulinen, T., Teppo, L., and Hakama, M. (1990). Cancer risk among glass factory workers: An excess of lung cancer? *Br. J. Ind. Med.* 47:815–818.
42. Ungers, L. H. J., Jones, J. H., McIntyre, A. J., and McHenry, C. R. (1985). Release of arsenic from semiconductor wafers. *Am. Ind. Hyg. Assoc. J.* 46:416–420.
43. Blot, W. J., and Fraumeni, J. F. (1975). Arsenical air pollution and lung cancer. *Lancet* 2:142–144.
44. Hughes, J. P., Polissar, L., and Van Belle, G. (1988). Evaluation and synthesis of health effects studies of communities surrounding arsenic producing industries. *Int. J. Epidemiol.* 17:407–413.
45. Greaves, W. U., Rom, W. N., Lyon, J. L., Varley, G., Wright, D. D., and Chiu, G. (1981). Relationship between lung cancer and distance of residence from nonferrous smelter stack effluent. *Am. J. Ind. Med.* 2:15–23.
46. Rom, W. W., Varley, G., Lyon, J. L., and Shopkow, S. (1982). Lung cancer mortality among residents near the El Paso smelter. *Br. J. Ind. Med.* 39:269–272.
47. Frost, F., Harter, L., Milham, S., Royce, R., Smith, A., Hartley, J., and Enterline, P. (1987). Lung cancer among women residing close to an arsenic emitting copper smelter. *Arch. Environ. Health* 42:148–152.
48. Cordier, S., Theriault, G., and Iturra, H. (1983). Mortality patterns in a population living near a copper smelter. *Environ. Res.* 31:311–322.
49. Brown, L. M., Pottern, L. M., and Blot, W. J. (1984). Lung cancer in relation to environmental pollutants emitted from industrial sources. *Environ. Res.* 34:250–261.
50. Pershagen, G. (1985). Lung cancer mortality among men living near an arsenic-emitting smelter. *Am. J. Epidemiol.* 122:684–694.
51. Matanoski, G., Landau, E., Tonascia, J., Lazar, C., Elliot, E., McEnroe, W., and King, K. (1981). Cancer mortality in an industrial area of Baltimore. *Environ. Res.* 25:8–28.
52. Wu, M., Kuo, T. Huang, Y., and Chen, C. (1989). Dose-response relation between arsenic concentration in well water and mortality from cancers and vascular diseases. *Am. J. Epidemiol.* 130:1123–1132.
53. Chen, C., and Wang, C. (1990). Ecological correlation between arsenic level in well water and age-adjusted mortality from malignant neoplasms. *Cancer Res.* 50:5470–5474.
54. Chen, C., Chuang, Y., You, S., Lin, T., and Wu, H. (1986). A retrospective study on malignant neoplasms of bladder, lung, and liver in blackfoot disease endemic area in Taiwan. *Br. J. Cancer* 53:399–405.
55. Hotta, N. (1989). Clinical aspects of chronic arsenic poisoning due to environmental and occupational pollution in and around a small refining spot. *Japan J. Constit. Med.* 53:49–70.
56. Cuzick, J., Sasieni, P., and Evans, S. (1992). Ingested arsenic, keratoses and bladder cancer. *Am. J. Epidemiol.* 136:417–421.
57. Reymann, F., Moeller, R., and Nielsen, A. (1978). Relationship between arsenic intake and internal malignant neoplasms. *Arch. Dermatol.* 114:378–381.
58. Robson, A. O., and Jelliffe, A. M. (1963). Medicinal arsenic poisoning and lung cancer. *Br. Med. J.* 2:207–209.

59. Leonard, A. (1985). Recent advances in arsenic mutation and carcinogenesis. *Curr. Top. Environ. Toxicol. Chem.* 8:443–451.
60. Okui, T., and Fujiwara, Y. (1986). Inhibition of human excision DNA repair by inorganic arsenic and the co-mutagenic effect in V79 Chinese hamster cells. *Mutat. Res.* 172:69–76.
61. Barrett, J. C., Lamb, P. W., Wang, T. C., and Lee, T. C. (1989). Mechanisms of arsenic induced cell transformation. *Biol. Trace Elem. Res.* 21:421–429.

10

Radon

SARAH C. DARBY

University of Oxford
Oxford, United Kingdom

JONATHAN M. SAMET

University of New Mexico School of Medicine
and the New Mexico Tumor Registry
Albuquerque, New Mexico

I. Introduction

Radon (radon-222) is an inert radioactive gas at usual environmental temperatures. It is a naturally occurring decay product of radium-226, the fifth daughter of uranium-238. Both uranium-238 and radium-226 are present in most soils and rocks, although the concentrations vary widely (1). When radon forms from the decay of radium-226, some atoms leave the soil or rock and enter the surrounding air or water. As a result, radon is ubiquitous in indoor and outdoor air and also in the air of underground passages and mines, and its concentration is increased by the presence of a rich source and by low ventilation of the air in contact with that source.

Radon decays with a half-life of 3.82 days into a series of solid, short-lived radioisotopes that are collectively referred to as radon daughters, radon progeny, or radon decay products (Fig. 1). Two of these decay products, polonium-218 and polonium-214, emit alpha particles—high-energy and high-mass particles consisting of two protons and two neutrons and highly effective in damaging tissues. When these emissions take place within the lung, as inhaled radon progeny decay, the genetic material of cells lining the airways may be damaged and lung cancer may ultimately result.

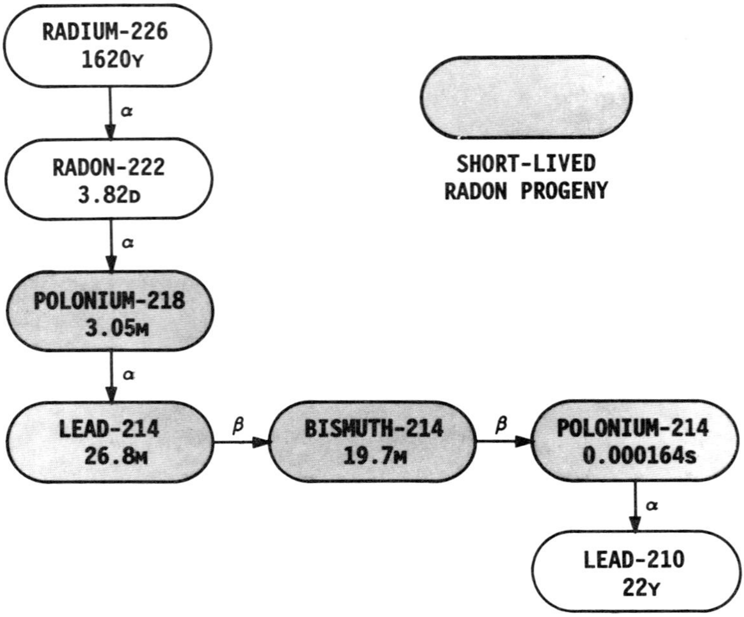

Figure 1 Decay pathway from radium-226 to lead-210. (Y = year, D = day, M = minute, S = second.) (From Ref. 2.)

The present chapter reviews the evidence that has established inhaled radon and its progeny as a cause of lung cancer. Further information is given elsewhere (3–5).

II. Radon as an Occupational Lung Carcinogen

As mentioned in Chapter 1, an increased risk of lung cancer in the miners of Schneeberg and Jachymov in the Erz mountains caused mining to be the first occupation associated with an increased risk of lung cancer. Ores had been mined there since the fifteenth century, and as early as the sixteenth century Agricola described exceptionally high mortality from respiratory diseases in this region (6). In 1879 Harting and Hesse described autopsy findings that documented an occupational risk of intrathoracic neoplasms in miners, which they classified as lymphosarcoma (7), although in retrospect most of these deaths were probably from small-cell lung cancer, and in the early years of this century case reviews established that the malignancy prevalent among the miners was primary cancer of the lung (8,9) (see Ref. 3 for further details).

Although the increased risk of lung cancer for miners in the Erz mountains has long been observed, identifying its cause has proved more elusive. Early theories favored dust exposure, metals in the ore, or the consequences of inbreeding in small mining communities. In 1924, it was reported that radioactivity could be measured in the air and water of the Schneeberg mines and might contribute to the development of lung cancer (10), but even in 1944 a review in the *Journal of the National Cancer Institute* argued that radon alone could not be the cause of the disease (11). Since then, however, the central role of radon as an occupational lung carcinogen has become clear. A number of studies of radon-exposed miners have shown rising lung cancer risk as cumulative exposure to radon decay products increases, while studies of other miners, such as coal miners, who also work in dusty conditions but who do not generally work in an atmosphere with a high concentration of radon, have shown that a raised risk of lung cancer is not necessarily a consequence of mining work. In 1988 the International Agency for Research on Cancer classified radon as a group I carcinogen (i.e., there is sufficient evidence that radon is carcinogenic to humans) (12). Animal studies have also shown a clear exposure-response relationship, thus providing strong experimental proof of the causal nature of the association of radon with lung cancer.

The risk of lung cancer has now been associated with exposure to radon decay products in about 20 different populations of underground miners in Czechoslovakia, the United States, Canada, Sweden, France, Britain, Norway, China, and Australia. These studies covered the mining of a variety of different substances, including uranium, iron, magnetite, fluorspar, zinc-lead, tin, and niobium. In most mines, the principal source of radon decay products is radon released from radium in the ore, but in some mines radon dissolved in water has made substantial contributions. The majority of the studies are cohort, or longitudinal, in design and involve the follow-up of miners and observation for deaths from lung cancer and other causes. At the present time the period of follow-up spans several decades in most of these studies, but none has as yet been continued until all or even the majority of the men included have died, and thus the full consequences of their exposures have not been studied.

The histopathology of the lung cancers has been characterized in some groups. Most of the studies are cross-sectional case series and have come from mining populations in which cigarette smoking was prevalent. In these studies about half the cases were of small-cell lung cancer, and this is about double the proportion expected based on patterns of lung cancer in the general population (4). Two studies of nonsmokers have indicated that the proportion of small-cell carcinomas in these groups also is higher than would be expected in populations of nonsmokers (13,14). Two further studies, of uranium miners in the Colorado Plateau and in Czechoslovakia, have described excess lung cancer occurrence by histological type. In the Colorado group, the distribution has changed markedly over time. In 1964, about three quarters of the lung cancers were small-cell tumors, but by the late 1970s the proportion had dropped to about one fifth, with a corresponding increase in the proportion of squamous cell carcinomas (15). The small-cell tumors in the early part of the follow-up were mostly in miners exposed to exceptionally high levels of radon (>1200 WLM), while in the later period there was very little difference in the histology of lung cancers in uranium miners compared with that of the general population, even though most of the cancers were still in excess. An analysis of lung cancers by cell type for the Czech cohort showed excesses of small-cell carcinoma, squamous carcinoma, and types other than adenocarcinoma, while adenocarcinoma itself was not increased (16). In this group also the ratio of observed to expected cases was greatest for small-cell carcinoma. Thus, the evidence on histological type of lung cancer in radon-exposed miners indicates an unusually high frequency of small-cell carcinoma in both smokers and nonsmokers. However, radon cannot be linked to small-cell carcinoma alone, as other histological types of lung cancer also occur in excess. It has been suggested that various histological types of lung cancers may arise from cells of origin that are in the same family (17), but the specific cells giving rise to lung cancers of the various types have not yet been identified. Thus neither the concentration of the excess in cancers of the small cell type, nor the shift with time in the distribution by cell type in the Colorado population can be fully explained at present. Thus, apart from the increased proportion of small-cell tumors and the decreased proportion of adenocarcinomas, lung cancers occurring in miners exposed to radon do not appear to differ greatly from those found in the general population (18).

The concentration of radon progeny in mines has traditionally been measured in terms of working levels (WL): 1 WL is any combination of radon progeny in 1 liter of air that ultimately releases 1.3×10^5 MeV of alpha particle potential energy during decay (19). The working level–month (WLM) was introduced as a measure of exposure to radon progeny that took into account both the concentration of the progeny in air and the duration of exposure at that concentration. The WLM is defined as the sum of the products of the WL multiplied by the durations of exposure at each WL value during some specified total time period. One WLM is equal to 170 WL-hours and would be the exposure received by a miner working in an atmosphere containing 1 WL for 170 h (approximately the number of hours worked in a month) (3).

In several studies it has proved possible to estimate the exposure of individual miners, usually by combining area measurements of radon or radon progeny with the worker's employment record documenting his underground experience. The availability of individual exposure estimates enables study of the quantitative relationships between exposure and risk, and in all cases where this has been possible a clear relationship between cumulative exposure and risk of lung cancer is seen. Estimates of the percentage excess relative risk (ERR) of lung cancer per WLM obtained from seven studies are summarized in Table 1.

Generally, the excess relative risk of lung cancer increases approximately

Table 1 Relative Risks and Average Exposure Rates in Cohorts of Miners Exposed to Radon

Cohort	Average exposure rate (WLM/year)	Relative risk (% per WLM)		
		Original[a]	BEIR IV[b]	Ref.
Beaverlodge	5[c]	3.3[c]	5.1[c]	20
Malmberget	5	3.6	3.6	21
Ontario	~10	1.3	1.8	22
New Mexico	~16	1.1	—	23
Newfoundland	~70	0.9	—	24
Port Radium	109	0.27	—	25
Colorado	124	—[d]	0.9[e]	26

[a]Estimate given by original authors.
[b]BEIR IV estimate, based on internal comparison but allowing the relative risk per WLM to vary between cohorts, for age 55–64, 5–14 years after exposure. When the relative risk is assumed to be the same for all cohorts, its estimated value is 2.5% per WLM.
[c]Under revision, see text.
[d]Original paper only gives estimates after allowing for exposure rate effect and are thus not directly comparable.
[e]Based on cumulative lagged exposures of less than 2000 WLM only.

linearly with estimated cumulative exposures in the range 0–500 WLM. In the study of Colorado Plateau uranium miners, however, exposures were very high and a considerable number of men had estimated cumulative exposures above 2000 WLM. In this study the excess relative risk per WLM was nonlinear and decreased at exposures above about 1000 WLM (Fig. 2). The decrease in excess risk at the higher exposures may reflect cell sterilization at these high doses, but bias from greater misclassification of higher exposures is an alternative explanation (3).

With so many epidemiological studies available, it is clearly more appropriate to base judgments on the quantitative consequences of occupational exposure to radon on data from several studies combined rather than on the results of any individual study. At the present time, the most extensive joint analysis has been carried out by the BEIR IV Committee (3). This committee obtained detailed information beyond that available in the published literature from the research workers who had studied four of the principal groups of exposed miners: uranium miners at Beaverlodge, Saskatchewan, and Ontario in Canada and in the Colorado Plateau in the United States, and iron ore miners at Malmberget in Sweden. The BEIR IV Committee concluded that, even though there were substantial differences between the individual studies, the data from them provided a good basis for estimating the effects of different exposures; they excluded from their analysis

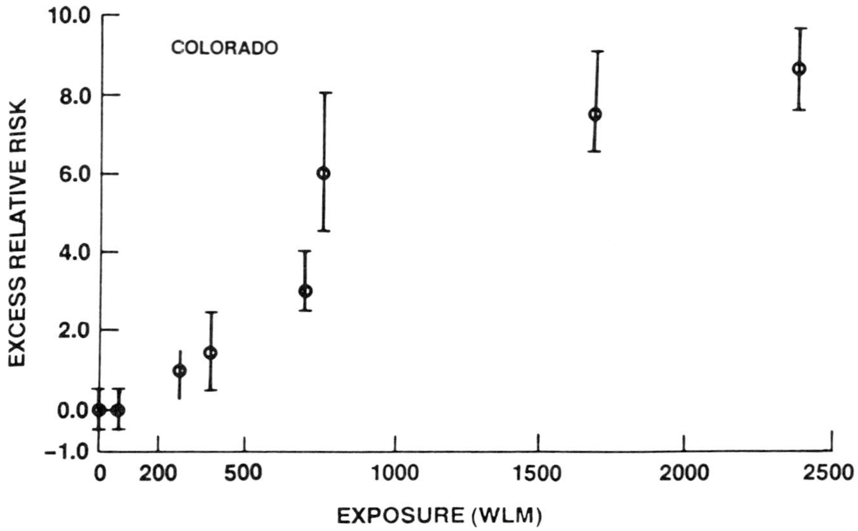

Figure 2 External relative risk and 67% confidence limits by exposure category as observed in the uranium miners on the Colorado Plateau. The comparison is to external population rates. Reprinted with permission from *Health Risks of Radon and Other Internally Deposited Alpha-Emitters*. ©1988 by the National Academy of Sciences. Published by the National Academy Press, Washington, D.C.

observations on the Colorado miners who had received cumulative exposures of more than 2000 WLM. From these data and other data on the effects of smoking the BEIR IV Committee concluded that radon and smoking acted synergistically in the production of lung cancer, the two factors multiplying each other's effect, and that the excess relative risk of lung cancer at age a could be summarized by the equation

$$\text{ERR} = b \times g_a \times (W_1 + 0.5W_2)$$

where $b = 0.025$, $g_a = 1.2$ for ages under 55 years; 1.0 for ages 55–64 years; 0.4 for ages 65 years and over, W_1 = cumulative dose in WLM 5–14 years before age a, and W_2 = cumulative dose in WLM 15 or more years before age a.

This relationship implies that the excess relative risk falls off with the passage of time after reaching a maximum a decade or so after exposure has occurred, although it provides little insight into the pattern of ERR as the interval since exposure lengthens beyond 15 years. Recent observations on the survivors of the atomic bombings of Hiroshima and Nagasaki, who were exposed primarily to gamma rays, and on patients with ankylosing spondylitis who were treated with x-rays also indicate that the ERR for lung cancer decreases with increasing time after exposure (27,28).

The BEIR IV Committee's report was published in 1988, and since then a number of additional studies have been published on the effects of radon in underground miners. This recent evidence suggests that two aspects of the BEIR IV model may need material modification: namely, the effects of exposure rate and the synergistic effect of exposure to radon and tobacco products.

III. Effect of Exposure Rate

Substantial evidence that higher excess relative risks per unit exposure are associated with lower average exposure rates among miners exposed to high concentrations of radon has emerged in recent years. The initial evidence arose from studies carried out at two Canadian uranium mines, both operated by Eldorado Resources Ltd. (20,25). In the first study, of workers at the Beaverlodge mine in Saskatchewan and for whom data were available to the BEIR IV Committee, the excess relative risk associated with one WLM increase in cumulative exposure was 3.28% (95% confidence interval 2.08–4.48). In the second study, of workers at the Port Radium mine in the Northwest Territories and which was not published until after the BEIR IV Committee's work was complete, the ERR per WLM was less than one-tenth of this value, at 0.27% (95% confidence interval 0.11–0.43). When expressed in terms of excess absolute risks the contrast between the findings for the two mines is just as striking, with an attributable risk per WLM of 20.8 per 10^6 person-years at Beaverlodge (95% confidence interval 11.8–29.8), while for Port Radium the corresponding figure was 3.10 (95% confidence interval 1.89–4.32). The chief difference between the mines seems to be in the average exposure rates, which are estimated in the initial reports as 5 WLM per year and 109 WLM per year at Beaverlodge and Port Radium, respectively. A subsequent reevaluation of a sample of the dosimetry data at the Beaverlodge mine has indicated that there was in fact considerable underestimation of the workers' exposures. However, there are still substantial differences between the results in the two mines (G. Howe, personal communication).

Evidence that higher relative risks per unit exposure are associated with lower average exposure rates in miners has also been reported within three other cohorts. First, a recent analysis of data from the study of uranium miners in the Colorado Plateau (26) found statistically significant evidence of a negative exposure rate effect, implying that among groups of miners receiving equivalent cumulative exposures, those exposed to lower levels for longer periods of time were at greater risk of lung cancer. They also found that this effect varied with cumulative exposure level, so that a miner with cumulative exposure in the range 0–834 WLM at a rate one tenth as great as another miner of the same age, smoking status, and cumulative exposure would have a 58% greater risk of lung cancer. Second, there was a significant decline in the excess relative risk per WLM in a cohort of Chinese tin miners with increasing exposure rate (29); and third, a similar effect has been reported within the cohort of Czech miners (30).

Additional evidence of an exposure rate effect comes from a comparison of the different estimates of risk derived from different cohorts of miners, including the four studied by the BEIR IV Committee, which are displayed in Table 1. The table shows the estimates of risk calculated by the original authors and, where available, also the estimates calculated by the Committee in one of their joint analyses, where the coefficient B in the basic BEIR IV model described in the previous section was allowed to vary between cohorts. The BEIR IV estimates given in Table 1 are specific to age 55–64 and to exposure in the period 5–14 years previously and thus take account of differences in the age structure and follow-up period between the different studies. Miners at Malmberget had exposure rates as low as the original estimates for Beaverlodge and also experienced high risks per WLM. Miners in the Colorado Plateau had exposure rates similar to those at Port Radium and experienced lower risks per WLM, while miners in the other three studies for which figures are available had intermediate exposure rates and experienced intermediate risks.

The above evidence clearly suggests that lower exposure rates lead to higher risks per unit dose. It is consistent with the results of much recent radiobiological data, both in vivo and in vitro, suggesting an increased effectiveness for oncogenic transformation at decreased dose rates of medium- and high-LET radiation (31). It is, however, hard to eliminate the possibility of an association between exposure rate and various confounders including total dose, smoking habits, the type of material mined (with more contaminants that are carcinogenic associated with lower exposure rates), or error rates (with larger errors in exposure estimates associated with higher exposure rates). At the present time such an investigation has been carried out only for the Beaverlodge mine, and this confirmed that confounding of cigarette smoking and other mining experience with radon exposure is unlikely to have contributed to the high relative risk coefficient seen in the Beaverlodge miners (32). Further evidence is needed to clarify the situation.

IV. Interaction with Cigarette Smoking

The BEIR IV Committee's assumption that radon and smoking act synergistically in the production of lung cancer in such a way that the relative risk following exposure to the two in combination is equal to the product of the relative risks following exposure to each separately was made in the light of evidence provided by two cohorts of uranium miners: one in the Colorado Plateau and one in New Mexico (23,26). This assumption fitted the data substantially better than the assumption that the two effects were additive, and the BEIR IV Committee assumed multiplicativity "for parsimony." Their analysis in fact suggested that something less than multiplicativity would provide the best fit to the data, although the improvement in fit over the multiplicative model was not significant statistically. The BEIR IV's conclusion does not, however, accord with the data summarized in Table 2, most of which were published after the Committee's analysis. The numbers of cases of lung cancer in nonsmokers are all small, but the consistency of the results is striking. The high relative risk in nonsmoking white miners in the Colorado Plateau compares with the much lower relative risk for all white miners in that area (4.82) (34). The similarity of the absolute risks in the Newfoundland fluorspar miners implies a much greater relative risk in nonsmokers than in smokers (24). Estimates for the Malmberget miners are based on many assumptions, and consequently are hard to understand (21), but there seems no reason to question their qualitative implication. The overall conclusion from the evidence now available seems to be that radon and smoking act more than additively but less than multiplicatively.

Further evidence that exposure to radiation does not simply multiply the effect of smoking is provided by the observations on the survivors of the atomic bombings at Hiroshima and Nagasaki. In this group women smoked very little, while men smoked a great deal more, and the effect of exposure to gamma radiation was to increase the relative risk of lung cancer in women more than in men (35). In addition, the results of animal experiments have shown that more lung cancers are induced when exposure to radon is followed by exposure to smoke than when the exposures were reversed (36).

Table 2 Interaction of Radon Exposure and Smoking from Cohort Studies of Miners Not Included in BEIR IV Analysis

Mine	Nonsmokers: Relative risk	Nonsmokers: Attributable risk (per 10^6 WLM-years)	Smokers: Relative risk	Smokers: Attributable risk (per 10^6 WLM-years)	Ref.
Colorado whites	12.7 (14)[a]	5.5 (14)			33
Czechoslovakia	10.0 (3)	16.6 (3)	1.6 (19)	26.1 (19)	30
Newfoundland		7.6 (7)		6.3 (57)	24
Malmberget, Sweden[b]	10.0 (18)	16.3 (18)	2.9 (32)	21.8 (32)	21

[a]Numbers of deaths in parentheses.

[b]Includes ex-smokers stopped more than 20 years with nonsmokers. Excluded from BEIR IV Committee's analyses of smoking effects because of complexity of the data.

V. Current Occupational Issues

In the United States, most underground uranium mines had shut down by the late 1980s, but uranium mining continues in several countries, including Canada, Australia, France, South Africa, and some other African countries. Furthermore, occupational exposure to radon progeny remains of concern for many other types of underground miners and other underground workers, and radon in underground miners remains a significant underground hazard as the end of the twentieth-century approaches. For many types of mine, and in most countries, occupational exposure to radon is controlled by legislation. In the United States, for example, complete individual exposure records are required for all employees entering areas with concentrations in excess of 0.3 WL. In addition, the current rules limit the concentration in active workings to 1 WL and annual exposure to 4 WLM (37), and this limit may in the future be lowered to 1 WLM. According to the estimates made by the BEIR IV Committee, exposure to 4 WLM per year for 40 years starting from age 20, such as would be incurred by a miner who spent most of his or her working life near the limit allowed by these regulations, would approximately double a person's lifetime risk of lung cancer. However, as indicated in the discussion in the preceding sections, there is considerable uncertainty in this estimate, and for a nonsmoking miner exposed at these rates the proportionate increase in risk could be considerably greater.

VI. Exposure to Radon in the General Environment

The hypothesis that radon in the general environment constitutes a hazard to the general public, albeit a small one, is not new. The possibility that it might do so began to be considered 40 years ago, when many towns in the United Kingdom were subject to intense atmospheric pollution from the domestic consumption of coal. The radon released was thought to contribute to the increasing mortality from lung cancer that was characteristic of urban life at the time, and one very crude calculation led to the conclusion that it might be responsible for about 1% of all cases (38).

No serious attention was, however, paid to the possible effects of radon progeny in the general environment until the late 1970s, when further understanding of the mechanism by which radon reaches indoor air began to be understood, and it began to be realized in several European countries that the concentration in the air of buildings such as homes, offices, and schools could vary more than 100-fold, and that the highest concentrations overlapped those in mines in which the workers had been shown to have an increased risk of lung cancer. In the United States, the problem did not receive great attention as a public health problem until a widely publicized incident in 1984. During the routine monitoring of workers in a Pennsylvania nuclear power plant, a worker in the plant was found to be contaminated with radioactivity, and the contamination was subsequently traced to a high concentration of radon in the worker's home.

Radon concentrations in homes are usually measured in terms of the number of disintegrations of radon gas in a fixed time period and in a given volume of air. In the International System concentrations are expressed in terms of Becquerels per cubic meter (Bq/m^3), where 1 Bq/m^3 corresponds to one disintegration per second per cubic meter. Concentrations of radon gas are also sometimes expressed in terms of picocuries per liter (pCi/L), where 1 pCi/L = 37 Bq/m^3. The relationship between the concentration of radon progeny and the concentration of radon gas is determined by the equilibrium between the two.

In several countries radon gas concentrations have been measured in a representative sample of homes, and, for example, in the United Kingdom such a survey has enabled the average concentration to be estimated at about 20 Bq/m^3 (39), while in Sweden the average is considerably higher, around 105 Bq/m^3 (40). Until quite recently when the Environmental Protection Agency (EPA) conducted a national radon survey, radon concentrations had not been measured in a large random sample of homes in the United States, although several smaller surveys had been carried out. Nero et al. (41) examined 35 such data sets and identified 22 that gave information on single family dwellings and were not biased by the approach used to select the dwellings. The average concentration of radon in the homes was 61 Bq/m^3. Preliminary findings from the U.S. EPA survey of about 6000 households estimate the annual average radon concentration to be 46 Bq/m^3, with 6% of households above 148 Bq/m^3. Most of the large-scale surveys that have been carried out indicate that the distribution of radon concentrations in homes is approximately lognormal, with a small proportion of homes having extremely high levels.

Up until the 1980s, estimates of the average annual effective dose equivalent received by the population from natural sources of ionizing radiation did not usually include a contribution from radon. However, the average concentrations found in samples of homes have been found to be so high that previous estimates of the average annual effective dose equivalent received from natural sources of ionizing radiation needed to be doubled or tripled in some countries. As a result the revised estimate of the average annual effective dose equivalent received in the United States is 3 mSv, made up as shown in Table 3, while the corresponding estimate in the United Kingdom is just over 2 mSv, with radon contributing about half (42).

In homes, the predominant source in indoor air is usually the soil beneath the structure, although building materials, water used within the home, and natural gas used for cooking and heating may also contribute (43–47). The concentration of radium in soil and rock varies over several orders of magnitude, and it is this variation in source strength that underlies most of the variation in radon

Table 3 Estimated Annual Average Dose Equivalents from Natural Radiation in the United States

Source of radiation	Average annual dose equivalent (mSv) to: Bronchial epithelium	Other soft tissues	Bone surface	Bone marrow	Annual effective dose equivalent whole body (mSv)
Cosmic	0.27	0.27	0.27	0.27	0.27
Terrestrial gamma	0.28	0.28	0.28	0.28	0.28
Cosmic radionuclides	0.01	0.01	0.01	0.03	0.01
Inhaled radio-nuclides[a] (mainly radon)	24.00	—	—	—	2.00
Other radionuclide in the body[a]	0.36	0.36	1.10	0.50	0.39
All sources	~25.0	0.9	1.7	1.1	~3.0

[a]Doses from radon to tissues other than the bronchial epithelium are included under "other radionuclides."
Source: Ref. 1.

concentration between dwellings. The rate of exchange of indoor with outdoor air also influences radon concentrations in indoor air and increased draft-proofing for energy efficiency may have lead to a small increase in domestic radon concentrations in recent years. However, air exchange rate is usually a less important determinant of variation in radon concentrations in homes than is the strength of the soil (44,45,48).

For the most part, building materials make only a small contribution to indoor radon. Certain materials, however, have high concentrations of radium and are strong sources of radon. These include granites, concrete made with alum shale, as has been used extensively in Sweden, and building materials made with wastes from industrial processes such as phosphogypsum, phosphate slag, and fly ash (44,46). Water from most sources contributes little to indoor radon, but water from some private wells may add significant amounts of radon to indoor air (47).

The movement of radon through building materials and soil is a complex process that involves molecular diffusion, gas flow, and transport via water (44,45). The entry of radon into a building is determined by the structural characteristics of, and the flow of radon-containing air into, the building. The flow is influenced by wind, temperature, barometric pressure, and soil moisture. Routes of entry include cracks and sump holes in basements, cracks in concrete floors, and crawl spaces. There is usually substantial diurnal and seasonal variation resulting from changes in air exchange rates and use of water and natural gas, and also from varying meteorological conditions.

VII. Prediction of Environmental Risks from Occupational Data

At the present time, estimates of the risk of lung cancer from radon in homes need to be derived from the effects observed in the studies of miners described in the earlier sections of this chapter. Several national and international groups have devised risk-projection models for this purpose (49–52). The models of the International Commission of Radiological Protection and the U.S. National Council for Radiation Protection and Measurements are based on risk estimates from miners. However, averages of published coefficients were used. The only model that is based on a joint analysis of the original data from several of the miners' studies is that provided by the BEIR IV Committee (3), and for this reason it seems preferable to the others at present.

Under usual conditions of equilibrium between radon and its decay products in a home, a concentration of 20 Bq/m^3 corresponds to about 0.02 WL. The BEIR IV Committee tentatively assumed that exposure to 1 WLM in a home and exposure to 1 WLM in a mine have equivalent potency in causing lung cancer, so that risk estimates could be transferred directly from an occupational setting to an indoor domestic environment. Application of the BEIR IV model separately to the smoking and nonsmoking populations of the United States yields estimates of the lifetime risk of lung cancer attributable to a cumulative dose of 1 WLM at 506×10^{-6} for males, 186×10^{-6} for females, and 350×10^{-6} for both sexes combined. Subsequent calculations, using the BEIR IV model, have led to the conclusion that radon in the general environment is responsible for about 10% of all lung cancers in the United States and 6% in the United Kingdom (42,53). On the assumptions made, the proportion would remain the same in the absence of smoking, but the absolute number would be less.

The ability that a given exposure to radon will have to cause lung cancer depends on the dose of alpha energy delivered to the epithelium of the airways. This relationship between dose and exposure is extremely complex and is dependent on both biological and nonbiological factors, including the physical characteristics of the inhaled air, the amount of air inhaled, breathing patterns, and the biological characteristics of the lung. In comparison with mines, the fraction of the decay products that remain unattached to particles in the air is higher in homes, and the size distribution of particles in the air may also differ between the two environments. The ventilation rates for working miners are also higher on average than for the general population during usual activities at home. The physical configuration of the airways of children differs from that of adults as well.

Table 4 K Factors for Bronchial Dose Calculated for Normal People in the General Environment Relative to Healthy Underground Miners

Subject	K factor[a] for target cells	
	Secretory	Basal
Infant, 1 month	0.74	0.64
Child, 1 year	1.00	0.87
Child, 5–10 years	0.83	0.72
Adult female	0.72	0.62
Adult male	0.76	0.66

[a]The K factor is the ratio of the dose of alpha energy delivered per unit exposure to an individual in the home to the dose per unit exposure to a male miner in a mine.
Source: Ref. 18.

Dosimetric models of the lung have proved useful in evaluating these effects, and since the BEIR IV Committee another National Research Council Committee has carried out a detailed comparison of the relations between exposure and dose in homes and in mines (18). This new committee used a new dosimetric model together with the most recent information on the parameter values. The findings were expressed as the ratio, termed K, of the dose of alpha energy delivered per unit exposure to an individual in the home to the dose per unit exposure to a male miner in a mine. These ratios, which were calculated for a variety of ages and for females as well as males, are summarized in Table 4. In no case did K take a value greater than unity, and the overall conclusion was that, under typical home conditions, the dose per WLM in homes is about 70% of mine value, with a corresponding reduction in the risk of lung cancer per WLM. In the light of this new dosimetry evaluation, estimates of the proportion of lung cancers attributable to radon need to be multiplied by a factor of about 0.7, but even when this is done the estimates place radon as the second most important cause of lung cancer in both the United States and the United Kingdom, after cigarette smoking.

VIII. Direct Studies of Environmental Risks

Dosimetric modeling can only address some of the difficulties in estimating the risks of environmental exposure to radon from the miners' data, and a number of major issues remain. These include the effect of exposure to radon progeny in childhood, differences between the effects of exposure between men and women over and above those caused by different smoking habits, differences in risk resulting from the different patterns of exposure experienced occupationally and environmentally, and differences caused by the different mix of other carcinogens and irritants in the mining compared with the general environment. In view of all these uncertainties, direct observations on the risks of environmental exposure to radon are essential. These can be made in three ways: (1) by ecological studies, correlating the incidence of lung cancer and the average concentration of radon in houses in different geographical areas; (2) by case-control studies, comparing the past exposure of men and women with lung cancer with those of control subjects without the disease; and (3) by cohort studies, following up the people who have lived in houses with different documented levels of exposure to determine the incidence of the disease in the different exposure groups.

At the present time, 15 ecological studies have been reported, the results of which are summarized in Table 5. In 8 of the 15 studies there was a significant positive association between radon exposure and lung cancer incidence or mortality, while in 2 further studies there was a positive correlation that did not reach significance statistically, in 2 there was no relation between lung cancer and radon concentration, and in 3 there was an inverse relation. The results of ecological studies are always difficult to interpret, and in the present case the difficulties are increased by the fact that very few of the studies were able to take account of differences in the prevalence of smoking and by the crudeness of the estimates of exposure. Stidley and Samet (54) have carried out a special study of the ecological method as a tool for assessing lung cancer risk due to indoor radon exposure and

Table 5 Correlation Between Lung Cancer Incidence in Geographic Regions and Indication of Level of Indoor Radon

	Number showing correlation			
	Positive			
Country	Significant	Nonsignificant	Absent	Inverse
United States	6	1		1
Canada			1	
United Kingdom				1
Sweden	1			
Norway	1			
France				1
Italy		1		
China			1	
All countries	8	2	2	3

have shown that, because of the difficulties mentioned above, ecological studies may well give unreliable results in assessing the lung cancer risk associated with indoor radon exposure. In spite of these limitations, two ecological studies in the Reading Prong area of the United States are of interest, because of the large number of homes in the area with high concentrations of radon (55,56). Both indicated that the mortality from lung cancer was increased in residents of the counties with the highest exposures. In contrast, the two ecological studies with the largest numbers of cases, covering 411 counties in the United States and all the counties of England and Wales, indicated the reverse (57,58), and their findings were probably due to the fact that most large cities and towns have higher smoking-induced lung cancer rates than rural areas and relatively low radon concentrations.

The association of radon and lung cancer has been much more directly tested in case-control and cohort studies, and 13 such studies have now been reported. Early studies tended to be small in size and did not always collect smoking histories on the individuals in the study. They also relied on surrogate measures of exposure, such as whether the houses were constructed of wood or stone or whether the residents lived on the ground or upper floors. Reliance on surrogate measures may introduce misclassification; that is, some subjects may be assigned higher or lower exposures than they actually received. If misclassification occurs randomly in cases and controls alike, the relative risk estimates will be biased toward unity, and an effect of exposure may not be found.

Later studies have tended to be larger, place greater emphasis on adjusting for smoking, and use more accurate measures of exposure. At the present time six case-control studies have been reported in which individual smoking histories have been collected and measurements have been made in some or all of the homes. In addition, one cohort study has been carried out based on homes with measured high exposures. These are summarized in Table 6.

Three of the case-control studies reported a significantly increasing trend in lung cancer risk with increasing exposure to domestic radon after adjusting for cigarette smoking (60,63,65). In these studies, lung cancer risks were approximately doubled among those living in homes with higher radon concentrations compared with those living in homes with lower concentrations. One further case-control study (61) also found risks of this order associated with living in a home with a high concentration, but as the study included only 27 cases and 49 controls, this increase was not significant statistically. The fifth case-control study (62) and the cohort study (64) found increases in some groups but not in others. Possible explanations for the apparent discrepancy between the results of these studies and the four case-control studies listed above include random variation, the fact that the available measurements of radon concentrations may still have allowed some misclassification of exposures to occur, and, in the case of the cohort study, confounding by cigarette smoking, as data were not available on smoking history so no adjustment could be made for it in the analysis.

Table 6 Case-Control and Cohort Studies of Domestic Exposure to Radon and Lung Cancer Based on Measured Concentrations of Radon

Location	Study design	Subjects	Exposure measure	Findings	Ref.
Oeland, Sweden	Case-control	23 cases and 202 controls	1-month measurement with alpha-sensitive film	Significant trend in risk of lung cancer with radon level after adjusting for smoking. Multiplicative interaction with smoking.	58, 59
Ontario, Canada	Case-control	27 cases and 49 controls	Reconstructed exposures based on measurements	RR = 2.4 (95% CI 0.8–7.1) with smoking adjustment for exposed vs. nonexposed.	60
Southern Sweden	Case-control	177 cases and 677 controls	Residence type and geology, all homes; 2-month measurement, some homes	After adjustment for smoking, exposure asociated with increased risk for rural, but not urban dwellers.	61
Stockholm, Sweden	Case-control	210 female cases, and 209 population and 191 hospital	Residence type and measurements lasting 2 weeks	Significant trend after adjusting for smoking, age, and degree of urbanization. RR – 1.8 (95% CI 1.2–2.9) comparing high and intermediate to low. RR highest for small-cell cancer.	62
New Jersey	Cohort	752 persons who had resided in 45 homes with documented contamination by radium waste	Measurements with carbon canister detectors. Residence for at least one year in one of the homes	SMR = 1.7 (95% CI 0.8–3.2) for lung cancer in white males. No excess for females. Smoking histories not obtained.	63
New Jersey	Case-control	433 female cases and 402 controls	Year-long alpha track measurements, some estimates	Significant trend in risk after adjusting for smoking, age, and occupation.	64
Shenyang, China	Case-control	308 cases and 356 controls	Year-long alpha track measurements	No association between radon and lung cancer, with or without adjustment for cigarette smoking.	65

RR, relative risk; CI, confidence interval; SMR, standardized mortality ratio.

In contrast, the results of the sixth case-control study (66) seem to be inconsistent with the others. This study includes 308 women with newly diagnosed lung cancer and 356 randomly selected women of similar ages in Shenyang, China, and it was carried out jointly by the U.S. National Cancer Institute and the public health authorities in Shenyang. Measurements were made for 1 year in two rooms in the houses in which the women lived (or in their previous residences if they had moved within 5 years), the median duration of reported residence being 24 years. Smoking histories were also obtained, and odds ratios were calculated separately for nonsmokers, light smokers, and heavy smokers. The results, which are summarized in Table 7, showed an increasing risk with amount smoked but no increase in risk with amount of exposure to radon in any category of smokers, despite the fact that the exposure categories varied from 4–74 Bq/m^3 (0.1–1.9 pCi/L) to 300 or more Bq/m^3 (8.0 or more pCi/L).

The Chinese study appears excellent methodologically and, due to the stability of the Chinese population, has the highest quality exposure data of all the studies published to date. Although there is at present no ready explanation for the difference between its findings and those of the other studies, Shenyang was specifically chosen for study because of the exceptionally high lung cancer rates experienced there by women. Indoor air pollution from home heating and cooking sources was found to be substantially greater than has been found in Western countries and was found to be a major risk factor for lung cancer, as well as cigarette smoking. Thus one possible explanation for the discrepancy between the findings of the Chinese study and those of the other studies is the predominance of other sources of indoor air pollution as a cause of lung cancer. Whatever the true explanation for the difference, the totality of the direct evidence must be inter-

Table 7 Risk of Lung Cancer by Smoking Status and Indoor Radon Level in China

	Odds ratios for radon levels (Bq/m^3)[a]				
Smoking history	4–74	75–149	150–299	⩾300	All levels
Never smoked (123)[b]	1.0	0.8	0.8	0.6	1.0
Light smoker (97)	3.0	1.5	1.4	1.7	2.2
Heavy smoker[c] (88)	1.9	4.3	6.8	2.3	4.2
All histories (308)	1.0	0.9	0.9	0.7	

[a]Approximate levels. The authors' units were given in pCi/L (i.e., 0.1–1.9, 2.0–3.9, 4.0–7.9, ⩾8.0)
[b]Number of women with lung cancer in parentheses.
[c]Smoked for ⩾40 years or ⩾20 cigarettes a day for 30 years.
Source: Ref. 67.

preted as providing support for the belief that radon in homes causes some lung cancer, but it is difficult at the present time to draw any precise conclusions about the size of the risk. Many new case-control studies are now in progress throughout the world. Most incorporate measurement of radon concentrations in current and former residences, and the sample sizes of these investigations are substantially greater than many of the completed studies. However, results of most of the newer studies will not be forthcoming for several years.

IX. Current Environmental Issues

In retrospect, both scientists and regulators allowed a remarkable length of time to pass following the realization that occupational exposure to radon in mines caused an increased risk of lung cancer before examining the implications of these conclusions for environmental exposure. In contrast, once attention had focused on the subject, government agencies in several countries were quick to act.

In 1986 the United States EPA published *Action Guidelines* for acceptable levels of radon indoors in its pamphlet *A Citizen's Guide to Radon* (67). This document recommended that the highest acceptable value for annual average exposure was 148 Bq/m^3 (4 pCi/L). In 1988 the EPA and the Centers for Disease Control issued an advisory urging that most houses in the United States be tested for radon, and an amendment to the Toxic Substances Control Act sets a national long-term goal of making the air in buildings "as free of radon as the ambient air outside."

In Britain, the National Radiological Protection Board (NRPB) devised a series of Action Levels in 1987 (68). For existing dwellings, if the concentration of radon gas was above 400 Bq/m^3 it was recommended that action be taken to reduce exposure within a few years, while for higher levels, such as 1000 Bq/m^3, it was recommended that remedial measures be carried out within a year. For future dwellings, it was thought that more stringent limits were appropriate, and an upper bound of 100 Bq/m^3 was recommended as the basis for implementing changes to building procedures in areas of the country where high levels of radon are likely. The NRPB revised its advice in 1990 and recommended a new Action Level of 200 Bq/m^3 for existing dwellings (69). It also designated parts of the country where present or future homes had a 1% or higher chance of being above the action level as Affected Areas. Within an Affected Area, it was recommended that present homes should be measured, and if the concentration proved to be above the new Action Level, remedial measures should be introduced before the occupants received a further time-integrated concentration of 1500 Bq/m^3 $\times$ y. For future homes it was recommended that all homes either be constructed with precautions against radon or else be tested for high radon levels after construction and remedied, if necessary.

Control of radon in indoor air poses a unique and unprecedented challenge. Sources of radon are largely natural, and radon is in the air of all public and private buildings. Levels of radon can be measured inexpensively and the costs of mitigation are generally not high. In view of the unquestionable evidence of the carcinogenicity of exposure to radon, there seems little doubt of the desirability of taking action to reduce radon levels in the small proportion of homes with extremely high levels. However, the population's total burden of exposure and of radon-related lung cancer reflects primarily the average concentration in homes, rather than the small proportion of homes with extremely high levels. For example, although it has been estimated using the BEIR IV model that approximately 14% of lung cancer deaths among residents of single-family homes in the United States are attributable to radon, the total elimination of all exposures in such homes currently above 296 Bq/m^3 could potentially affect only 2% of lung cancer deaths in this population, while elimination of all exposures in single-family homes currently above 148 Bq/m^3 (the EPA action level) could potentially affect a maximum of only 5% of such deaths (70).

The problems of determining an acceptable level of concentration with an acceptable associated level of lung cancer risk are compounded by the substantial uncertainty that remains concerning the risks of lower levels of exposure. Additional complexity is added by the lack of evidence about the effects of exposure in childhood and uncertainty over the way in which risks from radon interact with those from smoking. For example, as has been pointed out by Lubin and Boice (70), over 80% of the predicted radon-induced lung cancer deaths in the United States would occur among smokers under the BEIR IV model, because of its assumed multiplicative relationship of risk between smoking and radon. If this assumption were correct, then for all smokers the most important single action that could be taken to reduce an individual's risk of radon-induced lung cancer would be to stop smoking, and reduction of smoking in the population would greatly reduce the burden of radon-induced lung cancer in the population, as well as reducing the toll from smoking-induced diseases (71). If, however, the findings described for nonsmoking miners described in Sec. IV are confirmed in studies of environmental exposure to radon, reasoning along these lines would be incorrect. It is to be hoped that the large number of studies of the effects of environmental exposure to radon currently underway will provide evidence useful in guiding decisions about the control of radon in the environment.

References

1. National Council on Radiation Protection and Measurements. (1987). Ionizing radiation exposure of the population of the United States. NCRP Report No. 93, Bethesda, Maryland.
2. Samet, J. M. (1989). Radon and lung cancer. *JNCI* 81:745–756.

3. Committee on Biological Effects of Ionizing Radiation (BEIR IV). (1988). *Health Risks of Radon and Other Internally Deposited Alpha-Emitters*. United States National Academy of Sciences, National Research Council. Washington, D.C., National Academy Press.
4. Samet, J. Diseases of uranium miners and other underground miners exposed to radon. (In press.)
5. Darby, S. C., and Doll, R. (1990). Radon in houses; how large is the risk? *Radiat. Prot. Aust.* 8:83–88.
6. Agricola, G. (1556). *De Re Metallica*. Basel, New York, Dover Publications. English reprint, 1950.
7. Harting, F. H., and Hesse, W. (1979). Der Lungenkrebs, die Bergkrankheit in den Schneeberger Gruben. *Gesundheitswesen* 31:102–132, 313–337.
8. Arnstein, A. (1913). Sozialhygienische Untersuchungen über die Bergleute in den Schneeberget Kobaltgruben. *Wien. Arbeit. Geb. Soz. Med.* 5:64–83.
9. Rostoski, O., Saupe, E., and Schmorl, G. (1926). Die Bergkrankheit der Erzbergleute in Schneeberg in Sachsen ("Schneeberger Lungenkrebs"). *Z. Krebforsch.* 23:360–384.
10. Ludwig, P., and Lorenser, E. (1924). Untersuchungen der Grubenluft in den Schneeberger Gruben auf den Gehalt and Radiumemanation. *Strahlentherapie* 19:428–435.
11. Lorenz, E. (1944). Radioactivity and lung cancer; a critical review of lung cancer in the miners of Schneeberg and Joachimsthal. *JNCI* 5:1–13.
12. International Agency for Research on Cancer. (1988). IARC monographs on the evaluation of carcinogenic risks to humans. *Man-Made Mineral Fibres and Radon*. Volume 43. Lyon, IARC.
13. Saccomanno, G. S., Huth, G. C., Auerbach, O., and Kuschner M. (1988). Relationship of radioactive radon daughters and cigarette smoking in the genesis of lung cancer in uranium miners. *Cancer* 62:1402–1408.
14. Butler, C., Samet, J. M., Kutvirt, D. M., Key, C. R., and Black, W. C. (1986). Histopathologic findings of lung cancer in Navajo men: Relations to uranium mining. *Health Phys.* 51:365–368.
15. Saccomanno, G., Huth, G. C., Auerbach, O., and Kuschner, M. (1989). The histology of neoplasia in uranium miners with smoking and radon exposure evaluation. In *Proceedings of the 24th Annual Meeting* (N. H. Harley, ed.). Bethesda, MD, National Council on Radiation Protection and Measurements, pp. 53–62.
16. Kunz, E., Sevc, J., Placek, V., and Horacek, J. (1979). Lung cancer in man in relation to different time distribution of radiation exposure. *Health Phys.* 36:699–706.
17. Gatter, K. C., Dunnill, M. S., Pulford, K. A. F., Heryet, A., and Mason, D. Y. (1985). Human lung tumours: A correlation of antigenic profile with histological type. *Histopathology* 9:805–823.
18. National Research Council, Panel on Dosimetric Assumptions Affecting the Application of Radon Risk Estimates. (1991). *Comparative Dosimetry of Radon in Mines and Homes*. Washington, D.C., National Academy Press.
19. Holaday, D. A., Rushing, D. E., Coleman, R. D., Woolrich, P. F., Kusnetz, H. L., and Bale, W. F. (1957). *Control of Radon and Daughters in Uranium Mines and Calculations on Biologic Effects*. DHEW Publ. No. (PHS) 57-494. Washington, D.C., U.S. Government Printing Office.

20. Howe, G. R., Nair, R. C., Newcombe, H. B., Miller, A. B., Burch, J. D. and Abbatt, J. D. (1986). Lung cancer mortality (1950–80) in relation to radon daughter exposure in a cohort of workers at the Eldorado Beaverlodge uranium mine. *JNCI* 77:357–362.
21. Radford, E. P., and St. Clair Renard, K. G. (1984). Lung cancer in Swedish iron miners exposed to low doses of radon daughters. *N. Engl. J. Med.* 310:1485–1494.
22. Muller, J., Wheeler, W. C., and Gentleman, J. F. (1983). *Study of Mortality of Ontario Miners, 1955–57.* Part I. Report to Ontario Ministry of Labour, Ontario Workers' Compensation Board and Atomic Energy Control Board of Canada.
23. Samet, J. M., Pathak, D. R., Morgan, M. V., Marbury, M. C., Key, C. R., and Valdivia, A. A. (1989). Radon progeny exposure and lung cancer risk in New Mexico U miners: A case-control study. *Health Phys.* 56:415–421.
24. Morrison, H. I., Semenciw, R. M., Mao, Y., and Wigle, D. T. (1988). Cancer mortality among a group of fluorspar miners exposed to radon progeny. *Am. J. Epidemiol.* 128:1266–1275.
25. Howe, G. R., Nair, R. C., Newcombe, H. B., Miller, A. B., and Abbatt, J. D. (1987). Lung cancer mortality (1950–80) in relation to radon daughter exposure in a cohort of workers at the Eldorado Port radium uranium mine: Possible modification of risk by exposure rate. *JNCI* 79:1255–1260.
26. Hornung, R. W., and Meinhardt, T. J. (1987). Quantitative risk assessment of lung cancer in US uranium miners. *Health Phys.* 52:417–430.
27. Committee on Biological Effects of Ionizing Radiation (BEIR V). (1990). *Health Effects of Exposure to Low Levels of Ionizing Radiation.* United States National Academy of Sciences, National Research Council, Washington, D.C., National Academic Press.
28. Darby, S. C., Doll, R., Gill, S. K., and Smith, P. G. (1987). Long-term mortality after a single treatment course with X-rays in patients treated for ankylosing spondylitis. *Br. J. Cancer* 55:179–190.
29. Lubin, J. H., Qiao, Y., Taylor, P. R., Yao, S.-X., Schatzkin, A., Mao, B.-L., Rao, J.-Y., Xuan, X.-Z., and Li, J.-Y. (1990). Quantitative evaluation of the radon and lung cancer association in a case control study of Chinese tin miners. *Cancer Res.* 50: 174–180.
30. Sevc, J., Kunz, E., Tomasek, L., Placek, V., and Horacek, J. (1988). Cancer in man after exposure to radon daughters. *Health Phys.* 54:27–46.
31. Charles, M., Cox, R., Goodhead, D., and Wilson, A. (1990). CEIR forum on the effects of high-LET radiation at low doses dose-rates. *Int. J. Radiat. Biol.* 58: 859–885.
32. L'Abbé, K. A., Howe, G. R., Burch, J. D., Miller, A. B., Abbatt, J., Band, P., Choi, W., Du, J., Feather, J., Gallagher, R., Hill, G., and Matthews, V. (1991). Radon exposure, cigarette smoking, and other mining experience in the Beaverlodge uranium miners cohort. *Health Phys.* 60:489–495.
33. Roscoe, R. J., Steenland, K., Halperin, W. E., Beaumont, J. J., and Waxweiler, R. J. (1989). Lung cancer mortality among nonsmoking uranium miners exposed to radon daughters. *JAMA* 262:629–633.
34. Waxweiler, R. J., Roscoe, R. J., Archer, V. E., Thun, M. J., Wagoner, J. K., and Lundin, F. E. (1981). Mortality follow-up through 1977 of the white underground

uranium miners cohort examined by the United States Public Health Service. In *International Conference on Radiation Hazards in Mining: Control, Measurement, and Medical Aspects*. (M. Gomez, ed.). New York, American Institute of Mining, Metallurgical, and Petroleum Engineers.

35. Shimizu, Y., Kato, H., and Schull, W. J. (1988). Life Span Study Report 11, Part II: Cancer mortality in the years 1950–85 based on the recently revised doses (DS86). RERF TR/5–88, Hiroshima, Japan.
36. Gray, R. G., Lafuma, K., Parish, S. E., and Peto, R. (1986). Lung tumors and radon inhalation in over 2000 rats: Approximate linearity across a wide range of doses and potentiation by tobacco smoke. In *Life-span Radiation Effects Studies in Animals: What Can They Tell Us?* Edited by R. C. Thompson and J. A. Mahaffey. Office of Scientific and Technical Information, United States Department of Energy, pp. 592–607, Washington, D.C.
37. Morgan, M. V., and Samet, J. M. (1986). Radon daughter exposures of New Mexico U miners, 1967–1982. *Health Phys.* 50:656–662.
38. Doll, R. (1955). Etiology of lung cancer. In *Advances in Cancer Research*, Vol. 3, Edited by J. P. Greenstein and A. Haddow. New York, Academic Press.
39. Wrixon, A. D., Green, B. M. R., Lomas, P. R., Miles, J. C. H., Cliff, K. D., Francis, E. A., Driscoll, C. M. H., James, A. C., and O'Riordan, M. C. (1987). *Natural Radiation Exposure in UK Dwellings, NRPB-R190, 1987*. London, Her Majesty's Stationery Office.
40. Swedjemark, G. A., and Mjönes, L. (1984). Radon and radon daughter concentrations in Swedish homes. *Radiat. Prot. Dosim.* 7:341–345.
41. Nero, A. V., Schwehr, M. B., Nazaroff, W. W., et al. (1986). Distribution of air borne radon-222 concentrations in US homes. *Science* 234:992–997.
42. Clarke, R. H., and Southwood, T. R. E. (1989). Risk from ionizing radiation: A commentary. *Nature* 338:197.
43. National Council on Radiation Protection and Measurements. (1984). *Exposure from the Uranium Series with Emphasis on Radon and Its Daughters*. NCRP Rep No. 77. Bethesda, MD, MCRPP.
44. Nero, A. V., and Nazaroff, W. W. (1984). Characterizing the source of radon indoors. *Radiat. Prot. Dosim.* 7:23–29.
45. Nazaroff, W. W., Moed, B. A., and Sextro, R. G. (1988). Soil as a source of indoor radon: Generation, migration, and entry. In *Radon and Its Decay Products in Indoor Air*. Edited by W. W. Nazaroff and A. V. Nero, Jr. New York, Wiley, pp. 57–112.
46. Stranden, E. (1988). Building materials as a source of indoor radon. In *Radon and Its Decay Products in Indoor Air*. Edited by W. W. Nazaroff and A. V. Nero, Jr. New York, Wiley, pp. 113–130.
47. Nazaroff, W. W., Doyle, S. M., Nero, A. V., Jr., et al. (1988). Radon entry via potable water. In *Radon and Its Decay Products in Indoor Air*. Edited by W. W. Nazaroff and A. V. Nero, Jr. New York, Wiley, pp. 131–157.
48. Nero, A. V., Jr. (1988). Radon and its decay products in indoor air: An overview. In *Radon and Its Decay Products in Indoor Air*. Edited by W. W. Nazaroff and A. V. Nero, Jr. New York, Wiley, pp. 1–53.
49. National Council on Radiation Protection and Measurements. (1984). *Evaluation of*

Occupational and Environmental Exposure to Radon and Radon Daughters in the United States. NCRP Rep. No. 78. Bethesda, MD, NCRP.

50. International Commission on Radiological Protection. (1987). *Lung Cancer Risk from Indoor Exposures to Radon Daughters*. ICRP Publ. No. 50. Oxford, Pergamon Press.
51. U.S. Environmental Protection Agency. (1987). *Radon Reference Manual*. EPA Publ. No. 520/1-87-20. Washington, D.C., U.S. Government Printing Office.
52. National Institute for Occupational Safety and Health. (1987). *Radon Progeny in Underground Mines. A Recommended Standard for Occupational Exposure*. DHHS Publ. No. (NIOSH) 88-101. Washington, D.C., U.S. Government Printing Office.
53. Lubin, J. H., and Boice, J. D. (1989). Estimating Rn-induced lung cancer in the United States. *Health Phys.* 57:417.
54. Stidley, C. A., and Samet, J. M. An assessment of ecological and case-control methods for estimating lung cancer risk due to indoor radon. Proceedings of 1990 Hanford Symposium (in press).
55. Fleischer, R. L. (1986). A possible association between lung cancer and a geological outcrop. *Health Phys.* 50:823.
56. Archer, V. E. (1987). Association of lung cancer mortality with pre-Cambrian granite. *Environ. Health* 42:87–91.
57. Cohen, B. L. A test of the linear-no threshold theory of radiation carcinogenesis. *Environ Res.* (In press.)
58. Haynes, R. M. (1988). The distribution of domestic radon concentrations and lung cancer mortality in England and Wales. *Radiat. Prot. Dosim.* 25:93.
59. Edling, C. H., Kling, H., and Axelson, O. (1984). Radon in homes—a possible cause of lung cancer. *Scand. J. Work Environ. Health* 10:25–34.
60. Edling, C., Wingren, G., and Axelson, O. (1986). Quantification of the lung cancer risk from radon daughter exposure in dwellings—an epidemiological approach. *Environ. Int.* 12:55–60.
61. Lees, R. E. M., Steeles, R., and Roberts, J. H. (1987). A case-control study of lung cancer relative to domestic radon exposure. *Int. J. Epidemiol.* 16:7–12.
62. Axelson, O., Andersson, K., Desai, G., Fagerlund, I., Jansson, B., Karlsson, C., and Wingren, G. (1988). Indoor radon exposure and active and passive smoking in relation to the occurrence of lung cancer. *Scand. J. Work Environ. Health* 14: 286–292.
63. Svensson, C. G., Pershagen, G., and Klominek, J. (1988). Lung cancer in women and type of dwelling in relation to radon exposure. Section V: Lung cancer etiology in women. Dissertation, Stockholm, Karolinska Institute.
64. Klotz, J. B., Petix, J. R., and Zagraniski, R. T. (1989). Mortality of a residential cohort exposed to radon from industrially contaminated soil. *Am. J. Epidemiol.* 129: 1179–1186.
65. Schoenberg, J. B., Klotz, J. B., Wilcox, H. B., Nicholls, G. P., Gil-del-Real, M. T., Stemhagen, A., and Mason, T. J. (1990). Case-control study of residential radon and lung cancer among New Jersey women. *Cancer Res.* 50:6520–6524.
66. Blot, W. J., Xu, Z.-Y., Boice, J. D., Jr., Zhao, D.-Z., Stone, B. J., Sun, J., Jing, L.-B., and Fraumeni, J. F., Jr. (1990). Indoor radon and lung cancer in China. *JNCI* 82:1025–1030.

67. U.S. Environmental Protection Agency. (1986). *A Citizen's Guide to Radon—What It Is and What to Do About It*. EPA Publ. No. 86-0C4. Washington, D.C., U.S. Government Printing Office.
68. National Radiological Protection Board. (1987). *Exposure to Radon Daughters in Dwellings*. NRPB-G56, NRPB-ASP10. London, Her Majesty's Stationery Office.
69. National Radiological Protection Board. (1990). Human exposure to radon in homes. *Documents of the NRPB* 1:17–32.
70. Lubin, J. H., and Boice, J. D., Jr. (1989). Estimating Rn-induced lung cancer in the United States. *Health Physics* 57:417–427.
71. Ennever, F. K. (1990). Predicted reduction in lung cancer risk following cessation of smoking and radon exposure. *Epidemiology* 1:134–140.

11

Silica Exposure and Pulmonary Cancer

DAVID F. GOLDSMITH

Western Consortium for Public Health
Berkeley, California

I. Introduction

The carcinogenicity of crystalline silica, also known as free silica, quartz, alpha quartz, or silicon dioxide (SiO_2), has been debated since the 1930s. Silica dust exposures during the mining and smelting of metal ores have long been known to produce a frequently fatal pulmonary disease, now called silicosis, but given such diverse labels as "miners' phthisis," "potters' rot or asthma," and "consumption" in the past. In the first decades of the twentieth century, Collis demonstrated that the pulmonary disease affecting many dusty trades workers was silicosis (or silico-tuberculosis) caused by the inhalation of "free" or crystalline silica (1).

In 1934, Dible, a Liverpool pathologist, published a review of 14 autopsied cases of silicosis in which several cancers were found. On the basis of his findings, Dible suggested a link between silica exposure and cancer (2). From that time until the 1980s, many articles were published on the chronic disease risks among "dusty trades" workers, but the main concerns were the risks and sequelae of silicosis and its medicolegal implications, rather than the possible carcinogenicity of silica.

During the past decade, interest has been renewed in the link between silica exposure and the risk of lung cancer. The consensus in earlier and in some current publications is that silica exposure and silicosis are not risk factors for lung cancer (3–7,16,154). However, in 1982, Goldsmith and colleagues (8) questioned this view, and since then other researchers and agencies have judged silica to be a probable human carcinogen (9–12). This judgment is supported by findings of experimental rodent studies (13,14) and of epidemiological studies of pulmonary cancer risks among silica-exposed workers, particularly among workers who have developed silicosis (9,10,15).

This chapter reviews the newer literature on silica exposure and pulmonary cancer, including experimental evidence in laboratory animals and epidemiological data from studies of dusty trades workers and of persons with silicosis. The chapter also describes cancer risk assessments for silica, the current regulations regarding occupational and ambient exposures, and, finally, a review of the criteria for causation on silica exposure and lung cancer risks.

II. Laboratory Evidence

Silica in the form of Min-U-Sil (a commercial quartz of high purity used in glass making) was shown to be a pulmonary carcinogen in six studies of exposure in rats published during the 1970s and 1980s (17–22,24). Muhle and colleagues (14) and Spiethoff and co-workers (23) recently demonstrated that DQ 12 quartz inhaled by F344 and Wistar rats produced respiratory tumors at lower lifetime doses than those found in the older studies. Table 1 describes these experimental animal findings. These rodent studies were the first to demonstrate that silica can produce pulmonary tumors in animals without previous initiation by a carcinogen such as benzo[a]pyrene. Many of the findings were in animals exposed to silica as positive controls for the development of fibrosis; the animals were observed for 2 years or their full lifetimes, and the doses covered a wide range. Similar studies in hamsters failed to replicate the production of tumors (20,25). The rat studies were the first to produce pulmonary tumors by inhalation, paralleling the human route of exposure. With the exception of the studies by Muhle et al. (14) and Spiethoff et al. (23), these studies were the basis for the conclusion of the International Agency for Research on Cancer (IARC) that the evidence was sufficient to classify silica as an animal carcinogen (10).

III. Human Evidence

Because workers in many industries are exposed to silica dust, a substantial amount of information is available from occupational studies of silica exposure and cancer risk (9,11). Interpretation of these occupational studies should give consideration to the accuracy of the industrial hygiene data and to the potential for confounding by other workplace exposures and by cigarette smoking. For this review of the human evidence, we have grouped the worker studies into five categories: (1) general silica exposure; (2) mining and quarrying; (3) granite industry; (4) ceramics and glass industry; and (5) foundry industry.

A. General Silica Exposure

Dubrow and Wegman (26) examined the mortality of all silica-exposed workers in Massachusetts who died between 1971 and 1973. For ages 20–64 years, they reported a mortality odds ratio for respiratory cancer of 155, adjusted for social class.

From a survey of nearly 250,000 workers conducted from 1950 to 1960, Neuberger et al. (27) followed-up 1630 men employed in Vienna, Austria, in such dusty industries as foundries, metal working, glass, ceramics, brick, and stone. The authors compared lung cancer mortality in this group with that of the Viennese male population and of another male control group. The standardized mortality ratio (SMR) of the workers was 148 ($p < 0.001$), a significant increase compared with the control SMR of 110.

Siemiatycki et al. (28) described a case-control study undertaken in Montreal, Canada, that enabled the investigators to test the association among diverse silica-exposed occupations. Male cancer patients aged 35–70 years were interviewed to obtain detailed work histories, and industrial exposures to silica were identified from the interviews by industrial hygienists. The highest risks for silica exposure were among subjects with oat cell carcinomas (rate ratio [RR] = 1.4; 95% confidence interval [CI] = 0.9–2.4) and squamous cell carcinomas (RR = 1.5; 95% CI = 1.0–2.1)

B. Metal Ore Mining

Metal ores are often found in deposits that have high silica concentrations, and as a consequence underground mining operations can produce significant levels of respirable dust. For example, Beadle and Bradley (29) estimated that 60–80% of the mined ore rock in the gold mines of South Africa was quartz, and that the respirable mine dust contained approximately 30% free silica. Respirable silica dust concentrations ranged from 0.05 to 0.84 mg/m^3 in the South African underground gold mines and have been constant at these levels since the 1930s (30). Underground miners of metal ores may also be exposed to radon and its progeny, to diesel fumes, and to other occupational carcinogens, any of which may confound or modify associations of silica exposure with lung cancer.

Case Studies and Descriptive Studies of Metal Ore Miners

Descriptive studies using general population data have shown metal ore miners, excluding uranium miners, to have increased lung cancer risks. Based on a series of 37 African gold miners with lung cancer in Zimbabwe, Osburn (31) calculated

Table 1 Positive Tumor Bioassay Studies of Crystalline Silica

Author (year)	Animal species (type of silica)	Route of administration	Dose (% respirable)	Findings compared to controls (comments)
Wagner and Wagner (1972) (17)	95 SPF Wistar rats (alkaline-washed quartz from Safety in Mines Research Establishment [UK] [SMRE])	IP	Single 20 mg in 0.4 ml saline (100%)	25% vs. 0% HL
	94 standard Wistar rats (SMRE)	IP		32% vs. 0% HL
Wagner (1976) (18)	160 SPF Wistar rats (SMRE)	IP	Single 20 mg in 0.4 ml saline (100%)	14% vs. 0% HL
	64 SPF Wistar rats (Min-U-Sil)	IP		3% vs. 0% HL
Wagner et al. (1980) (19)	32 SPF Wistar rats (Min-U-Sil)	IP	Single 20 mg in 0.4 ml saline (100%)	25% vs. 0% HL
	32 ICI Alderly-Park rats (Min-U-Sil)	IP		34% vs. 0% HL
	32 ICI Alderly-Park rats (D and D)	IP		25% vs. 0% HL
	32 ICI Alderly-Park rats (Snowit)	IP		25% vs. 0% HL
	32 ICI Alderly-Park rats (DQ 12)	IP		16% vs. 0% HL
	24 PVG rats (Min-U-Sil)	IP		8.3% vs. 0% HL
	24 Agus rats (Min-U-Sil)	IP		5% vs. 0% HL
	32 SPF Wistar rats (Cristobalite from SMRE)	IP		40% vs. 0% HL
	32 ICI Alderly-Park rats (Cristobalite from SMRE)	IP		12.5% vs. 0% HL
	32 ICI Alderly-Park rats (Tridymite from SMRE)	IP		50% vs. 0% HL

Holland et al. (1983) (20)	40 Sprague-Dawley rats (Min-U-Sil)	IT	7 mg in 0.2 ml saline for 10 weeks (100% HL)	17% vs. 0% (LT)
Groth et al. (1986) (21)	85 male Fischer 344 rats (Min-U-Sil)	IT	20 mg in deionized water	45% vs. 1% (all adenocarcinomas) LT
	85 male Fischer 344 rats (No vaculite)	IT	20 mg in deionized water	29% vs. 1% (all but one were adenocarcinomas) LT
Dagle et al. (1986) (22)	144 Fischer 344 rats (Min-U-Sil)	IH	51.6 mg/m^3 (100% HL)	19% vs. 0% HL in female LT 2% vs. 0% HL in male (epidermoid carcinomas) LT
Holland et al. (1983; 1986) (20,24)	62 female Fischer 344 rats (Min-U-Sil)	IH	12 mg/m^3 (70% HL)	30% vs. 0% LT
Muhle et al. (1989) (14)	100 Fischer 344 rats (DQ 12)	IH	1 mg/m^3 (74%)	12% vs. 2% in male LT 24% vs. 4% in female LT
Spiethoff et al. (1992) (23)	82 female Wistar rats 82 male Wistar rats (DQ 12)	IH	6 mg/m^3 30 mg/m^3	45% vs. 0% LT 52% vs. 0% LT

IP = intrapleural injection; IT = intratracheal injection; IH = inhalation; HL = histiocytic lymphomas; LT = lung tumors.

that miners had a lung cancer incidence of 205.6 per 100,000 from 1957 through 1963, compared with 33.8 per 100,000 in adult men, a ratio of 6:1.

Bradshaw et al. (32) and McGlashan et al. (33) presented descriptive cancer incidence data for black gold miners in several countries of Southern Africa during two periods, 1964–1971 and 1972–1979. The reports indicated that the respiratory system and the esophagus were among the most common tumor sites. Sluis-Cremer (34) reported that white South African gold miners employed in mines with ore that had a high silica content had an elevated SMR for lung cancer (SMR = 161, $p < 0.10$).

Gylseth et al. (35) described two cases of lung cancer with pulmonary fibrosis among taconite miners in Norway. The authors examined dust samples and found that they contained 23–32% silica. Cummingtonite-grunerite (CG) fibers were also observed in both miners, with fibers and particles present in the lungs.

Icso and Szollosova (36) analyzed 384 cases of lung cancer diagnosed from 1965 to 1979 in a metal ore mining region of Czechoslovakia. In the general male population over 20 years of age, the pulmonary cancer incidence rate was 13.0 per 1000 persons, but for magnesite miners the rate was 21.3, and for workers in two iron ore mines the rates were 87.9 and 10.3 per 1000. The fraction of silica in the iron mines ranged from 13 to 30% and in the magnesite mine from 0.5 to 2%.

Based on examination of death certificates in Washington State for 1950–1971, Milham (37) reported a significant excess proportional mortality ratio (PMR) of 179 ($p < 0.05$) for cancers of the respiratory system. Peterson and Milham (38) reported that mine operatives and laborers dying in California from 1959 to 1961 had a PMR for lung cancer of 241. In a case-control study based on the U.S. Third National Cancer Survey, Williams et al. (39) calculated the odds ratio for lung cancer in miners to be 1.77 ($p < 0.05$) adjusted for smoking and other factors. White male miners and drillers in California during 1979–1981 had a SMR adjusted for smoking, alcohol, and socioeconomic status of 217 ($p < 0.05$) for cancers of the trachea, bronchus, and lung (40). Lynge et al. (41) used the Nordic census-based occupational registries to describe lung cancer incidence and mortality risks for miners in Norway, Sweden, and Finland. The Norwegian iron ore miners had a 36% excess risk; Swedish iron ore miners had a rate ratio (RR) of 3.19 (95% CI = 2.92–3.49), and other ore miners had a RR of 3.71 (95% CI = 3.1–4.44); and in Finland, iron ore miners had a 78% excess incidence (95% CI = 0.22–6.45) and non-ferrous-ore miners had a RR of 5.02 (95% CI = 3.11–7.68).

Epidemiological Studies of Metal Ore Miners

Costello (42) conducted a retrospective cohort study of mortality from 1958 to 1975 in U.S. metal ore miners employed in 50 different mines in 16 states. These men were originally identified in a cross-sectional silicosis study conducted by the U.S. Public Health Service and the U.S. Bureau of Mines between 1958 and

1961 (43). The original cohort consisted of 13,007 men involved in nonuranium metal ore mining. Costello (42) examined white miners at risk for silicosis who mined 11 different metal ores or combinations of ores. Although no ore-specific silica dust concentrations were presented, quartz constituted up to 40% of the airborne and settled particulates for all 50 mines surveyed (43).

Table 2 summarizes the overall results and the findings by type of ore mined. Miners who smoked at the time of the original survey had a much higher risk of dying from lung cancer than miners who did not smoke; the SMRs for never-smoking and ex-smoking miners were 35 and 57, respectively. Because 85.1% of the entire cohort had a history of smoking, the elevated SMRs for lung cancer in the cohort could reflect confounding by smoking. A matched, nested case-control analysis was used to assess the lung cancer risk by ore type, finding an increased risk for mercury, chromium, lead and zinc, and gold and silver miners and odds ratios below one for iron and copper ore miners. Matched analysis for lung cancer showed nonsignificantly increased risks associated with airways obstruction, diesel exhaust, and radon daughter exposure.

Amandus and Costello (15) divided the same cohort of white miners into two groups, 369 miners with silicosis and 9543 miners without silicosis, excluding those employed in mines with underground diesel equipment. The SMR for lung cancer in miners with silicosis was 1.73 (95% CI = 0.94–2.90); the SMR for miners without silicosis was 1.18 (95% CI = 0.98–1.42). As shown in Table 2, miners of every ore type except iron had elevated SMRs. The SMR for miners employed less than 20 years was 1.05, and for miners employed 20 or more years 1.52 (95% CI = 1.10–2.03). Employment in mines where radon levels were low showed a greater risk than employment in mines with higher concentrations, suggesting that radon exposure did not explain the association of lung cancer with underground mining.

Muller et al. (44) conducted a study in Ontario, Canada, of mortality of 50,201 miners followed from 1955 to 1977. The study evaluated cancer risk for miners of ores in Ontario other than gold, including nickel-copper, iron ore, "other ores," and "mixed ores." In this study, the cohort of 7125 full-time underground "mixed ore" miners had a significant excess of silicosis and other nonmalignant respiratory diseases, and the SMR for cancer of the trachea, bronchus, and lung was significantly elevated at 145 ($p = 0.00078$) (Table 2).

Two joint studies examined the mortality risks among South Central Chinese miners employed in 10 tungsten mines, six copper/iron mines, and four tin mines (45,46). The subjects had completed 1 year of employment between 1972 and 1974, and mortality was followed until 1989. For tungsten miners, the SMR was 53 ($p < 0.05$); for copper/iron miners, 104; and for tin miners, 198 ($p < 0.05$) (45). Using a case-control analysis to adjust for age and smoking, McLaughlin et al. (46) examined the risk by degree of cumulative exposure to respirable silica. There was a significant negative trend with exposure among tungsten miners, no

Table 2 Summary of Epidemiological Studies of Lung Cancer Risk Among Metal Ore Miners

Author (year)	Country	Ore type	Risk measures (p-value/95% CI)	Comment
Costello (1983) (42)	U.S.	All	SMR = 127 (117–137)	Only smokers show increased risk; no exposure measurements
		Lead-zinc	SMR = 134 (102–174)	
		Mercury	SMR = 355 (177–635)	
		Chromium	SMR = 347 (112–810)	
		Chromium	Match OR = 5.0 (0.6–24.9)	
		Gold and silver	Match OR = 9.0 (1.2–332.0)	
Amandus and Costello (1991) (15)	U.S.	All-solicotics	SMR = 173 (0.94–2.90)	No silica exposure measurements; significant excess for current smokers; no confounding by radon
		All-nonsilicotics (NS)	SMR = 118 (0.98–1.42)	
		All NS < 20 years	SMR = 105 (0.82–1.31)	
		All NS ⩾ 20 years	SMR = 152 (1.10–2.03)	
		Mercury	SMR = 266 (1.15–5.24)	Smoking explains risks of 1.3
		Copper	SMR = 120 (0.87–1.61)	
		Lead-zinc	SMR = 126 (0.86–1.29)	
Muller et al. (1983) (44)	Ontario, Canada	"Mixed ores," some gold and other metals; excluded uranium	SMR = 145 ($p < 0.001$)	No exposure measurements; no adjustment for smoking; assumed to have low radon levels
Chen et al. (1992) (45)	China	Tungsten	SMR = 53 ($p < 0.05$)	SMR for tin mines increased to 262 during 1985–1989; OR analysis adjusted for age and smoking; tin miners also correlated with arsenic exposure
		Copper/iron	SMR = 104	
McLaughlin et al. (1992) (46)		Tin	SMR = 198 ($p < 0.05$)	
		Low SiO_2 dust	OR = 1.5	
		Medium SiO_2	OR = 1.9	
		High SiO_2	OR = 3.1	

evident trend among copper/iron miners, and a significant positive trend (p = 0.004) among tin miners. The OR rose from 1.5 for low cumulative exposure to silica (0.1–8.69 μg/m³/year) to 1.9 for medium cumulative exposure (8.7–26.2 μg/m³/year) and to 3.1 for high cumulative exposure (>26.3 μg/m³/year). The authors also examined cumulative exposure to arsenic, polycyclic aromatic hydrocarbons, and radon decay products and found that arsenic alone was associated with a significant trend, but only among tin miners. The authors also found silicosis to be a significant risk factor for lung cancer among copper/iron miners (OR = 3.1) and among tin miners (OR = 2.0).

Studies of Iron Ore Miners

Jorgensen (47) examined the lung cancer risk among iron ore miners, using the death registry of the Swedish community of Kiruna from 1950 to 1970. With the general population of Swedish men as the basis for expected values, Jorgensen obtained a PMR of 308 (13 observed and 4.2 expected) for underground workers. He dismissed diesel fumes and smoking as explanations for this finding and considered iron oxide, quartz, and radon exposures as possible risk factors. Dust sampling data had shown the Kiruna mine to have total dust concentrations of between 3 and 9 mg/m³, with quartz being 7% of the particulate less than 5 μm.

Higgins et al. (48) examined the mortality from 1952 to 1976 of 5751 white male employees of Reserve Mining Company who were exposed to iron oxide/taconite dust. For overall mortality, the SMR was 87 in comparison with Minnesota males; for respiratory cancer, the SMR was 84. Estimates of total respirable and quartz dust concentrations were developed for all job codes. For respiratory cancers, trends of risk with cumulative silica exposure were not found, but a slight gradient in lung cancer risk with cumulative silica exposure was found.

Lawler and co-workers (49) conducted a retrospective cohort study of 10,403 white male miners employed in hematite iron ore extraction for at least 12 months prior to January 1, 1966, in Minnesota and followed from January 1, 1937, through December 31, 1978. Mortality in the study population was compared with expected numbers based on mortality rates for the U.S. white male population. Iron ore dust and silica dust made up approximately 20% and 24% of the dust exposure, respectively. The SMR for lung cancer was not elevated.

Boyd et al. (50) studied the mortality of Cumberland (U.K.) iron ore miners using death certificates of 5811 miners who died between 1948 and 1967. The observed values were compared to an external reference population of local and national men not involved in mining. Radon concentrations were found to be well below permissible levels at the time. Silica constituted 10–12% of the local iron-ore deposits, but there was no specific information on dust concentrations in any of the mines surveyed. Deaths from lung cancer were significantly increased, with a SMR of 152 (95% CI = 129–177).

Radford and St. Clair Renard (51) investigated cancer mortality from 1951 to

1976 among 1415 Swedish iron miners in Malmberget in relation to radon progeny exposure. The SMR for all cancers was increased to 156 ($p < 0.01$), and that for lung cancer to 342 ($p < 0.01$). An exposure-response relationship of lung cancer risk with radon progeny exposure was evident. There was no association of lung cancer with a prior diagnosis of tuberculosis or silicosis. Silica dust levels were not assessed.

Chen and co-workers (52) examined mortality risks during the years 1970–1982 of 5406 male underground hematite miners and 1038 surface mine workers employed in Longyan and Taochong, China. Forty-two percent of the deaths were due to silicosis, and 20% to cancer. Compared with Chinese men, the RRs were 3.7 for lung cancer in underground workers and 1.2 in surface miners. A greater risk (RR = 4.8) occurred among miners first employed before the introduction of improved ventilation and wet drilling. The RR was 4.2 for heavy exposure to silica dust and radon. Miners with a previous history of silicosis had a RR of 5.3, and those with a history of silicotuberculosis had a RR of 6.6. For smokers, the risk rose with level of exposure to silica dust.

In general, iron ore miners have had excess lung cancer (47,50–52). The excess has been attributed primarily to radon progeny, but a contribution of silica is plausible (53,54).

Studies of Gold Ore Miners

Table 3 summarizes the lung cancer epidemiology studies of gold ore miners. Three studies have been conducted of workers employed at the Homestake gold mine in Lead, South Dakota. The miners were exposed to silica dust and to cummingtonite-grunerite (CG), an amphibole crystalline silicate fiber. Gillam et al. (55) conducted a retrospective cohort study of 440 male miners from the mine who were identified during 1958–1961, employed for at least 5 years underground, and had never worked in another underground mine. Follow-up from 1960 to 1973 showed lung cancer mortality to be increased (SMR = 370, $p < 0.01$). Crystalline silica concentrations were not apparently elevated; arsenic, chromium, and nickel were present only in trace concentrations; and radon progeny were not detected. Therefore, the authors postulated that the lung cancer excess was related to asbestos-like CG fibers and cigarette smoking. A possible additive role for free silica was proposed (55).

McDonald and colleagues (56) conducted an enlarged follow-up study from 1937 to 1973 of the Homestake Veterans Association cohort that included 1321 men with at least 21 years of employment at the mine. For the years 1937–1955, the SMR was 176 for respiratory cancer, but during 1937–1973 it was not elevated. Using Homestake dust exposure data from midget impinger samples McDonald et al. examined the mortality risks in three categories of dustiness. The risks showed striking gradients for tuberculosis and pneumoconiosis but no gradient for respiratory cancers (56).

Brown et al. (57) conducted a study of 3328 white male miners employed at

Table 3 Summary of Epidemiologic Studies of Lung Cancer Risk Among Gold Ore Miners

Author (year)	Country	Risk measure (95% CI)	Comment
Gillam et al. (1976) (55)	South Dakota (U.S.)	SMR = 370 (260–521)	No exposure measurements or smoking adjustment
McDonald et al. (1978) (56)	All Only 1937–1955	SMR = 103 (79–133) SMR = 176	Used SD rates as expected values; no risk gradient from dustiness
Brown et al. (1986) (57)		SMR = 100 (73–133) SMR = 500 based on 3 deaths from other parts of the respiratory system	No trends for latency or dust exposure
Katsnelson and Mokronosova (1979) (61)	Sverdlovsk (Russia) Removing silicotics	RR = 7.9 for men ($p < 0.001$) RR = 3.1 ($p < 0.001$)	No smoking or exposure data
Armstrong et al. (1979) (62)	Kalgoorlie, Western Australia	SMR = 140 (127–165)	Silicosis predicts modest lung cancer risk; risk remained after adjustment for smoking among underground miners
Muller et al. (1983) (44)	Ontario, Canada	SMR = 145 (135–156)	No dust measurements and no smoking information
Shannon et al. (1987) (58)	Expanded follow-up of Muller's cohort	SMR = 141 (131–151)	Risk greatest for those employed before 1936, with positive gradient for time since first dust exposure
Miller et al. (1987) (59)	Expanded follow-up of Muller's cohort	SMR = 156 (145–167) Employed < 1935–1936 SMR = 164 1936–1944 SMR = 142 >1944 SMR = 110	Smoking did not confound the results; gradient for degree of silicosis
Kusiak et al. (1991) (155)	Expanded follow-up of Muller's cohort	SMR = 140 (122–159) employed before 1946 and never mined nickel SMR = 181 (109–283) mining both nickel before 1936 and gold before 1946	Smoking and mineral fibers unlikely to explain excess; equally possible that silica dust and/or arsenic-radon exposures could explain this excess
Wyndham et al. (1986) (60)	South Africa (white miners only)	SMR = 161 (137–190)	Cumulative dust exposure had RR = 1.77 per 10 particle-years underground, adjusted for smoking
Hnizdo and Sluis Cremer (1991) (30)		Smoking adjusted RR for silica particle-years/1000 (SPY) <15 SPY RR = 1.00 15–30 SPY RR = 1.54 31–40 SPY RR = 2.07 ≥41 SPY RR = 2.92	Dose-related gradient; apparent synergy between smoking and silica exposure, with greatest effect among those with 35 pack-years and >30 SPY

least 1 year by Homestake between 1940 and 1965 and followed up until June 1, 1977. An index of dust exposure by job location was assembled for the purpose of assessing dose-response gradients. The SMR for malignant neoplasms of trachea, bronchus, and lung was 100, with no trends in risk by dust exposure or length of employment.

Katsnelson and Mokronosova (61) examined the mortality experience of male underground miners at a gold mine in Sverdlovsk, Russia. The authors presented sex-specific mortality relative risks (RR) for the years 1948–1974, comparing the results for the miners with the death rates from a neighboring town. The observed and expected numbers were not provided, nor were dust exposure or smoking data available. Overall, the RR from pulmonary tumors was 7.9 ($p < 0.001$). The RR dropped to 3.1 ($p < 0.02$) with exclusion of miners with silicosis.

Armstrong et al. (62) studied 1974 gold miners from Kalgoorlie, Western Australia, who were first surveyed in 1961 and 1962 for silicosis and then followed until 1975. The SMR for respiratory cancer was 145 (95% CI = 127–165); with adjustment for cigarette smoking, underground miners had a SMR of 141. A diagnosis of silicosis in the early 1960s was demonstrated to be a modest predictor of mortality from respiratory cancer. The authors evaluated radon and arsenic levels in the gold ore and concluded that the concentrations were low and did not confound the results.

Muller and colleagues (44) conducted a retrospective cohort study of 6972 underground gold miners (excluding miners with uranium and asbestos employment) from the Province of Ontario, Canada, who were employed at least 60 months from 1955 to 1977. Dust exposures were not incorporated into this analysis, although silica concentrations in Ontario gold mines have been known to be high. No information on the smoking habits of the miners was available, although later analysis demonstrated that smoking was not a confounder in the mortality rates (63). The SMR for cancers of the trachea, bronchus, and lung was elevated (SMR = 145).

In a report to the Ontario Workers' Compensation Board (OWCB), two additional analyses were undertaken of the lung cancer risk among the Province's gold miners (63). Shannon et al. (58) defined a larger cohort than Muller et al., including 2183 deaths of gold miners with a minimum of 5 years in gold mining. Previous exposure to asbestos or uranium eliminated the miner from entry to the expanded cohort. Paralleling the findings of Muller et al. (44), the lung cancer SMR was 141 ($p < 0.001$). The data suggested that the lung cancer risk was greatest for those first exposed before 1936, and a clear gradient emerged with time since first dust exposure, including a weighted duration of dust-years.

A second evaluation of Muller and co-workers' findings by Miller et al. (59) accompanied the 1987 OWCB report. Miller and colleagues combined cohorts of gold miners including those who had worked less than 85% of the time in gold ore mining. Miller and colleagues confirmed the overall excess of lung cancer and showed that year of first employment was a risk factor for lung cancer in a pattern reflective of high silica dust exposures extant in the mines before 1945. Uncontrolled confounding by smoking was rejected as an explanation for the excess lung cancer because pulmonary cancer risk was not elevated among other Ontario miners with similar smoking histories.

The most recent determination of the lung cancer risk among Ontario gold miners included follow-up on 13,603 men from 1955 to 1986 (155). This analysis included some sampling data for silica, radon daughters, arsenic, and asbestiform fibers and also examined smoking status. The authors found that gold miners who began work before 1946 and never mined nickel had a lung cancer SMR of 140 (95% CI = 122–159); for men who mined gold before 1946 and nickel before 1936 had a SMR of 181 (95% CI = 109–283). Poisson regression model of experience before 1945 showed significant linear trends for arsenic exposure (lagged by 20 years) and for radon decay products (lagged by 5 years). The best fitting models were found for joint exposure to arsenic and to radon, but the model with duration of exposure to high silica dust and employment before 1945 explains greater variance in the regression. Smoking and exposure to fibrous mineral dusts were evaluated and found to be unlikely explanations for the lung cancer excess.

Wyndham et al. (60) found excess lung cancer in a cohort of 3971 white South African gold miners, born between 1916 and 1930 and alive and actively employed in 1970, who were followed for 9 years. The authors used a case-referent approach to examine risk factors, including cumulative dust exposure and length of service. The smoking-adjusted cumulative dust exposure rate ratio (RR) was 1.77 per 10 particle years of underground exposure (95% CI = 0.94–3.31). In addition, the smoking-adjusted RR was 1.14 per 10 years of underground employment (95% CI = 0.632–2.05). The findings suggest that degree of silica exposure is a stronger risk factor than length of underground employment.

Hnizdo and Sluis-Cremer (30) presented a benchmark study of 2209 South African white male gold miners who began mining during the years 1936–1943. The men were examined for pulmonary disease risk during the years 1968–1971 and then followed for mortality from 1968 to 1986. The study objectives were to describe the dose-response relationship between silica dust and lung cancer risk, the combined effect of silica dust and smoking, and the association between lung cancer and silicosis at necropsy (addressed below). The selection criteria for the 1968–1971 sample were age between 45 and 54 years and a minimum of 10 years of underground gold mining experience. Vital status was ascertained using South African sources, and causes of death were determined from the best available evidence, including the extensive postmortem records maintained for medicolegal purposes.

The authors classified the gold mine jobs into 11 groups based on the average respirable silica dust concentrations (64). Cumulative dust measures (in respirable particles-years/1000) were calculated for each miner based on the number of shifts and occupations for each decade worked. Smoking information had been obtained in the 1968–1971 survey, and changes in smoking status were obtained from the miners' longitudinal medical files. In contrast with the other cohort members, the 77 lung cancer patients had higher cumulative levels of silica exposure, were more often smokers, had lower pulmonary function, and had more symptoms of pulmonary disease.

In Cox proportional hazards models that adjusted for age and cigarette equivalent pack-years, the following four cumulative dust variables were statistically significant: silica particle years (SPY) to 1949/1000 ($p < 0.01$); SPY to 1959/1000 ($p < 0.05$); SPY to start of follow-up in 1968/1000 ($p < 0.01$); and SPY up to 1986/1000 ($p < 0.05$). The smoking-adjusted RR increased with cumulative silica particulate exposure (Table 3). The proportional hazards model estimated the RR for lung cancer per 1000 SPY as 1.023 (95% CI = 1.005–1.042) with adjustment for smoking, year of birth, and age. Miners exposed to 50,000 SPY have 3.2 times greater likelihood of dying from lung cancer than those exposed to only 15,000 SPY. In analyses of the combined effects of smoking and silica exposure, the two exposures appeared to act synergistically.

With the exception of the studies of the Homestake miners by Brown et al. (57) and McDonald et al. (56), studies have found lung cancer risks to be increased in populations of gold ore miners throughout the world (30,44,55,58–60,62). The increased risk does not appear to result from confounding by smoking and shows a positive association with degree of silicosis. Wyndham et al. (60) and Hnizdo and Sluis-Cremer (30) have demonstrated that indexes of cumulative exposure to respirable silica are significantly associated with lung cancer risk, even after adjusting for smoking. The study of Hnizdo and Sluis-Cremer (30) indicated that smoking and silicosis act synergistically, supporting a hypothesis advanced by Goldsmith and Guidotti (65).

C. Granite Industry and Stone and Construction Work

Studies of workers employed in the granite, stone, and tunneling industries have proved informative on the relationship between silica exposure and cancer. Few of the potentially confounding exposures to such agents as radon and diesel fumes, found in some metal ore mines, or polycyclic aromatic hydrocarbons, found in foundries, are present in these industries.

Case Reports and Descriptive Studies

Boiler scalers, who clean the insides of steam generators, are exposed to dust with a silica concentration ranging from 6.4 to 26.4%. Harding et al. (66) described a case of pneumoconiosis with typical silicotic fibrosis and squamous cell carcinoma of the bronchus; smoking history was not provided. Craighead and Vallyathan (67) conducted postmortem examinations of 15 Vermont granite workers who died without radiological evidence of pneumoconiosis. Evidence of crystalline silica and fibrotic lesions was found in all lung samples, and in 6 of 15 cases, the cause of death was bronchogenic carcinoma.

Kennaway and Kennaway, (68) using data from the Registrar-General's Statistical Review of England and Wales for the years 1921–1932 and 1933–1938, examined lung and larynx cancer mortality according to occupation listed on the death certificates (Table 4). In general, the SMRs suggest that street masons, stonemasons, and sandblasters had elevated risks for lung cancer. There was a 40% elevated risk for laryngeal cancer among street masons; however, street pavers were exposed to asphalt fumes in addition to silica dust.

Guralnick (69) examined the 1950 U.S. mortality among men aged 20–64 years and found that stonemasons had a SMR for lung cancer of 148, while operatives in stone, clay, and glass products had a SMR of 117. Milham (37) reported that Washington brick masons, stonemasons, and like workers had a PMR of 141 ($p < 0.05$) for cancer of the trachea, bronchus, and lung. Milham also reported that sandblasters who died during the years 1950–1979 in Washington had a PMR of 348 ($p < 0.01$) for ages 20–64 years (70). Dubrow and Wegman (26) calculated social-class-adjusted mortality odds ratios (MOR) for Massachusetts residents from 1971 to 1973. For brick masons and stonemasons, the MOR was 143 for cancers of the trachea, bronchus, and lung. Lynge et al. (41) used the Nordic occupational mortality and cancer incidence registers to assess the lung cancer risk for granite, stone, and construction workers. For Norway, the authors reported elevated RRs for other construction workers and for stone quarrying; for Sweden, an increased risk for workers in the sand and clay pits; for Finland, a significant risk for excavating and highway construction (RR = 1.97; 95% CI = 1.32–2.83), an elevated RR for limestone quarrying, and a RR of 1.75 for stonecutting; and for Denmark, a RR of 2.10 for stonecutting and a RR of 2.9 (95% CI = 1.17–5.98) for self-employed stonecutters.

Table 4 Mortality Risks for Granite, Stone, and Construction Occupations, UK, 1921–1938

	SMR 1921–1932		SMR 1933–1938		Overall SMR 1921–1938	
Occupation	Lung	Larynx	Lung	Larynx	Lung	Larynx
Pavers, street masons, concretors, asphalters	109	154	137	116	164	140
Stonemasons, cutters, and dressers	149	125	140	48	143	96
Sandblasters	201	—	103	—	136	—
Stone miners and quarriers	105	73	49	98	70	82

Source: Kennaway and Kennaway (68).

Epidemiological Studies of Granite Workers, Tunnelers, and Sandblasters

Table 5 summarizes the epidemiological studies of granite workers, tunnelers, and sandblasters. Vermont granite workers are exposed to quartz dust having approximately 30% free silica; the workers do not have other potentially confounding exposures such as metal oxide fumes, radiation, or asbestiform fibers. Davis et al. (71) conducted a PMR study of 969 deceased white granite workers whose x-rays were on file at the Vermont Division of Industrial Hygiene and who died between 1952 and 1978. The authors developed a dust index for estimating exposures and excluded persons with tuberculosis and silicosis. The PMR was 1.3 for all respiratory cancers (95% CI = 1.0–1.6). A trend of respiratory cancer risk with dust exposure categories was not found, but statistical power was low. Smoking data were not available for the subjects. Because participation in the x-ray program before 1951 was voluntary, the study may have been affected by "volunteer bias" (see Ref. 77), with healthier subjects tending to enter the cohort.

Costello and Graham (72) conducted a cohort study of 5414 Vermont granite workers from 1950 and 1982 based on personnel information from the Occupational Hygiene Division of the Vermont State Health Department. Overall, the risk of lung cancer was not increased, but there was an approximately 25% excess mortality from lung cancers among workers hired before 1940.

Steenland and Beaumont (78) conducted a proportional mortality study of 1905 white members of the U.S. Granite Cutters Union using U.S. deaths for comparison. Lung cancer mortality (PMR = 119) was elevated but not significantly, and lung cancer risk did not increase with duration of exposure. In a case-control analysis, mention of silicosis or silicotuberculosis on the death certificate was associated with increased lung cancer risk (OR = 3.16, $p < 0.001$).

Kurppa et al. (79) and Koskela et al. (73,80) assessed cancer risks among a cohort of Finnish granite workers. The geometric mean quartz dust levels ranged from 1.0 to 1.5 mg/m^3, with the highest concentrations found in drilling jobs. Koskela et al. (80) demonstrated a maximum SMR of approximately 350 after 27 years of follow-up. Koskela et al. (73) continued the follow-up to 1985, finding that the SMR for lung cancer was 156 ($p < 0.05$). With increasing years since entry into granite work, the SMR rose from 156 to 281 ($p < 0.001$) for employment of 25 years or more, and to 226 for 30 years or more. Although smoking information was not available for the subjects, tobacco use by granite workers was reported to be comparable to that of all Finnish men.

Selikoff (5) examined a 932-member cohort of unionized New York City tunnel workers from 1955 to 1972. These men were exposed to siliceous dusts containing sizable amounts of quartz, schists, and gneisses and were unlikely to have been exposed to asbestos. The overall SMR for lung cancer was 160, and the risk of respiratory cancer increased with the number of years worked, with a minimum of 20 years employment before elevated cancer risk was demonstrated.

Table 5 Summary of Epidemiological Studies of Lung Cancer Risk Among Granite Workers, Tunnelers, and Sandblasters

Author (year)	Country	Type of exposure	Risk measure (95% CI)	Comment
Davis et al. (1983) (71)	Vermont, U.S.	Granite	PMR = 1.3 (1.0–1.6)	No apparent trends for dust index
Costello and Graham (1986) (72)	Vermont, U.S.	Granite	SMR – 104	Excess observed among workers hired before 1940 when dust levels were high
Steenland and Beaumont (1986) (78)	U.S.	Members of Granite Workers Union	PMR = 119	No time trends or gradients for duration; no dust exposures
			OR = 3.16 ($p < 0.001$)	Mention of silicosis on the death certificate; no smoking data
Koskela et al. (1990) (73)	Finland	Granite workers	SMR = 156 ($p < 0.05$)	No individual dust levels; no smoking data
		≥25 yrs	SMR = 281 ($p < 0.001$)	
Selikoff (1978) (5)	New York City, U.S.	Unionized tunnel workers	SMR = 160	No smoking data
		Employed <20 years	SMR = ~100	
		20–29 years	SMR = 210	
		≥30 years	SMR = 430	
Puntoni et al. (1979) (74)	Genoa, Italy	Sandblasters	RR = 3.76 ($p < 0.05$)	No smoking or dust exposure data; possible confounding by solvents and asbestos
Guenel et al. (1989) (75)	Denmark	Stone workers	SIR = 200 (149–189)	No smoking data; no exposure data; national incidence rates adjusted for region
	Copenhagen	All skilled stone workers	SIR = 306 (181–482)	
	Copenhagen	Sandstone workers	SIR = 808 (323–1657)	
	Copenhagen	Granite workers	SIR = 404 (202–723)	
	Bornholm	Mixed skilled and unskilled	SIR = 119 (51–235)	
	Other Denmark	Skilled workers	SIR = 192 (167–303)	
Mehnert et al. (1990) (76)	Germany	Slate quarryworkers	SMR = 109	Positive risk gradient for time since first exposure and duration of employment; no smoking data
		with silicosis	SMR = 183	

Sandblasting produces a large quantity of silica dust, and workers often blast in confined spaces where exposures can be very high. Puntoni et al. (74) compared the lung cancer risk among 190 sandblasters, employed in a cohort of 2190 Genoa, Italy, shipyard workers, with the general male population of Genoa. The sandblasters had RRs of 3.76 ($p < 0.05$) for lung cancer and 5.04 ($p < 0.05$) for laryngeal cancer (based on only three cases). Smoking information was not available.

The study by Lynge et al. (41) of Nordic dusty trades indicated that stonecutting doubled the lung cancer mortality risk in Denmark. To further explore that association, Guenel et al. (75) studied a cohort of 2071 Danish stone workers from 1943 to 1984. For the whole cohort, the age- and region-standardized incidence ratio (SIR) for lung cancer was 200 (95% CI = 149–269); for Copenhagen, the SIR was 306 (95% CI = 181–482); for Bornholm (a center of road and building materials industry and stonecutting), the SIR was 119 (95% CI = 51–235); and for other regions of Denmark, the SIR was 192 (95% CI = 167–303). Among skilled trades from Copenhagen, sandstone workers had a SIR of 808 (95% CI = 323–1657) and granite workers a SIR of 404 (95% CI = 202–723). Among unskilled workers, the overall SIR was 181 (95% CI = 116–270), while the road building materials industry showed a significantly increased SIR of 246 (95% CI = 143–394).

Mehnert et al. (76) evaluated the mortality risks of 2483 German slate quarry workers employed at least 1 year between 1953 and 1985 and followed-up from 1970 to 1985. The SMR for lung cancer mortality for all workers was non-significantly increased to 109, but was 183 for workers with silicosis. For slate workers who survived 20 years after first exposure, lung cancer mortality showed a positive risk-response gradient with time since first exposure and an increase with duration of employment. The positive association of exposure measures with lung cancer risk was present among workers with and without silicosis.

These studies show a pattern of generally increased lung cancer risk among granite workers and tunnelers that is apparent only after decades of work. The studies of Selikoff (5) and Mehnert et al. (76) indicate a gradient of risk associated with duration of employment. This group of studies is limited by a lack of information on individual silica exposure levels.

D. Ceramics, Porcelain, and Glass Industries (Including Potteries, Cement, and Tile and Brick Workers)

Descriptive Studies of Ceramics and Pottery Industries

Kennaway and Kennaway (68) reported that potters had elevated risks for lung and larynx cancer in addition to dramatic elevations for silicosis and tuberculosis; the risks for brick workers were lower (Table 6). Brick kiln workers clean and repair refractory brick, which contains very high levels of silica dust. Using the records of the U.K. National Health Service Central Register and the Office of Popu-

Table 6 Mortality Risks for Ceramic and Pottery Occupations, U.K., 1921–1938

	SMR 1921–1932		SMR 1933–1938		Overall SMR 1921–1938	
Occupation	Lung	Larynx	Lung	Larynx	Lung	Larynx
Potters, mill workers, etc.	96	—	218	—	174	—
Potters, waremakers, casters	152	184	132	118	140	160
Brick kiln and ovenmen	23	71	121	123	85	90
Brick and plain tile makers	49	106	47	0	48	67

Source: Kennaway and Kennaway (68).

lation Censuses and Surveys, McDowall (81) examined the risk of death among 607 cement workers employed in three areas in North Kent from 1948 to 1981. The SMR for lung cancer was 85. Dubrow and Wegman (26) reported that Massachusetts glass workers had a social-class-adjusted MOR of 314 for trachea, bronchus, and lung. Lynge et al. (41) reported the RR for lung cancer in the following Nordic countries as—Norway: glass, ceramic, and clay workers, 1.79 (95% CI = 1.00–2.95), and ceramic modelers and formers 1.75; Sweden: glass makers, 1.23; Finland: glass, ceramic, and clay workers, 1.27, and glass molders, 1.16; Denmark: glass makers, 1.62, and unskilled glass workers, 1.75 (95% CI = 1.09–2.68).

Epidemiological Studies of Glass, Ceramic, and Pottery Workers

A lung cancer excess among glass, ceramic, and pottery workers has been found in several studies. Sankila et al. (82) studied cancer incidence from 1953 to 1986 in two cohorts of Finnish glass workers. Overall, the SIR for lung cancer for men was 130 (95% CI = 100–167) and for women 111 (95% CI = 45–229). Glassblowers from one cohort had a SIR of 85 (95% CI = 28–198) and all other glass workers had a SIR of 133 (95% CI = 93–183), approximately the same as the SIR of 134 of the other cohort (95% CI = 88–194).

Thomas (83) examined the mortality of members of the U.S. Pottery and Allied Workers Union from 1955 to 1977 and found a significant ($p < 0.01$) increase in the PMR for lung cancer. Because the lung cancer excess appeared to be confined to workers in sanitary-ware production, Thomas and Stewart (84) conducted a mortality study of 2055 white male sanitary-ware workers employed between 1939 and 1966 and followed until 1980. Although lacking specific industrial hygiene data, the authors were able to categorize qualitatively the exposure to silica and nonfibrous talc. Overall, the SMR was 143, with the lung cancer excesses occurring in workers in the high silica exposure jobs (SMR = 181; $p < 0.05$) and in jobs characterized by high silica and high exposure to nonfibrous talc (SMR = 254; $p < 0.05$). Further analysis suggested that risk increased more steeply with years exposed to talc than with years exposed to silica (85).

Forastiere et al. (86) used the death registry of Civitacastellana, Italy, for the years 1968–1984 to examine lung cancer risk among pottery workers, using matched case-referent methods. The study subjects were 72 lung cancer patients and 319 matched controls; next-of-kin of the subjects were interviewed on smoking and occupational histories by public health nurses blinded to study objectives. The presence of disability from silicosis was ascertained for all subjects from the Italian National Institute for Compensation of Occupational Diseases. The time-, age-, and smoking-adjusted Mantel-Haenszel RR was 1.0 for quarry work and 2.0 (95% confidence intervals = 1.1–3.5) for ceramics. For workers with silicosis, the risk of lung cancer (OR = 3.9, 95% CI = 1.8–8.3) was greater than for those without silicosis (OR = 1.4; 95% CI = 0.7–2.8). Further analysis by Lagorio et al. (87) suggested that the combination of silicosis and smoking enhances the lung cancer risk compared with the risk among subjects either unexposed to ceramics or without silicosis. Firing and repairing and cleaning jobs were associated with significantly increased RRs of 2.2 and 3.1, respectively.

Winter and co-workers (88) examined mortality in 6187 British pottery workers who were surveyed in 1970–1971 and followed from 1970 to 1985. For men younger than 60 years old at the time of the survey, the SMR for lung cancer comparison was significantly increased (SMR = 140, 95% CI = 107–180). Although employment in several ceramic products or job groups was associated with increased SMRs, the increase was significant only for employment in glazing and decorating jobs (SMR 282, 95% CI = 103–613).

Chen et al. (45) and McLaughlin and colleagues (46) examined the risk in workers in eight pottery factories in southern China. The SMR for lung cancer in pottery workers from 1972 to 1989 was 58 ($p < 0.05$). In a case-control analysis, the OR (adjusted for age and smoking) did not vary significantly with cumulative exposure to respirable silica or with estimates of cumulative exposures to all dusts, arsenic, polycyclic aromatic hydrocarbons (PAH), or radon. Furthermore, the OR was 0.5 for a previous history of silicosis among pottery workers.

Katsnelson and Mokronosova (61) examined lung cancer at two aluminosilicate fireclay plants and at a silica firebrick plant. Although the firebrick and fireclay dusts contain high levels of quartz, dust samples were not collected. At the two fireclay plants, the RRs for lung cancer in men were 4.0 ($p < 0.01$) and 4.5; women at the first plant had a nonsignificant RR for respiratory cancer of 5.1. At the firebrick plants the RR was 2.0 ($p < 0.05$) for male workers and 0.8 for women.

Refractory brick manufacture uses extensive amounts of silica. Merlo et al. (89) examined the lung cancer risk among 1022 refractory brick workers. Overall, the lung cancer SMR was 151 (95% CI = 100–218) with an additional SMR of 193 (95% CI = 63–451) for laryngeal cancer. These investigators found an increasing lung cancer risk for more than 19 years latency (SMR = 178; 95% CI = 75–346), and greater risk for workers hired before 1957 (SMR = 177; 95% CI = 103–284).

Puntoni et al. (90) conducted a follow-up study of 211 workers employed in a refractory silica brick plant near Genoa. The mortality of these workers from 1960 to 1979 was compared to that of the age-specific male population of Genoa from 1960 to 1980. For the respiratory tract, the SMR was 208 for lung cancer (95% CI = 113–349) and 405 for laryngeal cancer, based on small numbers of deaths. The excess respiratory tract cancer risk was similar in the subjects with and without silicosis.

E. Foundry Work and Metallurgical Industries

Metal foundries use large quantities of sand and binders to make molds into which molten metal is poured during the manufacture of cast parts. After the metal cools, the mold is broken (the "knockout" process), and the molded piece is cleaned of sand on its surface with abrasive grinders. Although this section emphasizes the potential causal role of silica in lung cancer in foundry workers, metallurgy production also entails exposures to many other agents, including known and suspect carcinogens such as benzo[a]pyrene, metal oxide fumes, arsenic, and acid mists.

Case Series and Descriptive Studies of Foundry Workers

Kennaway and Kennaway (68) reported that both metal grinders and foundry sandblasters had elevated lung cancer SMRs. McLaughlin and Harding (91) presented the pathological findings in two series of male steel foundry workers from the Sheffield, U.K., area who were autopsied between 1949 and 1954. Of 64 patients with pneumoconiosis (silicosis and mixed-dust fibrosis) from 1950, three had concomitant carcinomas of the bronchus. A 1956 series included 85 cases, 76 with pneumoconiosis, and 13 with bronchial carcinomas.

Guralnick (69) reported that for deaths among steel workers classified as blacksmiths or forgemen, aged 20–64 years, the SMR was 190 ($p < 0.05$); for metal molders, the SMR was 227 ($p < 0.05$); and for operatives and kindred workers in primary metal industries, the lung cancer SMR was 159 ($p < 0.05$). Milham (37) reported that Washington State metal molders aged 20–64 years had a PMR of 312 for cancer of the bronchus and lung. Peterson and Milham (38) found California metal molders to have a PMR of 192 ($p < 0.05$) for cancer of the respiratory system. Williams et al. (39) reported smoking-adjusted ORs of 2.97 for laryngeal cancer for those from the metal industry; the pulmonary cancer risks were less than the null value for metal and fabricated metal industries. Dubrow and Wegman (26) reported that foundry workers had striking excesses of cancer for trachea, bronchus, and lung. Lynge and co-workers (41) reported that in Norway, foundry workers had a RR of 1.73 (95% CI = 1.12–2.25) and in Sweden, a RR of 1.38 (95% CI = 1.16–1.64); in Finland, workers in metallurgical smelting had a RR of 1.56 (95% CI = 1.31–1.86); and in Denmark, skilled molders had a RR of 1.6.

Gallagher and Threlfall (92) examined the cancer risk among metal workers in British Columbia, Canada, from 1950 to 1978. The lung cancer PMR was 134 (95% CI = 123–145). The authors examined occupational groups of metal workers and showed that metal mill workers had a significant PMR of 168 for pulmonary cancers. Boilermakers and structural iron workers had a significant PMR of 157 for lung cancer.

Epidemiological Studies of Foundry Workers

Table 7 summarizes the epidemiological studies of foundry workers. In a comprehensive examination of the Finnish foundry industry, Siltanen et al. (103) documented levels of silica and total dust concentrations in work areas, finding exposures of varying intensity throughout the industry. Koskela et al. (93) studied lung cancer in 3876 iron, steel, and nonferrous Finnish foundry workers, reporting an overall SMR of 151 ($p < 0.05$). The excess was confined to iron foundries, particularly to molders with more than 5 years of experience. Although the smoking habits of the full cohort were not obtained, surveys of employed workers showed that smoking among foundrymen was comparable to that of the general population, suggesting that the excess could not be attributed solely to smoking.

Tola et al. (94) conducted an expanded study of 3425 Finnish iron foundry workers with at least 1 year's employment and reported an overall PMR of 144 for lung cancer. In a nested case-control study, the molders alone and the molders and casters together had significant increases of 4.2 and 4.6, respectively. Dust exposure and smoking were not directly considered.

Gibson and co-workers (95) conducted a retrospective cohort study of Dofasco steel mill workers in Hamilton, Ontario, from 1967 to 1976. The authors compared foundry workers to nonfoundry workers, finding the overall lung cancer relative risk to be 5.0 ($p < 0.0005$). Lung cancer excesses were found for crane operators, finishers, molders, coremakers, and furnace operators. The authors noted that the finishing, molding, and furnace areas had the highest mean levels of total suspended particulates, much of them being silica, respirable particulates, and a benzene-soluble fraction of total suspended particulates. Surveys taken in the 1970s showed that the foundry workers smoked no more than the general male population. The authors proposed that smoking and exposure to particulate containing adsorbed organic material might be an explanation for the lung cancer excess. In a later study, Gibson et al. (104) demonstrated that foundry particulate was mutagenic and that a gradient of mutagenicity correlated well with particulate samples from the foundry where the elevated lung cancer SMRs were noted. The excess findings for crane operators were not supported by data from a study in the U.S. steel industry (105).

Redmond (96) and Redmond et al. (97) have conducted two major cancer mortality studies among nearly 59,000 members of the United Steelworkers of America, initially studied in 1953 and followed until 1975. Using deaths from

1953 to 1966, Redmond and co-workers first found elevated SMRs for pulmonary cancer among white men employed in the foundry, mason, and blacksmithing departments; complete follow-up to 1975 indicated that only blacksmithing showed a consistent lung cancer excess (97). Workers in the mason department remove, clean, and repair silica brick linings in the blast furnaces. No smoking data were available in these studies, but the rest of the steelworker cohort not employed in the department under study was used as the comparison group, which provided internal adjustment for smoking and social class.

Although the findings by Redmond et al. (97) do not show an overall excess mortality from employment in the foundry department, several smaller studies support the view that foundry workers have excess lung cancer RRs that range from 1.5 to 2 (98–101). Despite showing similar risks, these studies lacked smoking data, most of them lacked dust estimates, and several had small sample sizes.

Blot et al. (102) conducted a case-control study of lung cancer among white men in eastern Pennsylvania to assess the association with employment in the steel industry. The authors demonstrated a smoking-adjusted OR of 2.2 for usual employment (95% CI = 1.5–3.3). For the job category "foundry worker, mold maker," there was an odds ratio of 7.1 (95% CI = 1.2–5.8) based on only six cases. Although the authors obtained smoking histories, the next-of-kin respondents were able to provide only a surrogate measure of silica exposure by naming the subjects' departments.

Sherson and Iversen (106) evaluated the lung cancer risk among a cohort of 5579 Danish male foundry workers who were examined in national surveys from 1967 to 1974. Job exposures were ranked by industrial hygienists so that work histories could be scored for exposures to dust, PAH, and carbon monoxide. The authors observed a slight excess of lung cancer (SMR = 115), which was greatest for workers with more than 25 years of employment. Sherson and Iversen (106) also reported that there were eight deaths from lung cancer among 163 foundrymen with extant silicosis, suggesting a possible synergistic or additive effect between quartz and PAH either from the foundry environment or from smoking.

Fletcher (107) and Fletcher and Ades (108) conducted three studies of U.K. foundry workers. The first of these was a cohort study of 11,048 workers from nine steel foundries who began work between 1946 and 1965, worked at least 12 months, and were followed until 1978 (108). Overall, there was a significantly increased SMR of 149 ($p < 0.001$) for lung cancer, a level of risk shared by many dusty occupations in the plant. In the second study, Fletcher (107) sorted occupations into groups: a "silica group" that included sand preparation, molding coremakers, furnace repair, mold knockout men, shotblasters, and dressers. The overall risk for lung cancer among the silica group was increased (SMR = 171, $p < 0.001$). Lacking any direct data on past particulate exposures, Fletcher used the length of employment, which was considered an estimate of dust "dose." The overall SMR was 89 for an unexposed group, and 180 ($p < 0.001$) for the silica

Table 7 Summary of Epidemiological Studies of Lung Cancer Among Foundry Workers

Author (year)	Country	Occupation or source of SiO_2 exposure	Risk measure (95% CI)	Comments
Koskela et al. (1976) (93)	Finland	Iron, steel, and nonferrous foundry workers	SMR = 151 ($p < 0.05$)	Excess centered on iron foundries with ≥5 years
		Iron foundries only	SMR = 270 ($p < 0.05$)	employment; neither smoking nor exposure data available
Tola et al. (1979) (94)	Finland	Iron foundry workers	PMR = 144	No smoking or dust exposure information
		Molders	OR = 4.2 ($p < 0.01$)	
		Molders and casters	OR = 4.6 ($p < 0.01$)	
Gibson et al. (1977) (95)	Ontario, Canada	Foundry workers	RR = 5.0 ($p < 0.0005$)	Compared with nonfoundry
		Steel casting	SMR = 250 ($p < 0.05$)	workers; no smoking information
		Crane operators	SMR = 714 ($p < 0.01$)	
		Finishers	SMR = 314	Highest mean total suspended
		Molders	SMR = 255	particulates
Redmond, (1975); (96) Redmond et al. (1981) (97)	U.S., members of United Steelworkers of America employed in 7 plants	Foundry dept. (whites only)	SMR = 162	Elevated for 1953–1966 only;
		Mason dept. (whites only)	SMR = 212	indirect adjustment for smoking; no exposure data
		Blacksmith dept. (whites only)	SMR = 242	Consistent excess for 1953–1975

Decoufle and Wood (1979) (98)	U.S.	Foundry workers with 5 years of employment	SMR = 200	No smoking or exposure information
Egan et al. (1979) (99)	U.S., members of International Molders and Allied Workers	Union member for ⩾11 yrs	PMR = 147 ($p < 0.05$)	No smoking or exposure information
Egan-Baum et al. (1981) (100)	Expanded follow-up of 1979 study	For whites	PMR = 144 ($p < 0.05$)	No smoking or exposure information
		For blacks	PMR = 176 ($p < 0.05$)	
		Iron foundries among those aged 42–64 years	OR = 2.36 (1.0–5.5)	Compared to steel and nonferrous metal workers
Mirer et al. (1986) (101)	U.S., United Autoworkers Union members employed in ferrous foundry	For whites	PMR = 146 ($p < 0.05$)	White workers with longest employment in finishing had PMR of 179; no smoking or exposure data
		For blacks	PMR = 106	
Blot et al. (1983) (102)	U.S., Pennsylvania	Steel industry	OR = 1.8	Adjusted for smoking, age, education, other hazard employment; no exposure data
		Usual industry for 15 years as foundry workers and mold makers	OR = 7.1 (1.2–42.3)	

group, with a significant test for trend for 20 or more years of employment. A survey conducted in 1964 showed that the number of foundrymen in the United Kingdom who smoked was about the same as the national average of 70%, thus making this factor less likely to be a confounder. The third study presented standardized PMRs for death benefits paid to British foundry union members from 1979 to 1982 (107). In this study, Fletcher (107) listed four job categories: skilled molders, semiskilled molders, dressers, and laborers. The findings indicated that lung cancer was either constant or increasing among foundry molders.

Foundry workers may have substantial quartz exposure, particularly in such jobs as mason and fettling work, where there are high levels of silica particulate. Some studies show increased lung cancer in these highly exposed workers (107). However, the potential role of silica cannot be readily separated from the risk of other hazardous agents in the metallurgy environment, for example, polycyclic aromatic hydrocarbons, heavy metal fumes, and other chemicals; potential confounding by cigarette smoking was not directly controlled in most of the studies.

IV. Studies of Workers' Risk after Diagnosis with Silicosis

When the potential for silica to be a respiratory carcinogen was raised again by Goldsmith and colleagues in 1982 (8), the supportive evidence included animal studies, studies of selected dusty trades workers, and epidemiological studies of persons with silicosis. Heppleston (4) responded that silica was not a carcinogen and pointed to evidence from studies of coal miners and hematite miners and autopsy studies of persons with silicosis. Although there is general agreement that coal workers and iron ore miners are not at excess risk for pulmonary malignancies from occupational silica exposure, interpretations of the findings on lung cancer risk in persons with silicosis have varied. Why do the results of autopsy and epidemiology studies of silicotics seem to differ? This section examines the evidence from both types of studies and the potential biases that may underlie the apparent differences between the two sets of data.

A. Autopsy Study Results

The initial concern that silica exposure might be associated with lung cancer arose from autopsies of silicosis cases. During the 1930s, investigators in England, Canada, and South Africa compared the proportion of lung cancers in autopsied silicosis cases with that in nonsilicosis cases from the same dusty industries and also with that in general population series of autopsies. Although these early studies did not consider smoking, the descriptive findings suggested a link between silicosis and lung cancer.

In his 1934 report, Dible (2) described four cancer cases, including two with lung cancer, among 14 autopsied silicotics from East Lancashire, U.K., and from his findings proposed that silicosis and cancer could be associated. A subsequent study in Liverpool compared the silica content of lungs of 48 control subjects with that of 70 subjects dying from lung cancer, of whom 12 had silicosis or other fibrotic lung disease (109). The lungs of the silicotics with lung cancer had a mean silica content of 2.29 g, whereas the 48 controls and remaining 58 cancer patients had mean levels of 0.26 g [$p < 0.0001$ (calculated by the author)].

Table 8 provides a summary of autopsy series cited by Heppleston (4). Klotz (110) found respiratory tumors to be more common in 50 cases of silicosis (8.0%) than in 4500 deaths from other causes (1.2%) in Toronto, Ontario, Canada. A more recent study of porcelain workers in Germany (119) found lung cancer to be 2.1 times more common in persons with silicosis.

However, most other autopsy studies have shown less lung cancer in persons with silicosis than in comparison series (Table 8). In 1938, J. C. Bridge, the Senior Medical Inspector for the United Kingdom, compared the percentages of pulmonary tumors among 943 autopsies in silicosis patients with 347 necropsies in patients deceased from other causes (cited in Ref. 68). Of cases with silicosis, 2.4% had lung cancer compared with 4.9% in the controls, a mortality ratio (MR) of 0.5. Several series have been published from South Africa, including the report of Irvine (111) from the South African Miners' Phthisis Medical Bureau based on 6046 necropsies performed from 1920 to 1938, and later reports for the years 1948–1951 from the South African Institute for Medical Research (112,113). Meiklejohn reported on autopsies in the British pottery industries and on various dusty trades workers (114,115). Roadhouse Gloyne (116) also described necropsies of persons with silicosis in the United Kingdom. In 1949, Rüttner (117) reported that 1.1% of 271 silicotics had bronchogenic cancers compared with 2.0% in the general male population of Switzerland. Two decades later, Rüttner and Heer (118) and Rüttner (120) reported that among 684 autopsies of silicotics, 2.2% had lung cancer compared with 4.0% among the male population of Switzerland.

B. Epidemiological Study Results

Tables 9, 10, and 11 summarize contemporary epidemiological studies of lung cancer among workers with silicosis in Sweden, Ontario, Canada, Switzerland, Austria, Finland, South Africa, Italy, Japan, China, Singapore, and the United States. Table 9 presents the studies that used SMR or SIR to examine the cancer risks among silicotics. Table 11 presents studies using other measures of effect to assess cancer risk: PMR, MOR, and Mantel-Haenszel odds ratio (M-HOR).

Westerholm et al. (121) conducted a follow-up study from 1961 to 1980 of 712 silicotics and 810 controls from the same industries, matched for age, industry, and occupation. For silicotics from mining, quarrying, and tunneling industries, the

Table 8 Summary of Autopsy and Lung Cancer Studies

Author (year)	Country (Industry)	Mortality ratio (Years)	Comment
Bridge (1938) (cited in Ref. 68)	U.K.	0.5 (1938)	No adjustment for age, sex, or smoking
Klotz (1939) (110)	Toronto, Canada	6.7 (1925–1936)	No adjustment for age, sex, or smoking
Irvine (1939) (111)	South Africa (Miners' Phthisis Medical Bureau—gold mining)	0.58 miners without silicosis 0.57 miners with silicosis (1920–1938)	No adjustment for age or smoking
Becker and Chatgidakis (1959) (112)	South Africa (Inst. for Med. Research)	0.88 (1948–1951)	No adjustment for age or smoking
Chatgidakis (1963) (113)			
Meiklejohn (1949a) (114)	Stoke-on-Trent, U.K.	0.34 (1931–1946)	No adjustment for age, sex, or smoking
Meiklejohn (1949b) (115)	(pottery) (sandstone occupations)	0.21 (1931–1946)	
Roadhouse Gloyne (1951) (116)	U.K. (mineral dust workers)	0.83 (1929–1949)	No adjustment for age, sex, or smoking
Rüttner (1949) (117)	Switzerland	0.55	No adjustment for age or smoking
Rüttner and Heer (1969) (118)	Switzerland	0.55 (1960–1967)	No adjustment for age or smoking
Otto and Hinüber (1972) (119)	German (porcelain workers)	2.10	No adjustment for age, sex, or smoking

Table 9 Summary of the Lung Cancer Epidemiology Studies Using Standardized Mortality Ratios and Standardized Incidence Ratios

Author (year)	Country (industry)	SMR (significance)	Comment
Westerholm et al. (1986) (121)	Sweden	441 ($p < 0.05$)	Matched for occupation, age, year of first exposure to silica; indirect adjustment for smoking
	(Mining, quarrying, tunneling)	538 ($p < 0.05$) 529 ($p < 0.05$) SIR	
	(Mining, quarrying, tunneling)	385 ($p < 0.05$) 182 SIR	
	(Foundries)		
Finkelstein et al. (1982) (122)	Ontario, Canada (Underground miners)	198 ($p < 0.01$)	No adjustment for smoking, although authors estimate that 20% of excess explained by smoking
Finkelstein et al. (1987) (123)	(Above-ground occupations)	302 (173–489)	
Neuberger et al. (1986) (27)	Austria (All ocupations)	140 ($p < 0.05$)	No adjustment for smoking
Gudbergsson et al. (1984) (124)	Finland	3.0 (1.5–5.3) SIR	CIs are 99%
Kurppa et al. (1986) (125)	Finland	312 (230–414)	No adjustment for smoking; all CIs are 99%; all categories of radiographic findings show significant SMRs
	(Mining)	436 (246–670)	
	(Rock and stone)	271 (112–549)	
	(Steel casting)	184 (54–451)	
	(Foundries)	225 (88–464)	
	(Other)	343 (168–628)	
Zambon et al. (1986) (126)	Veneto Region, Italy	228 (169–302)	Smoking explains part of the excess; apparent dose-response for years since first exposure with 20 years minimum
	(Mining)	156 (68–871)	
	(Tunneling)	239 (145–376)	
	(Quarrying)	569 (200–1187)	
	(Mixed mine)	190 (90–347)	
	(Others)	279 (78–732)	

Table 9 Continued

Author (year)	Country (industry)	SMR (significance)	Comment
Chiyotani (1984) (127)	Japan—All	653 ($p < 0.05$)	Elevated risks for all smoking categories including 2.22 for never-smokers; inverse association for category of pneumoconiosis
Chiyotani et al. (1990) (128)	All	603 (529–677)	
	(Mining)	1.83 [Nested case/control (NCC)]	
	(Mining/tunneling)	1.75 NCC	
	(Ceramics)	∞ ($p < 0.05$) NCC	
	(Quarrymen)	1.33 NCC	
	(Quarrymen/coal miners)	0.57 NCC	
	(Kilnmen or casters)	∞ ($p < 0.05$) NCC	
Miller et al. (1987) (59)	Ontario, Canada (Goldminers)	156 (145–167)	Employment before 1945; smoking examined, but not thought to confound results
Infante-Rivard et al. (1989) (129)	Quebec, Canada	347 (311–390)	Smoking data unavailable
	(Mining)	378 (253–543)	
	(Granite)	204 (75–444)	
	(Foundries)	304 (255–369)	
	(Pottery)	499 (162–1166)	
	(Miscellaneous)	694 (332–1273)	

Amandus and Costello (1991) (15)	U.S.	173 (94–290)	Risk 2–3 times greater for smokers; radon levels do not explain the risk
	(Metal ore miners)	1.96 (1.19–3.20)#	#Compared to nonsilicotics and adjusted for age and smoking
	(Copper ore)	0.96 (0.20–2.81)	
	(Lead-zinc ore)	2.42 (0.66–6.21)	
	(Iron ore)	1,77 (0.21–6.38)	
	(Mercury ore)	14.03 (2.89–40.99)	
	(Other ores)	1.01 (0.12–3.68)	
Amandus et al. (1991) (130)	North Carolina, U.S	2.60 (1.80–3.60) 3.9 (2.4–6.4) when compared to nonsilicotic metal ore miners	Risks not explained by smoking
Chia et al. (1991) (131)	Singapore residents of Chinese ancestry (Granite and gravel work)	201 (92–381) SIR	No adjustment for smoking; risk increases with length of employment
	(Mild silicosis)	140 SIR	
	(Moderate silicosis)	279 SIR	
	(Severe silicosis)	511 SIR	
Merlo et al. (1991) (89)	Genoa, Italy	685 (447–1000)	Indirect adjustment for smoking explains 12 and 30% of risk
Ng et al. (1990) (132)	Hong Kong, China	203 (135–293)	All deaths were among smokers, but only 50% of the risk was due to unadjusted confounding

Table 10 Lung Cancer Risk Related to X-Ray Evaluation Among Ontario Gold Miners Employed Before 1945

X-ray rating[a]	Obs/exp.	SMR	95% CI
A (silicosis free)	118/88.0	134	122–147
B (mild silicosis)	53/26.3	201	175–232
C (severe silicosis)	21/8.7	242	191–303
Total	192/123.1	156	145–167

[a]Based on Ontario pneumoconiosis criteria.
Source: Miller et al. (59).

SMR was 538 ($p < 0.05$), and for the steel and iron industry, the SMR was 385 ($p < 0.05$).

Finkelstein et al. (122) conducted a follow-up study of 1190 Ontario, Canada, silicotics who had been employed underground from 1940 to 1975, comparing the lung cancer risk to that of Ontario men. The authors reported an overall SMR of 198 ($p < 0.01$) with SMRs of 303 ($p < 0.01$) and 195 ($p < 0.05$) for silicotics diagnosed from 1940 to 1949 and from 1950 to 1959, respectively. In another Canadian study, lung cancer risk from 1940 to 1985 among 276 silicotics employed in above-ground industries (excluding foundries) was elevated (SMR = 302, 95% CI = 173–489) (123).

Miller et al. (59) obtained x-rays of Ontario gold miners and demonstrated that lung cancer risk increased with the severity of radiographic silicosis, but this association was limited to miners employed before 1945 (see Table 10). Infante-Rivard et al. (129) assessed the lung cancer risk among 1165 silicotics in Quebec who were diagnosed from 1938 to 1985 and followed until 1986; they found an overall increase in lung cancer risk (SMR = 350, $p < 0.05$) and an increase in all industries together, mining, quarrying and tunneling, metallurgy, and ceramics, with SMRs that ranged from 200 to 690.

Lung cancer mortality has been examined in a number of European cohorts. Neuberger et al. (27) found increased risk for lung cancer among Austrian silicotics, using death certificate data from 1955 to 1979 (SMR = 140, $p < 0.05$). Gudbergsson et al. (124) examined cancer incidence among 331 silicotics identified from the Finnish Registry of Occupational Diseases who were compensated between 1964 and 1974 and followed through 1975. Compared to the general population of Finnish men, the SIR was 3.0 (95% CI = 1.5–5.3). In another Finnish study, Kurppa and colleagues (125) examined lung cancer mortality among 961 cases of silicosis diagnosed from 1935 to 1977; 80 lung cancer deaths were observed, with 25.5 expected from Finnish men (SMR = 312, 99% CI = 230–414). Silicotics from the mining industry had a SMR of 436 (99% CI = 246–

670); the rock and stone industry, 271 (99% CI = 112–549); steel casting, 184 (99% CI = 54–451); and iron foundries, 225 (99% CI = 88–455). Zambon et al. (126) followed a cohort of 1234 silicotics from the Veneto Region of Italy diagnosed from 1959 to 1963 and followed through 1980. Overall, the SMR for lung cancer was 228 (95% CI = 169–302). For the mining industry, the SMR was 156 (95% CI = 68–871); for tunneling, 239 (95% CI = 145–376); and for quarrying, 569 (95% CI = 200–1187).

Merlo and co-workers (89) conducted a follow-up study of 520 male silicotic patients seen at San Marco Hospital in Genoa, Italy, from 1961 to 1981. The SMR for respiratory tract cancers was 685 (26 observed, 3.8 expected based on Italian national mortality for men) with 95% CI = 447–1000. Using Axelson's method for indirect adjustment for smoking (140,142), the authors estimated that between 12% and 30% of the excess cancer risk could be attributed to unadjusted confounding from smoking.

Tornling et al. (141) examined lung cancer incidence and mortality among 280 silicotic men employed in the Swedish ceramics industry. Follow-up was from 1958 to 1983; the SMR for lung cancer was 188, with 95% CI = 85–356. For those subjects whose lung cancer occurred >10 years following diagnosis of silicosis, the SMR was 236 (95% CI = 107–448).

Carta et al. (143) reported SMR of 129 (95% CI = 80–200) for lung cancer for a cohort of 724 silicotics from Sardinia. The authors reported a SMR of 411 among heavy smokers and a SMR of 283 among cases with airflow obstruction. There was no association with severity of silicosis or with cumulative silica exposure.

In Japan, Chiyotani (127) showed that the SMR for lung cancer among silicotics rose from 178 to 573 for the periods 1971–1975 to 1976–1981. Chiyotani calculated the risk for lung cancer for the years 1979–1981 using patients from 11 pneumoconiosis clinics throughout Japan and found the SMR to be 575 (48 observed, 8.35 expected); for silicotics, the SMR was 653; and for anthracosilicosis, the SMR was 491. With extension of follow-up for 2 additional years, Chiyotani et al. (128) found the SMR to be 603 (95% CI = 529–677). In a case-control analysis (matching on hospital, age, and smoking), the odds ratios were elevated for mining, quarry work, and ceramics manufacture.

Amandus and Costello (15) examined the lung cancer risk among silicotics diagnosed in the 1959–1961 U.S. Public Health Service study of metal ore miners. Overall, these men had a SMR of 173 (95% CI = 94–290). Although the numbers of deaths were small, risks were elevated for lead-zinc, iron, and mercury ores. Compared with nonsilicotics and adjusting for age and smoking, silicotics had a RR of 1.96 (95% CI = 1.19–3.23).

Amandus et al. (130) published a seminal paper on the lung cancer risk among 760 silicotics from the North Carolina Dusty Trades surveillance program who were diagnosed after 1939 and followed for vital status until 1983. The authors compared the mortality rates of the silicotics with those of the United States and of North Carolina and with the nonsilicotics in the U.S. Public Health survey of metal ore miners described above. Among whites with silicosis, the SMR was 260 (95% CI = 180–360) based on U.S. rates and 300 (95% CI = 200–420) based on North Carolina rates. Cigarette smokers had a SMR of 340 (95% CI = 200–530) and nonsmokers a SMR of 170 (95% CI = 50–390). Compared to metal ore miners, North Carolina silicotics had a lung cancer RR of 3.9 (95% CI = 2.4–6.4), adjusted for smoking. In a comparison of silicotics with metal ore miners, never-smokers had a RR of 8.6, and smokers a RR of 3.2.

Chia and colleagues (131) examined the lung cancer incidence in 159 cases of silicosis among Chinese men registered between 1970 and 1984 in Singapore. All subjects had been employed in granite excavation and gravel crushing. The risk of lung cancer rose from 1.76 for 20–40 years of employment to 2.54 for more than 40 years; it also increased with the degree of radiographic silicosis: category 1 (mild silicosis) SIR = 1.4; category 2 (moderate profusion) SIR = 2.79; and category 3 (severe silicosis) SIR = 5.11.

Ng and colleagues (132) conducted a follow-up study of 1419 men registered as silicotics in Hong Kong, China. They reported a SMR of 203 (95% CI = 135–293), and the classification of radiographic capacities showed an increasing trend associated with lung cancer risk. All pulmonary cancer deaths occurred among smokers. Using Axelson's (142) approach for estimating degree of confounding from smoking, the authors suggested that 50% of the risk may have been from confounding by tobacco.

Table 11 presents the results of the studies using effect measures other than SMR or SIR. Westerholm (133) used a proportional mortality approach to examine lung cancer risk among silicotics enrolled in the Swedish Pneumoconiosis Register. He found the overall PMR to be 2.7 ($p < 0.05$); for subjects with silicosis arising from employment in mining, quarrying, and tunneling between 1931 and 1948, the PMR was 5.9 ($p < 0.01$); and for those with pneumoconiosis diagnosed between 1949 and 1969, the PMR was 3.8 ($p < 0.01$). For silicotics employed in the steel and iron industry and whose condition presented between 1949 and 1969, the PMR was 2.2 ($p < 0.05$).

Hessel and Sluis-Cremer (134) tested the association of underground exposure and silicosis in a matched case-control study of lung cancer among white South African gold miners. The authors used 127 lung cancer deaths and an equal number of controls from the files of the gold miners' pension fund for January 1979–October 1983. The pulmonary cancers were verified by autopsy or biopsy record. Matched-pairs analysis revealed that there was no association between silicosis (or cumulative dust exposure) and lung cancer; the matched OR was 1.1. Hessel et al. (135) conducted an expanded case-control study of necropsied miners that included 231 primary lung tumors and 318 controls who died from 1975 to 1986 (excluding those in the prior study). Their findings showed no differences in cumulative dust exposure, dust intensity, shifts employed underground, and shifts in high-dust jobs. The OR (adjusted for age, smoking, and cumulative dust exposure by conditional logistic regression) for silicosis of the parenchyma was 1.10 (95% CI = 0.79–1.60); for silicosis of the pleura, 0.80 (95% CI = 0.54–1.20); and for silicosis of the hilar lymph glands, 1.29 (95% CI = 0.83–2.00). Hnizdo and Sluis-Cremer (30) also examined the association between silicosis and lung cancer in a nested case-control study of their study cohort of miners (see above for details). They reported that the OR (adjusted for age, cumulative dust particle-years, and cigarette smoking) for silicosis of the lung was 0.9 (95% CI = 0.5–1.6); for silicosis of the pleura, 1.2 (95% CI = 0.7–2.0), and for silicosis of the hilar lymph glands, 3.9 (95% CI = 1.2–12.7). There was a significant trend of risk ($p = 0.035$) with the degree of silicosis of the hilar glands (comparing slight, moderate, and marked with no silicosis).

Schüler and Rüttner (136) used the mortality odds ratio in a study of the mortality from 1960 to 1978 of 2399 cases of silicosis in Switzerland. The overall lung cancer risk was 2.2 ($p < 0.05$); for mining, the MOR was 2.3 ($p < 0.001$); for stone and quarrying work, 1.2; for the foundry industry, 3.3 ($p < 0.001$); and for the ceramic industry, 2.0.

Rubino et al. (137) conducted a PMR study of 746 silicotics from the Piedmont area of Italy during the years 1970–1985. They reported a significant PMR of 1.4 for lung cancer ($p < 0.05$).

Forastiere et al. (86) demonstrated that among Italian ceramic workers with silicosis there was a smoking- and age-adjusted Mantel-Haenszel OR of 3.9 (95% CI = 1.8–8.3). A more recent report of the lung cancer risk among 595 Latium region silicotics showed a MOR of 1.5 (95% CI = 1.1–1.9), with significant risks demonstrated for mining and for pottery work (138)

Steenland and Beaumont (78) conducted a nested case-control study in a cohort study of the mortality of granite workers that showed a 3.2-fold OR ($p < 0.001$) when comparing lung cancer cases with other cancers for mention of silicosis on the death certificate.

Goldsmith et al. (139) reported a PMR of 2.22 (95% CI = 139–337) for white pneumoconiosis claimants identified from 1945 to 1963 in the California Silicosis Registry and followed until 1984. There was no adjustment for smoking.

McLaughlin et al. (46) reported ORs of 0.5 for tungsten ore miners, 2.0 ($p < 0.05$) for tin miners, and 3.1 for copper/iron ore miners. These findings among Chinese silicotics were adjusted for age and smoking.

C. Biases in Autopsy Studies

The mortality ratios from the autopsy findings are calculated as:

[# lung cancers/silicotics autopsied]/[# lung cancers/nonsilicotics autopsied]

Table 11 Summary of Lung Cancer Epidemiology Studies Using Other Study Methods

Author (year)	Country (industry)	Measure of effect (Test of significance)	Comment
Westerholm (1980) (133)	Sweden (All)	PMR = 2.7 ($p < 0.05$)	No smoking information
	(Mining, quarrying, and tunneling 1931–1948)	PMR = 5.9 ($p < 0.01$)	
	(Mining, quarrying, and tunneling 1949–1969)	PMR = 3.8 ($p < 0.01$)	
	(Steel and iron foundries 1949–1969)	PMR = 2.2 ($p < 0.05$)	
	(Ceramics)	PMR = 1.3	
	(Other)	PMR = 3.3	
Hessel and Sluis-Cremer (1986) (134)	South Africa (White gold miners)	OR = 1.1 ($p = 0.87$)	Matched for year of birth, tobacco consumption, and minimum number of dusty shifts
Hessel et al. (1990) (135)	(Parenchymal silicosis)	OR = 1.10 (0.79–1.60)	Matched only on age and minimum number of dusty shifts;
	(PS)	OR = 0.80 (0.54–1.20)	Adjusted for smoking, age, and dust exposure
	(SHG)	OR = 1.29 (0.83–2.00)	

Hnizdo and Sluis-Cremer (1991) (30)	(White gold miners surveyed 1968–1971 aged 45–54 with 10 years minimum underground)	OR = 0.9 (0.5–1.6) for silicosis of lung OR = 1.2 (0.7–2.0) for PS OR = 3.9 (1.2–12.7) for SHG	Adjusted for age, smoking, and cumulative dust exposure; gradient for degree of SHG
Schüler and Rüttner (1986) (136)	Switzerland	MOR = 2.0 ($p < 0.001$)	No smoking data
	(Mining)	MOR = 2.3 ($p < 0.001$)	
	(Stone and quarry)	MOR = 1.2 ($p > 0.6$)	
	(Ceramics)	MOR = 2.0 ($p = 0.25$)	
	(Foundry)	MOR = 3.3 ($p < 0.001$)	
	(Others and ceramics)	MOR = 2.4 ($p < 0.05$)	
Steenland and Beaumont (1986) (78)	U.S. (members of Granite Workers Union)	OR = 3.2 ($p < 0.001$) Nested case-control study	No smoking data
Rubino et al. (1985) (137)	Piedmont Region, Italy	PMR = 1.54 ($p < 0.05$)	No smoking information
Forastiere et al. (1986) (86)	Civitacastellana, Italy (Ceramics)	OR = 3.9 (1.8–8.3)	Adjusted for smoking
Forastiere et al. (1989) (138)	Latium Region, Italy	MOR = 1.5 (1.1–1.9)	
Goldsmith et al. (1990) (139)	California, U.S.	PMR = 2.2 (1.4–3.4)	No adjustment for smoking
McLaughlin et al. 1992 (46)	China		
	(Tungsten)	OR = 0.5	Adjusted for age and smoking
	(Tin)	OR = 2.0 ($p < 0.05$)	
	(Copper/iron)	OR = 3.1	

PS = pleural silicosis, SHG = silicosis of hilar glands

As Heppleston has argued (4), the mortality ratio (MR) for the autopsy studies is approximately 1.0. However, bias from failure to adjust for age and smoking could contribute to this null finding. If the age of patients with silicosis tends to be less than the age of comparison persons, or smoking is greater in the comparison group, the MR would be biased toward the null value of unity. Undoubtedly, selection bias affects both the numerator and denominator of the autopsy ratio. Subjects labeled as having silicosis have different degrees of disability [without standardized criteria for definition, such as those developed by the International Labor Organization (144)] and different levels of compensation. Depending on the significance of silicosis to the patient and the physician, the silicotic may be monitored with chest x-rays and examinations, and as a result, lung cancers may be more likely to be diagnosed (10). The probability of autopsy may depend on cultural and clinical practices that vary among societies, by cause of death, and by occupational characteristics. Most autopsy series used for the denominators in MR studies were convenience samples and were not drawn systematically from defined populations. Because smoking is a powerful cause of mortality, smokers are likely to be overrepresented in autopsy series compared to all deaths, and the proportion of cases with lung cancer to be exaggerated as a result. There is also the possibility of misclassifying subjects as "silicotic" when they actually have another pulmonary condition, such as coal workers' pneumoconiosis, asbestosis, or mixed-dust fibrosis (145).

Webster (146) described concerns about autopsy evidence, noting the following characteristics of necropsies among white South African miners:

> (a) That according to the [South African] Pneumoconiosis Act of 1956, if any medical practitioner consider[s] that his patient is suffering from pneumoconiosis or suspect[s] that he has worked in a controlled dust occupation, should his patient die, he is obliged to remove the cardiorespiratory organs of the deceased and submit them to the Miners' Medical Bureau, *provided the nearest relative gives consent to the autopsy*.
> (b) Should a miner be classified as [having] pneumoconiosis with more than 20% disability, it is most *unlikely* that the results of an autopsy examination will add to the monetary compensation which she or her family will obtain. Miners with this type of certification are often in the age group with the higher incidence of bronchogenic carcinoma. In a recent survey . . . it appears that for the last few years before (1969) in approximately *20% of the miners who die, the cardiorespiratory organs are not received by the Miners' Medical Bureau* [emphasis added].

The likelihood of this sort of selection bias in autopsies among South African miners has been reiterated by Hessel et al. (135).

Because many studies have used data from the 1930s, another explanation for the lack of positive association exists: silicotics suffered heavily from the sequelae of fibrotic lung disease, such as tuberculosis, silicotuberculosis, and pneumonia (7). In the light of these major competing causes of death, the probability of lung cancer was reduced, and it emerged only when silicotics survived long enough to be at higher risk for this malignancy.

D. Biases in Epidemiological Studies

In the epidemiological studies of silicosis and lung cancer, the observed number of cases is compared with that expected on the basis of some reference population. The data in Tables 9 and 11 show increased risk of lung cancer for persons with silicosis in sharp contrast to the findings from autopsy studies. Of the 24 epidemiological studies reviewed, only two reports (134,135), both involving the same cohort, did not show association between silicosis and pulmonary cancer.

In parallel with autopsy studies, there are several sources of bias with the potential to affect epidemiological studies. Smoking was not controlled in many of the earlier studies, but smoking rates were probably not high in the early studies and the comparison series may have overrepresented smokers, tending to bias toward the null. Axelson's (142) assessment of the consequences of confounding suggests that smoking could account for 12–50% of the excess relative risk but not the full excess. Smoking has been considered in many recent reports (15,30,130), and yet lung cancer risk remains two to three times greater than expected. Epidemiological studies of lung cancer among silicotics, like the autopsy studies, may be subject to detection bias. It is possible that subjects may have been mislabeled as silicotics when they suffered from other pulmonary conditions, such as asbestosis. It is also difficult to attribute the excess solely to silica; the work environments of the occupational groups were contaminated by many other agents, some associated with lung cancer. However, lung cancer risk was elevated among silicotics having relatively "pure" quartz exposures, such as those in granite work, rock quarrying, or tunneling (78,125,126,136). Some studies also show gradients of risk with degree of silicosis, as demonstrated by findings of Ng et al. (132), Miller et al. (59), Chia et al. (131), and Hnizdo and Sluis-Cremer (30).

V. Cancer Risk Assessment for Crystalline Silica

Cancer risks have been assessed for ambient environmental exposures to quartz particulate as for other airborne respiratory carcinogens, such as arsenic, asbestos, coke oven emissions, and radon. At present, risk assessment requires extrapolation of the risks from animal studies, using the cancer potency slope or the geometric means of several slope lines and the methods recommended by an environmental regulatory agency (147). Cancer risk assessment for quartz was an outgrowth of two determinations of the carcinogenicity of silica by the International Agency for Research on Cancer (10) and by the Science Advisory Board for California's Proposition 65 (12). IARC reviewed the evidence for carcinogenicity of silica and concluded that there was *sufficient* evidence for carcinogenicity in laboratory animals and *limited* evidence for carcinogenicity in humans, and therefore silica was a probable human carcinogen. The Proposition 65 Science Advisory Board also reviewed the animal and human evidence and judged that airborne respirable silica was a carcinogen known to the state of California.

Because silica was judged to be a carcinogen, a risk assessment was required under California's Air Toxics law, AB2588 (148). This section will describe the three cancer risk assessment extrapolations used in California and other governmental regulations of quartz.

Data from three positive inhalation studies in Table 1 were selected for risk assessment purposes: Holland et al. 1983, Dagle et al. 1986, and Muhle et al. 1989 (14,20,22). The linearized multistage model developed by Howe and co-workers (149) was used to estimate the excess lifetime cancer risks from exposure to 1 $\mu g/m^3$ of respirable silica dust. The cancer risk is expressed as the unit cancer risk or cancer potency slope and is regarded as the upper limit of the estimated risk because of the nonthreshold assumption for carcinogens at low doses. The cancer risks estimated by Goldsmith et al. (150) ranged from 2.3×10^{-5} to 6.0×10^{-3}, and by the California EPA Office of Health Hazard Evaluation and Assessment, from 4.4×10^{-5} to 2.9×10^{-4} (148). Brantner and Klein (151) derived a unit cancer risk of 3.6×10^{-5}. There are many uncertainties involved in these risk assessments, including the use of worst-case assumptions and the practice of assuming that no thresholds exist for carcinogens.

Cancer risk assessments based on experimental animal data, like these studies, embody extrapolations to ambient residential exposure levels. Some uncertainties in this risk assessment could be reduced if epidemiological studies, such as studies of gold miners (30) or silicotics (59) provide exposure-response data at relevant dose levels. Use of human data would reduce uncertainties from extrapolating across species (156). Furthermore, epidemiological findings represent risks in the realm of human experiences and biological processes, while there have been no demonstrated pulmonary cancer risks from ambient silica exposures.

Although the National Institute for Occupational Safety and Health (NIOSH) regards silica exposure as potentially carcinogenic, the Occupational Safety and Health Administration (OSHA) disagrees. The OSHA permissible exposure limit (PEL) over an 8-h workday for silica is 0.1 mg/m^3, and for tridymite and cristobalite 0.05 mg/m^3 (157). In California, airborne, respirable crystalline silica is considered carcinogenic under proposition 65, and thus a cancer warning label is required on certain silica-containing materials.

VI. Does Silica Exposure or Silicosis Cause Lung Cancer?

In determining whether silica causes lung cancer, evaluation of the evidence against standard criteria for determining causation provides guidance. Such assessments were performed by the International Agency for Research on Cancer (10) and by the State of California (12). This review uses the modified criteria of Hill (152), considering silica exposure and silicosis separately, and evaluates whether the evidence meets the following criteria: strong relative risk, dose-response, consistency, control for confounding, temporal cogency, biological specificity, valid exposure data, and overall coherence. Table 12 compares these criteria for both silica exposure and silicosis.

A. Strong Relative Risk

For silica-exposed workers, the relative risk levels are consistently elevated across studies but within the range of 1.3–1.7. The relatively low relative risks for granite workers, tunnelers, and sandblasters are noteworthy (see Table 7). Gold miners throughout the world, with the exception of Homestake miners in South Dakota, have elevated lung cancer risks (Table 4). Foundry workers have elevated lung cancer risks, but with the exception of the study by Fletcher (107), the linkage with silica exposure remains elusive.

For persons with silicosis, the reported relative risks from the epidemiological studies are higher. Although the autopsy studies do not show increased risk, 22 of 24 epidemiology studies of silicotics throughout the world show increased risks that range from 1.4 in Austria (27) to 6.5 in Japan (128). Only the studies by Hessel and co-workers (134,135) did not find an association between silicosis and lung cancer. In the same mining population, Hnizdo and Sluis-Cremer (30) found a relative risk of 3.9 in subjects with silicosis of hilar lymph glands. Also noteworthy are the recently published elevated risks for silicotics in North Carolina and among a national sample of metal ore miners reported by Amandus et al. (130) and by Amandus and Costello (15).

B. Consistent Findings

The relative risks for silica-exposed workers and for silicotics have been consistent between investigations and across national boundaries; positive associations have

Table 12 Criteria for Causation for Silica Exposure and for Silicosis

Point of evidence	Silica-exposed workers	Workers with silicosis
Strong relative risk	√	√√√
Consistent findings	√√	√√√
Dose-response gradients	√√	√
Controlled confounding	√	√
Reliable exposure data	√	±
Biological specificity	√√	±
Temporal cogency	√	√
Overall coherence	Yes	Yes

√ = yes for that factor
± = needs more research

been found in studies in Europe, Asia, and North America. An exception appears to be iron ore miners, who have not shown the elevated risks found in other silica-exposed groups. The consistency of the findings among epidemiological studies of silicotics is impressive, and these associations hold true in Europe, Asia, and North America.

C. Dose-Response Gradients

The finding of a dose-response relationship strengthens the biological argument for causality. Among the studies of silica-exposed workers, dose-response relationships have been found, but primarily with indirect measures of exposure, such as length of employment (5) or working in dustier jobs (107). However, the work of Hnizdo and Sluis-Cremer (30) demonstrating a dose-response relationship with cumulative respirable particle exposure confirms the previous indirect associations and strengthens the link between silica dust and lung cancer. Among silicotics, there are only indirect data linking workplace silica concentrations to lung cancer risk. However, four positive studies show a relationship between the degree of silicosis disability and risk for lung cancer (30,59,131,132). To the extent that severity of silicosis reflects silica exposure, silicotics share the dose-related gradients demonstrated in studies of silica exposure.

D. Controlled for Confounding

Smoking was the most important potential confounder in the early studies. However, adjustment for smoking did not remove the association in the studies with smoking data. In studies of foundry workers, other environmental exposures may continue to confound a suggestive link with silica dust. A report published by IARC (10) observed that selection bias may play a role in the elevated risk for silicotics because, having chronic pulmonary disease, they are more likely to have medical evaluation and thus lung tumors are more likely to be detected. However, given the consistency of the findings, selection bias is unlikely to explain the results.

E. Accurate Exposure Data

The occupational/industrial groups reviewed in this chapter all have a history of high dust exposure to crystalline silica. The best exposure data exist for the quartz-exposed workers and the gold miners; data for other groups of silicotics tend to be inaccurate because obtaining individual dust exposures has not been possible. An exception are the historical sampling data from the North Carolina Dusty Trades monitoring program; unfortunately, Amandus et al. (15) did not present the data in their report. The most accurate exposure data are those presented for respirable quartz in the South African gold mines by Wyndham et al. (60) and Hnizdo and

Sluis-Cremer (30); both studies found measurable lung cancer risks to be correlated with cumulative silica exposures after adjustment for smoking habits.

F. Biological Specificity

Effects of respirable silica on pulmonary tissue were considered by Goldsmith et al. (8) to be the pathway by which silica increases lung cancer risk. Silica exposure causes silicosis, a diffuse pulmonary disease, increases risk for tuberculosis, and may cause nephritis (158). Goldsmith et al. (8) suggested that quartz could act directly as a carcinogen or increase risk by promoting fibrogenesis. These two mechanisms have not yet been sufficiently evaluated. Saffiotti (25) suggested that release of mediators during the fibrotic process could stimulate cell proliferation in adjacent tissue and ultimately cause neoplasia. Based on experimental work in his laboratory, Saffiotti suggested that silica's complex biological and neoplastic capability requires host susceptibility via the production of, or access to, reactive oxygen species (153).

There is ample animal evidence to support the biological specificity of silica, as recognized in the IARC (10) review. In 1989, Muhle et al. (14) reported that lifetime exposure to DQ 12 quartz is carcinogenic with inhalation at 1 mg/m^3. It is also clear that quartz produces fibrosis in the lung, and that the fibrosis either precedes or appears simultaneously with respiratory tumors. Positive animal results show some species specificity; rats exposed to silica develop fibrosis and neoplasia, while other rodents (such as hamsters and guinea pigs) do not. These species differences have perplexed Saffiotti (25,153), who has developed several lines of research to try to explain the paradox and the mechanisms of carcinogenesis. The experimental inhalation studies of silica have been sufficiently consistent for risk assessment extrapolations to be undertaken (148,150,151).

G. Temporal Cogency

In both silica-exposed workers and silicotics, the data support appropriate time-related events. That is, cancer risk is not elevated until at least 20 years of employment, a pattern consistent with other workplace carcinogens such as asbestos and arsenic. The lung cancer excesses among silicotics have arisen after the diagnosis of silicosis (not coincidentally) and usually after decades of employment/exposure to silica.

H. Overall Coherence

For silica-exposed workers, there is a moderate relative risk: the risk is consistent across industries, countries, and investigators, and there is evidence of dose-response in data from South Africa. After adjusting for age and smoking, the risk of lung cancer remains elevated; evidence for dose-response has been found, even in the face of some limitations of the available exposure data; the temporal sequence between exposure and response is appropriate; and the animal findings are confirmatory. The weight of evidence supports the conclusion that occupational silica exposure is carcinogenic for humans.

For silicotics, the relative risks for lung cancer are relatively high and consistent between countries and investigators, and among the dusty industries associated with this fibrotic lung disease. Several studies show an increased risk according to severity of fibrosis; the association cannot be accounted for by bias, including selection bias and confounding from smoking or other factors. Adequate animal models have not yet been developed and the mechanisms by which fibrosis may increase lung cancer risk need additional research. Nevertheless, the epidemiological evidence makes clear that chronic silicosis predisposes to an increased lung cancer risk, and that risk is due either to high silica exposure or to the fibrotic process or to both factors.

Acknowledgments

This work was supported by a grant, 5 R01 OH02726-02, from the National Institute for Occupational Safety and Health, and by contracts from the Monterey Bay Unified Air Pollution Control District.

References

1. Collis, E. L. (1919). *Industrial Pneumoconioses with Special Reference to Dust Phthisis*. Milroy Lectures, 1915. London, His Majesty's Stationery Office.
2. Dible, J. H. (1934). Silicosis and malignant disease. *Lancet* ii:982–983.
3. Hueper, W. C. (1966). Occupational and environmental cancers of the respiratory system. *Recent Results Cancer Res.* 3:1–159.
4. Heppleston, A. G. (1985). Silica, pneumoconiosis, and carcinoma of the lung. *Am. J. Indust. Med.* 7:285–294.
5. Selikoff, I. J. (1978). Carcinogenic potential of silica compounds. In *Biochemistry of Silicon and Related Problems*. Edited by G. Benz and I. Lindquist. New York, Plenum Press, pp. 331–336.
6. National Institute for Occupational Safety and Health, Silicosis and Silicate Disease Committee. (1988). Diseases associated with exposure to silica and nonfibrous silicate materials. *Arch. Pathol. Lab. Med.* 112:673–720.
7. Ziskind, M., Jones, R. N., and Weill, H. (1976). Silicosis. *Am. Rev. Respir. Dis.* 113: 643–655.
8. Goldsmith, D. F., Guidotti, T. L., and Johnston, D. R. (1982). Does occupational exposure to silica cause lung cancer? *Am. J. Indust. Med.* 3:423–440.
9. Goldsmith, D. F., Winn, D. M., and Shy, C. M., eds. (1986). *Silica, Silicosis, and Cancer: Controversy in Occupational Medicine*. New York, Praeger.

10. International Agency for Research on Cancer (1987). *Evaluation of the Carcinogenic Risk of Chemicals to Humans—Silica and Some Silicates*. IARC Monograph #42, Lyon.
11. Simonato, L., Fletcher, A. C., Saracci, R., and Thomas, T. L., eds. (1990). *Occupational Exposure to Silica and Cancer Risk*. Lyon, International Agency for Research on Cancer (IARC), Scientific publication no. 97.
12. Scientific Advisory Board. Hearings of the Scientific Advisory Board for Proposition 65, State of California Safe Drinking Water and Toxic Enforcement Act of 1986. *Chemicals Known to the State (of California) to Cause Cancer or Reproductive Toxicity*. Davis, CA, September 15, 1958.
13. Saffiotti, U., and Stinson, S. F. (1988). Lung cancer induction by crystalline silica: relationships to granulomatous reactions and host factors. *J. Environ. Sci. Health* 6: 197–222.
14. Muhle, H., Takenaka, S., Mohr, U., Dasenbrock, C., and Marmelstein, R. (1989). Lung tumor induction upon long-term low-level inhalation of crystalline silica. *Am. J. Indust. Med.* 15:343–346.
15. Amandus, H., and Costello, J. (1991). Silicosis and lung cancer in U.S. metal miners. *Arch. Environ. Health* 46:82–89.
16. Pairon, J. C., Brochard, P., Jaurand, M. C., and Bignon, J. (1991). Silica and lung cancer: a controversial issue. *Eur. Respir. J.* 4:730–744.
17. Wagner, M. M. F., and Wagner, J. C. (1972). Lymphomas in the Wistar rat after intrapleural inoculation of silica. *J. Natl. Cancer Inst.* 41:908–917.
18. Wagner, M. M. F. (1976). Pathogenesis of malignant histiocytic lymphomas induced by silica in a colony of specific pathogen-free Wistar rats. *J. Natl. Cancer Inst.* 57: 509–518.
19. Wagner, M. M. F., Wagner, J. C., Davies, R., and Griffiths, D. M. (1980). Silica-induced malignant histocytic lymphoma: incidence linked with strain of rat and type of silica. *Br. J. Cancer* 41:908–917.
20. Holland, L. M., Gonzales, M., Wilson, J. S., and Tillery, M. I. (1983). Pulmonary effects of shale dusts in experimental animals. In *Health Issues Related to Metal and Nonmetal Mining*. Edited by W. L. Wagner, W. N. Rom, and J. A. Merchant. Boston, Butterworth, pp. 485–496.
21. Groth, D. H., Stettler, L. E., Platek, S. F., Lal, J. B., and Burg, J. R. (1986). Lung tumors in rats treated with quartz and other minerals by intratracheal instillation. In *Silica, Silicosis, and Cancer*. Edited by D. F. Goldsmith, D. M. Winn, and C. M. Shy. New York, Praeger, pp. 243–254.
22. Dagle, G. E., Wehner, A. P., Clark, M. L., and Buschbom, R. L. (1986). Chronic inhalation exposure of rats to quartz. In *Silica, Silicosis, and Cancer*. Edited by D. F. Goldsmith, D. M. Winn, and C. M. Shy. New York, Praeger, pp. 255–266.
23. Spiethoff, A., Wesch, H., Wegener, K., and Klimisch, H-J. (1992). The effects of thorotrast and quartz on the induction of lung tumors in rats. *Health Phys.* 63: 101–110.
24. Holland, L. M., Wilson, J. S., Tillery, M. I., and Smith D. M. (1986). Lung cancer in rats exposed to fibrogenic dusts. In *Silica, Silicosis, and Cancer*. Edited by D. F. Goldsmith, D. M. Winn, and C. M. Shy. New York, Praeger, pp. 267–279.

25. Saffiotti, U. (1986). The pathology induced by silica in relation to fibrogenesis and carcinogenesis. In *Silica, Silicosis, and Cancer*. Edited by D. F. Goldsmith, D. M. Winn, and C. M. Shy. New York, Praeger, pp. 287–307.
26. Dubrow, R., and Wegman, D. H. (1984). *Occupational Characteristics of Cancer Victims in Massachusetts: 1971–1973*. NIOSH, Division of Surveillance, Hazard Evaluations, and Field Studies. 1984. DHHS (NIOSH) publication no. 94–109, 185 pp.
27. Neuberger, M., Kundi, M., Westphal, G., and Grundorfer, W., (1986). The Viennese dusty worker study. In *Silica, Silicosis, and Cancer*. Edited by D. F. Goldsmith, D. M. Winn, and C. M. Shy. New York, Praeger, pp. 415–422.
28. Siemiatycki, J., Gerin, M., Dewar, R., Lakhani, R., Begin, D., and Richardson, L. (1990). Silica and cancer associations from a multicancer and occupational exposure case-referent study. In *Occupational Exposure to Silica and Cancer Risk*. Edited by L. Simonato, A. C. Fletcher, R. Saracci, and T. L. Thomas. Lyon, International Agency for Research on Cancer (IARC), Scientific publication no. 97, pp. 29–42.
29. Beadle, D. G., and Bradley, A. A. (1970). The composition of airborne dust in South African gold mines. In *Pneumoconiosis, Proceedings of the International Conference, Johannesburg, 1969*. Edited by H. A. Shapiro. Cape Town, Oxford University Press, pp. 462–466.
30. Hnizdo, E., and Sluis-Cremer, G. K. (1991). Silica exposures, silicosis, and lung cancer: a mortality study of South African gold miners. *Br. J. Indust. Med.* 48:53–60.
31. Osburn, H. S. (1969). Lung cancer in the mining district of Rhodesia. *S. Afr. Med. J.* 43:1307–1312.
32. Bradshaw, E., McGlashan, N. D., Fitzgerald, D. J., and Harrington, J. S. (1982). Analysis of cancer incidence in black gold miners from Southern Africa (1964–79). *Br. J. Cancer* 46:737–748.
33. McGlashan, N. D., Harrington, J. S., and Bradshaw, E. (1982). Eleven sites of cancer in black gold miners from Southern Africa: a geographic enquiry. *Br. J. Cancer* 46:947–954.
34. Sluis-Cremer, G. K. (1986). Silica exposure and silicosis in Witwatersrand gold miners in South Africa. In *Silica, Silicosis, and Cancer*. Edited by D. F. Goldsmith, D. M. Winn, and C. M. Shy. New York, Praeger, pp. 67–70.
35. Gylseth, B., Norseth, T., and Skaug, V. (1981). Amphibole fibers in a taconite mine and the lungs of the miners. *Am. J. Indust. Med.* 2:175–184.
36. Icso, J., and Szollosova, M. (1984). The incidence of lung cancer in the miners of iron-ore mines. *Pracov. Lek.* 36:294–298.
37. Milham, S. J. (1976). *Occupational Mortality in Washington State, 1950–1971*. DHEW publication no. (NIOSH) 76-175-A, Cincinnati Ohio, p. 87.
38. Peterson, G. R., and Milham, S. J. (1980). *Occupational Mortality in the State of California, 1959–1961*. DHEW (NIOSH) publication no. 80-104, Bethesda, MD.
39. Williams, R. R., Stegens, N. L., and Goldsmith, J. R. (1977). Associations of cancer site and type with occupation and industry from the Third National Cancer Survey interview. *J. Natl. Cancer Inst.* 59:1147–1185.
40. Singleton, J. A., and Beaumont, J. J. (1989). *COMS I, California Occupational Mortality, 1979–1981, Adjusted for Smoking, Alcohol, and Socioeconomic Status*. Sacramento, California Department of Health Services.

41. Lynge, E., Kurppa, K., Kristofersen, L., Malker, H., and Sauli, H. (1990). Occupational groups potentially exposed to silica dust: a comparative analysis of cancer mortality and incidence based on the Nordic occupational mortality and cancer incidence registers. In *Occupational Exposure to Silica and Cancer Risk*. Edited by L. Simonato, A. C. Fletcher, R. Saracci, and T L. Thomas. Lyon, International Agency for Research on Cancer (IARC), Scientific publication no. 97, pp. 7–20.
42. Costello, J. (1983). Mortality of metal miners—a retrospective cohort and case-control study. In *Health Issues Related to Metal and Nonmetal Mining*. Edited by W. L. Wagner, W. N. Rom, and J. A. Merchant. Boston, Butterworth, pp. 226–240.
43. U.S. Department of Health, Education, and Welfare. (1963). *Silicosis in the Metal Mining Industry: A Re-Evaluation, 1958–1961*. Washington, DC, U.S. Public Health Service, publication no. 1076.
44. Muller, J., Wheeler, W. C., Gentleman, J. F., Suranyi, G., and Kusiak, R. A. (1983). *Study of Mortality of Ontario Miners 1955–1977*. Part I, p. 84. Ontario Ministry of Labour, Workers Compensation Board, Atomic Energy Control Board of Canada.
45. Chen, J., McLaughlin, J. K., Zhang, J-Y., Stone, B. J., Luo, J., Chen, R. A., Dosemeci, M., Rexing, S. H., Wu, Z., Hearl, F. J., McCawley, M. A., and Blot, W. J. (1992). Mortality among dust-exposed Chinese mine and pottery workers. *J. Occup. Med.* 34:311–316.
46. McLaughlin, J. K., Chen, J. Q., Dosemecci, M., Chen, R-A., Rexing, S. H., Zhien, W., Hearl, F. J., McCawley, M. A., and Blot, W. J. (1992). A nested case-control study of lung cancer among silica exposed workers in China. *Br. J. Indust. Med.* 49:167–171.
47. Jorgensen, H. S. (1973). A study of mortality from lung cancer among miners in Kiruna 1950–1970. *Work Environ. Health* 10:126–133.
48. Higgins, I. T., Glassman, J. H., Oh, M. S., and Cornell, R. G. (1983). Mortality of reserve mining company employees in relation to taconite dust exposure. *Am. J. Epidemiol.* 118:710–719.
49. Lawler, A. B., Mandel, J. S., Schuman, L. M., and Lubin, J. H. (1985). A retrospective cohort mortality study of iron ore (hematite) miners in Minnesota. *J. Occup. Med.* 27:507–517.
50. Boyd, J. P., Doll, R., Faulds, J. S., and Keiper, J. (1970). Cancer of the lung in iron ore (haematite) miners. *Br. J. Indust. Med.* 27:97–105.
51. Radford, E. P., and St. Clair Renard, K. G. (1984). Lung cancer in Swedish iron miners exposed to low doses of radon daughters. *N. Engl. J. Med.* 310:1485–1494.
52. Chen, S. Y., Hayes, R. B., Liang, S. R., Li, Q. G., Stewart, P. A., and Blair, A. (1990). Mortality experience of haematite mine workers in China. *Br. J. Indust. Med.* 47:175–181.
53. National Research Council, Panel on Dosimetric Assumptions Affecting the Application of Radon Risk Estimates (1991). *Comparative Dosimetry of Radon in Mines and Homes*. Companion to Beir IV Report. Washington, DC, National Academy Press.
54. Abelson, P. H. (1991). Mineral dusts and radon in uranium mines (editorial). *Science* 254:777.

55. Gillam, J. D., Dement, J. M., Lemen, R. A., Wagoner, J. R., Archer, V. E., and Blejer, H. P. (1976). Mortality patterns among hard rock gold mines exposed to an asbestiform mineral. *Ann. NY Acad. Sci.* 271:335–344.
56. McDonald, J. C., Gibbs, G. W., Liddell, F. D. K., and McDonald, A. D. (1978). Mortality after long exposure to cummingtonite-grunerite. *Am. Rev. Respir. Dis.* 118:271–277.
57. Brown, D. P., Kaplan, S. D., Zumwalde, R. D., Kaplowitz, M., and Archer, V. E. (1986). Retrospective cohort mortality study of underground gold mine workers. In *Silica, Silicosis, and Cancer*. Edited by D. F. Goldsmith, D. M. Winn, and C. M. Shy. New York, Praeger, pp. 335–350.
58. Shannon, H., Heller, J. G., Pron, G., Gallina, P., and MacRae, J. (1987). *Report of the Special Panel on the Ontario Gold Mining Industry, Appendix A of Industrial Disease Standards Panel Report to the Workers Compensation Board on the Ontario Gold Mining Industry*. Toronto, Ontario Ministry of Labour, pp. 11–63.
59. Miller, A. B., Scarpelli, D., and Weiss, N. S. (1987). *Report of the Scientific Panel on Mortality from Cancer Among Ontario Gold Miners 1955–1977. Appendix C of Industrial Disease Standards Panel Report to the Workers' Compensation Board of the Ontario Gold Mining Industry*. Toronto, Ontario Ministry of Labour, pp. 64–86.
60. Wyndham, C. H., Bezuidenhout, B. N., Greenacre, M. J., and Sluis-Cremer, G. K. (1986). Mortality of middle aged white South African gold miners. *Br. J. Indust. Med.* 43:677–684.
61. Katsnelson, B. A., and Mokronosova, K. A. (1979). Non-fibrous mineral dusts and malignant tumors. *J. Occup. Med.* 21:15–20.
62. Armstrong, B. K., McNulty, J. C., Levitt, L. J., Williams, K. A., and Hobbs, M. S. T. (1979). Mortality in gold and coal miners in Western Australia with special reference to lung cancer. *Br. J. Indust. Med.* 36:199–205.
63. Industrial Disease Standards Panel (IDSP) (1987). *IDSP Report to the Workers' Compensation Board on the Ontario Gold Mining Industry*. Toronto, Ontario Ministry of Labour.
64. Beadle, D. G. (1971). The relationship between the amount of dust breathed and the development of radiological signs of silicosis: an epidemiological study of South African gold miners. In *Inhaled Particles*, vol. III. Edited by W. H. Walton. Oxford, Pergamon Press, pp. 953–964.
65. Goldsmith, D. F., and Guidotti, T. L. (1986). Combined silica exposure and cigarette smoking: a possible synergistic effect. In *Silica, Silicosis, and Cancer*. Edited by D. F. Goldsmith, D. M. Winn, and C. M. Shy. New York, Praeger, pp. 451–459.
66. Harding, H. E., McRae Tod, L., McLaughlin, A. I. G. (1944). Disease of lungs in boiler scalers. *Br. J. Indust. Med.* 1:247–251.
67. Craighead, J. E., and Vallyathan, N. V. (1980). Cryptic pulmonary lesions in workers occupationally exposed to dust containing silica. *JAMA* 244:1939–1941.
68. Kennaway, E. L., and Kennaway, N. M. (1947). A further study of the incidence of cancer of the lung and larynx. *Br. J. Cancer* 1:260–298.
69. Guralnick, L. *Mortality by Occupation and Cause of Death Among Men 20 to 64 Years of Age: United States, 1950*. U.S. Department of Vital Statistics, Special Reports, vol. 53, no. 3, Washington, DC.

70. Milham, S. J. (1983). *Occupational Mortality in Washington State, 1950–1979.* Cincinnati, Ohio, PHS Publication No. (NIOSH) 83-116, p. 167.
71. Davis, L. K., Wegman, D. H., Monson, R. R., and Froines, J. (1983). Mortality experience of Vermont granite workers. *Am. J. Indust. Med.* 4:705–723.
72. Costello, J., and Graham, W. G. B. (1986). Vermont granite workers' mortality study. In *Silica, Silicosis, and Cancer*. Edited by D. F. Goldsmith, D. M. Winn, and C. M. Shy. New York, Praeger, pp. 437–440.
73. Koskela, R. S., Klockers, M., Jarvinen, E., Rossi, A., and Kolari, P. J. (1990). Cancer mortality of granite workers 1940–1985. In *Occupational Exposure to Silica and Cancer Risk*. Edited by L. Simonato, A. C. Fletcher, R. Saracci, and T. L. Thomas. Lyon, International Agency for Research on Cancer (IARC), Scientific publication no. 97, pp. 43–53.
74. Puntoni, R., Vercelli, M., Merlo, F., Valerio, F., and Santi, L. (1979). Mortality among shipyard workers in Genoa, Italy. *Ann. NY Acad. Sci.* 330:353–377.
75. Guenel, P., Hojberg, G., and Lynge, E. (1989). Cancer incidence among Danish stone workers. *Scand. J. Work Environ. Health* 15:265–270.
76. Mehnert, W. H., Staneczek, W., Mohner, M., Konwtzke, G., Muller, W., Ahlendorf, W., Beck, B., Winkelmann, R., and Simonato, L. (1990). A mortality study of a cohort of slate quarry workers in the German Democratic Republic. In *Occupational Exposure to Silica and Cancer Risk*. Edited by L. Simonato, A. C. Fletcher, R. Saracci, and T. L. Thomas. Lyon, International Agency for Research on Cancer (IARC), Scientific publication no. 97, pp. 55–64.
77. Sackett, D. L. (1979). Bias in analytic research. *J. Chronic Dis.* 32:51–63.
78. Steenland, K., and Beaumont, J. (1986). A proportionate mortality study of granite cutters. *Am. J. Indust. Med.* 9:189–201.
79. Kurppa, K., Koskela, R. S., and Gudbergsson, H. (1982). Gastrointestinal cancer in workers exposed to quartz (letter). *Lancet* 2:150.
80. Koskela, R. S., Jarvinen, E., and Kolari, P. J. (1984). Effect of cohort definition and follow-up length on occupational mortality rates. *Scand. J. Work Environ. Health* 10: 311–316.
81. McDowall, M. E. (1984). A mortality study of cement workers. *Br. J. Indust. Med.* 41:179–182.
82. Sankila, R., Karjalainen, S., Pukkala, E., Oksanen, H., Hakulinen, T., Teppo, L., and Hakama, M. (1990). Cancer risk among glass factory workers: an excess of lung cancer? *Br. J. Indust. Med.* 47:815–818.
83. Thomas, T. L. (1982). A preliminary investigation of mortality among workers in the pottery industry. *Int. J. Epidemiol.* 11:175–180.
84. Thomas, T. L., and Stewart, P. A. (1987). Mortality from lung cancer and respiratory disease among pottery workers exposed to silica and talc. *Am. J. Epidemiol.* 125: 35–43.
85. Thomas, T. L. (1990). Lung cancer mortality among pottery workers in the United States. In *Occupational Exposure to Silica and Cancer Risk*. Edited by L. Simonato, A. C. Fletcher, R. Saracci, and T. L. Thomas. Lyon, International Agency for Research on Cancer (IARC), Scientific publication no. 97, pp. 75–81.
86. Forastiere, F., Lagorio, S., Michelozzi, P., Cavariani, F., Arca, M., Borgia, P.,

Perucci, C., and Axelson, O. (1986). Silica, silicosis and lung cancer among ceramic workers: a case-referent study. *Am. J. Indust. Med.* 10:363–370.

87. Lagorio, S., Forastiere, F., Michelozzi, P., Cavariani, F., Perucci, C. A., and Axelson, O. (1990). A case-referent study on lung cancer mortality among ceramic workers. In *Occupational Exposure to Silica and Cancer Risk.* Edited by L. Simonato, A. C. Fletcher, R. Saracci, and T. L. Thomas. Lyon, International Agency for Research on Cancer (IARC), Scientific publication no. 97, pp. 21–28.
88. Winter, P. D., Gardner, M. J., Fletcher, A. C., and Jones, R. D. (1990). A mortality follow-up study of pottery workers: preliminary findings on lung cancer. In *Occupational Exposure to Silica and Cancer Risk.* Edited by L. Simonato, A. C. Fletcher, R. Saracci, and T. L. Thomas. Lyon, International Agency for Research on Cancer (IARC), Scientific publication no. 97, pp. 83–94.
89. Merlo, F., Costantini, M., Reggiardo, G., Ceppi, M., and Puntoni, R. (1991). Lung cancer risk among refractory brickworkers exposed to crystalline silica: a retrospective cohort study. *Epidemiology* 2:299–305.
90. Puntoni, R., Goldsmith, D. F., Valerio, F., Vercelli, M., Bonassi, S., DiGiorgio, F., Ceppi, M., Stagnaro, E., Filiberti, R., Santi, L., and Merlo, F. (1988). A cohort study of workers employed in refractory brick plant. *Tumori* 74:27–33.
91. McLaughlin, A. I. G., and Harding, H. E. (1956). Pneumoconiosis and other causes of death in iron and steel foundry workers. *Arch. Indust. Health* 14:350–378.
92. Gallagher, R. P., and Threlfall, W. J. (1983). Cancer mortality in metal workers. *Can. Med. Assoc. J.* 129:1191–1194.
93. Koskela, R. S., Hernberg, S., Karava, R., Jarvinen, E., and Nurminen, M. (1976). A mortality study of foundry workers. *Scand. J. Work Environ. Health* 2(Suppl 1): 73–89.
94. Tola, S., Koskela, R. S., Hernberg, S., and Jarvinen, E. (1979). Lung cancer mortality among iron foundry workers. *J. Occup. Med.* 21:753–760.
95. Gibson, E. S., Martin, R. H., and Lockington, J. N. (1977). Lung cancer mortality in steel foundries. *J. Occup. Med.* 19:807–812.
96. Redmond, C. K. (1975). Comparative cause-specific mortality patterns by work area within the steel industry. DHEW (NIOSH) publication no. 75-157, Rockville, MD.
97. Redmond, C. K., Weiland, H. S., Rockette, H. E., Sass, R., and Weinberg, G. (1981). Long-term mortality experience of steelworkers. DHHS (NIOSH) publication no. 81-120, Cincinnati, OH.
98. Decoufle, P., and Wood, D. J. (1979). Mortality patterns among workers in a gray iron foundry. *Am. J. Epidemiol.* 109:667–675.
99. Egan, E., Waxweiler, R. J., Blade, L., Wolfe, J., and Wagoner, J. K. (1979). A preliminary report of mortality patterns among foundry workers. *J. Environ. Pathol. Toxicol.* 2:259–272.
100. Egan-Baum, E., Miller, B. A., and Waxweiler, E. J. (1981). Lung cancer and other mortality patterns among foundrymen. *Scand. J. Work Environ. Health* 7(Suppl 4): 147–155.
101. Mirer, F., Silverstein, M., Maizlish, N., Park, R., Silverstein, B., and Brodsky, L. (1986). Dust measurements and cancer mortality at a ferrous foundry. In *Silica,*

Silicosis, and Cancer. Edited by D. F. Goldsmith, D. M. Winn, and C. M. Shy. New York, Praeger, pp. 29–44.

102. Blot, W. J., Brown, L. M., Pottern, L. M., Stone, B. J., and Fraumeni, J. F., Jr. (1983). Lung cancer among long-term steel workers. *Am. J. Epidemiol.* 117:706–716.
103. Siltanen, E., Koponen, M., Kokko, A., Engstrom, B., and Reponen, J. (1976). Dust exposure in Finnish foundries. *Scand. J. Work Environ. Health* 2(Suppl 1):19–31.
104. Gibson, E. S., McCalla, D. R., Kaiser-Farrell, C., Kerr, A. A., and Lockington, J. N. (1986). Industrial mutagenicity testing: assessing silica's role in lung cancer among foundry workers. In *Silica, Silicosis, and Cancer*. Edited by D. F. Goldsmith, D. M. Winn, and C. M. Shy. New York, Praeger, pp. 167–176.
105. Lerer, T. J., Redmond, C. K., Breslin, P. P., Salvin, L., and Rush, H. W. (1974). Long-term mortality study of steelworkers. VII. Mortality patterns among crane operators. *J. Occup. Med.* 16:608–614.
106. Sherson, D., and Iversen, E. (1986). Mortality among foundry workers in Denmark due to cancer and respiratory and cardiovascular diseases. In *Silica, Silicosis, and Cancer*. Edited by D. F. Goldsmith, D. M. Winn, and C. M. Shy. New York, Praeger, pp. 403–414.
107. Fletcher, A. C. (1986). The mortality of foundry workers in the United Kingdom. In *Silica, Silicosis, and Cancer*. Edited by D. F. Goldsmith, D. M. Winn, and C. M. Shy. New York, Praeger, pp. 385–401.
108. Fletcher, A. C., and Ades, A. (1984). Lung cancer mortality in a cohort of English foundry workers. *Scand. J. Work Environ. Health* 10:7–16.
109. Anderson, C. S., and Dible, J. H. (1938). Silicosis and carcinoma of the lung. *J. Hyg.* 38:185–204.
110. Klotz, M. O. (1939). Association of silicosis and carcinoma of the lung. *Am. J. Cancer* 35:38–49.
111. Irvine, L. G. (1939). *Rep Miners' Phthisis Medical Bureau 1935–1938*. Pretoria, Government Printer, Union of South Africa (cited in Ref. 4).
112. Becker, B. J. P., and Chatgidakis, C. B. (1959). The heart in silicosis. In *Proceedings of the International Conference on Pneumoconiosis, Johannesburg*. Edited by A. J. Orenstein. London, Churchill, pp. 205–216.
113. Chatgidakis, C. B. (1963). Silicosis in South African white gold miners. *S. Afr. J. Adv. Med. Sci.* 9:383–392.
114. Meiklejohn, A. (1949). Silicosis in the potteries. *Br. J. Indust. Med.* 6:230–240.
115. Meiklejohn, A. (1949). Silicosis in sandstone workers. *Br. J. Indust. Med.* 6: 241–244.
116. Roadhouse Gloyne, S. (1951). Pneumoconiosis, a histological survey of necropsy material in 1205 cases. *Lancet* 1:810–814.
117. Rüttner, J. R. (1949). Kann der silikose eine etiologischee bedeutung fur die geschwulstbildung zugesprochen werden? *Oncologia* 2:115–122.
118. Rüttner, J. R., and Heer, H. R. (1969). Silikose und Lungenkarzinom. *Schweiz. Med. Wochenschr.* 99:245–249.
119. Otto, H. V., and Hinüber, G. (1972). Sur haufigkeit des emphysems, der tuberculose und des bronchuskarzinoms bei staublungenerkrankungen. *Prax. Pneumol.* 26:145–158 (cited in Ref. 4).

120. Rüttner, J. R., (1970). Silicosis and lung cancer in Switzerland. In *Pneumoconiosis, Proceedings of the International Conference, Johannesburg 1969, Cape Town.* Edited by H. A. Shapiro. Oxford, Oxford University Press, pp. 512–513.
121. Westerholm, P., Ahlmark, A., Maasing, R., and Segelberg, I. (1986). Silicosis and lung cancer—a cohort study. In *Silica, Silicosis, and Cancer*. Edited by D. F. Goldsmith, D. M. Winn, and C. M. Shy. New York, Praeger, pp. 327–333.
122. Finkelstein, M., Kusiak, R., and Suranyi, G. (1982). Mortality among miners receiving workmen's compensation for silicosis in Ontario: 1940–1975. *J. Occup. Med.* 24:663–667.
123. Finkelstein, M. M., Liss, G. M., Kramer, F., and Kusiak, R. A. (1987). Mortality among surface-industry workers receiving Workers' Compensation awards for silicosis in Ontario: 1940–1984. *Br. J. Indust. Med.* 44:588–594.
124. Gudbergsson, H., Kurppa, K., Koskenin, H., and Vasama, M. (1984). An association between silicosis and lung cancer, a register approach. In *Proceedings of the VI International Conference on Pneumoconiosis, Bochum, 1983*. Geneva, ILO, pp. 212–216.
125. Kurppa, K., Gudbergsson, H., Hannunkari, I., Koskinen, H., Hernberg, S., Koskela, K. S., and Ahlman, K. (1986). Lung cancer among silicotics in Finland. In *Silica, Silicosis, and Cancer*. Edited by D. F. Goldsmith, D. M. Winn, and C. M. Shy. New York, Praeger, pp. 311–319.
126. Zambon, P., Simonato, L., Mastrangelo, G., Winkelmann, R., Saia, B., and Crepet, M. (1986). A mortality study of workers compensated for silicosis during 1959 to 1963 in the Veneto region of Italy. In *Silica, Silicosis, and Cancer*. Edited by D. F. Goldsmith, D. M. Winn, and C. M. Shy. New York, Praeger, pp. 643–665.
127. Chiyotani, K. (1984). Excess risk of lung cancer deaths in hospitalized pneumoconiotic patients. In *Proceedings of the VI International Conference on Pneumoconiosis, Bochum, 1983*. Geneva, ILO, pp. 228–236.
128. Chiyotani, K., Saito, K., Okubo, T., and Takahashi, K. (1990). Lung cancer risk among pneumoconiosis patients in Japan, with special reference to silicotics. In *Occupational Exposure to Silica and Cancer Risk*. Edited by L. Simonato, A. C. Fletcher, R. Saracci, and T. L. Thomas. Lyon, International Agency for Research on Cancer, Scientific publication no. 97, pp. 95–104.
129. Infante-Rivard, C., Armstrong, G., Petitclerc, M., Cloutier, L. G., and Theriault, G. (1989). Lung cancer mortality and silicosis in Quebec, 1930–85. *Lancet* 2:23–30.
130. Amandus, H. E., Shy, C. M., Wing, S., Blair, A., and Heineman, E. F. (1991). Silicosis and lung cancer in North Carolina dusty trades workers. *Am. J. Indust. Med.* 20:57–70.
131. Chia, S. E., Chia, K. S., Phoon, W. H., and Lee, H. P. (1991). Silicosis and lung cancer among Chinese granite workers. *Scand. J. Work Environ. Health* 17: 170–174.
132. Ng, P. N., Chan, S. L., and Lee, J. (1990). Mortality of a cohort of men in a silicosis register: further evidence of an association with lung cancer. *Am. J. Indust. Med.* 17: 163–171.
133. Westerholm, P. (1980). Silicosis—observation on a case register. *Scand. J. Work Environ. Health* 6(Suppl 2):1–86.

134. Hessel, P. A., and Sluis-Cremer, G. C. (1986). Case-control study of lung cancer and silicosis. In *Silica, Silicosis, and Cancer*. Edited by D. F. Goldsmith, D. M. Winn, and C. M. Shy. New York, Praeger, pp. 351–355.
135. Hessel, P. A., Sluis-Cremer, G. K., and Hnizdo, E. (1990). Silica exposure, silicosis, and lung cancer: a necropsy study. *Br. J. Indust. Med.* 47:4–9.
136. Schüler, G., and Rüttner, J. R. (1986). Lung cancer and silicosis in Switzerland. In *Silica, Silicosis, and Cancer*. Edited by D. F. Goldsmith, D. M. Winn, and C. M. Shy. New York, Praeger, pp. 357–366.
137. Rubino. G. F., Scansett, G., Coggiola, M., Pira, E., Piolatto, G., and Coscia, G. C. (1985). Epidemiologic study of the mortality of a cohort of silicotics in Piedmont. In *Silice, Silicosi e cancro Padua*. Edited by E. I. Deutsch, and A. Marcato. University of Padua, pp. 121–132.
138. Forastiere, F., Lagorio, S., Michelozzi, P., Perucci, C. A., and Axelson, O. (1989). Mortality patterns of silicotic subjects in the Latium region Italy. *Br. J. Indust. Med.* 46:877–880.
139. Goldsmith, D. F., Beaumont, J. J., Lutzenhiser, S., and Schenker, M. B. (1990). Silicosis and lung cancer: preliminary results from the California Silicosis Registry. In *Proceedings of the 7th International Conference on Pneumoconioses, 1988*. Vol. I. DHHS publication no. 90-108, pp. 421–425.
140. Axelson, O., and Sundell, L. (1978). Mining, lung cancer and smoking. *Scand. J. Work Environ. Health* 4:46–52.
141. Tornling, G. Hogstedt, C., and Westerholm, P. (1990). Lung cancer incidence among Swedish ceramic workers with silicosis. In *Occupational Exposure to Silica and Lung Cancer*. Edited by L. Simonato, A. C. Fletcher, R. Saracci, and T. L. Thomas. Lyon, International Agency for Research on Cancer (IARC), Scientific publication no. 97, pp. 75–81.
142. Axelson, O. (1978). Aspects of confounding in occupational health epidemiology. *Scand. J. Work Environ. Health* 4:85–88.
143. Carta, P., Cocco, P. L., and Casula, D. (1991). Mortality from lung cancer among Sardinian patients with silicosis. *Br. J. Indust. Med.* 48:122–129.
144. International Labor Office (1980). *Guidelines for the Use of the ILO International Classification of Pneumoconiosis*. Geneva, International Labor Office.
145. Copeland, K. T., Checkoway, H., Holbrook, R. H., and McMichael, A. J. (1977). Bias due to misclassification in the estimate of relative risk. *Am. J. Epidemiol.* 105:488–495.
146. Webster, I. (1970). Bronchogenic carcinoma in South African gold miners. In *Pneumoconiosis, Proceedings of the International Conference, Johannesburg, 1969, Cape Town*. Edited by H. A. Shapiro. Oxford, Oxford University Press, pp. 572–574.
147. U.S. Environmental Protection Agency. (1989). *Risk Assessment Guidance for Superfund—Human Health Evaluation Manual*, Part A. Washington, DC, U.S. Environmental Protection Agency, (OS-230), 9285 701A.
148. California Air Pollution Control Officers Association (1991). *Air Toxics "Hot Spots" Program*, AB 2588, Risk Assessment Committee, Risk Assessment Guidelines, CAPCOA, January 1991.

149. Howe, R. B., Crump K. S., Van Landingham C. (1986). *GLOBAL86. A Computer Program to Extrapolate Quantal Animal Toxicity Data to Low Doses*. Ruston, LA, K. S. Crump and Company.
150. Goldsmith, D. F., Collins, J. F., and Klein, C. (1991). Cancer risk assessment from airborne silica exposure. Paper presented at the Society for Occupational and Environmental Health Conference—Health Effects of Air Pollution: Impact of Clean Air Legislation, Crystal City, VA, March 25–27, 1991.
151. Brantner, J. H., and Klein, A. K. (1991). Carcinogenic risk assessment for silica. Paper presented at the Society of Toxicology meeting, Dallas, TX, February 1991.
152. Hill, A. B. (1965). The environment and disease: association or causation? *Proc. Roy. Soc. Med.* 58:295–300.
153. Saffiotti, U. (1992). Lung cancer induction of crystalline silica. In *Relevance of Animal Studies to the Evaluation of Human Cancer Risk*. Edited by R. D'Amato, T. J. Slaga, W. H. Farland, and C. Henry. New York, Wiley-Liss, pp. 51–69.
154. McDonald, J. C. (1989). Silica, silicosis and lung cancer (editorial). *Br. J. Indust. Med.* 46:289–291.
155. Kusiak, R. A., Springer, J., Ritchie, A. C., and Muller, J. (1991). Carcinoma of the lung in Ontario gold miners: possible aetiological factors. *Br. J. Indust. Med.* 48:808–817.
156. Goldsmith, D. F., and Hertz-Picciotto, I. (in press). Comparing the epidemiology and toxicology for environmental risk assessments for silica. *J. Exp. Analysis Environ. Epidem.*
157. U.S. Department of Labor (1989). Occupational Safety and Health Administration, 29CFR Part 1910, Air Contaminants; Final Rule, *Federal Register* 54:2521–2523.
158. Goldsmith, J. R., and Goldsmith, D. F. (1993). Fiberglass or silica exposure and increased nephritis or end-stage renal disease (ESRD). *Am. J. Indust. Med.* 23: 873–881.

12

Other Occupational Carcinogens

DAVID B. COULTAS

University of New Mexico School
of Medicine
and the New Mexico Tumor Registry
Albuquerque, New Mexico

I. Introduction

Based on animal exposure studies and in vitro testing, hundreds of agents and industrial processes have been identified as possible carcinogens in humans (1); however, far fewer have been shown by epidemiological data to cause lung cancer (Table 1). Chemicals and industrial processes have been assessed and categorized as causes of cancer in humans by the International Agency for Research on Cancer (IARC) of the World Health Organization (WHO) since 1969 (1) and subsequently by agencies of the U.S. government, including the National Institute for Occupation Safety and Health, the Occupational Safety and Health Administration, the Mine Safety and Health Administration, and the Environmental Protection Agency (2), as well as agencies of other governments. Committees of the IARC evaluate available scientific literature including animal experiments, epidemiological studies of humans, and other relevant information, and based on this evidence assign carcinogenicity of chemicals or industrial processes to one of five categories (Table 2).

Several methodological problems, reviewed extensively by Doll (3), may affect epidemiological investigations of occupational exposures and lung cancer. A detailed review of these potential problems is beyond the scope of this chapter;

Table 1 Occupational Agents Associated with Lung Cancer, Categorized by the Criteria of the International Agency for Research on Cancer

Known Carcinogens (Group 1)	Probable Carcinogens (Group 2A)
Arsenic	Acrylonitrile
Asbestos	Beryllium
Bis(chloromethyl)ether	Cadmium
Chromium, hexavalent	Formaldehyde
Nickel and nickel compounds	Possible carcinogens (Group 2B)
Polycyclic aromatic compounds	Acetaldehyde
Radon	Man-made fibers
Vinyl chloride	Silica
	Welding fumes

Source: Ref. 1.

however, the following brief summary of the main factors, study design, exposure assessment, and confounders is provided as background for interpreting the available studies.

The retrospective cohort design has been used most often to study occupa-

Table 2 Categories of Carcinogenicity Used by the International Agency for Research on Cancer

Known Carcinogens (Group 1): There is *sufficient evidence* of carcinogenicity in humans. That is, a positive relationship has been observed between exposure to the agent and cancer in human studies in which chance, bias, and confounding could be ruled out with reasonable confidence.

Probable Carcinogens (Group 2A): There is *limited evidence* of carcinogenicity in humans and *sufficient evidence* of carcinogenicity in experimental animals. In human studies if a positive association between exposure to an agent and cancer is considered credible, but chance, bias or confounding cannot be ruled out then the evidence is limited.

Sufficient evidence for carcinogenicity in animals includes increased incidence of malignant neoplasms or of an appropriate combination of benign and malignant neoplasms in (a) two or more species of animals or (b) in two or more independent studies in one species.

Possible Carcinogens (Group 2B): There is limited evidence in humans in the absence of sufficient evidence in experimental animals. This category may also apply if there is inadequate or nonexistent data in humans, but sufficient evidence in experimental animals.

Not Classifiable (Group 3): Agents are placed in this category when they do not fall into any other group.

Probably Not Carcinogenic (Group 4)

Source: Ref. 1.

tional lung cancer. This design compares incidence of disease or causes of death in a historical cohort of workers with the expected frequency in a reference population, which may be national, regional, local, or from within the industry. The ratio of observed numbers of deaths in the cohort of workers to the expected numbers of deaths from the reference population defines the standardized mortality ratio (SMR). Because mortality in the reference population may also include deaths from exposures among workers, the SMR may underestimate the true risk associated with the exposure being investigated (4). The magnitude of the SMR may be highly dependent upon the reference population chosen for comparison; a nonexposed group of workers, comparable to the exposed population in other respects, would provide the optimal reference group. Moreover, SMRs from different worker populations are not directly comparable (4).

Other aspects of study design to be considered in interpreting epidemiological data on occupational carcinogens include the approach used to estimate exposure and the availability of information on possible confounders (e.g., cigarette smoking). Exposure estimates are usually based on the categorization of workers by subjective evaluation of specific jobs, or on inferences from measures of air contaminants in the general area where specific jobs are preformed. Cumulative exposures may be estimated from the job descriptions and the duration of employment at different jobs. These methods of estimating the intensity and duration of exposure have great potential for misclassifying a worker's actual personal exposure.

Workers frequently may be exposed to multiple agents which are possible causes of lung cancer (see Table 1), but information on some of the exposures may be lacking. Lack of information on all relevant exposures may compromise assessment of associations as to causality. For example, because cigarette smoking is the most important known cause of lung cancer, any investigation of other causes of lung cancer would ideally examine the potential role of smoking as a confounder and as an effect modifier. Unfortunately, many epidemiological investigations have not included information on cigarette smoking, and evidence on risks in nonsmokers and on interaction between the occupational agent and cigarette smoking is limited for many agents. Lack of information on smoking or other exposures does not necessarily negate findings of increased risk for lung cancer in an occupational cohort, but the results should be interpreted cautiously with increases in risk of 40% or less (5).

This review considers agents that are known or probable carcinogens according to the IARC scheme for categorization of carcinogenic potential (see Tables 1 and 2) which are not discussed in other chapters of this volume. Agents that are known causes of lung cancer and are discussed in other chapters include arsenic, asbestos, and radon. Silica, a possible cause of lung cancer, is also considered in another chapter. Other possible causes of lung cancer, acetaldehyde and welding fumes, are not considered in this volume but are discussed elsewhere (1,6).

II. Known Carcinogens

A. Chloromethyl Ethers

The chloromethyl ethers, bis(chloromethyl)ether and chloromethyl methyl ether, are found primarily as chemical intermediates in the production of other organic chemicals (7). Use of these chemicals began in 1948, with production of ion-exchange resins as the single largest product. During the chemical production process workers were frequently exposed to fumes containing bis(chloromethyl)-ether and chloromethyl methyl ether (8). As the industrial process for production of chloromethyl ethers evolved, exposures lessened, and in 1971 the entire process was maintained in a closed system (9). The changes in the industrial process have markedly reduced exposures to these chemicals in the workplace today.

Chloromethyl ethers were identified as possible carcinogens following discovery of excess lung cancer among employees at a chemical manufacturing plant in Philadelphia in 1962 (8). A subsequent epidemiological investigation of 125 workers resulted in the identification of bis(chloromethyl)ether and chloromethyl methyl ether as the agents associated with the excess risk of lung cancer. Further investigations at the same plant (9–14), other U.S. plants (15,16), and plants in other countries (17) have confirmed the risk of lung cancer associated with exposure to these chemicals (Table 3) and provided strong evidence of a causal relation between chloromethyl ethers and lung cancer. The causal nature of this relation is further supported by the demonstration of increasing risk with increasing intensity and duration of exposure. Maher and DeFonso (13) examined the association of intensity and duration of exposure with risk among 2857 chemical production workers, using job classification to estimate dose and time in each job to estimate duration. These researchers found an observed/expected ratio of 1.02 among workers with the lowest cumulative exposure and a ratio of 11.69 among workers with the highest cumulative exposure. They also observed a decline in the risk of lung cancer from 1960 to 1981, years associated with improved control of workplace exposure to chloromethyl ethers.

Further support for a causal relation may also be provided by finding an association between a specific histologic type of lung cancer and exposure to chloromethyl ethers. Among 28 cases of lung cancer reported by Weiss et al. (11), 20 occurred in workers with moderate to high levels of exposure, and 85% of these were small-cell carcinomas. Of eight workers with lung cancer and low levels of exposure, the proportion of small-cell carcinomas was similar to that seen in nonexposed workers and in the general population.

Although most studies have not included data on smoking habits, the available information shows that workers who developed lung cancer were usually cigarette smokers. Of the five cases of lung cancer reported by Lemen et al. (15), four were smokers and the smoking status of the fifth was unknown. The most detailed information about smoking status was provided by Weiss et al. (11) in an investigation of 1446 chemical production workers. Of 28 lung cancers that were observed, five occurred in nonsmokers who had moderate to high levels of cumulative exposure to chloromethyl ethers. Weiss (9) examined the interaction between smoking and moderate to high exposure to chloromethyl ethers among 11 workers with lung cancer, and found the highest standardized mortality ratio in the category of nonsmokers, which included never smokers, cigar smokers, and smokers who had quit for a year or more. Although these findings suggest antagonism between smoking and chloromethyl ethers, the results should be interpreted cautiously because of the small number of never smokers ($n = 3$).

B. Chromium

Chromium, identified as a metal in 1798 by the French chemist Vauquelin (18), had early industrial use in chromium compounds serving as pigments and tanning agents for hides. Today, chromium and chromium compounds are produced from chromite ore and used in numerous materials and industrial processes, including stainless steels, heat- and corrosion-resistant materials, special purpose alloys, alloy cast iron, pigments, metal plating, leather tanning, chemicals, and refractory materials for metallurgical furnaces. A survey by the U.S. National Institute for Occupational Safety and Health reported in 1977 estimated that about 2 million U.S. workers were exposed to chromium and chromium compounds (18).

Case reports of lung cancer in chromate production workers appeared in the mid- to late 1930s. Subsequent epidemiological investigations have confirmed a strong relation between lung cancer and chromium compounds (18) in studies of workers exposed through chromate production, production of chromate pigments, chromium plating, production of ferrochromium alloys, and other processes (Table 4). These processes are discussed separately in this section.

Chromate Production

In the production of chromium compounds from chromite ore, workers are exposed to trivalent and hexavalent chromium compounds. Available experimental and epidemiological data suggest that the hexavalent compounds have the greatest carcinogenic potential (18). For example, a case-control study of 20 Japanese workers showed that the two production stages involving hexavalent chromium exposure had the highest risk of lung cancer (38).

Investigations of chromate production workers have consistently shown a strong relation between working in this industry and the development of lung cancer (18) (see Table 4). Although expected numbers of lung cancers in these studies were based on national data and little information was available on the frequency of smoking, these potential sources of bias do not alter the conclusion

Table 3 Selected Investigations of Occupational Exposures to Chloromethyl Ethers and Risk of Lung Cancer

Author/Country	Study population	Industrial process	Exposures	Findings	Comments
Lemen et al. (15), United States	136 males employed at least 5 years between 1955–1972	Anion-exchange resin production	Chloromethyl ethers	Number of lung cancers observed: 5 expected: 0.54	1. SMR based on rates from Connecticut (study plant in California) 2. 4/5 smokers, one unknown 3. mean latent period 15 years 4. 4/5 small-cell carcinoma 5. follow-up period 1955–1972
Pasternack et al. (16), United States	1827 exposed workers and 8870 nonexposed workers from six U.S. firms from 1948–1972	Chemical production	Chloromethyl ethers	Number of respiratory cancers (ICD-8 160–163[a]) nonexposed observed: 115 expected: 119.1 exposed observed: 26 expected: 9.3	1. SMR based on rates from U.S. population 2. no smoking data 3. the increased frequency of lung cancer resulted from one firm 4. follow-up period 1948–1972

Weiss et al. (11)[b] United States	465 exposed and 981 unexposed males employed between 1948–1960	Chemical production	Chloromethyl ethers	Number of lung cancers nonexposed observed: 15 expected: 13.3 exposed observed: 24 expected: 4.8	1. SMR based on rates from local general population 2. five lung cancers in nonsmokers occurred with moderate-heavy exposure 3. lung cancers in moderate to heavy exposure occurred at young ages 4. small cell carcinomas predominant cell type at moderate-heavy exposure 5. follow-up period 1960–1975
McCallum et al. (17), United Kingdom	670 exposed males, 1097 nonexposed males employed at two factories 1948–1980	Chemical production	Chloromethyl ethers	Number of lung cancers Factory A nonexposed: 1 exposed: 10 Factory B nonexposed: 8 exposed: 1	1. SMR based on rates from local general population 2. no smoking data 3. Factory A had higher exposures with strong dose response 4. follow-up period 1948–1980
Maher and DeFonso (13)[b], United States	737 exposed, 2120 unexposed white males employed between 1948–1971	Chemical production	Chloromethyl ethers	Number of respiratory cancers (ICDA 160–163[a]) nonexposed observed: 25 expected: 23.75 exposed observed: 32 expected: 11.45	1. SMR based on rates from local population 2. no smoking data 3. strong dose-response 4. latent period 10–20 years from first exposure 5. follow-up period 1948–1981

[a]160 = nose/sinus, 161 = larynx, 162 = trachea/bronchus/lung, 163 = pleura/mediastinum/other.
[b]Same study population.

Table 4 Selected Investigations of Occupational Exposures to Chromates and Risk of Lung Cancer

Author/ Country	Study population	Industrial process	Exposures	Findings	Comments
Enterline (19), United States	1200 workers employed 1937–1940, ages 20–64 years	Chromate production	Chromates	Number of respiratory cancers (ICD 160–164[a]) observed: 69 expected: 7.3	1. SMR based on rates from national population 2. no smoking data 3. risk declined from 1941 to 1960 4. 2 of 69 cancers neoplasm of maxillary sinuses 5. follow-up period through 1960
Ohsaki et al. (20), Japan	554 workers employed 1936–1973	Chromate production	Chromates	Annual incidence of lung cancer observed: 658×10^{-5} expected: 13×10^{-5}	1. expected based on national population 2. incidence based on 14 cases in workers 3. 86% smokers 4. 24 years average duration of exposure

Alderson et al. (21), United Kingdom	2715 males employed one or more years between 1948 and 1977 at three factories	Chromate production	Chromates	Number of lung cancers observed: 116 expected: 47.96	1. SMR based on rates from national population 2. no smoking data 3. risk increased with duration of employment 4. risk declined with changes in production process
Satoh et al. (22), Japan	896 males employed for one or more years between 1918 and 1975	Manufacturing	Chromium compounds	Number of lung cancers (ICD 162[a]) observed: 26 expected: 2.7	1. SMR based on rates from national population 2. no smoking data 3. risk of respiratory cancer increased with duration of employment 4. follow-up period through 1978
Sheffet et al. (23), United States	1946 males employed for greater than one month between 1940 and 1970	Pigment production	Chromates	Number of lung cancers observed white: 21 nonwhite: 10 expected white: 16 nonwhite: 7	1. SMR based on rates from US population 2. smoking histories available for 14 lung cancer patients, 93% smoked 3. mean latent period >30 years 4. follow-up period 1940–1979

Table 4 Continued

Author/ Country	Study population	Industrial process	Exposures	Findings	Comments
Frentzel-Beyme (24), Germany and Netherlands	978 workers at five plants in Germany and the Netherlands	Pigment production	Chromates	Number of lung cancers plant / observed / expected 1 / 5 / 2.2 2 / 2 / 0.8 3 / 3 / 0.8 4 / 2 / 1.3 5 / 7 / 4.3	1. SMR based on rates from national populations 2. no smoking data 3. no clear relation to duration of exposure 4. risk highest in medium to high exposure levels
Langard and Vigander (25), Norway	133 male workers employed between 1948 and 1972	Pigment production	Chromates	Number of lung cancers in 18 employed >5 years observed: 6 expected: 0.1	1. SMR based on rates from national population 2. 83% of lung cancer patients smoked 3. follow-up period 1948–1980

Davies (26), United Kingdom	1152 male workers at three plants employed for at least one year from 1930s or 1940s until 1975	Pigment production	Chromates	Number of respiratory cancers (ICD-9 162–165[a]) observed / expected plant A low[b]: 2 / 2.69 high/med[c]: 21 / 9.45 plant B low: 0 / 0.23 high/med: 11 / 2.5 plant C low: 1 / 0.38 high/med: 1 / 3.10	1. SMR based on rates from national population 2. of lung cancer cases, 61% unknown smoking status, 36% ever smokers, 3% nonsmokers 3. risk highest with ≥10 years employment but falls with ≥30 years employment 4. plants A and B produced primarily zinc chromate, plant C primarily lead chromate
Axelsson et al. (27), Sweden	1932 workers employed ≥1 year between 1930 and 1975	Ferrochromium production	Chromium	Number of respiratory cancers (ICD 162–163[a]) observed: 7 expected: 5.9	1. SMR based on rates from local county populations 2. no smoking data 3. workers also exposed to asbestos—three of the seven cancers were mesotheliomas 4. follow-up period 1951–1975

Table 4 Continued

Author/ Country	Study population	Industrial process	Exposures	Findings	Comments
Langard et al. (28), Norway	379 workers employed ≥1 year between 1928 and 1965	Ferrochromium production	Chromium	Number of respiratory cancers (ICD 162–163[a]) observed: 10 expected: 6.5	1. SMR based on rates from national population 2. no smoking data 3. all cancers occurred in those employed before 1960 4. follow-up period 1953–1985
Moulin et al. (29), France	2269 workers employed for ≥1 year between 1952 and 1982	Ferrochromium and stainless steel production	Chromium, nickel, PAH	Number of lung cancers (ICD-8 162[a]) nonexposed observed: 1 expected: 3.15 exposed observed: 11 expected: 5.40	1. SMR based on rates from national population 2. smoking habits determined for 67% of workers—74% exposed eversmokers and 79% of nonexposed eversmokers 3. see text for discussion of nested case-control study 4. follow-up period 1952–1982

Silverstein et al. (30), United States	238 hourly workers with ⩾10 years of employment who died between 1974 and 1978	Production of zinc castings plated with chrome, nickel, and copper for automobiles	1. metal fumes 2. organic combustion products 3. fumes from nickel and chrome-plating	Number of respiratory cancers (ICD-8 162–163[a]) observed white males: 28 white females: 10 expected white males: 14.68 white females: 2.7	1. PMR based on mortality distributions of national population 2. no smoking data 3. increased risk with duration of employment 4. workers exposed to several compounds that may cause cancer
Franchini et al. (31), Italy	178 male workers who worked ⩾1 year at one of nine plants between 1951 and 1981	Electroplating: 3 hard plating, 6 bright plating plants	Chromium	Number of lung cancers (ICD-8 162[a]) observed: 6 expected: 1.7	1. SMR based on rates from national population 2. no smoking data 3. all lung cancers were in hard chrome platers who had highest exposures 4. follow-up period through 1981
Sorahan et al. (32), United Kingdom	3085 workers employed ⩾6 months between 1946 and 1975	Chrome plating of automobile parts	Chromium, nickel	Number of lung cancers (ICD-8 162–163[a]) observed / expected males: 63 / 40.0 females: 9 / 8.1	1. SMR based on rates from national population 2. no smoking data 3. positive association of duration of employment and risk of lung cancer 4. positive association with higher exposure 5. follow-up period 1946–1983

Table 4 Continued

Author/ Country	Study population	Industrial process	Exposures	Findings	Comments
Takahashi et al. (33), Japan	1195 male workers employed ≥6 months between 1970 and 1976	Metal plating	Chromium, other metals	Number of lung cancers (ICD-9 162[a]) observed chromium platers: 8 nonchromium platers: 8 expected chromium platers: 4.3 nonchromium platers: 4.7	1. SMR based on rates from national population 2. no smoking data 3. employment prior to 1960 associated with highest risk 4. follow-up period 1976–1987
Chiazze et al. (34), United States	4760 decedents from 10 plants who died between 1970 and 1976	Spray painting automobiles	Chromate pigments	Number of lung cancers (ICD-8 162[a]) observed: 21 expected: 14.92	1. PMR based on mortality distributions of counties of plants 2. no smoking data 3. no effect of duration of spray painting experience 4. a case-control study was performed with OR = 1.43 ($p > 0.05$) for spray painting

Dalager et al. (35), United States	977 male workers employed prior to 1959 at two aircraft bases	Spray painting aircraft	Zinc chromate pigments	Number of respiratory cancers (ICD-7 160–164[a]) observed: 21 expected: 11.4	1. PMR based on mortality distributions of national population 2. no smoking data 3. increased risk with increased length of employment 4. follow-up period through 1977
Pippard et al. (36), United Kingdom	260 workers employed in 1939	Leather tanning	Chromium compounds	Number of lung cancers observed: 13 expected: 12.0	1. SMR based on rates from England and Wales 2. no smoking data 3. follow-up period 1939 1982
Constantini et al. (37), Italy	2926 workers employed for ≥6 months between 1950 and 1981	Leather tanning	Hexavalent chrome salts	Number of lung cancers (ICD-8 162[a]) observed: 29 expected: 22.04	1. SMR based on rates from national population 2. no smoking data 3. follow-up period 1950–1983

[a]160 = nose/sinus, 161 = larynx, 162 = trachea/bronchus/lung, 163 = pleura, 164 = mediastinum, 165 = other.
[b]low = low levels of exposure.
[c]high/med = high and medium levels of exposure.

that chromate production causes lung cancer. Further associations of risk with duration of employment and changes in production that limited exposure provide additional evidence for a causal relation. Alderson et al. (21) found in an investigation of three chromate-producing plants in the United Kingdom that risk of lung cancer was increased with longer duration of employment and employment prior to changes in the production process from 1957 through 1959 that limited workers' exposure.

Pigment Production

As in chromate production, production of chromate pigments may be associated with exposure to numerous chromium compounds. However, of two major pigments, zinc chromate and lead chromate, only zinc chromate is associated with an increased risk of lung cancer (26) (see Table 4).

Chromium Electroplating

Electroplating involves the application of a layer of chromium onto a metal surface to provide a protective, nontarnishable finish. Two types of electroplating provide either a thin (decorative) or a thick (hard) surface. Hard electroplating is associated with the highest exposure to chromium compounds (31). In addition to chromium, electroplaters may be exposed to other agents that cause lung cancer, including organic combustion products and nickel (30).

Among male electroplaters there is a consistent increase in the risk of lung cancer, with available data suggesting a dose-response relation between chromium exposure and risk of lung cancer (see Table 4). However, little information is available on the role of other cancer-causing agents among workers in the electroplating industry. In a multivariate analysis Sorahan et al. (32) found that duration of employment at nickel baths used in electroplating was not significantly associated with lung cancer.

Ferrochromium Alloy Production

Ferrochromium production involves the electrothermal reduction of chromite ore with coke. Workers in the area of the furnaces are exposed to fumes containing chromium and polycyclic aromatic hydrocarbons. In addition, workers may be exposed to asbestos used to insulate the furnaces.

Studies of ferrochromium production workers have not shown a consistent increase in the risk of lung cancer (see Table 4). Axelsson et al. (27) did not find a statistically significant increase in cancers of the trachea, bronchus, lung, or pleura among Swedish workers (see Table 4). Of the seven cancers Axelsson and coworkers did find, three were mesotheliomas, suggesting significant asbestos exposure. In contrast, Langard et al. (39) found seven lung cancers among a group of Norwegian ferrochromium workers, with 1.8 expected from local rates. In a follow-up study of these ferrochromium workers and of ferrosilicon workers, Langard et al. (28) again found an increased risk of lung cancer among the ferrochromium workers (see Table 4) that was limited to workers employed prior to 1960. The risk of lung cancer was not increased in the ferrosilicon workers, who probably had similar exposures to asbestos and other particulate materials, suggesting that asbestos was not an important confounder.

To explore the effects of other exposures on the development of lung cancer among ferrochromium workers, Moulin et al. (29) conducted a case-control study with 12 lung cancer cases in workers and 58 age-matched controls selected randomly from the same cohort of workers. For those who were exposed only to chromium and/or nickel ($n = 4$ cases, 32 controls), the relative risk for lung cancer was 2.75 (95% confidence interval 0.29–26.30). The relative risk for workers exposed only to polycyclic aromatic hydrocarbons (certain, possible, or intermittent) ($n = 7$ cases, 4 controls) was 14.86 (95% confidence interval 3.04–75.52). This pattern of associations suggests that exposures other than chromium may underlie the elevated risk of lung cancer associated with ferrochromium production.

Other Industrial Exposures to Chromium

Compared with the industrial processes that produce chromium-containing products, the risks associated with use of these products have received little attention. Two proportional mortality studies were made of painters who sprayed chromate pigments (34,35). Both investigations showed small increases in the proportional mortality ratio (PMR) for respiratory cancer deaths, but these results must be interpreted cautiously as the PMR may be increased because of limitations of this study design and because no smoking data were available.

Chrome salts may be used in the leather tanning industry. Several investigations have been conducted among workers in this industry (36,37,40,41) with conflicting results (see Table 4). The small increases in risk for lung cancer that have been observed could be explained by smoking or other confounding factors.

Welding is a complex process that involves the joining of pieces of metal. Exposure to chromium compounds will result if chromium-containing alloys are welded. However, metal alloys frequently contain nickel (discussed below), and other cancer-causing agents such as asbestos may be found in the working environment of welders. To date, results from epidemiological investigations of lung cancer risk in welders have been inconsistent (6).

Exposure to chromium and chromium compounds is associated with an increased risk of developing lung cancer that is probably greatest among chromate production workers. Unfortunately, little information is available on smoking habits and the interaction between smoking and chromium exposure has not been examined.

C. Nickel and Nickel Compounds

In 1751 a Swedish chemist first isolated nickel from arsenosulfide ore (18). Today, nickel is produced from sulfide ores by flotation and magnetic separation and from silicate-oxide ores by chemical means. Nickel has long been used in combination with other metals and with nonmetals to form alloys characterized by strength and corrosion resistance. Currently, the primary uses of nickel are in the production of stainless and heat-resistant steels, nonferrous alloys, and superalloys. Nickel is also used in electroplating, in catalysts, nickel-cadmium batteries, coins, welding products, pigments, and electronic products. Based on a survey conducted by the National Institute for Occupational Safety and Health from 1972 through 1974 (42), researchers estimated that 1.5 million workers in the U.S. were exposed to nickel and nickel compounds.

Epidemiologic investigations of the association of nickel exposure with lung cancer have been conducted in mining operations, smelting, refining, nickel alloy manufacturing, and other manufacturing operations (Table 5). The greatest risk of lung cancer has been found with mining, smelting, and refining. Several changes in industrial processes that have limited workers' exposures to nickel have been followed by decreased risk of lung cancer. For example, among 967 men employed at a nickel refinery in South Wales, Doll et al. (45) found SMRs for lung cancer of 6.2 among workers first employed before 1930 and 1.5 among workers first employed between 1930 and 1944. Changes in the refinery process and the use of face masks in 1924 began to reduce workers' exposure to dust. To further characterize the risk for lung cancer among these workers in South Wales, Kaldor et al. (50) conducted a case-control study and found that mortality from lung cancer increased with increasing exposure to nickel in the workplace.

Two investigations from New Caledonia provide inconsistent results on the risk of lung cancer associated with nickel mining and refining (51,52). During the period 1970–1974, Lessard et al. (51) identified 92 cases of lung cancer among New Caledonia residents. Using a case-control design with hospital-based controls they found a relative risk of 3.0 associated with employment in the nickel industry. In a subsequent investigation in New Caledonia, Goldberg et al. (52) identified 49 cases of lung cancer during the period 1978 through 1981 among nickel workers employed for 10 or more years in the nickel industry. Goldberg and coworkers also used a case-control design, with controls selected from all men working for the nickel company, and they found no increase in risk among nickel workers. The negative findings in this study may be due to selection bias: cases included only men who had worked for 10 or more years in the nickel industry, and controls included only men who also worked in the nickel industry.

The risk of lung cancer with work in the nickel industry has been associated primarily with exposure to specific nickel compounds (53). Results from a collaborative investigation of 10 cohorts of nickel workers from the United States,

Table 5 Selected Investigations of Occupational Exposures to Nickel and Risk of Lung Cancer

Author/Country	Study population	Industrial process	Exposures	Findings	Comments
Chovil et al. (43), Canada	495 workers employed ⩾5 years between 1948 and 1962	Sinter plant[a]	Nickel PAHs	Number of lung cancers observed: 37 expected: 4.56	1. SMR based on rates from Ontario population 2. no smoking data, anecdotes suggest >90% smoked 3. risk of cancer increased with duration of employment 4. follow-up period 1963–1978
Shannon et al. (44), Canada	11,594 workers employed ⩾6 months between 1950 and 1976	Mining, milling, smelting	Nickel	Number of lung cancers (ICD-8 162–163[b]) observed: 46 expected: 37.5	1. SMR based on rates from Ontario population 2. no smoking data 3. lung cancer risk highest in miners and service workers 4. lung cancer risk increased with length of employment 5. confounding by radon exposure from work in uranium mines or diesel exposure unlikely 6. follow-up period 1950–1976

Table 5 Continued

Author/ Country	Study population	Industrial process	Exposures	Findings	Comments
Doll et al. (45), United Kingdom	967 men employed ≥5 years before 1945	Refining	Nickel	Number of lung cancers <1930 / 1930–44 observed: 137 / 8 expected: 21.98 / 5.46	1. SMR based on rates from population of England and Wales 2. no smoking data 3. small amount of arsenic also present in process 4. follow-up period 1934–1971
Magnus et al. (46), Norway	2247 men employed ≥3 years before 1966	Refining	Nickel	Number of lung cancers observed: 82 expected: 22.0	1. SMR based on rates from national population 2. smoking data available for 97% of study population (see text for discussion) 3. risk highest in processing departments 4. follow-up period 1954–1979

Enterline et al. (47), United States	1855 men employed ≥1 year before 1947 1354 men employed ≥1 year between 1947 and 1959	Refining	Nickel chromium grinding dust	Number of respiratory cancers (ICD-7 162–163) <1947 ≥1947 observed 55 10 expected 50.44 7.27	1. SMRs based on rates from national, state, and local populations 2. no smoking data 3. weak increase in risk with increase in exposure 4. nickel concentration lower at this plant than others 5. follow-up period 1948–1977
Cox et al. (48), United Kingdom	1925 men employed ≥5 years between 1953 and 1978	Metal manufacturing	Metallic, nickel, chrome, molybdenum, copper, iron	Number of lung cancers (ICD-8) observed: 15 expected: 18.21	1. SMR based on rates from local population 2. no smoking data 3. slight increase in risk for men with highest exposures to nickel 4. follow-up period 1958–1978
Godbold and Tompkins (49), United States	814 males employed between 1948 and 1953, with median duration of 3.75 years 1600 males not exposed	Manufacturing	Metallic nickel powder	Number of lung cancers exposed nonexposed observed 3 21 expected 6.68 19.42	1. SMR based on rates from national population 2. smoking status unknown for about 34% exposed and 52% of unexposed 3. follow-up period 1948–1972

[a]Sinter plant is part of smelter.
[b]160 = nose/sinus, 161 = larynx, 162 = trachea/bronchus/lung, 163 = pleura, 164 = mediastinum.

Canada, the United Kingdom, Norway, Finland, and New Caledonia suggest that most respiratory cancers may be attributed to oxidic and sulfidic nickel. Furthermore, the soluble forms of nickel are associated with an increased risk for developing these cancers at concentrations of 1 mg/m^3 or greater. Less soluble forms of nickel may result in an excess risk of respiratory cancer at nickel levels greater than 10 mg/m^3. In contrast, exposure to metallic nickel has not been associated with an increased risk of lung cancer (48,49).

Cigarette smoking and other exposures in the nickel industry may affect the association between lung cancer and exposure to nickel. Although little data are available on the smoking habits of nickel workers, two investigations from Norway (46,54) and one from New Caledonia (51) provide some insight into smoking and the risk for lung cancer. Between 1948 and 1974, Kreyberg (54) identified 39 cases of lung cancer among workers at a nickel refinery; 82% were smokers, 10% nonsmokers, and 8% possible nonsmokers. Magnus et al. (46) compared the incidence of lung cancer among 2247 employees at a nickel refinery with the incidence from a population-based sample in Norway (see Table 5). The relative risk for lung cancer among nonsmokers working at the nickel refinery was approximately 8.4 (five cases) compared with 2.9 (39 cases) among smoking nickel workers. During the period 1970 through 1974, Lessard et al. (51) identified 29 cases of lung cancer among nickel workers, and 97% were smokers.

Workers in the nickel industry may also be exposed to other agents that are known causes of lung cancer. For example, chrysotile asbestos has been found in rock mined for nickel in New Caledonia (55), and the nickel-smelting process results in generation of polycyclic aromatic compounds (see discussion in next section). The role of both of these agents and others in causing lung cancer in nickel workers has received little attention.

D. Polycyclic Aromatic Compounds

The polycyclic aromatic compounds result primarily from pyrolysis or incomplete combustion of organic matter; polycyclic aromatic hydrocarbons (PAHs) comprise a major subgroup of the polycyclic aromatic compounds (56,57). A large fraction of PAHs are associated with or adsorbed to particles produced by combustion. As mentioned previously, these chemicals may result from ferrochromium production and smelting of nickel-containing ores. Other occupational exposures to PAHs may result from aluminum production (1,59), iron and steel founding (1,59), coke production (1,59), and coal gasification (1,59). Agents containing polycyclic aromatic compounds used in workplace settings include coal tars (1,60), coal tar pitches (1,60), and untreated and mildly treated mineral oils (1,58). Soots from combustion (1,60) and diesel exhaust also contain PAHs (61). Although exposures to PAHs are prevalent, few data are available on exposures to specific compounds or on quantitive exposures to these compounds (57).

Worldwide, over 2 million workers are estimated to be exposed to polycyclic aromatic compounds in aluminum production, iron and steel founding, coke production, and coal gasification (59). In addition to polycyclic aromatic compounds, work in aluminum production may result in exposure to a complex mixture of gases and particles, with known carcinogens in the mixture. Based on review of the experimental and epidemiological evidence for lung cancer, an IARC committee (59) concluded that work in aluminum production probably increases risk of cancer. However, the epidemiological evidence is not strong, with relative risks ranging from 1.0 to 2.0. Limited evidence suggests a dose-response relation. A mortality study of 5891 aluminum smelter workers from Canada demonstrated increased mortality from lung cancer (62), which was highest among workers with 21 or more years of exposure in the industry. The effects of smoking have not been examined in the investigations of aluminum production workers.

As in aluminum production, work in iron and steel founding may result in exposure to a complex mixture of gases and particles. Although the mixture contains agents known to cause lung cancer, results of epidemiological studies provide limited evidence for an association between work in iron and steel founding and lung cancer, with relative risks ranging from 1.5 to 2.5 (59).

Although coal gasification and coke production are two different processes, they both involve the heating of coal under various conditions at varying temperatures and lengths of time (59), and they both produce many by-products including combustible gases, coke, and hydrocarbons (tar). Available occupational studies provide sufficient evidence of work in coal gasification and coke production as risk factors for development of lung cancer. The highest risk for lung cancer occurs with work on the topside of coke ovens, and the risk increases with duration and intensity of exposure to coke oven emissions. In a study of steelworkers, relative risks of respiratory cancers for topside oven workers compared to non–oven workers increased from 9, with 5 or more years of employment, to 16 with 15 or more years of employment (63). To estimate the lifetime risk for lung cancer associated with work as a coke oven worker, Dong et al. (64) used data from cohorts of U.S. and Canadian steelworkers and modeled lifetime risk of lung cancer accounting for competing causes of death. For a worker starting at age 20 years and exposed to high levels of coke oven emissions for 40 years, the probability of developing lung cancer by age 85 years or later was estimated at 40%, 15 times that for unexposed men.

Coal tars, also known as asphalts, are by-products from the destructive distillation of coal for coal gasification and coke production Coal tars are used in paving, roofing, and other industrial applications. Mortality studies of the roofing industry suggest a slight excess in mortality from lung cancer among roofers, but the role of smoking has not been examined (60). A recent case-control study at a metal stamping plant addressed the risk of cancer associated with specific jobs in the plant (65) and found an odds ratio of 13.2 (95% confidence limits, 1.1–

154.9) for lung cancer among maintenance welders and millwrights at the plant. These workers were exposed to coal tar volatiles and welding fumes.

Numerous case reports and epidemiological investigations have documented an increased risk for skin cancer among workers exposed to mineral oils, but the evidence for lung cancer has been inconsistent (58). The major occupations with such exposures that have been examined for risk of lung cancer include metal workers and printing press workers. Mortality statistics have shown excess lung cancer deaths among mechanics and repairmen, tool and die makers and setters, oilers and greasers, and pressmen and plate printers.

Soots are unintentional by-products of incomplete combustion of organic material. The risk of lung cancer associated with exposure to soots has been examined primarily in chimney sweeps (60). Mortality studies of chimney sweeps from Denmark and Sweden have documented an excess number of lung cancer deaths (66,67). However, the role of smoking has not been adequately examined in these workers.

A major source of soots in the general environment and selected occupational environments is engine exhaust. The use of diesel engines in certain occupations and evidence from experimental studies in several species of animals (61) makes diesel exhaust of particular concern as a risk for lung cancer in humans. Because of their exposures to diesel exhaust, epidemiological investigations have been conducted in railroad workers, mine workers, bus garage and other bus workers, truck drivers, fork lift operators, and firefighters (61).

The largest epidemiological investigations of exposure to diesel exhaust and lung cancer have been conducted in railroad workers from Canada (68) and the United States (69). Howe et al. (68) conducted a mortality study of 43,826 pensioners of the Canadian National Railway Company and found that the relative risks for lung cancer among workers possibly exposed or probably exposed to diesel fumes were 1.2 and 1.35, respectively, compared with workers not exposed. Similar results were obtained by Garshick et al. (69) among a cohort of 55,407 U.S. railroad workers. Those workers with the longest possible duration of exposure to diesel exhaust had a relative risk for lung cancer of 1.45 (95% confidence interval, 1.11–1.89). In an earlier case-control study of 1256 deaths from lung cancer among these railroad workers, Garshick et al. (70) found an odds ratio for lung cancer of 1.41 (95% confidence interval, 1.06–1.88) for those working in a job exposed to diesel exhaust for 20 years after controlling for smoking and asbestos exposure.

Although information on the risk for lung cancer with exposure to specific polycyclic aromatic compounds in the occupational setting are limited, selected examples are available. Dioxin (2,3,7,8-tetrachlorodibenzo-*p*-dioxin) is generated as a contaminant in the production of chemicals used as defoliants, herbicides, insecticides, and bactericides. Fingerhut et al. (71) conducted a mortality study of 5172 male workers from 12 U.S. chemical plants where production processes may have caused dioxin contamination. Overall, the standardized mortality ratio for lung cancer was 111 (95% confidence interval, 89–137). For workers with a year or more of exposure to high levels of dioxin and a latency of 20 or more years from first exposure, the SMR for lung cancer was 142 (95% confidence interval, 103–192). More information is needed on the risk of lung cancer associated with exposures to specific polycyclic aromatic compounds.

E. Vinyl Chloride

Following the recognition of vinyl chloride as a cause of angiosarcoma of the liver (72) several epidemiological investigations were conducted on the relation of vinyl chloride exposure to other cancers (73–76). Buffler et al. (73) examined mortality of 464 white male employees from 1948 through 1975 at a vinyl chloride monomer production plant in Texas. SMRs were calculated using statewide cause-specific death rates for comparison. The SMR for malignant neoplasms of the respiratory system was 289 ($p = 0.032$, one-tailed test). Of five workers who died from respiratory cancer, four were cigarette smokers.

To determine whether exposure to vinyl chloride or to other chemicals was associated with an increased risk of lung cancer, Waxweiler et al. (74) conducted an investigation of 4806 men employed at a synthetic plastics plant from 1942 through 1973. The SMR for respiratory system cancers in this cohort was 149. Exposure to polyvinyl chloride dust was determined to be the most likely cause of the elevated lung cancer mortality.

At a plant producing vinyl chloride and polyvinyl chloride in Norway, Heldaas et al. (75) determined the causes of death among 454 male workers from 1953 through 1979. During this period five cases of lung cancer were observed with 2.8 expected. Information on smoking habits of these workers was not available.

Mortality for a cohort of 4835 men employed at a polyvinyl chloride polymerization plant between 1942 and 1986 was examined by Wu et al. (76). For lung cancer, 115 deaths were observed with 94 expected (SMR, 90% confidence interval, 104–142). A nested case-control study to examine risk for lung cancer associated with specific exposures to vinyl chloride monomer and polyvinyl chloride showed no significant risk.

III. Probable Carcinogens

A. Acrylonitrile

Acrylonitrile is a chemical used in manufacturing plastics, synthetic rubber, and fibers. An association between exposure to acrylonitrile and lung cancer was first reported by O'Berg in 1980 (77). Subsequent reports provide further support for this association, but are based on small numbers of cases and lack information on smoking and other possible confounding factors (78–80).

B. Beryllium

Beryllium is a metal used as a hardening agent in several alloys and in other industrial applications. Occupational exposures may occur during mining, refining, alloy manufacturing, ceramics manufacturing, and in various parts of the electronic industry (81).

Beryllium compounds were the first nonradioactive agents found to cause lung cancer by inhalation in experimental animals (82), and several epidemiological investigations provide limited evidence that exposure to beryllium is a cause of lung cancer in humans (81). The epidemiological data are based on workers at two beryllium production plants in Ohio and Pennsylvania (83) and the U.S. Beryllium Case Registry (84,85). Mancuso (83) compared mortality patterns among 3685 workers at the two beryllium factories with those of 5929 rayon viscose workers, and found a 40% increase in lung cancer mortality (n = 80) among the beryllium workers. However, the role of smoking was not examined.

The Beryllium Case Registry was started in 1952 at the Massachusetts General Hospital. Cases for the registry are identified by referral. Using the Registry data base, Infante et al. (84) determined the frequency of lung cancer among all white males who were alive and enrolled in the Registry from 1952 through 1975. During this period, a total of 7 lung cancer deaths was observed with 3.3 expected. Of these deaths, six occurred among patients who had an acute respiratory illness attributed to beryllium exposure. A higher fatality rate from nonmalignant respiratory diseases among patients with chronic versus acute beryllium-related respiratory illness may partly explain the high proportion of lung cancer deaths in those with acute respiratory disease.

The risk of lung cancer in beryllium-exposed workers was recently reexamined by Steenland and Ward (85) among 685 patients in the Beryllium Case Registry. This investigation extended the work of Infante et al. (84) by including females, adding 13 years of follow-up, and examining the effects of smoking. Based on 28 cases of lung cancer, the SMR was 2.00 (95% confidence interval, 1.33–2.89) and was elevated in both sexes and unaffected by smoking.

C. Cadmium

Occupational exposure to cadmium may result from work in several industrial processes including cadmium production, metal plating, plastics production, pigment production, and other manufacturing processes (e.g., nickel-cadmium batteries, alloys) (86). Occupational exposure to cadmium and risk for lung cancer has been examined among cadmium production workers (87) and among workers producing nickel-cadmium batteries (88,89). Patterns of mortality among 602 workers from a U.S. cadmium production plant were examined by Thun et al. (87), who found 20 lung cancers with 11.43 expected. All of these lung cancers occurred among workers with more than 2 years of employment. Furthermore, mortality from lung cancer was found to increase with increasing cumulative exposure to cadmium. The excess mortality could not be explained by a concomitant exposure to arsenic for some of the workers. Although smoking data were not included in the analysis, interviews with 70% of survivors or next of kin, suggested that the prevalence of smoking was similar to that of the general population of U.S. males.

Compared with lung cancer mortality in the cadmium production workers, the production of nickel-cadmium batteries has been associated with smaller excesses of lung cancer, but the association has been confounded by exposure to nickel (88,89). Among 522 workers at a Swedish plant, Elinder et al. (88) observed 8 lung cancers with 6 expected. Although Elinder and coworkers found only one case of nasopharyngeal cancer, this case suggests a possible role of nickel in the development of cancer among these workers. At a nickel-cadmium battery factory in the United Kingdom, Sorahan (89) determined patterns of mortality for 3025 workers and found 110 lung cancers with 84.5 expected. However, a consistent increase in lung cancer mortality with increases in cumulative exposure was not observed.

D. Formaldehyde

Formaldehyde and its compounds are used in a wide variety of applications including adhesives for production of plywood, particleboard, and other products, and manufacturing rubber, photographic film, leather, explosives, dyes, cosmetics, corrosion inhibitors, and embalming fluids (90). The health effects of exposure to formaldehyde have been examined among pathologists, anatomists, and morticians, and among chemical workers (90). Investigations of pathologists, anatomists, and morticians have not shown relationships between these occupations and mortality from lung cancer, although some of these studies had limited statistical power because of small numbers of subjects.

The findings of epidemiological studies of chemical workers have created controversy about the risk of lung cancer from formaldehyde exposure in this industry (91–93). In one of the largest studies reported to date, Blair et al. (91) assembled a cohort of 26,561 workers from 10 formaldehyde-producing or -using facilities and examined patterns of mortality. Based on national mortality experience, the overall SMR for lung cancer in white men was 111; a significant exposure-response relationship was found with intensity of formaldehyde exposure. However, a clear dose-response relationship was not found between cumulative levels of exposure to formaldehyde and lung cancer mortality. The cause-and-effect relationships of these findings have been argued (91–93). However, available evidence of genotoxic effects and from animal studies provides sufficient information to classify formaldehyde as a suspected human carcinogen (94).

IV. Conclusions

Although accurate estimates on the number or workers exposed worldwide to the agents discussed in this chapter are not available, it is clear that millions of workers may be exposed in a wide variety of occupational settings and thereby placed at increased risk for developing lung cancer. For some carcinogenic agents, such as the chloromethyl ethers, the industrial processes have been modified to virtually eliminate workers' exposures. Exposures to other agents may have been decreased, but have not been eliminated, and the need remains to evaluate the risk associated with the lower levels of exposure that persist.

Despite the development and application of numerous experimental systems for determining potential carcinogenic risks of substances, epidemiological studies are still needed to assess carcinogenic risks in humans. As methods become available to measure personal exposure and, possibly, dose of exposure more precisely, more accurate estimates of risk will be possible in epidemiological investigations. In addition, assessment of risk from multiple exposures has received little attention and requires investigation. As new industrial processes are developed, exposures to new agents or mixtures of substances may occur, and surveillance of workers will remain important to detect previously unrecognized hazards.

Cigarette smoking is a well-recognized hazard for lung cancer that has received little attention in occupational exposure studies, except studies of exposure to asbestos and radon, and requires greater attention in future investigations of occupational exposures and lung cancer. Based on current epidemiological studies, lung cancer is relatively uncommon among never smokers compared with former or current cigarette smokers in most occupational settings (95). Excluding occupational exposures to radon decay products among miners and chloromethyl ethers, about 5% of the lung cancers in various occupational settings occur in nonsmokers (95). This figure is similar to the proportion of nonsmokers in case series derived from the general population (96). For the mining occupations involving exposure to radon decay products, about 12% of the cases occurred in nonsmokers.

The proportion of lung cancers in the general population caused by occupational and other environmental agents has been the topic of several investigations and a continuing source of controversy (97,98). The controversy has centered on the wide variation in estimates of the role of occupation in the cause of lung cancer. Such estimates, however, have not been offered for smokers and nonsmokers separately. A federal report released in the late 1970s projected a surprisingly high burden of occupational lung cancer; from 61,000 to 98,000 cases annually were attributed to asbestos and four other agents alone (99). Many estimates followed, some much more conservative. For example, Doll and Peto (97), in their 1981 review of causes of cancer, estimated that 5% of lung cancers in women and 15% in men were related to occupational exposures. A population-based case-control study in New Mexico empirically documented that about 10% of lung cancer cases in men could be attributed to occupation (100). In a recent literature review, Vineis and Simonato (101) cited attributable risk estimates for occupation and lung cancer that ranged from 4 to 40%. Although these estimates can be expected to vary across locations and over time; nevertheless, they indicate that occupation is still an important factor among causes of lung cancer.

Prevention of lung cancer mortality among workers exposed to agents or industrial processes that cause lung cancer may involve several strategies including eliminating or reducing exposures, smoking cessation, screening, and chemoprevention. For example, changes in industrial processes that have eliminated or reduced exposures to chloromethyl ethers (13) and nickel compounds (45) have provided evidence of reduced risk of lung cancer following the reduction. Of the other potential strategies for prevention of lung cancer among workers, smoking cessation is clearly the most important.

Acknowledgments

This chapter was supported in part by a Preventive Pulmonary Academic Award, K07HL02474, National Heart, Lung, and Blood Institute, and by Contract NO1-CN-55426 from the Biometry Branch, National Cancer Institute.

References

1. International Agency for Research on Cancer. (1987). *Overall evaluations of carcinogenicity: An Updating of IARC Monographs Volumes 1 to 42*. Supplement 7. Lyon, France, IARC.
2. U.S. Congress, Office of Technology Assessment. (1987). *Identifying and Regulating Carcinogens*. Washington, D.C., U.S. Government Printing Office, OTA-BP-H-42.
3. Doll, R. (1985). Occupational cancer: A hazard for epidemiologists. *Int. J. Epidemiol.* 14:22–31.
4. Hennekens, C. H., and Buring, J. E. (1987). *Epidemiology in Medicine*. Boston, MA, Little, Brown, and Company.
5. Siemiatycki, J., Wacholder, S., Dewar, R., Cardis, E., Greenwood, C., and Richardson, L. (1988). Degree of confounding bias related to smoking, ethnic group, and socioeconomic status in estimates of the associations between occupation and cancer. *J. Occup. Med.* 30:617–625.

45. Doll, R., Mathews, J. D., and Morgan, L. G. (1977). Cancers of the lung and nasal sinuses in nickel workers: A reassessment of the period of risk. *Br. J. Ind. Med.* 34: 102–105.
46. Magnus, K., Andersen, A., and Hogetveit, A. (1982). Cancer of respiratory organs among workers at a nickel refinery in Norway. *Int. J. Cancer* 30:681–685.
47. Enterline, P. E., and Marsh, G. M. (1982). Mortality among workers in a nickel refinery and alloy manufacturing plant in West Virginia. *J. Natl. Cancer Inst.* 68: 925–933.
48. Cox, J. E., Doll, R., Scott, W. A., and Smith, S. (1981). Mortality of nickel workers: Experience of men working with metallic nickel. *Br. J. Ind. Med.* 38:235–239.
49. Godbold, J. H., and Tompkins, E. A. (1979). A long-term mortality study of workers occupationally exposed to metallic nickel at the Oak Ridge gaseous diffusion plant. *J. Occup. Med.* 21:799–806.
50. Kaldor, J., Peto, J., Easton, D., Doll, R., Hermon, C., and Morgan, L. (1986). Models for respiratory cancer in nickel refinery workers. *J. Natl. Cancer Inst.* 77: 841–848.
51. Lessard, R., Reed., D., Maheux, B., and Lambert, J. (1978). Lung cancer in New Caledonia, a nickel smelting island. *J. Occup. Med.* 20:815–817.
52. Goldberg, M., Goldberg, P., Leclerc, A., Chastang, J. F., Fuhrer, R., Brodeur, J. M., Segnan, N., Floch, J. J., and Michel, G. (1987). Epidemiology of respiratory cancers related to nickel mining and refining in New Caledonia (1978–1984). *Int. J. Cancer* 40:300–304.
53. Report of the International Committee on Nickel Carcinogenesis in Man. (1990). *Scand. J. Work Environ. Health* 16(special issue):1–82.
54. Kreyberg, L. (1978). Lung cancer in workers in a nickel refinery. *Br. J. Ind. Med.* 35:109–116.
55. Langer, A. M., Rohl, A. N., and Selikoff, I. J. (1980). Asbestos as a cofactor in carcinogenesis among nickel-processing workers. *Science* 209:420–422.
56. International Agency for Research on Cancer. (1983). IARC monographs on the evaluation of the carcinogenic risk of chemicals to humans. *Polynuclear Aromatic Compounds, Part 1, Chemical, Environmental and Experimental Data*. Volume 32, Lyon, France, IARC.
57. Matanoski, G., Fishbein, L., Redmond, C., Rosenkranz, H., and Wallace, L. (1986). Contribution of organic particulates to respiratory cancer. *Environ. Health Perspect.* 70:37–49.
58. International Agency for Research on Cancer. (1984). IARC monographs on the evaluation of the carcinogenic risk of chemicals to humans. *Polynuclear Aromatic Compounds, Part 2, Carbon Blacks, Mineral Oils and Some Nitroarenes*. Volume 33. Lyon, France, IARC.
59. International Agency for Research on Cancer. (1984). IARC monographs on the evaluation of the carcinogenic risk of chemicals to humans. *Polynuclear Aromatic Compounds, Part 3, Industrial Exposures in Aluminum Production, Coal Gasification, Coke Production, and Iron and Steel Founding*. Volume 34. Lyon, France, IARC.
60. International Agency for Research on Cancer. (1984). IARC monographs on the evaluation of the carcinogenic risk of chemicals to humans. *Polynuclear Aromatic*

Compounds, Part 4, Bitumens, Coal-Tars and Derived Products, Shale-Oils and Soots. Volume 35. Lyon, France, IARC.

61. International Agency for Research on Cancer. (1989). IARC monographs on the evaluation of the carcinogenic risks to humans. *Diesel and Gasoline Engine Exhausts and Some Nitroarenes*. Volume 46. Lyon, France, IARC.
62. Gibbs, G. W. (1985). Mortality of aluminum reduction plant workers, 1950 through 1977. *J. Occup. Med.* 27:762–770.
63. Redmond, C. K. (1983). Cancer mortality among coke oven workers. *Environ. Health Perspect.* 52:67–73.
64. Dong, M. H., Redmond, C. K., Mazumdar, S., and Costantino, J. P. (1988). A multistage approach to the cohort analysis of lifetime lung cancer risk among steelworkers exposed to coke oven emissions. *Am J. Epidemiol.* 128:860–873.
65. Silverstein, M., Maizlish, N., Park, R., and Mirer, F. (1985). Mortality among workers exposed to coal tar pitch volatiles and welding emissions: An exercise in epidemiologic triage. *Am. J. Public Health* 75:1283–1287.
66. Hogstedt, C., Andersson, K., Frenning, B., and Gustavsson, A. (1982). A cohort study on mortality among long-term employed Swedish chimney sweeps. *Scand. J. Work Environ. Health* 8(Suppl):72–78.
67. Hansen, E. S. (1983). Mortality from cancer and ischemic heart disease in Danish chimney sweeps: A five-year follow-up. *Am. J. Epidemiol.* 117:160–164.
68. Howe, G. R., Fraser, D., Lindsay, J., Presnal, G., and Yu, S. Z. (1983). Cancer mortality (1965–1977) in relation to diesel fume and coal exposure in a cohort of retired railway workers. *J. Natl. Cancer Inst.* 70:1015–1019.
69. Garshick, E., Schenker, M. B., Munoz, A., Segal, M., Smith, T. J., Woskie, S. R., Hammond, S. K., and Speizer, F. E. (1988). A retrospective cohort study of lung cancer and diesel exhaust exposure in railroad workers. *Am. Rev. Respir. Dis.* 137: 820–825.
70. Garshick, E., Schenker, M. B., Munoz, A., Segal, M., Smith, T. J., Woskie, S. R., Hammond, S. K., and Speizer, F. E. (1987). A case-control study of lung cancer and diesel exhaust exposure in railroad workers. *Am. Rev. Respir. Dis.* 135:1242–1248.
71. Fingerhut, M. A., Halperin, W. E., Marlow, D. A., Piacitelli, L. A., Honchar, P. A., Sweeney, M. H., Greife, A. L., Dill, P. A., Steenland, K., and Suruda, A. J. (1991). Cancer mortality in workers exposed to 2,3,7,8-tetrachlorodibenzo-p-dioxin. *N. Engl. J. Med.* 324:212–218.
72. Creech, J. L., and Johnson, M. N. (1974). Angiosarcoma of liver in the manufacture of polyvinyl chloride. *J. Occup. Med.* 16:150–151.
73. Buffler, P. A., Wood, S., Eifler, C., Suarez, L., and Kilian, D. J. (1979). Mortality experience of workers in a vinyl chloride monomer production plant. *J. Occup. Med.* 21:195–203.
74. Waxweiler, R. J., Smith, A. H., Falk, H., and Tyroler, H. A. (1981). Excess lung cancer risk in a synthetic chemicals plant. *Environ. Health Perspect.* 41:159–165.
75. Heldaas, S. S., Langard, S. L., and Andersen, A. (1984). Incidence of cancer among vinyl chloride and polyvinyl chloride workers. *Br. J. Ind. Med.* 41:25–30.
76. Wu, W., Steenland, K., Brown, D., Wells, V., Jones, J., Schulte, P., and Halperin, W.

(1989). Cohort and case-control analyses of workers exposed to vinyl chloride: An update. *J. Occup. Med.* 31:518–523.

77. O'Berg, M. T. (1980). Epidemiologic study of workers exposed to acrylonitrile. *J. Occup. Med.* 22:245–252.
78. Werner, J. B., and Carter, J. T. (1981). Mortality of United Kingdom acrylonitrile polymerisation workers. *Br. J. Ind. Med.* 38:247–253.
79. Delzell, E., and Monson, R. R. (1982). Mortality among rubber workers: VI. Men with potential exposure to acrylonitrile. *J. Occup. Med.* 24:767–771.
80. O'Berg, M. T., Chen, J. L., Burke, C. A., Walrath, J., and Pell, S. (1985). Epidemiologic study of workers exposed to acrylonitrile: An update. *J. Occup. Med.* 27:835–840.
81. Saracci, R. (1985). Beryllium: Epidemiologic evidence. *IARC Sci. Publ.* 65: 203–219.
82. Groth, D. H. (1980). Carcinogenicity of beryllium: Review of the literature. *Environ. Res.* 21:56–62.
83. Mancuso, T. F. (1980). Mortality study of beryllium industry workers' occupational lung cancer. *Environ. Res.* 21:48–55.
84. Infante, P. F., Wagoner, J. K., and Sprince, N. L. (1980). Mortality patterns from lung cancer and nonneoplastic respiratory disease among white males in the Beryllium Case Registry. *Environ. Res.* 21:35–43.
85. Steenland, K., and Ward, E. (1991). Lung cancer incidence among patients with beryllium disease: A cohort mortality study. *J. Natl. Cancer Inst.* 83:1380–1385.
86. International Agency for Research on Cancer. (1976). IARC monographs on the evaluation of the carcinogenic risk of chemicals to man. *Cadmium, Nickel, Some Epoxides, Miscellaneous Industrial Chemicals and General Considerations on Volatile Anesthetics*. Volume 11. Lyon, France, IARC.
87. Thun, M. J., Schnorr, T. M., Smith, A. B., Halperin, W. E., and Lemen, R. A. (1985). Mortality among a cohort of U.S. cadmium production workers—an update. *J. Natl. Cancer Inst.* 74:325–333.
88. Elinder, C-G., Kjellstrom, T., Hogstedt, C., Andersson, K., and Spang, G. (1985). Cancer mortality of cadmium workers. *Br. J. Ind. Med.* 42:651–655.
89. Sorahan, T. (1987). Mortality from lung cancer among a cohort of nickel cadmium battery workers: 1946–1984. *Br. J. Ind. Med.* 44:803–809.
90. Nelson, N., Levine, R. J., Albert, R. E., Blair, A. E., Griesemer, R. A., Landrigan, P. J., Stayner, L. T., and Swenberg, J. A. (1986). Contribution of formaldehyde to respiratory cancer. *Environ. Health Perspect.* 70:23–35.
91. Blair, A., Stewart, P., O'berg, M., Gaffey, W., Walrath, J., Ward, J., Bales, R., Kaplan, S., and Cubit, D. (1986). Mortality among industrial workers exposed to formaldehyde. *J. Natl. Cancer Inst.* 76:1071–1084.
92. Sterling, T. D., and Weinkam, J. J. (1988). Reanalysis of lung cancer mortality in a National Cancer Institute study on mortality among industrial workers exposed to formaldehyde. *J. Occup. Med.* 30:895–901.
93. Sterling, T. D., and Weinkam, J. J. (1989). Reanalysis of lung cancer mortality in a National Cancer Institute study of "mortality among industrial workers exposed to formaldehyde": Additional discussion. *J. Occup. Med.* 31:881–883.

94. Leikauf, G. D. (1991). Formaldehyde and other aldehydes. In *Critical Reviews of Environmental Toxicants—Human Exposures and Their Health Effects*. Edited by M. Lippman. New York, Van Nostrand Reinhold.
95. Samet, J. M., and Coultas, D. B. (1990). Epidemiology of lung disease. In *Problems in Respiratory Care*. Edited by T. J. Witek, Jr., and E. N. Schachter. Current Issues in Respiratory Public Health: I. Volume 3, Number 1. Philadelphia, PA, J. B. Lippincott Company.
96. National Research Council. (1988). *Health Risks of Radon and Other Internally Deposited Alpha-Emitters*. BEIR IV. Committee on the Biological Effects of Ionizing Radiation. Washington, D.C., National Academy Press.
97. Doll, R., and Peto, R. (1981). The causes of cancer. *J. Natl. Cancer Inst.* 66:1191–1308.
98. Samet, J. M., and Lerchen, M. L. (1984). Proportion of lung cancer caused by occupation: A critical review. In *Occupational Lung Disease*. Edited by J. B. L. Gee, W. K. C. Morgan, and S. M. Brooks. New York, Raven Press. pp. 55–67.
99. Bridbord, K., Decoufle, P., Fraumeni, J. F., Hoel, D. G., Hoover, R. N., Rall, D. P., Saffiotti, U., Schneiderman, M. A., and Upton, A. C. (1981). *Estimates of the Function of Cancer in the United States Related to Occupational Factors*. Prepared by NCI, NIEHS, and NIOSH. Published in an appendix of the Banbury Report 9. Quantification of Occupational Cancer. Cold Spring Harbor Laboratory.
100. Lerchen, M. L., Wiggins, C. L., and Samet, J. M. (1987). Lung cancer and occupation in New Mexico. *J. Natl. Cancer Inst.* 79:639–645.
101. Vineis, P., and Simonato, L. (1991). Proportion of lung and bladder cancers in males resulting from occupation: A systematic approach. *Arch. Environ. Health* 46:6–15.

13

Diet as a Factor in the Etiology and Prevention of Lung Cancer

TIM BYERS

Centers for Disease Control
Atlanta, Georgia

I. Introduction

We have known for more than 30 years that cigarette smoking is the leading preventable cause of cancer in the United States, yet substantial numbers of people continue to smoke cigarettes. Consequently, lung cancer, though on the decline, continues to take more lives than any other kind of cancer in the United States (1). Other lung carcinogens in the environment, including radon, asbestos, and various chemicals in the workplace, also contribute to these deaths. Although we have made considerable progress in reducing our exposures to environmental carcinogens and in motivating people to avoid tobacco smoke, additional measures are needed in the overall strategy to prevent lung cancer. In particular, we need to more carefully consider cofactors that might predispose individuals to lung cancer after exposure to carcinogens.

Considerable evidence indicates that diet may be a significant cofactor in the cause of lung cancer. The dietary factors most intensively studied in lung cancer

---

The opinions expressed in this paper are those of the author and do not necessarily reflect those of the U.S. government.

are the retinoids, in the form of either preformed vitamin A (retinol) or its precursor carotenoids (2–5). Both laboratory and epidemiological studies strongly suggest that carotenoids may produce a substantial protective effect. Dietary fat, dietary cholesterol, vitamin C, vitamin E, and other dietary factors have also been hypothesized to affect lung cancer risk, though findings for these nutrients have been equivocal. Because none of the relationships between diet and lung cancer have yet been conclusively proven, agencies that have formally reviewed the evidence on the link between diet and cancer (e.g., the American Cancer Society, the National Research Council, and the National Cancer Institute) have refrained from recommending that smokers modify their diet to reduce lung cancer risk (6–8). In this chapter we will review scientific evidence related to the possible association between diet and lung cancer and discuss the potential for reducing lung cancer risk in the United States through dietary modification and/or supplementation.

II. Studies in Laboratory Animals

No completely satisfactory animal models for human lung cancer exist (9). Consequently, animal models now in use have limited utility for improving our understanding of the relationship between diet and lung cancer in humans. Nonetheless, animal experiments and laboratory studies can help us to elucidate possible mechanisms and generate hypotheses about relationships between diet and human cancer risk. Data from the laboratory support the hypotheses that dietary fat may promote cancer (10) and that dietary antioxidants may protect against cancer (11).

Experimental studies involving animal models have provided evidence in support of a protective effect of retinoids against cancer. As early as 1925, Wolbach and Howe demonstrated that vitamin A–deficient diets created widespread epithelial abnormalities in rats (12). Among these effects were a profound disturbance of the epithelium of the respiratory tract, loss of normal cellular architecture, and metaplasia. More recently, investigators have examined the ability of retinoids to protect the integrity of the respiratory epithelium in the presence of chemical carcinogens (13). While these studies have provided some evidence that low levels of dietary or circulating retinol are associated with increased tumor yield, that association has not been demonstrated in all tumor model systems, and its pathophysiology has not been clearly delineated. We do know that vitamin A is necessary both to maintain proper differentiation of epithelial cells and to inhibit the proliferation of neoplastic cells after transformation. Carotenes, which are precursor compounds for vitamin A (beta-carotene is enzymatically cleaved to form two retinol molecules), may therefore act as anticarcinogenic agents through their conversion to vitamin A. However, dietary intakes of retinol and carotenoids are correlated with circulating blood levels of vitamin A only in the context of severe dietary deprivation. In well-nourished animals and people, circulating levels of retinol are highly buffered by large liver stores, and the conversion of carotenoids to retinol is a highly controlled enzymatic process (14). These homeostatic mechanisms account for the almost complete lack of correlation between dietary intake of either retinol or carotenoids and blood retinol levels. In contrast, circulating levels of carotenoids are correlated with carotene intake in the diet (15). The protective effect of carotenoids may therefore be mediated by a mechanism independent of their conversion to vitamin A. Because carotenoids are potent antioxidants, they may be anticarcinogenic via their ability to neutralize free radicals and excited oxygen (16–18). This antioxidant property of the carotenoids may be a much more plausible mechanism for protection against cancer than would their effect on vitamin A levels in well-nourished populations such as persons in the United States.

There appears to be a relationship between fat intake and lung cancer risk in animal models (9,10). Using animal models, researchers have shown that high intake of dietary fat can promote chemically induced pulmonary tumors (9,19). Again, however, the relevance of these models to lung cancer in humans can be questioned (20).

Vitamin C is an important human nutrient, being crucial in many metabolic systems and a major antioxidant protecting against lipid peroxidation. The possible relevance of vitamin C to human cancer risk has been extensively reviewed (21). In many animal carcinogenesis models, vitamin C reduces tumor yield, acting both at the initiation and promotion phases, but little work on vitamin C and pulmonary tumors in animal models has been done (11). Vitamin E, another important antioxidant in human nutrition, is highly fat soluble and is therefore found in high concentrations in lipid components of cell membranes, where it serves as the major compound protecting against oxidative damage (22). As with vitamin C, however, little work has been done to study the role of vitamin E in experimental animal pulmonary tumor systems.

III. Epidemiological Dietary Studies

Many epidemiological studies have probed the relationship between diet and lung cancer in humans. Various types of epidemiological research have been conducted, including ecological, case-control, and prospective studies, as well as randomized controlled trials. In ecological (or correlational) studies, dietary intake in different populations is correlated with lung cancer incidence and mortality. In case-control (or retrospective) studies, the diet of cancer cases, as ascertained retrospectively by interview, is compared with similarly collected information about diets of noncases (controls). In prospective (or cohort) studies, investigators interview or administer questionnaires to large groups of individuals to ascertain their diets and/or measure their blood nutrient levels at one or more points in time; they later examine cancer incidence related to those (prediagnostic) nutritional measures. In randomized controlled trials, micronutrient intake is manipulated experimentally by supplementation with random assignment to intervention and placebo groups; cancer incidence is later examined according to the randomized groups.

Very few ecological studies of diet and lung cancer have been conducted, largely because of concern about potential confounding by cigarettes, the factor of overriding importance in lung cancer etiology. In ecological studies, the ability to control for potential confounding factors is very limited, and findings are difficult to interpret, particularly when strong known risk factors have uncontrolled confounding influences on much weaker factors under study (23).

Case-control studies have by far been the design most commonly employed in diet and lung cancer studies. In these studies, investigators can control for smoking exposures and other lung cancer risk factors by measuring these factors for specific individuals. The biggest weakness of case-control studies is that the assessment of diet through retrospective interviews yields imperfect measures of usual diet prior to disease (24). Biased misclassification of diet can create artificial associations, whereas random misclassification of diet can bias risk estimates toward the null. If, for instance, individuals who have been diagnosed as having lung cancer (cases) were more likely to erroneously recall their past intake of a particular food than were well individuals (controls), then the estimate of the association between that food and cancer risk would be stronger than the true association due to recall bias. The possibility of recall bias in dietary reports should be carefully considered when associations are observed only in case-control studies. On the other hand, random error in diet reports by both cases and controls can serve to hide true associations. If both cases and controls report their past diet equally poorly, then the estimate of the association between that food and lung cancer would be weaker than the true association. Even strong relationships between diet and disease could be reduced to nil by high levels of random error in dietary reports.

Several prospective studies have been conducted with lung cancer as an end-point. Although prospective studies are not subject to dietary measurement errors biased by subjects' experiences after diagnosed disease, the possible effects of random measurement error from erroneous diet reports are the same as in case-control studies. Many prospective studies have limited power because they include small numbers of lung cancer cases. Some prospective studies have included the collection and storage of blood samples from subjects many years before diagnosis. These studies are particularly informative because they can elucidate nutrition–lung cancer relationships both by assessing diet and by examining nutrient levels in the blood before diagnosis.

No randomized controlled trials of micronutrient supplementation for lung cancer prevention have yet been completed, but several are now in progress, and the results from many are expected within the next 5 years (25). The advantage of randomized trials is that exposure to the dietary factor need not be inferred from self-reports, but can be controlled in a random, blinded fashion. Dietary factors that can be experimentally manipulated by administering supplements (such as micronutrients) can be studied best by randomized trials because compliance is relatively easy to monitor, and the trials can be blinded to both the participants and the investigators. Dietary interventions that necessitate behavioral change, however, such as reducing dietary fat or increasing the intake of fruits and vegetables, are much more difficult to affect, and cannot be blinded. All experimental trials now underway for lung cancer prevention are therefore blinded trials of micronutrient supplementation (25).

Studies that have examined the role of vitamin A and/or carotene in lung cancer have yielded findings that are much more consistent than for studies of other cancer sites (2–5,26). These studies are summarized in Table 1 (27–53). In each of these selected 27 studies, researchers have found evidence of a protective effect for dietary vitamin A and/or carotene. In most of these studies, cigarette smoking was carefully controlled in the analysis. The vitamin A index examined in many of the older studies included foods containing retinol as well as provitamin A carotenoids from fruits and vegetables. Most investigators who examined both retinol and carotenoids in the diet found that dietary carotenes were more protective against lung cancer than was retinol (42–45,50,52) Conversely, studies have consistently indicated an increased risk of lung cancer with low intake of dietary carotenes (see Table 1).

Considered together, these 27 studies indicate that there is roughly a 50–100% increase in lung cancer risk for persons below the (approximate) 25th percentile of carotene intake as compared with those above the (approximate) 75th percentile. Table 2 displays findings regarding the dose-response relationship between dietary carotene and lung cancer in those studies that have presented that detail (41–45,48,50–52). The slope of the dose-response relationship is linear in most studies, but not in all. Some studies indicate a gradient of risk across the entire range of intake (41,47,50,51), while others suggest a threshold effect somewhat at or below the population's median (42–45).

Studies that have examined the diet–lung cancer relationship in men and women separately have tended to indicate a weaker association in women (37,41, 45,48). Whether dietary factors may affect lung cancer risk differently in women is not yet clear, however (44,50). This difference between the sexes may be partially the result of different distributions of histologic types of lung cancer in men and women. There is a stronger protective effect of dietary carotenes on squamous cell and small-cell lung cancers, while lung adenocarcinomas tend to show weaker associations with dietary carotenes in some studies (38,42,48,54), but not all (44,45,50,52). Because lung cancer in women is more likely to be of adenocar-

Table 1 Association Between Lung Cancer and Indicators of Dietary Vitamin A or Carotene in Selected Studies

Sex	Location	Design[a]	Dietary factor	Relative risk for low intake[b]	Ref.
M	Singapore	c:c	Vegetables	2.2	27
M	Japan	pro	Vegetables	1.3[d]	28
F	Japan	pro	Vegetables	1.5[d]	
F	Massachusetts	pro	Vegetables	3.3	29
M	China	c:c	Vegetables	2.3	30
M	Italy	c:c	Carrots	1.8	31
M, F	California	pro	Fruits	3.2	32
M, F	United States	pro	Fruits	1.8	33
F	Iowa	pro	Fruits/vegetables	1.7	34
M	Norway	pro	Vit A index[c]	2.6	35
M	Buffalo	c:c	Vit A index	1.7	36
M	England	c:c	Vit A index	2.4[d]	37
F	England	c:c	Vit A index	0.5[e]	37
M	Norway	pro	vit A index	1.5	38
F	Italy	c:c	Carotene	3.3	39
M	Chicago	pro	Carotene	7.2[d]	40
M	Hawaii	c:c	Carotene	2.2	41
F	Hawaii	c:c	Carotene	0.6	
M	New Jersey	c:c	Carotene	1.3	42
M, F	New Mexico	c:c	Carotene	1.5	43
F	Los Angeles	c:c	Carotene	2.5	44
M	Buffalo	c:c	Carotene	1.8	45
F	Buffalo	c:c	Carotene	1.3	
M	Netherlands	pro	Carotene	1.5	46
M	Michigan	c:c	Carotene	1.2	47
M	New Orleans	c:c	Carotene	1.2	48
F	New Orleans	c:c	Carotene	1.0	
M	Los Angeles	pro	Carotene	1.4	49
F	Los Angeles	pro	Carotene	1.5	
M	Hawaii	c:c	Carotene	1.9	50
F	Hawaii	c:c	Carotene	2.7	
M, F	Buffalo	c:c	Carotene	2.0	51
M, F	Toronto	c:c	Carotene	1.1	52
M	France	c:c	Carotene	4.1	53

[a]Pro = prospective study; c:c = case:control study.
[b]In most studies, the low-intake group included persons in the approximate lowest quartile of intake in the population.
[c]An index of vitamin A activity from foods, including both vitamin A and carotene.
[d]Relative risk estimates are not adjusted for smoking.
[e]Based on only 22 cases.

Table 2 Dose-Response Relationships Between Dietary Carotene Intake and Lung Cancer Risk in Selected Studies[a]

Subjects' sex	Location	Relative risk according to percentile rank of the population's dietary carotene intake: Lowest intake (0–25)	(25–50)	Median intake (50)	(50–75)	Highest intake (75–100)	Ref.
M	Hawaii	1.7	1.4		1.2	1.0	41
F	Los Angeles	2.5	3.3		2.0	1.0	44
M	Buffalo	1.7	1.7		1.0	1.0	45
F	Buffalo	1.2	1.2		1.7	1.0	
M	Hawaii	1.9	2.4		1.5	1.0	50
F	Hawaii	2.7	2.4		1.9	1.0	
M, F	Toronto	1.1	1.3		1.1	1.0	52
M	New Jersey	1.2		1.0		1.0	42
M, F	New Mexico	1.4		1.0		1.0	43
M, F	New Orleans	1.1		1.0		1.0	48
M, F	Buffalo	2.0	1.7	1.2	1.1	1.0	51
M	Michigan	2.5		1.4		1.0	47

[a]Studies varied in definitions of dietary carotene; some examined total dietary carotenoids, while others examined beta carotene specifically. Only those studies presenting dose-response relationships for more than 100 cases are included.

cinoma histology, the difference in the carotene–lung cancer association between men and women may be in part due to differences between the sexes in histologic types of tumors.

Despite these repeated observations of an apparent protective effect of dietary carotene against lung cancer, the question of whether this effect is modified by cigarette smoking has not yet been clearly answered. Whether current heavy smokers respond differently to dietary carotene than do ex-smokers or never-smokers is a question of considerable importance both to biological science and to public health. Table 3 summarizes the findings from selected studies on the association of dietary vitamin A and carotene with lung cancer risk at different levels of cigarette-smoking exposure. Bjelke's study showed a 4.1-fold increase in the risk of lung cancer with low dietary intake of vitamin A among those who were ex-smokers at baseline, but only a 2.6-fold increase for low vitamin A intake in those who were actively smoking at baseline (35). A Norwegian study by Kvale et al. showed contrasting results, however, with the strongest association

Table 3 The Association Between Lung Cancer and Indicators of Dietary Vitamin A or Carotene at Different Levels of Cirgarette Smoking in Selected Studies[a]

Subjects' sex	Dietary factor	Relative risk estimates: Persons who have never smoked	Former smokers	Current light smokers		Current heavy smokers	Ref.
M, F	Vegetables	2.2	3.0	—	1.2	—	28
M, F	Fruits	4.3	NP[c]	—	4.5[b]	—	32
M	Carrots	0.8	0.9	2.9		NP	31
M	Vit A Index	1.0	4.1	2.3		2.8	35
M	Vit A Index	NP	NP	1.4[d]		2.4	36
M	Vit A Index	1.1	1.3	1.1		2.0	38
M	Carotene	NP	2.6	1.1		NP	43
M	Carotene	NP	1.9[e]	1.8		1.3	45
F	Carotene	NP	3.3	0.8		0.8	
M	Carotene	1.3	NP	0.3		NP	49
M	Carotene	NP	1.6	0.9		1.7	50
F	Carotene	NP	2.4[e]	8.8		0.9	

[a]Numbers in the table are relative risk estimates for the lowest levels of dietary consumption, as compared to the highest levels presented in each analysis.
[b]Includes former and current smokers.
[c]Not Presented.
[d]Includes never and light smokers.
[e]Includes never and former smokers.

between lung cancer and low vitamin A consumption in those who were current, heavy smokers at baseline (38). Hirayama's prospective study of about 250,000 Japanese over a 10-year period showed that among ex-smokers, those who consumed green or yellow vegetables in low amounts experienced a threefold increase in lung cancer mortality compared with those who consumed high amounts, whereas no such association was seen in current smokers (28). Studies in New Mexico and New York showed that the increased risk associated with low carotene intake was greater in ex-smokers than in current smokers (43,45).

Although most studies of diet and lung cancer have focused on the carotenoids, several studies have analyzed other antioxidant micronutrients. Low levels of vitamin C have been associated with increased lung cancer risk in some studies (41,46,48,50), but not all (45,52). One study demonstrated an apparent protective association between vitamin C and lung cancer that was statistically independent of carotene (48); however, separating the effects of vitamin C and carotenoids is very difficult, as they are found in similar foods and therefore tend to vary together in the population. Epidemiological evidence that vitamin E may play a role in lung cancer is very scant. The observation that foods and food groups often are more strongly associated with lung cancer risk than are micronutrient indices supports the concept that the beneficial effects of fruit and vegetable consumption on lung cancer risk may not be due to a single micronutrient, but may instead be the result of a combined effect of many micronutrients (34,50,52).

If dietary micronutrients such as beta-carotene do protect against lung cancer, properly conducted randomized controlled trials would be the most definitive way to demonstrate that effect. Four such studies are now under way. Each study involves daily micronutrient supplementation in a placebo-controlled design in men. Three of these trials involve men at high risk for lung cancer (Chinese tin miners who are exposed to high doses of radon, heavy smokers, and asbestos workers), and one trial focuses on a group at relatively low risk (physicians in the United States) (55). The agents being used in these trials are various combinations of beta-carotene, vitamin A, retinoic acid, and vitamin E. Although these randomized trials may provide definitive proof that micronutrients can reduce the risk of lung cancer, several important limitations need to be considered. The micronutrients being tested are those considered to be good candidates for explaining the observed diet-lung cancer relationships. Even if the randomized controlled trials reveal no benefit to supplementation, the strong and consistent protective associations observed between carotene-containing foods and lung cancer cannot be denied, and we may well then conclude that we have tested the wrong compounds. The strong impression that eating plenty of fruits and vegetables reduces lung cancer risk (see Table 1) will then still remain to be explained.

Animal experiments (9) and international correlational studies (10) provide some support for the hypothesis that diets high in fat may be associated with increased lung cancer risk. Only a few epidemiological studies have made comprehensive enough measures of diet to allow us to examine the role of dietary fat in lung cancer. Some studies have shown greater risk among people with higher levels of fat (45,51) or cholesterol (52,56) intake in their diets, though other studies (40) have not made such observations (40). The interaction of diets high in fat and also low in fruits and vegetables has not been well studied.

IV. Blood Nutrient Studies

In at least eight prospective studies, levels of retinol and/or carotene in blood samples, frozen and stored at baseline, were compared for persons who later developed lung cancer with those who did not (Table 4) (57–64). Most studies have found similar levels of vitamins A, C, and E in individuals who subsequently developed cancer and in those who remained cancer-free. In contrast, studies have more consistently shown lower serum carotene levels to be associated with lung cancer.

Table 4 Dietary Micronutrient Levels in Plasma Samples Collected Prospectively from People Who Later Developed Lung Cancer as Compared with Those who Remained Free of Lung Cancer[a]

Subjects' sex	Location	Nutrient	Nutrient level[b]	Ref.
M	Switzerland	Beta-carotene	69	57
		Vitamin A	100	
		Vitamin C	99	
		Vitamin E	97	
M	Hawaii	Beta-carotene	69	58
		Vitamin A	107	
		Vitamin C	104	
M, F	Maryland	Beta-carotene	86	59
		Vitamin A	99	
		Vitamin E	88	
M	England	Beta-carotene	78	60
		Vitamin A	99	61
	California	Vitamin A	100	62
M	United States	Carotene	78	63
		Vitamin A	96	
		Vitamin E	96	
M, F	Finland	Vitamin E	96	64

[a]Only studies including more than 20 lung cancer cases are included.
[b]Expressed as percent of level in persons remaining free of lung cancer.

These observations support the hypothesis that low intake of carotenoids increases lung cancer risk, because the laboratory assessment of carotene levels is not subject to the same uncertainties inherent in self-reported dietary exposures. The interpretation of these findings is not entirely straightforward, however. There are many determinants of circulating carotene levels apart from diet. Because smoking can profoundly reduce circulating carotene levels (see Table 4), smoking may have a residual confounding effect on the association between lung cancer and carotene levels, even in prospective studies. For instance, if the frequency and intensity of cigarette smoking at the time of blood drawing were not precisely measured, tobacco exposure could still confound the blood carotene-lung cancer association even though tobacco exposure were included as an adjustment factor in the statistical analysis. The absence of an association between vitamin C and lung cancer in the study that examined both carotene and vitamin C (58) argues against this, however, because smoking also profoundly reduces circulating levels of vitamin C. More importantly, because of within-person variations in diet and because of the effects of nondietary factors on nutrient levels in the circulating serum collected at a single point in time, a single blood assay may be less representative of nutritional intake of vitamins A, C, E, and carotene than is a self-report of dietary intake as estimated by questionnaires or interviews.

Many investigators have found that cigarette smokers have lower levels of circulating carotene than do nonsmokers (Table 5) (60,63,65–71). These reductions in serum carotene cannot be explained by differences in dietary intake of carotene. Even in an intervention trial in which beta-carotene intake was increased more than 10-fold, substantial differences in circulating beta-carotene levels were observed between smokers and nonsmokers (72). We do not know whether low levels of carotene in smokers are due to differences in absorption or to a high turnover of carotene as it quenches free radicals. In any case, smokers (and perhaps also ex-smokers for some period of time) may need to consume more carotene than do nonsmokers to maintain similar circulating levels. This observation of lower blood levels of carotene in smokers therefore creates a very plausible biological mechanism whereby low dietary carotene intake might increase lung cancer risk. Because cigarette smoking reduces circulating carotene levels, low levels of intake may place smokers at high risk for having low circulating carotene levels, either considered as low average levels or as intermittently low levels. Oxidative damage to DNA and/or cellular membranes resulting from very low circulating levels could then result in the initiation and/or the promotion of respiratory epithelial neoplasia.

Table 5 Plasma Beta-Carotene Levels According to Smoking Status in Selected Studies

		Beta-carotene levels (× g/dl)				
Subjects' sex	Location	Current smokers	Current nonsmokers	Never smokes	Former smokers	Ref.
M	United States	24.9	28.8			65
M	Japan	25.0		39.0	35.0	66
F	Japan	42.0		75.0	54.0	
M	England	18.5		25.5	22.8	60
M	Maryland	25.0		35.7	32.4	67
F	Maryland	30.3		42.4	39.5	
M, F	Seattle	19.4	27.6			68
M, F	United States	12.8		20.1	17.7	69
F	New York	10.5	16.8			70
M	Japan	22.1	31.7			71
F	Japan	35.0	54.6			
M	Maryland	11.2	16.8			63

V. Lung Cancer Prevention and Diet

Clearly, quitting or never smoking are the most important strategies for preventing lung cancer. Nonetheless, because many people continue to smoke and because the risk of lung cancer in former smokers returns to baseline only after a decade or more, we must consider additional means of lung cancer prevention.

In epidemiological studies of the effect of diet on the risk of lung cancer, investigators have consistently suggested that smokers with lower intakes of carotene appear to be at higher risk, even after accounting for the possible confounding effects of cigarette smoking. Even though researchers have not yet conclusively proven that low dietary or circulating carotene levels are causally related to lung cancer, the consistency of the epidemiological observations, the inability to explain the association as confounding by either cigarettes or another lung cancer risk factor, the supportive evidence from animal cancer research, the apparent depressant effect of smoking on circulating carotene levels, and the biologic plausibility of such a relationship demand that we carefully consider the public health implications of diet and lung cancer.

If low intake of carotene (even just the lowest quartile of the population distribution) increases the risk of lung cancer by only 50%, then 20% of lung cancer cases might be preventable by diet modification (the population attributable risk). This 20% estimate would be high if the association between carotene (or fruits and vegetables) results from measurement bias or is due to confounding by an unmeasured causal factor. Both these possibilities are reduced considerably by the remarkably consistent observation of the diet–lung cancer association in studies of many different populations, using different designs and different methods of dietary assessment. Biased measures are particularly unlikely in prospective studies, and residual confounding by a subtle underestimate of smoking that is correlated with diet is unlikely to have occurred in so many different populations. Therefore, the conclusion that there is truly a causal association between lung cancer and low levels of fruits and vegetables in the diet (perhaps in conjunction with high-fat diets) is supportable. Because imperfect dietary assessment creates random error in dietary exposure classification, we may have considerably underestimated the magnitude of the association between diet and lung cancer. This factor, along with the likelihood that there are effects of diet across the entire range of intake (not only the lowest quartile), leads us to conclude that an attributable risk estimate of 20% may be far lower than the true potential that could be achieved.

What should we be advising smokers about diet and lung cancer? One fact is clear: if there is a protective effect of dietary carotene, it is very weak in comparison with the risk-enhancing effect of cigarettes. Consequently, the health-behavioral implications of targeting dietary advice to smokers must be carefully considered. Currently, the general U.S. population is being urged to increase consumption of carotene-containing fruits and vegetables for cancer risk reduction (6–8), but no special advice has been directed either to current smokers or to ex-smokers, the populations at greatest risk of lung cancer. A recent review of prevention strategies by a Canadian task force, however, concluded that smokers should be given specific dietary advice to lower their lung cancer risk: "Smokers and ex-smokers should be advised to eat foods rich in beta carotene (e.g., carrots) once daily on average" (73). U.S. smokers have been advised to consume more vitamin C than nonsmokers (100 mg vs. 60 mg) in the most recent release of the Recommended Daily Allowances (74). This recommendation was based on the observation of considerably lower levels of circulating vitamin C in smokers. The diet of smokers appears to be somewhat less healthful than the average American's diet, as indicated by its higher fat content and lower fruit and vegetable content, but differences are relatively small (75–77). The U.S. health objectives for the year 2000 include a goal to double the average frequency of consumption of fruits and vegetables in the coming decade, from 2.5 to 5 servings per day (78). Though this recommendation is partially based on the assumption that such dietary changes may prevent smoking-related diseases, smokers have not been specified as a high-risk target for dietary intervention.

We do not yet know whether current heavy cigarette smokers may benefit from increases in dietary intake of vitamin A or carotene, or whether the beneficial effect might be limited to ex-smokers. Nonetheless, the best evidence now available suggests that if we were to advise current smokers and ex-smokers to substantially increase their consumption of fruits and vegetables rich in carotene, their risk of lung cancer would be reduced. We lack the data to specify an explicit amount of carotene-containing food that smokers should consume because the dose-response relationships have not been well quantified. However, the amount of carotene that divides the upper and lower categories of intake is often very small (see Table 1). For instance, in one study the difference between the extreme quartiles was estimated to be only about one carrot per day (39). Therefore, the dietary modification necessary to reduce risk may not require a major dietary change. Advice to take carotene (or any other micronutrient supplements) in pill form may well be premature at this time, however, because substances other than carotene in fruits and vegetables may be the true protective factors. Even if carotene is really responsible for the reduced risk observed in these studies, we have no guarantee that beta-carotene alone will reduce risk, as compared with any of the hundreds of other compounds found naturally in whole foods.

We cannot give smokers dietary advice intended to reduce their lung cancer risk without carefully considering the possibility that such advice could do more harm than good. Even if increasing dietary fruits and vegetables could reduce lung cancer risk by as much as one half for smokers in the lowest quartile of consumption, those who continue to smoke cigarettes will still have more than 10 times the lung cancer risk of nonsmokers. If smokers perceive that they are substantially neutralizing the harmful effects of cigarettes by making a dietary change, then this may reduce their propensity to quit smoking. On the other hand, the process of quitting smoking may be aided by the concurrent attention to dietary change. The question of the relationship between dietary change and smoking cessation deserves careful health-behavioral research as soon as possible.

Current smokers and ex-smokers should substantially increase their intake of fruits and vegetables. The U.S. health objectives for the year 2000 calling for all Americans to eat five servings of fruits and vegetables per day (78) would be a particularly important target for smokers, as would be the advice given to Canadian smokers to eat a carotene-rich food at least once a day (73). It is imperative, however, that we present such recommendations in a way that does not interfere with the more important recommendation to stop smoking.

References

1. American Cancer Society. (1991). *Cancer Facts and Figures—1991*. Atlanta, GA, American Cancer Society.
2. Ziegler, R. (1989). A review of epidemiologic evidence that carotenoids reduce the risk of cancer. *J. Nutr.* 119:116–122.
3. Willett, W. (1990). Vitamin A and lung cancer. *Nutr. Rev.* 48(5):201–211.
4. Morrison, B., and Woolf, S. (1989). In *Lung Cancer, in Preventing Disease, Beyond the Rhetoric*. Edited by R. B. Goldbloom and R. S. Lawrence. New York, Springer-Verlag.
5. Miller, A. B., and Risch, H. A. (1989). Diet and lung cancer. *Chest* 96 (Suppl.):8–9.
6. Committee on Diet, Nutrition, and Cancer, Assembly of Life Sciences, National Research Council. (1982). *Diet, Nutrition, and Cancer*. Washington, DC, National Academy Press.
7. National Cancer Institute. (1986). *Diet, Nutrition, and Cancer Prevention: the Good News*. NIH publication no. 87-2878. Washington, D.C., U.S. Government Printing Office.
8. American Cancer Society. (1984). Nutrition and cancer: Cause and prevention, American Cancer Society special report. *CA* 34:5–10.
9. Kroes, R., Beems, M., Bosland, G. S., Bunnik, S. J., and Sinkeldam, E. J. (1986). Nutritional factors in lung, colon, and prostate carcinogenesis in animal models. *Fed. Proc.* 45:136–141.
10. Wynder, E. L., Hebert, J. R., and Kabat, G. C. (1987). Association of dietary fat and lung cancer. *J. Natl. Cancer. Inst.* 79:631–637.
11. Dorgan, J. F., and Schatzkin, A. (1991). Antioxidant micronutrients in cancer prevention. *Nutr. Cancer* 5:1.
12. Wolbach, S. B., and Howe, P. R. (1925). Tissue changes following deprivation of fat-soluble vitamin A. *J. Exp. Med.* 42:753–777.
13. Sporn, M. B., and Roberts, A. B. (1984). Role of retinoids in differentiation and carcinogenesis. *J. Natl. Cancer Inst.* 73:1381–1386.
14. Underwood, B. (1974). The determinants of vitamin A and some aspects of its

distribution, mobilization, and transport in health and disease. *World Rev. Nutr. Diet.* 19:123–172.

15. Willett, W. C., Stampfer, M. J., Underwood, B. A., et al. (1983). Validation of a dietary questionnaire with plasma carotenoid and alpha tocopherol levels. *Am. J. Clin. Nutr.* 38:631–639.
16. Peto, R., Doll, R., Buckley, J. D., and Sporn, M. B. (1981). Can dietary beta-carotene materially reduce human cancer rates? *Nature* 290:201–208.
17. Moon, T. E., and Micozzi (eds.). (1989). *Nutrition and Cancer Prevention, Investigating the Role of Micronutrients*. New York, Marcel Dekker, Inc.
18. Moon, R. (1989). Comparative aspects of carotenoids and retinoids as chemopreventative agents for cancer. *J. Nutr.* 119:127–134.
19. Birt, D. F., and Pour, P. M. (1985). Effects of the interaction of dietary fat and protein on N-nitrosobis (2-oxopropyl) amine-induced carcinogenesis and spontaneous lesion in Syrian golden hamsters. *J. Natl. Cancer Inst.* 74:1121–1127.
20. Byers, T., Haughey, P., Marshall, J., et al. (1988). Diet and lung cancer risk: Findings from the western New York diet study (letter). *Am. J. Epidemiol.* 127:417.
21. Henson, D., Block, G., and Levine, M. (1991). Ascorbic acid: Biologic functions and relation to cancer. *J. Natl. Cancer Inst.* 83:547–550.
22. Bjorneboe, A., Bjorneboe, G. E., and Drevon, C. A. (1990). Absorption, transport, and distribution of vitamin E. *Am. J. Clin. Nutr.* 120:233–242.
23. Greenland, S., and Morgonstern, H. (1987). Ecological bias, confounding, and effect modification. *Int. J. Epidemiol.* 18:269–274.
24. Willett, W. (1990). Reproducibility and validity of food frequency questionnaires. In *Nutritional Epidemiology*, Chapter 6. New York, Oxford University Press.
25. Cullen, J. (1988). The National Cancer Institute's intervention trials. *Cancer* 62: 1851–1864.
26. Byers, T. (1988). Diet and cancer: Any progress in the interim? *Cancer* 62(Suppl.): 41–52.
27. MacLennan, R., DaCosta, J., Day, N. E., et al. (1977). Risk factors for lung cancer in Singapore Chinese, a population with high female incidence rates. *Int. J. Cancer* 20: 854–860.
28. Hirayama, T. (1979). Diet and cancer. *Nutr. Cancer* 1:67–81.
29. Colditz, G. A., Branch, L. G., Lipnick, R. J., et al. (1985). Increased green and yellow vegetable intake and lowered cancer deaths in an elderly population. *Am. J. Clin. Nutr.* 41:32–36.
30. Forman, M. R., Yao, S. X., Graubard, B. I., et al. (1991). The effect of dietary intake of fruits and vegetables on the odds ratio of lung cancer among Yunnan tin miners (abstract). Presented at 24th Annual Meeting of the Society for Epidemiologic Research, Buffalo, NY, June 1991.
31. Pisani, P., Berrino, F., Macaluso, M., et al. (1986). Carrots, green vegetables and lung cancer: A case-control study. *Int. J. Epidemiol.* 15:4.
32. Fraser, G. E., Beeson, W. L., and Phillips, R. L. (1991). Diet and lung cancer in California Seventh-Day Adventists. *Am. J. Epidemiol.* 133:7.
33. Long-de, W., and Hammond, E. C. (1985). Lung cancer, fruit, green salad and vitamin pills. *Chin. Med. J.* 98:206–210.
34. Steinmetz, K. A., Potter, J. D., and Folsom, A. R. (1991). Lung cancer, vegetables

and fruit: The Iowa Women's Health Study (abstract). Presented at the 24th Annual Meeting of the Society for Epidemiologic Research, Buffalo, New York, June 1991.

35. Bjelke, E. (1975). Dietary vitamin A and human lung cancer. *Int. J. Cancer* 15: 561–565.
36. Mettlin, C., Graham, S., and Swanson, M. (1979). Vitamin A and lung cancer. *J. Natl. Cancer Inst.* 62:1435–1438.
37. Gregor, A., Lee, P. N., Roe, F. J. C., et al. (1980). Comparison of dietary histories in lung cancer cases and controls with special reference to vitamin A. *Nutr. Cancer* 2: 93–97.
38. Kvale, G., Bjelke, E., and Gart, J. J. (1983). Dietary habits and lung cancer risk. *Int. J. Cancer* 31:297–405.
39. Pastorino, U. Pisani, P., Berrino, F., et al. (1987). Vitamin A and female lung cancer: A case-control study on plasma and diet. *Nutr. Cancer* 10:171–179.
40. Shekelle, R. B., Raynor, W. J., Jr., Lepper, M., et al. (1982). Dietary vitamin A and risk of cancer in the Western Electric study. *Lancet* 2:1185–1190.
41. Hinds, M. W., Kolonel, L. N., Hankin, J. H. (1984). Dietary vitamin A, carotene, vitamin C and risk of lung cancer in Hawaii. *Am. J. Epidemiol.* 119:227–237.
42. Ziegler, R. G., Mason, T. J., Stemhagen, A., et al. (1984). Dietary carotene and vitamin A and risk of lung cancer among white men in New Jersey. *J. Natl. Cancer Inst.* 73:1429–1434.
43. Samet, J. M., Skipper, B. J., Humble, C. G., and Pathak, D. R. (1985). Lung cancer risk and vitamin A consumption in New Mexico. *Am. Rev. Respir. Dis.* 131:198–202.
44. Wu, A. H., Henderson, B. E., Pike, M. C., and Yu, M. C. (1985). Smoking and other risk factors for lung cancer in women. *J. Natl. Cancer Inst.* 74:747–751.
45. Byers, T. E., Graham, S., Haughey, B. P., Marshall, J. R., and Swanson, M. K. (1987). Diet and lung cancer risk: Findings from the western New York diet study. *Am. J. Epidemiol.* 125:351–363.
46. Kromhout. (1987). Essential micronutrients in relation to carcinogenesis. *Am. J. Clin. Nutr.* 45:1361–1367.
47. Bond, G. G., Thompson, F. E., and Cook, R. R. (1987). Dietary vitamin A and lung cancer: Results of a case-control study among chemical workers. *Nutr. Cancer* 9: 109–121.
48. Fontham, E. T., Pickle, L. W., Haenszel, W., Correa, P., Lin, Y., and Falk, R. T. (1988). Dietary vitamins A and C and lung cancer risk in Louisiana. *Cancer* 62:2267–2273.
49. Paganini-Hill, A., Chao, A., Ross, R. K., et al. (1987). Vitamin A, β-carotene and the risk of cancer: A prospective study. *J. Natl. Cancer Inst.* 79:3.
50. Le Marchand, L. L., Yoshizawa, C. N., Kolonel, L. N., et al. (1989). Vegetable consumption and lung cancer risk: A population-based case-control study in Hawaii. *J. Natl. Cancer Inst.* 81:1158–1164.
51. Mettlin, C. (1989). Milk drinking, other beverage habits, and lung cancer risks. *Int. J. Cancer* 43:608–612.
52. Jain, M., Barch, J. D., Howe, G. R., et al. (1990). Dietary factors and risk of lung cancer: Results from a case-control study, Toronto, 1981-85. *Int. J. Cancer* 45: 287–293.

53. Dartigues, J. F., Dabis, F., Gros, N., et al. (1990). Dietary vitamin A, beta carotene and risk of epidermoid lung cancer in south-western France. *Eur. J. Epidemiol.* 9: 261–265.
54. Byers, T., Vena, J., Mettlin, C., Swanson, M., and Graham, S. (1984). Dietary vitamin A and lung cancer risk: An analysis by histologic subtypes. *Am. J. Epidemiol.* 120:769–776.
55. Taylor, P. R., Dawsey, S. S., and Albanes, D. (1990). Cancer prevention trials in China and Finland. *Ann. Epidemiol.* 1:195–203.
56. Hinds, M. W., Kolonel, L. N., Lee, J., and Hankin, J. H. (1983). Dietary cholesterol and lung cancer risk among men in Hawaii. *Am. J. Clin. Nutr.* 37:192–193.
57. Stahelin, H. B., Gey, F. K., Eichholzer, M., et al. (1991). Plasma antioxidant vitamins and subsequent cancer mortality in the 12-year follow-up of the prospective Basel study. *Am. J. Epidemiol.* 133:8.
58. Nomura, A. M., Stemmermann, G. N., Heilbrun, L. K., et al. (1985). Serum vitamin levels and the risk of cancer of specific sites in men of Japanese ancestry in Hawaii. *Cancer Res.* 45:2369–2372.
59. Menkes, M. S., Comstock, G. W., Vuilleumier, J. P., Helsing, K. J., Rider, A. A., and Brookmeyer, R. (1986). Serum beta-carotene, vitamins A and E, selenium, and the risk of lung cancer. *N. Engl. J. Med.* 315:1250–1254.
60. Wald, N., Thompson, S., Densem, J., Boreham, J., Bailey, A. (1988). Serum beta-carotene and subsequent risk of cancer: Results from the BUPA study. *Br. J. Cancer* 57:428–433.
61. Wald, N., Boreham, J., and Baily, A. (1986). Serum retinol and subsequent risk of cancer. *Br. J. Cancer* 54:957–961.
62. Friedman, G., Bloner, W., Volgelman, J., et al. (1986). Serum retinol and retinol-finding proteins levels do most predict subsequent lung cancer. *Am. J. Epidemiol.* 123: 781–789.
63. Connett, J. E., Kuller, L. H., Kjelsberg, M. O., et al. (1989). Relationship between carotenoids and cancer. *Cancer* 64:126–134.
64. Knekt, P., Aromaa, A., Maatela, J., et al. (1988). Serum vitamin E and risk of cancer among Finnish men during a 10-year follow-up. *Am. J. Epidemiol.* 127:1.
65. Russell-Briefel, R. M., Bates, M. W., and Kuller, L. H. (1985). The relationship of plasma carotenoids to health and biochemical factors in middle-aged men. *Am. J. Epidemiol.* 122:741–749.
66. Aoki, K., Ito, Y., Sasaki, M., et al. Smoking, alcohol drinking, and serum carotenoid levels. *Jpn. J. Cancer Res.* 78:1049–1056.
67. Comstock, G., Menkes, M., Schober, S., Vuilleumier, J., and Helsing, K. (1988). Serum levels of retinol, beta-carotene, and alpha-tocopherol in older adults. *Am. J. Epidemiol.* 127:114–123.
68. Riodt, L., White, E., Goodman, G., et al. (1988). Association of food frequency questionnaire estimates of vitamin A intake with serum vitamin levels. *Am. J. Epidemiol.* 128:645–654.
69. Nierenberg, D. W., Stukel, T., Baron, J., Dain, B., and Greenberg, E. (1989). Determinants of plasma levels of beta-carotene and retinol. Skin cancer prevention study group. *Am. J. Epidemiol.* 130:511–521.

70. Palan, P. R., Romney, S. Vermund, S., Mikhail, M., and Basu, J. (1989). Effects of smoking and oral contraception on plasma beta-carotene levels in healthy women. *Am. J. Obstet. Gynecol.* 161:881–885.
71. Shibata, A., Saskai, R., Ito, Y., et al. (1989). Serum concentration of beta-carotene and intake frequency of green-yellow vegetables among healthy inhabitants of Japan. *Int. J. Cancer* 44:48–52.
72. Nierenberg, D. W., Stakel, T. A., Baron, J. A., et al. (1991). Determinants of increase in plasma concentration of β-carotene after chronic oral supplementation. *Am. J. Clin. Nutr.* 53:1443–1449.
73. Canadian Task Force on the Periodic Health Examination. (1990). Periodic health examination, 1990 update: 3. Interventions to prevent lung cancer other than smoking cessation. *Cancer Med. Assoc. J.* 143:269–271.
74. Food and Nutrition Board. (1989). *Recommended Daily Allowances*, 10th Edition. Washington, DC, National Academy Press.
75. Subar, A. F., Harlan, L. C., and Mattson, M. E. (1990). Food and nutrient intake differences between smokers and non-smokers in the U.S. *Am. J. Public Health* 80: 1323–1329.
76. Morabia, A., and Wynder, E. L. (1990). Dietary habits of smokers, people who never smoked, and exsmokers. *Am. J. Clin. Nutr.* 52:933–937.
77. Smith, A. H., and Waller, K. D. (1990). Serum beta-carotene in persons with cancer and their immediate families. *Am. J. Epidemiol.* 133:661–671.
78. Public Health Service. (1991). *Health People 2000: National Health Promotion and Disease Prevention Objective*. Full Report, with commentary. DHHS Publication no. (PHS) 91-50212. Washington, DC, U.S. Department of Health and Human Services, Public Health Service.

14

Familial and Genetic Factors in the Pathogenesis of Lung Cancer

PETER ECONOMOU

University of New Mexico School
of Medicine
Albuquerque, New Mexico

JOHN F. LECHNER

Inhalation Toxicology Research Institute
Albuquerque, New Mexico

JONATHAN M. SAMET

University of New Mexico School
of Medicine
and the New Mexico Tumor Registry
Albuquerque, New Mexico

I. Introduction

Lung cancer, the major cause of cancer-related deaths in the United States, is often cited as a disorder that is solely environmentally induced. However, it is now becoming increasingly evident that lung cancer has a genetic basis in addition to the well-known contribution of environmental factors. A variety of research approaches including genetic epidemiology, metabolic phenotyping, cytogenetic analysis, and examination of oncogene and autocrine growth factor expression all support the conclusion that lung cancer is a genetic disease. The series of events that occur during the transformation of normal lung epithelial cells to malignant cells and the subsequent development of lung cancer in a susceptible individual is incompletely understood. The purpose of this chapter is to review the current state of knowledge of the familial and genetic factors involved in the pathogenesis of lung cancer.

Since Watkins' first description of familial inheritance of cancer (1), a number of family cancer syndromes and clusters have been reported. In each of these, host susceptibility to cancer is inherited. This genetic predisposition can be the result of individual differences in metabolism, DNA repair, genetic instability, or, alternatively, altered oncogene expression (2). Examples of the latter include the Li-Fraumeni syndrome, in which germline transmission of a mutated p53 gene predisposes individuals to tumors at multiple sites (3,4), or familial retinoblastoma (Rb), in which loss of the retinoblastoma gene, a tumor suppressor gene, predisposes carriers to ocular and other malignancies (5,6).

It has been well established that smoking and other environmental exposures are linked to the development of lung cancer (7). However, not all smokers and others exposed to potent lung carcinogens develop lung cancer. Therefore, investigators have long hypothesized that individuals differ in their susceptibility to these environmental exposures. This premise, however, has been difficult to test definitively because indicators of genetic predisposition have not been available. Conventional epidemiological methods may not be sensitive for detecting familial aggregation. Using genetic modeling, Peto showed that a cancer may have a major genetic component yet show little evidence of familial clustering, unless a specific marker is present (8). This methodologic problem can be explained by three factors: (1) not all cancer patients are susceptible; (2) even fewer of their relatives are susceptible; and (3) the general population contains both susceptibles and nonsusceptibles. Thus, familial clustering or the ratio of the incidence of the cancer in relatives of known cases to that in age-matched controls will be substantially "diluted." Furthermore, using Peto's genetic model of a common recessive cancer gene, which increases the risk of cancer 50- to 100-fold with a gene frequency of 0.01–0.10, the relative risk of developing cancer in children and siblings of probands would be between 1.0 and 8.0.

II. Genetic Epidemiology

Several epidemiologic studies have examined lung cancer aggregation in family members of lung cancer patients and found evidence of family susceptibility to development of this malignancy (Table 1). The studies have all been case-control in design, with various methods used to verify diagnoses. Most controlled for cigarette smoking, which does aggregate in families.

Tokuhata and Lilienfeld used a case-control approach to assess familial aggregation of lung cancer in two separate studies (9,10). In the first study, conducted at Roswell Park Memorial Institute, an approximate doubling of lung cancer mortality was found in the relatives of cases, but cigarette smoking was not considered in the analysis. In the second study, conducted in Baltimore and using neighborhood controls, a significant excess of lung cancer mortality was found in both nonsmoking (fourfold) and smoking (twofold) relatives. Ooi et al. examined 336 families of deceased lung cancer probands in Louisiana (11). Using the probands' spouses as controls and controlling for confounding variables, including cigarette smoking, Ooi and coworkers found a 2.4-fold greater risk of lung cancer among the probands' relatives. Lynch et al. studied 254 lung cancer probands and

231 probands with other smoking-related cancers (12). This study showed a significant ($p < 0.001$) increased risk for cancers of all anatomic sites, but not for lung cancer when considered separately, among the relatives of lung cancer probands. This increased risk was not evident for relatives of probands with other smoking-associated cancers. Samet et al. showed that personal lung cancer risk was significantly increased ($p < 0.001$ odds ratio (OR) = 5.3, 95% confidence interval 2.2–12.8) if at least one parent had lung cancer (13). Shaw et al. found a modest increase in lung cancer risk associated with reported cancer in first-degree relatives (14). This risk was greatest for those subjects with first-degree relatives with lung cancer (OR = 2.8) followed by first-degree relatives with other tobacco-related cancers (OR = 1.5). Sellers et al. reported an increased familial risk for nonlung cancer among relatives of lung cancer patients (OR = 2.16, $p < 0.05$) (15). In a subsequent study applying segregation analyses to these data, the results indicated compatibility of the data with Mendelian codominant inheritance of a rare major autosomal gene that produces earlier age of onset of the cancer (16). Several studies have examined female probands only. Horwitz et al. performed a case-control study on female lung cancer probands to assess the possible role of family history and its interrelationship with cigarette smoking (17). An ecogenetic relationship of cigarette smoking and family history was supported by a gradient in the odds ratio created by the two variables: patients who never smoked but had a positive family history had an odds ratio of 5.7; patients who smoked but had a negative family history had an odds ratio of 15.1; patients who smoked and had a positive family history had an odds ratio of almost 30. Osann confirmed these results in a subsequent study (18).

Also of interest is a recent study by Sanders et al., who examined nonocular cancer incidence in relatives of retinoblastoma patients (19). Sanders and co-workers found that relatives who are carriers of the mutated Rb gene are about 15 times more likely to die from lung cancer, particularly small-cell lung cancer, in comparison with the general population. Another study also observed a significant excess of lung cancer in relatives of retinoblastoma patients under age 55 (20). These studies support the premise that inactivation of the Rb gene may be important in the development of lung cancer, as will be discussed later.

Studies of selected families have also indicated familial aggregation (21–24). Goffman et al. reported two families with familial respiratory tract cancer; in one of the families there was an associated syndrome of limb and dental anomalies (25). Two members of the family were also carriers of a balanced translocation between chromosomes 13 and 14. Paul et al. reported a family with three siblings who developed alveolar carcinoma (26). Interestingly, all three affected patients expressed HLA-A28, while an uninfected sibling did not. Finally, Joisy et al. described alveolar cell carcinoma in identical male twins with similar age of onset, histopathologic features, and site of metastasis (27).

Other relevant evidence for a genetic basis for lung cancer includes the

Table 1 Case-Control Studies of Familial Risk of Lung Cancer

Location	Odds ratio for familial history	Comments	Ref.
Nine major hospitals in Baltimore, Maryland	2.6	Limited to white population Neighborhood controls Death certificates reviewed for diagnoses Index subjects and immediate family interviewed directly by mail or telephone Control for smoking status	9
Roswell Park Memorial Institute, Buffalo, NY	2.5	Limited to white population Noncancer hospital controls Questionnaires mailed to subjects and immediate families Death certificates reviewed (92%) Smoking status not controlled	10
Oncology clinics at 2 Omaha, Nebraska, medical schools	No significant increase	Controls were relatives of other probands of smoking-related cancers Family history obtained by interview, questionnaire and death certificate review Control for smoking status	12
Death records of Louisiana Office of Public Health Statistics	2.4 4.4 (parental)	Controls were probands' spouses and first-degree relatives Limited to white population History obtained by interview (direct and telephone and questionnaire Reliability of interview data confirmed by a death certificate review and further family interview of a 20% random sample Control for smoking status and occupational exposure	11
Records of New Mexico Tumor Registry	5.3 (parental)	Limited to white population Controls chosen from random telephone lists and Medicare recipients Cases or surrogates were interviewed in person or by telephone Smoking status controlled	13
Yale-New Haven (Connecticut) Tumor Registry	2.8	Limited to females Controls were hospital patients admitted to medical and surgical services of Yale-New Haven (cancer and noncancer) History obtained from record review Smoking status controlled	17

Table 1 Continued

Location	Odds ratio for familial history	Comments	Ref.
Saskatchewan Cancer Foundation, Canada	1.96	Community controls History obtained by direct interview, mailed questionnaire and Provincial Tumor Registry review Smoking status and occupational exposure controlled	
State health department records and hospitals in the Texas Gulf Coast region	1.8	Limited to white population Random controls chosen from drivers' license files, Medicare recipients and State health department mortality tapes History obtained from direct interview and record review Smoking status and occupational exposure controlled	14
Northern California Kaiser hospitals and California Tumor Registry	1.4	Limited to females All cases had completed self-administered questionnaire concerning history prior to diagnosis Controls were chosen from Kaiser screening program Smoking status controlled	18

observation that patients apparently cured of lung cancer have an elevated risk of developing another lung cancer (28–30) or cancer at a different site (31–33). Admittedly this risk may be related to cigarette smoking or another environmental exposure; genetic predisposition may also contribute. The finding of similar chromosomal abnormalities in the first and second malignancies also suggests genetic predisposition. In this regard, two patients with an apparent complete remission of small-cell lung cancer developed erythroleukemias, which exhibited the 3p14-23 deletion, which is commonly seen in small-cell carcinoma and is uncommon in erythroleukemias arising after other malignancies (34). Unfortunately, cytogenetic analysis was not performed on the primary lung tumors.

The association between human ABO blood groups and the risk of developing lung cancer has been investigated in several studies (35–42). The majority of the studies did not show any difference in the distribution of ABO blood groups in lung cancer patients compared with the general population. However, Lee et al. recently examined 253 patients with non–small-cell lung cancer undergoing surgical resection (43). They found that patients with blood type A or AB who had primary tumors negative for blood group antigen A had a significantly shorter survival than that of patients with antigen A–positive tumors ($p < 0.001$) and of patients with blood type B or O ($p = 0.002$). They interpreted these results by suggesting that loss of expression of blood group antigen A in non–small-cell tumors is a possible marker for the multistage process of tumor regression in patients with type A or AB blood.

Associations between HLA antigens and lung cancer has also been investigated. Tongio et al. showed an increase in B12 antigen in patients with bronchial carcinoma (44). Markan et al. found this same allele significantly overrepresented in a study population of 50 white patients with small-cell carcinoma of the lung (45). Other studies, however, have failed to show this association (46–48). A number of studies have also shown differences in survival in subgroups of patients possessing the HLA-A1, HLA Aw19, and/or HLA B5 phenotype (45,49–51).

In summary, although associations between lung cancer, blood types, and HLA antigens have been observed, many of the statistical associations have been weak, and conflicting data have emerged. Much of this disparity can be explained by the observation that when multiple comparisons are made without a prior hypothesis, some associations will be statistically significant by chance alone (52). However, some of the associations could exist, but further and larger confirmatory studies are needed to validate their biological significance.

III. Metabolic Phenotypes

Although 90% of the lung cancer cases in the United States can be attributed to cigarette smoking, only approximately 10% of smokers develop a bronchial malignancy (7). This observation implies that host factors or other environmental agents also influence individual susceptibility to tobacco smoke. One such host factor is the pleiotropic genes of the cytochrome P-450 system that control the oxidative metabolism of some environmental carcinogens.

There are two phases to the metabolism of a compound (Fig. 1) (53). In phase I, which is mediated by cytochrome P-450 monooxygenases, a reactive intermediate is formed. This intermediate is then conjugated with an endogenous compound in phase II to become water soluble and thus readily excreted. Numerous products in tobacco smoke, including polycyclic aromatic hydrocarbons and nitrosamines, are inducers of the P-450 enzymes, but specific carcinogens are less well defined. Occasionally, phase I intermediate compounds covalently bind to nucleic acids and proteins and form carcinogen-DNA adducts, which may initiate carcinogenesis. In support of this supposition, Phillips et al., using the ^{32}P-postlabeling technique, have shown that cigarette smokers have higher adduct levels than nonsmokers and that there is a linear relationship between adduct levels and cigarette consumption (54).

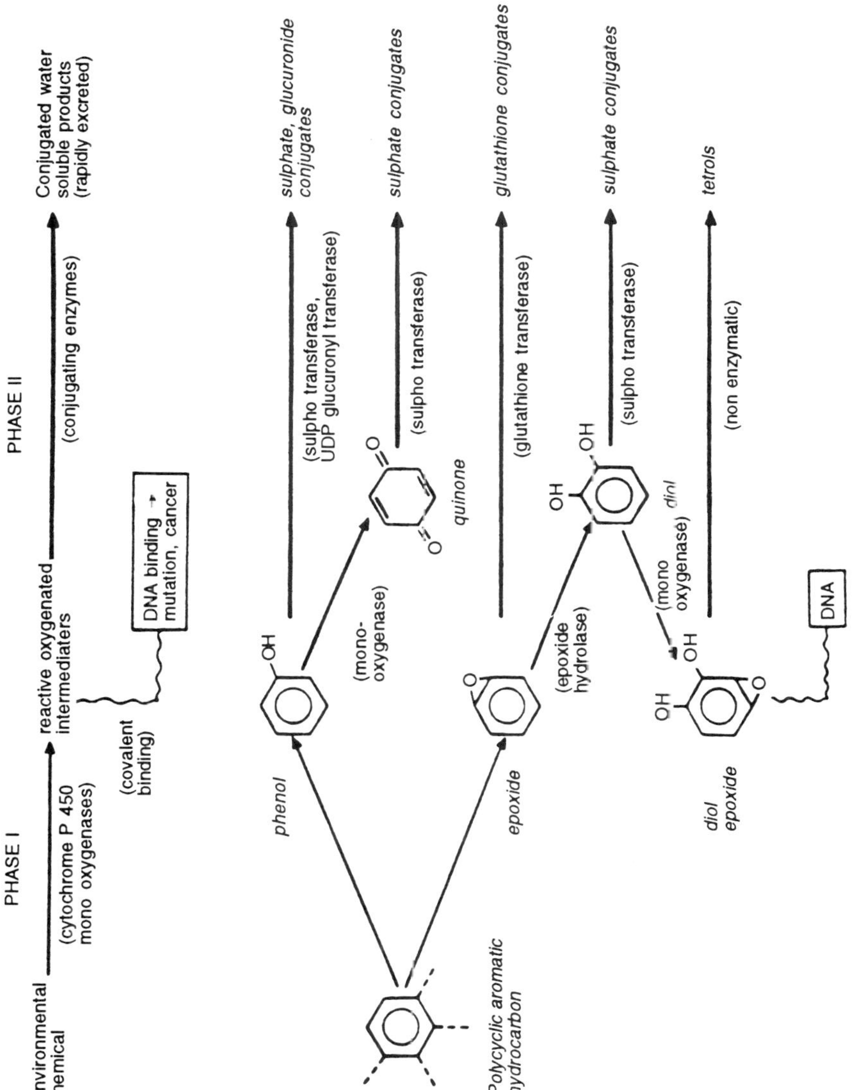

Figure 1 Metabolism of foreign chemicals, specifically polycyclic aromatic hydrocarbons. (From Ref. 53.)

It has been hypothesized that genetic factors must contribute to lung cancer risk because it is the metabolites of carcinogens (not the carcinogens themselves) that usually initiate a cancer, and the activation of these metabolic pathways is genetically determined (55,56). This assumption, however, oversimplifies a complex phenomenon in which the metabolism of many compounds involves the action of a number of enzymes, each with different environmental and genetic determinants of activity. Furthermore, the effect of one gene may dominate the other determinants and so produce a large variation of the entire metabolic pathway.

Early studies of metabolic markers focused on aryl hydrocarbon hydroxylase (AHH), an inducible mixed-function oxidase. AHH catalyzes the first step in the metabolism of benzopyrene and other polycyclic aromatic hydrocarbons, the metabolites of which are known to cause DNA mutations and malignant transformation of cells (57–59). The regulatory locus of AHH is believed to be on chromosome 2 (60,61), although other P-450 subfamilies that also contribute to its activity have been assigned to other chromosomes (62). Most studies have observed a unimodal distribution of AHH activity consistent with polygenic control (63,64), but the findings of some investigations have been divergent (65,66).

AHH is found in most human tissues. Most human studies, however, have for convenience measured activity in peripheral lymphocytes rather than lung tissue (67). McLemore et al. (67) compared AHH activity in lymphocytes and in lung tissue. Correlation between activity at these two sites was high ($r = 0.98$) in normal subjects but poor ($r = 0.62$) in subjects with lung cancer. Kellerman et al., measuring lymphocyte AHH activity, first reported that high and intermediate metabolizers had 36 and 16 times, respectively, the lung cancer risk of low metabolizers (68). Numerous subsequent studies have shown conflicting results (69–72). Most studies of AHH activity in human lung tissue have either been negative or inadequately controlled for a number of relevant factors including other concurrent medications, the status and amount of cigarette smoking, the metabolic effects of the malignancy, and changes in diet and activity (67,73–75).

More recently, debrisoquine metabolism has been examined as a model of phase I monooxygenation. Debrisoquine has only one metabolite, 4-hydroxydebrisoquine (76); its metabolism correlates with that of many other drugs and chemicals, some of which may be carcinogens in tobacco smoke (77). Debrisoquine hydroxylation appears to be under Mendelian autosomal genetic control (78). The gene (CYP 2D6), located on chromosome 22, has been cloned (79,80). There appear to be two phenotypes in humans: the poor metabolizer phenotype, which is an autosomal recessive trait, and the extensive metabolizer, which is either heterozygous or homozygous dominant (78). The metabolic ratio (i.e., either poor or extensive) can easily be determined by measuring 4-hydroxydebrisoquine concentration in urine after an oral dose (81). The description of phenotypes by this test provides a good reflection of the distribution of genotypes in the population. In addition, a method for genotyping poor metabolizers of debrisoquine using specific polymerase chain reaction (PCR) amplification of mutants and wild-type alleles is now available (82). Finally, assessment of debrisoquine hydroxylation does not appear to have many of the biases potentially affecting the AHH model (78,83).

Several recent studies have measured debrisoquine metabolism in lung cancer cases and controls (Table 2). Most of these studies have confirmed a higher risk of lung cancer in extensive metabolizers (odds ratio range 0.61–6.1) (42,83–86). Caporaso et al. noted that this risk applies particularly to squamous cell and small-cell subtypes but, interestingly, not to adenocarcinoma (the subtype least associated with cigarette smoking) (85). In addition, they found a synergistic risk between the ability to extensively metabolize debrisoquine and occupational exposure to lung carcinogens (relative risk = 18). One recent study comparing lung cancer patients and controls showed no difference in the degree of metabolization although historical controls were used (87). Finally, Sugimura et al. investigated human debrisoquine hydroxylase gene polymorphisms in lung cancer patients and controls (88). They found that no single mutant CYP2D6 allele as determined by EcoRI appears to be associated with lung cancer risk.

Crespi et al. have recently shown that p4502D6 activates 4-(methylnitrosamino)-1-(3 pyridyl)-1-butanone (NNK), a tobacco smoke–specific nitrosamine and potent carcinogen in animal studies (89). These data do not, however, establish that NNK activation by p4502D6 is solely responsible for the increased lung cancer risk. In fact, other cytochrome p-450–dependent monooxygenases (CYP1A2, CYP2A3, and CYP2E1) activate NNK. An alternative possibility for the association of debrisoquine metabolism and lung cancer is that the gene regulating debrisoquine hydroxylation is in linkage disequilibrium with a different gene (i.e., an oncogene) that does influence susceptibility.

Kawajiri et al. reported the association of lung cancer with DNA polymorphisms of a second gene, P450IAI, which is responsible for the metabolic activation of benzopyrene and other presumed carcinogens in cigarette smoke (90). In a further study, Nakachi et al. found that individuals with a "susceptible genotype" had an increased lung cancer risk with an odds ratio of 7.31 at low smoking levels and that the difference in susceptibility between genotypes decreased at high levels (91). This gradient in the odds ratio was postulated to indicate a dose-response relationship of the enzymatic reaction causing metabolic activity saturation.

Phase II conjugation activity is also believed to influence cancer risk. Roots et al. showed, however, that acetylation was not associated with lung cancer risk (42). In addition, Oesch et al. did not find a significant difference in monooxygenase, epoxide hydrolase, and glutathione-S-transferase activities in lung cancer patients and controls (74). On the other hand, Seidegard et al. found that lung cancer patients underexpressed glutathione transferase in peripheral monocytes compared with controls ($p < 0.01$) (92). In a later study they showed that the

Table 2 Comparison of Extensive Versus Poor Debrisoquine Metabolic Phenotypes in Lung Cancer Cases and Controls

Location	Odds ratio	Comments	Ref.
Hospitals in London, England	Not given	Limited to white population Controls were patients with COPD Smoking controlled Patients excluded if confounding variables present No occupational exposure history given	84
Cases of German extraction	0.61	Controls were noncancer hospital patients Smoking controlled Patients excluded if confounding variables present	42
Outpatient chest clinics in London, England	4.0	All patients of northern European extraction Controls were patients with asthma and COPD Smoking status controlled Occupational exposure controlled Patients excluded if confounding variables present	85
Hospital in London, England	4.8	Limited to white population Controls were veterans, noncancer hospital inpatients and hospital employees Smoking status controlled Patients excluded if possible confounding variables present	83
Hospitals in Baltimore, Maryland	6.1	Both white and black population represented Controls were patients with COPD and noncancer malignancies Smoking status controlled Occupational exposure controlled Patients excluded if possible confounding variables present	86
Hospitals in London, England	Not given	Historical controls used Patients excluded if potential confounding variables present Smoking status recorded Occupational exposure not recorded	87

class Mu isoenzyme of glutathione transferase was underexpressed in lung cancer patients (36.6%) versus controls (58.3%) ($p < 0.0001$) and concluded that the gene controlling expression of this isoenzyme may be a host determinant of genetic susceptibility to lung cancer among smokers (93). These findings, however, have not been confirmed.

IV. Multistep Carcinogenesis

The foundations of our current knowledge of carcinogenesis processes derive from experimental animal models. These studies have led to the understanding of carcinogenesis as a multistep process driven by carcinogen-induced genetic and epigenetic damage in suspicious cells (94,95). Traditionally, this process is considered to proceed through three stages referred to as initiation, promotion, and progression (Fig. 2). The first stage, initiation, is the exposure of a normal cell to an agent that causes a genetic change resulting in the cell having an altered responsiveness to its microenvironment. As a consequence, the cell is no longer subject to normal (growth and/or programmed cell death) regulation controls. Tumor promotion results from the initiated cell dividing chaotically and thereby enhancing the probability of accumulating additional genetic damage. Progression is the culmination of these changes toward the malignant phenotype.

While these stages of carcinogenesis were primarily described as the basis of experimental studies in vivo, they appear compatible with evidence of the pathogenesis of lung cancer. The age-incidence patterns for lung cancer, which show that the rates usually increase as a power of age, are consistent with a multistage process (96–98). There is also pathologic evidence consistent with a multistep process. Saccomanno et al. showed that the bronchial epithelia of sustained smokers show a progression of abnormality from squamous metaplasia to invasive bronchogenic carcinoma (99). In addition, cytogenetic studies show that chromosomal losses in lung cancer increase with the stage of the disease (100). Finally, other, better characterized models of multistep carcinogenesis involving epithelial surfaces such as colorectal tumorigenesis have been developed (101,102), and there is no reason to suspect that respiratory carcinogenesis is a distinct process.

V. Cytogenetics

Cytogenic abnormalities are common in lung cancer. Many of these are probably random events that reflect the chromosomal instability inherent in cancer. Some, however, are nonrandom events which play a direct role in the pathogenesis of lung cancer. Identifying consistent cytogenetic changes in the background of numerous random abnormalities has been the subject of much investigation because such

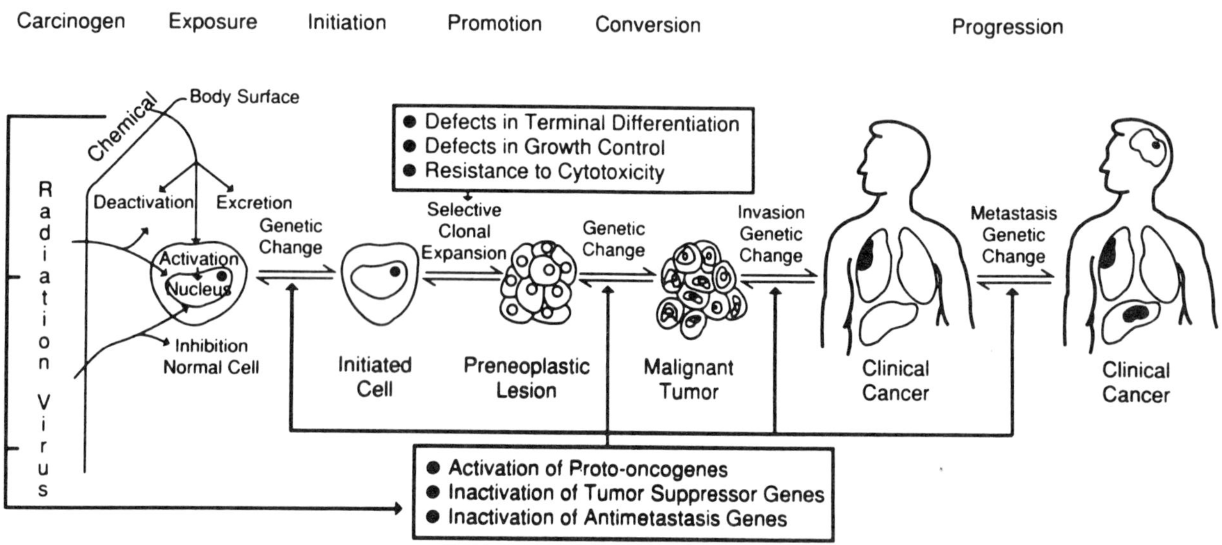

Figure 2 Simplistic model of multistage lung carcinogenesis. (From Ref. 2.)

changes might provide insight into the pathogenesis of lung cancer. Numerous studies have found abnormalities in the chromosome number in lung cancer. DNA analysis has revealed that lung cancer tumor specimens or cell lines can be either hypodiploid, hyperdiploid, or tetraploid (103–107). Some of these studies have suggested that the degree of hyperploidy or aneuploidy may be associated with tumor progression and hence with prognosis (108–111). The absence of chromosomes 13 and 15, and aberrations of a number of others, including 1, 2, 9, 10, 14, and X, in addition to the presence of double minutes and homogeneously staining regions have also been noted (112).

By far the most common chromosomal abnormality found in lung cancer is a 3p(14-23) deletion (Fig. 3). Whang-Peng et al. examined 16 small-cell lung cancer (SCLC) cell lines and three tumor specimens and found a 3p deletion to be present in all cases, but not in lymphoblastoid cell lines or peripheral lymphocytes (112). This pattern implies that the deletion is somatically acquired. Further analysis revealed a shortest region of overlap corresponding to bands 3p14-23. This result has been confirmed in numerous subsequent studies of SCLC, with the reported prevalence of the abnormality ranging from 21 to 100% (113–121). Other lines of evidence, however, also support this finding. DNA probes that detect restriction fragment length polymorphisms within 3p14-23 have shown loss of heterozygosity (i.e., loss of alleles) in this region in 95% of SCLCs (122–124). In addition, reduced or undetectable activity of aminoacylase-1, an enzyme encoded by 3p23, was found in 10 of 18 SCLC cell lines studied (125). These results are consistent with loss or inactivation of genes in this region.

In their 1982 report, Whang-Peng et al. did not find this deletion in the five non–small-cell lung cancer (NSCLC) cell lines studied (112). Several subsequent studies of SCLS have documented its presence, but found it less common than in SCLC (118,122,126–128). Karyotypic analysis has demonstrated a 3p14-23 deletion in five adenocarcinoma cell lines (118,129) and two primary adenocarcinoma (130) and isolated squamous cell and large cell lines (118). DNA probes have shown loss of 3p alleles in 3 of 10 adenocarcinomas and one of two squamous cell carcinomas (122). Buys et al. found loss of 3p21 alleles in five adenocarcinomas and four squamous cell carcinomas (131). In addition, 3p14-23 deletions are well documented in a variety of neoplasms including renal cell carcinoma (132). Finally, the deletion has been found in a variety of specimens, including primary tumors, pre- and posttreatment specimens, and metastases, supporting the premise that inactivation of one or more genes within this region is a critical, and perhaps early, step in the pathogenesis of lung cancer and other malignancies.

In addition to 3p14-23 deletions, several other nonrandom chromosomal abnormalities have been described. Wurster-Hill et al. found absent or hypodiploid numbers of chromosome 13 in 17 out of 21 SCLC lines in one cytogenetic study (114). Fan and Li found deletions or rearrangements of the short arm of chromosome 1 in four human lung adenocarcinoma cell lines (129). Interestingly,

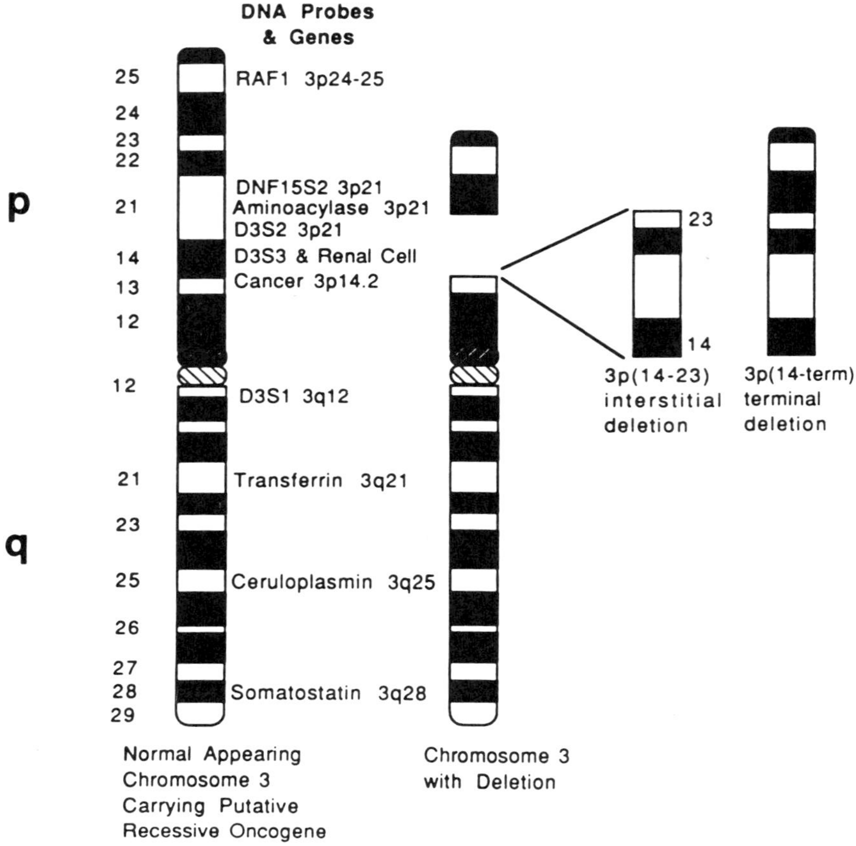

Figure 3 Deletions in chromosome 3 found in lung cancer. (From Ref. 148.)

the breakpoints occurred at 1P12-1p22, coincident with the location of N-*ras*, a cellular oncogene. Yokota et al. demonstrated loss of heterozygosity in chromosomes 3, 13, and 17 in both SCLC and NSCLC (133). Weston et al. found differential DNA sequence deletions from chromosomes 3, 11, 13, and 17 in cases of NSCLC (134). This deletion was especially noted from chromosome 17 in squamous cell carcinoma (8 of 9 cases). Skinner et al. found loss of heterozygosity for genes on 11p in 9 of 39 cases of NSCLC (135).

Other observed chromosomal abnormalities in NSCLC have been observed. Lee et al., using karyotypic analysis, found trisomy 7 in two adenocarcinomas and three squamous cell carcinomas as well as normal lung tissue in four of these cases (136). They hypothesized that trisomy 7 may be an early premalignant finding in

NSCLC. Isochromes (8q and 9q) have also been described in adenocarcinomas of the lung (130,137). Finally, Liang et al. describe trisomy 12 in a primary culture of a human adenosquamous carcinoma of the lung (138). They also found a 10-fold increase in the level of p21, the K-*ras* oncogene protein product. Since K-*ras* is located on chromosome 12, they speculated a causal relationship between trisomy 12 and K-*ras* activation.

Cytogenetic studies also supply the evidence that multiple genetic lesions are involved in the development of lung cancer. They also suggest several possible mechanisms of carcinogenesis. Deletions (especially 3p14-23) could uncover an otherwise recessive mutation residing on the cytogenetically normal chromosome as occur in retinoblastoma and Wilms' tumor. The genes inactivated by these deletions are thought to be tumor suppressor genes, which are thought to inhibit turmorigenesis. On the other hand, translocations could activate dominant proto-oncogenes and thus promote transformation.

Also of interest are studies involving fragile sites, which are unstable portions in the human genome (139,140). Common fragile sites occur in all individuals, but their expressions show great individual differences, which implies some type of genetic influence. Folic acid or thymidine deprivation induces the expression of fragile sites in DNA. There is a very high significant statistical association between human fragile sites and cancer breakpoints (areas where chromosome rearrangements in neoplasia occur) (141) (chi-square test value = 15.8 [$p < 0.001$]). Interestingly, one of the most common fragile sites found in human DNA is 3p14.2. Kao-shan et al. showed that cigarette smokers have an increased number of fragile sites, especially at 3p14.2 in peripheral lymphocytes and bone marrow precursor cells (142). Liu et al. showed a significantly higher expression frequency of common fragile sites, including 3p14, in lung cancer patients and their relatives than in control subjects ($p < 0.01$) (143). Unfortunately, cigarette smoking was not considered. Thus the expression of fragile sites, specifically 3p14, may play an important role in oncogenesis and perhaps in determining genetic susceptibility to lung cancer; obviously, further studies are needed to confirm this preliminary evidence.

VI. Oncogenes

A number of oncogenes have been implicated in the pathogenesis of lung cancer. Oncogenes are functionally or structurally aberrant forms of normal cellular genes termed proto-oncogenes (144–147). Proto-oncogenes participate in normal cell growth and proliferation, especially during fetal development. They encode for a variety of proteins, which function as growth regulators, and are highly conserved across species. Under normal conditions, proto-oncogenes are strictly regulated by other genes, which control their transcription. However, when this regulatory influence becomes impaired, proto-oncogenes become activated or oncogenic and their protein products can stimulate the cell in an uncontrolled fashion. Activation can occur by the increased production of a normal regulatory protein (i.e., amplification that causes an increased number of gene copies or genetic rearrangements that disrupt normal regulatory gene expression) or by the production of an abnormal regulatory protein (through point mutation within the gene or genetic rearrangements within the coding sequence of the gene). These genes are referred to as dominant oncogenes because of their transforming ability and because only one of the maternal or paternal alleles is affected (100,148–151).

Unlike oncogenes, antioncogenes or tumor-suppressor genes function as inhibitors of cell growth and proliferation (152–157). These genes are thought to act as a balance to proto-oncogene function. In contrast to the dominant oncogenes, both the maternal and paternal alleles are affected and hence inactivated. As might be expected, loss of anti-oncogene function may also be oncogenic. Both oncogene and anti-oncogene abnormalities have been observed in lung cancer and are therefore thought to play a fundamental role in lung carcinogenesis.

Several different families of dominant oncogenes have been shown to undergo genetic changes in lung cancer. Of these, perhaps the most studied are the nuclear oncogenes c-*myc*, N-*myc*, and L-*myc*, which encode nuclear phosphoproteins thought to be involved in growth regulation (158,159). Each share a three-exon and two-intron structure with extensive regions of homology (160–162). In addition, *myc* genes are activated by overexpression, either by gene amplification or disruption of the normal control of gene expression (163). Each member can also cooperate with an activated *ras* gene to transform primary rat embryo cells (164–166).

C-*myc* deregulation has been found in a variety of human tumors, perhaps the best example being Burkitt's lymphoma (167). The role of c-*myc* deregulation in lung cancer was not appreciated until cytogenetic studies of SCLC cell lines showed double minute chromosomes and homogenous staining regions, findings suggestive of gene amplification (112). Consequently, Little et al. studied c-*myc* oncogene expression in a series of human lung cancer lines and found evidence of c-*myc* amplication in 8 of 18 cell lines (168). Five of these cell lines (all SCLC) had a high degree of c-*myc* DNA amplification (20- to 76-fold) in addition to greatly increased levels of c-*myc* RNA. Of interest is the fact that all of these cell lines were of the variant class characterized by altered morphology, shorter doubling times, decreased neuroendocrine differentiation, and more malignant behavior than classic SCLC cell lines (169,170). In another study, Johnson et al. showed that transfection of c-*myc* genes into classic SCLC cell lines resulted in the development of some of the phenotypic properties of variant cell lines (171). This data suggests a key role for c-*myc* in the growth characteristics and hence cellular phenotype of SCLC.

Although c-*myc* amplification appears to be common in SCLC cell lines (172–177), it appears to be much less frequent in fresh tumor specimens. Brooks et al. did not find any evidence of c-*myc* amplification in 20 SCLC tumor specimens obtained at autopsy (178). Wong et al. found only two instances of c-*myc* gene amplification in 96 DNA preparations of paraffin-embedded tissues from 45 patients (179). In another study, Morstyn et al. showed that c-*myc* amplification was not found in any of 10 SCLC cell lines cultured for short periods (i.e., several months) (180).

The important clinical question of whether *myc* amplification influences patient progress was addressed by Johnson et al. (181) They examined 44 SCLC cell lines established from 227 patients and found that (1) the ability to establish cell lines in vitro portended a poorer prognosis (14 vs. 48 week survival) ($p < 0.001$); (2) *myc* family DNA amplification was more common in tumor cell lines established from treated than untreated patients (44% vs. 11%); and (3) c-*myc* amplification in treated patients' tumor cell lines was associated with shortened survival (33 vs. 53 weeks) ($p = 0.04$).

It appears that c-*myc* amplification is not an early critical event in the pathogenesis of SCLC. Rather, c-*myc* amplification may offer a growth advantage for an already transformed cell, perhaps allowing it to become the dominant population in a heterogeneous tumor. Finally, chemotherapy may select out clones that amplify c-*myc* and become resistant to further therapy.

N-*myc* amplification and expression has also been demonstrated in SCLC cell lines. Nau et al. found that 6 of 31 SCLC cell lines displayed 5- to 170-fold amplification of N-*myc* gene sequences (182). They observed that N-*myc* amplification was present in both classic and variant SCLC cell lines. Amplified N-*myc* expression was also found in SCLC tumor samples from metastases at autopsy and from a primary SCLC tumor at resection, while normal tissue from these patients did not show these changes. Other studies have also confirmed N-*myc* amplification in SCLC, though with less frequency than c-*myc* (172,176–179,181).

While investigating c-*myc* and N-*myc* amplification in SCLC cell lines, a third *myc*-related gene (L-*myc*) was identified. Nau et al. found 10- to 20-fold L-*myc* sequence amplification in four SCLC cell lines and one SCLC tumor specimen (161). They also reported expression of L-*myc* in the absence of gene amplification in some SCLC cell lines. Kawashima et al. examined restriction fragment length polymorphisms (RFLP) of the L-*myc* gene (using ECoRI) in 51 patients with lung cancer (183). They observed that patients who were homozygous for the 10-Kb alleles (L-L) were less likely to have lymph node metastases at the time of surgery than heterozygotes (L-S) or 6.6-Kb homozygotes (S-S). Tamai et al. performed a similar study, but found no association between the L-*myc* allelic frequencies and lung cancer risk or disease status (184).

In summary, one member of the *myc* gene family is amplified and/or overexpressed in approximately 60% of SCLC cell lines. Such changes in *myc* genes have been rarely found in NSCLC cell lines or tumor specimens (168,185). In addition, no one SCLC tumor or cell line has been reported to exhibit amplification of more than one of the *myc* oncogenes. Thus, deregulation of the *myc* family of oncogenes appears to offer a selective growth advantage to cell lines and appears to be associated with a more aggressive tumor. Although our knowledge of these events has increased, our understanding of the *myc* genes in normal and malignant growth is still very limited.

The *ras* family of oncogenes (H-*ras*, N-*ras*, and Ki-*ras*), which are expressed in a wide variety of cells, have also been implicated in the pathogenesis of lung cancer (186). These genes encode a membrane-associated 21-kd protein, p21, thought to be involved in signal transduction pathways (187). P21 is activated by the binding of guanine triphosphate (GTP). Point mutations of these genes (especially at codons 12, 13, and 61) abolish GTPase activity and result in a molecule unable to convert GTP to its inactive state, guanine diphosphate (GDP). Thus, these mutated genes remain continually "activated" and acquire transforming potential.

The mutated *ras* gene, in cooperation with other dominantly acting oncogenes, can transform normal cells (164). In addition, transfection of the V-Ha-*ras* gene into SCLC cell lines produces more features of neuroendocrine differentiation (188) and other characteristics typical of NSCLCs (189). These data suggest an important role of the mutated *ras* gene in the phenotypic expression of certain features of cell lines and also imply a critical role in tumor progression in vitro.

Ras mutations have been observed in a number of human NSCLC cell lines and tumor specimens (190–197). The great majority of these were found in lung adenocarcinomas at the 12th codon position of K-*ras*. Rodenhuis et al. examined K-*ras* mutations in 39 untreated NSCLC tumors (194). They found that the K-*ras* gene was activated by point mutations in codon 12 in 5 of 10 adenocarcinomas, whereas all other lung cancer types did not show this mutation ($p < 0.001$). Interestingly, all five patients whose tumors displayed the K-*ras* mutation were heavy smokers, while two of the patients with a K-*ras*–negative adenocarcinoma had never smoked. In a further study, Rodenhuis and coworkers found that K-*ras* mutations occurred in about one third of adenocarcinomas (195). Furthermore, Slebos et al. studied 69 patients with adenocarcinoma of the lung, 19 of whom had a tumor with a K-*ras* mutation in codon 12 (196). These tumors tended to be smaller and less differentiated than those without mutations. The presence of tumors positive for K-*ras* mutations tended to be associated with a poorer prognosis ($p = 0.001$), shorter disease-free survival ($p = 0.038$), and a larger number of deaths due to cancer ($p = 0.001$). Slebos et al. also investigated the possible relationship between the exposure to tobacco smoke and the presence of *ras* point mutations from lung adenocarcinoma samples from 27 smokers and 27 nonsmokers (197). Point mutations in K-*ras* codon 12 were found in 8 of 27 smokers' samples vs. only 2 of 27 nonsmokers' ($p = 0.044$). These studies suggest that K-*ras* mutation is an essential step in the pathogenesis of adenocarcinoma of the lung. The observation that K-*ras* point mutations are more common in heavy smokers than in nonsmokers with adenocarcinoma is particularly intriguing, since this is the histological type of lung cancer most frequently seen in nonsmokers.

Finally, genetic predisposition to human lung cancer has been suggested by RFLP analysis of the human c-Ha-*ras* gene. Heighway et al. examined the allele frequencies in 132 lung cancer patients and controls (198). Using DNA extracted from white blood cells, they found that a specific allele (a4Aa-*ras*) occurred in 29% of patients with NSCLC but in only 16% of controls ($p = 0.03$). However, smoking history and ethnicity were not controlled. In another study, Sugimura et al. performed an age-, race-, and smoking-matched case-control study in 74 lung cancer patients and 67 controls (either patients with COPD or cancer at sites other than the lungs) (199). They found the frequency of rare alleles was significantly higher in blacks with either squamous cell carcinoma or small-cell carcinoma. A similar trend was observed in whites, but this did not reach statistical significance. Further support of c-Ha-*ras* as a genetic marker for lung cancer is that loss of this allele is associated with a more aggressive tumor in NSCLC (200). C-Ha-*ras* is located on chromosome 11p and is frequently reduced to homozygosity in Wilms' tumor, suggesting that c-Has-*ras* may act as a marker for a putative tumor suppressor gene on 11p (201).

Several other cellular proto-oncogenes have been found to be expressed in lung cancer. C-*jun*, a nuclear oncogene, encodes a transcription factor AP-1, which is involved with the regulation of transcription and with the mediation of tumor promotor effects (202,203). C-*jun* is also located in the same chromosomal region as L-*myc* (1p31-32) (204). Alone, C-*jun* can also transform Rat-1a cells (205). The gene also cooperates with activated c-Ha-*ras* to transform primary rat embryo cells. In addition, Schütte et al. found a 4- to 12-fold increase in c-*jun* expression in 5 of 12 SCLC cell lines and 5 of 26 NSCLC cell lines (206).

C-*raf*-1 encodes for a cytoplasmic serine theronic protein kinase involved in signal transduction pathways (207). Constitutive expression of c-*raf*-1 has been found in SCLC and NSCLC cell lines as well as in NSCLC tumor specimens (208,209). This finding is interesting because this gene is assigned to chromosome region 3p25, an area frequently involved in the terminal deletions in lung cancer (210). In fact, Sithanandum et al. found that one c-*raf*-1 allele was deleted in approximately 80% of SCLC cell lines examined and that the kinase activity of the c-*raf* protein appears to be constitutively activated in these cells (211). Overexpression of c-*raf*-1 and *myc*-family proto-oncogenes is associated with SCLC (212). Recently, Pfeifer et al. showed that transformation of a SV40 T-antigen gene expressing human bronchial epithelial cells (BEAS-2B) with either c-*raf*-1 or c-*myc* resulted in cell lines that expressed these genes but failed to cause tumorigenic conversion (212,213). On the other hand, BEAS-2B cells that had been dual infected with retroviral vectors containing both proto-oncogenes were tumorigenic, and the tumors resembled the multidifferentiated phenotype of SCLC. Interestingly, when other oncogenes were introduced into the genome of BEAS-2B cells, the resultant tumors expressed different histopathologies. Specifically, the phenotypes of v-Ki-*ras* transformants were described as poorly differentiated adenocarcinomas (214), whereas v-Ha-*ras*–expressing cells developed large cell undifferentiated tumors (215). Thus, the same cell can be the progenitor of tumors with differing histopathologies and the nature of the histotype can be affected by the oncogene(s) expressed. C-*myb* is another oncogene implicated in the pathogenesis of lung cancer. Griffin and Baylin found differential expression of c-*myb* in 7 of 8 SCLC cell lines but not in 5 of 5 NSCLC cell lines (216).

Amplification and overexpression of the c-*erb*B-1 proto-oncogene, which encodes the epidermal growth factor receptor (EGF), have been found in NSCLC cell lines and tumor specimens. Cline and Battifora found amplification of c-*erb*B-1 in 5 of 27 NSCLC tumor specimens (217). Sakiyama et al. found overexpression of c-*erb*B-1 in 6 of 11 NSCLC cell lines (218). Shiraishi et al. found amplification of c-*erb*B-1 in 10 of 114 tumor specimens (219); all amplifications occurred in NSCLCS. Thus, amplification of c-*erb*B-1 results in overexpression of the EGF receptor, which may provide epidermal cells with a proliferative advantage. HER2/new (also referred to as c-*erb*B-2) is a proto-oncogene that codes for a 185-kd membrane bound receptor with tyrosine kinase activity and sequence homology with the EGF receptor (220,221). Excess of the protein product is a common feature of NSCLC. In particular, Kern et al. reported that 5 of 16 squamous cell carcinomas and adenocarcinoma cells overexpressed this gene product (222). In a second study, 7 of 7 NSCLC lines demonstrated increased expression of c-*erb*B-2, whereas SCLC lines had considerably lower transcription levels (223). Finally, a number of the protooncogenes, including c-*fes*, c-*fos*, v-*abl*, v-*fms*, v-*sis*, and v-*src* have been found to be expressed in lung cancer cell lines and tumor specimens. Their occurrence, however, appears to be less frequent than other protooncogenes, and little is known of their role in the pathogenesis of lung cancer (176,208,217,219).

Anti-oncogenes or tumor-suppressor genes are also implicated in the pathogenesis of lung cancer. Unlike dominant oncogenes, these tumor-suppressor genes have a negative regulatory role on growth, and it is their inactivation through deletions or mutations that allows the expression of the malignant phenotype (144–157). In addition, inactivation of both the maternal and paternal alleles is required for their effect.

The first tumor-suppressor gene to be identified was the Rb gene (224–227). This gene, assigned to chromosomal region 13q14.1, was found to determine susceptibility to human retinoblastoma (228–230). The gene's tumor-suppressor effects have been demonstrated by the introduction of the Rb gene into retinoblastoma or osteosarcoma cells that had inactivated Rb copies and the subsequent suppression of the malignant phenotype (231). The presence of deletions and chromosomal rearrangements involving chromosome 13 in SCLC cell lines prompted investigators to examine the involvement of the Rb gene in lung cancer. Harbour et al. found structural abnormalities within the Rb gene in 4 of 22 SCLC cell lines, 1 of 8 primary SCLC tumors, and 1 of 4 pulmonary carcinoids, but not in 20 NSCLC cell lines examined (232). In addition, absent or trace Rb mRNA expression was found in 60% of SCLC lines and only 10% of NSCLC lines. In another study, Horowitz et al. found absent or aberrant Rb protein in 8 of 9 SCLC cell lines (233). Other studies have confirmed that inactivation of the Rb gene is a frequent event in SCLC (234–236).

p53 is another recently identified tumor suppressor gene, assigned to chromosome region 17p13 and frequently deleted in lung cancer (237). p53 was originally considered to be a dominant oncogene because mutated p53 alleles in cooperation with an activated ras gene could transform primary rat embryo fibroblasts (238,239). Further studies showed that cotransfection of wild-type p53 reduced transformation efficiency by many other oncogenes (240) and suppresses the growth of transformed cells in culture (241) and the tumorigenic potential of cells in animals (242). Current evidence suggests, however, that the wild-type p53 gene acts as a tumor suppressor gene and that a mutant p53 gene promotes transformation by inactivating normal p53 function in a dominant negative fashion (243,244). Moreover, the normal allele of this autosomal gene encodes a 53-kd nuclear phosphoprotein involved in cell proliferation (245,246). The mutant alleles, on the other hand, code for proteins with aberrant growth regulatory characteristics, which are believed to be seminal in transformation (240,243,244).

p53's role in lung cancer was first investigated following the discovery of 17p allele loss by RFLP analysis and the further assignment of human p53 to this region. Takahashi et al. reported p53 abnormalities in 17 of 30 lung cancer cell lines (247). These included homozygous deletions, point mutations, gene arrangements, and absent or abnormally sized mRNAs. Takahashi and coworkers also examined 50 lung cancer tumor samples and found abnormalities in approximately 20% of the specimens. In another study, Chiba et al. examined 51 primary resected NSCLC specimens and found mutations in 23, but not in the corresponding normal lung (248). These mutations thus appear to be somatically acquired and not inherited. Chiba and coworkers also observed a lack of clinical and pathologic correlations, suggesting a role independent of tumor progression. Other human studies also support the role of mutant p53 in lung cancer and in human cancer in general (249–252).

Thus, it appears that mutations of the Rb and p53 genes are common in lung cancer. However, these genetic abnormalities are not mutually exclusive. A number of cell lines show alterations of the Rb and p53 genes in addition to other abnormalities, suggesting a series of sequential genetic lesions during different stages of tumor progression. Furthermore, other tumor-suppressor genes that are involved in the pathogenesis of lung cancer are likely to exist. Candidates at the present time include putative genes located within the 3p deletion site. Perhaps the most likely of these is PTP-γ, the gene for protein-tyrosine phosphatase γ. LaForgia et al. found loss of one PTP-γ allele in 3 of 5 renal carcinoma cell lines and 5 of 10 lung carcinoma tumor samples tested (253). In addition, they localized the PTP-γ gene to human chromosome region 3p21 using filter and in situ hybridization. This observation is of interest because one of the functions of the protein-tyrosine phosphatases is control of the level of phosphorylation within the cell (254,255). The protein-tyrosine phosphatases serve to balance the protein-tyrosine kinases, many of which are oncogenes and growth factor receptors and are involved in the control of cell growth and differentiation. Thus, the PTP-γ gene is implicated as a possible tumor-suppressor gene in the pathogenesis of lung cancer. Other putative tumor-suppressor genes located within the 3p deletion site include ErbA, which encodes a thyroid hormone receptor (256–258), and Hap-1, which encodes a retinoic acid receptor (259). Although little is known about their roles in lung carcinogenesis, it is speculated that inactivation of these genes causes deregulation of hormone receptor functions, which transmit signals for differentiation. Another candidate tumor-suppressor gene thought to be involved in the pathogenesis of lung cancer is the Wilms' tumor gene located in the chromosome region 11p13 (260,261). Lung cancer frequently shows loss of heterozygosity in this area, suggesting that inactivation of this gene is probable. Further careful studies to detect subtle mutations are needed to confirm these hypotheses.

VII. Growth Factors

A variety of growth factors are considered to be involved in the pathogenesis of lung cancer. Growth factors are polypeptides that control and regulate cellular growth and differentiation, and also control expression of specific genes, some of which are oncogenes. Growth factors act upon a target cell at specific receptors at the cell surface and are extremely biologically active. Both oncogenes and growth factors are involved in a hierarchical control of cell proliferation and in the development of the malignant phenotype during carcinogenesis.

Growth factors can be either stimulatory or inhibitory and can act through an endocrine, paracrine, or autocrine mechanism. Autocrine growth factor stimulation refers to the ability of cells to both produce and respond to their own growth factors (262,263). Such stimulation was shown to occur in a number of tumor systems. Two observations suggested that autocrine growth factor stimulation may occur in lung cancer: (1) SCLC cell lines were grown in serum-free media (i.e., in media without exogenous growth factors) (264,265), and (2) SCLC cell lines secrete a number of peptide hormones (266–268). The finding that SCLC cell lines both produce and exhibit a mitogenic response to gastrin-releasing peptide (GRP) solidified this hypothesis.

GRP, the mammalian analog of bombesin, is an important regulator peptide during normal lung growth and development. SCLC cell lines have been found to secrete GRP, possess GRP receptors, increase Ca^{2+} mobilization under GRP stimulation, and increase growth rate in the presence of GRP (269,270). Carney et al. found that GRP stimulated clonal growth of SCLC in vitro up to 150-fold but not growth of NSCLC cell lines (271). In another study, Cuttitta et al. found that a monoclonal anti-GRP antibody could inhibit the clonal growth of SCLC cell lines in vitro and SCLC xenografts in vivo (269). Other studies have also confirmed GRP's role as an autocrine growth factor in SCLC (272–276).

Smokers have high levels of bombesinlike immunoreactivity in bronchial lavage samples (277). In addition, GRP has been found to stimulate the growth of normal bronchial epithelial cells supporting its role as a paracrine growth factor (278). This places GRP-mediated events early in the pathogenesis of lung cancer. It is hypothesized that GRP may promote genetic lesions caused by carcinogens and allow for the accumulation of multiple lesions (i.e., multistage carcinogenesis).

Epidermal growth factor (EGF) is another growth factor that has been examined in lung cancer. EGF is found in normal human plasma and almost all body fluids, and EGF receptors are present in a wide range of normal epithelial tissues (279,280). Its biologic activity appears to be primarily mitogenic. Sherwin et al. found that five of six NSCLC cell lines expressed EGF receptors, while none of 11 SCLC cell lines were found to possess the receptor (281). In another study, Cerny et al. examined 63 lung tumor specimens with a monoclonal antibody to the EGF receptor. They found that 80% of NSCLC specimens were positive, while none of the SCLC samples had detectable EGF receptors. Other studies have also confirmed this finding (282,283). Dazzi et al. found no relationship between EGF receptor status and size of primary tumor or lymph node status in 152 NSCLC thoracotomy specimens (284). Thus, although EGF appears implicated in NSCLC, its primary role remains poorly understood.

SCLC cell lines have been found to express a variety of other growth factors and peptides. These include insulinlike growth factor-1 (IGF-1), platelet-derived growth factor (PDGF), transferrinlike peptides, vasopressin, neurotensin, ACTH, physalamin, calcintonin, and atrial nutriuretic factor (285–288). The role these hormones play in the transformed state of SCLC is unknown. Recently, new autocrine and paracrine regulatory systems involving opioid and nicotine receptors have been identified. Maneckjee et al. found that lung cancer cell lines expressed multiple, high-affinity membrane receptors for opioid agonists and for nicotine and expressed various combinations of opioid peptides (289). Opioid agonists at low concentrations inhibited lung cancer growth in vitro, while nicotine reversed this inhibition in 9 of 14 lung cancer cell lines. The authors believe that opioids may function as "tumor suppressors" and that nicotine may circumvent this in the pathogenesis of lung cancer. Further studies are necessary to clarify these effects.

VIII. Conclusion

Human lung cancer is a complex environmental and genetic disease involving the accumulation of a series of genetic defects. The sequence of events that occurs during lung carcinogenesis is becoming apparent. Multistep progression from normal cell to malignant tumor involves both activation of cellular proto-oncogenes and the inactivation of tumor-suppressor genes (Fig. 4). Each step probably enhances the likelihood of the next by producing cells that escape the normal growth-controlling mechanisms. Oncogene expression appears to influence the histopathology and biologic behavior of the tumor. Autocrine growth factors act as promoting agents, clonally expanding cells from each stage. Most of the observed genetic defects appear to be somatically acquired during adult life and are probably related to carcinogen exposure. However, there is mounting circumstantial evidence that some of these genetic changes or the likelihood of their occurrence are inherited in a Mendelian fashion.

The strong association between the inheritance of the extensive metabolic phenotype of debrisoquine and the development of lung cancer offers compelling evidence for genetic predisposition to lung cancer. Alternatively, a yet unidentified

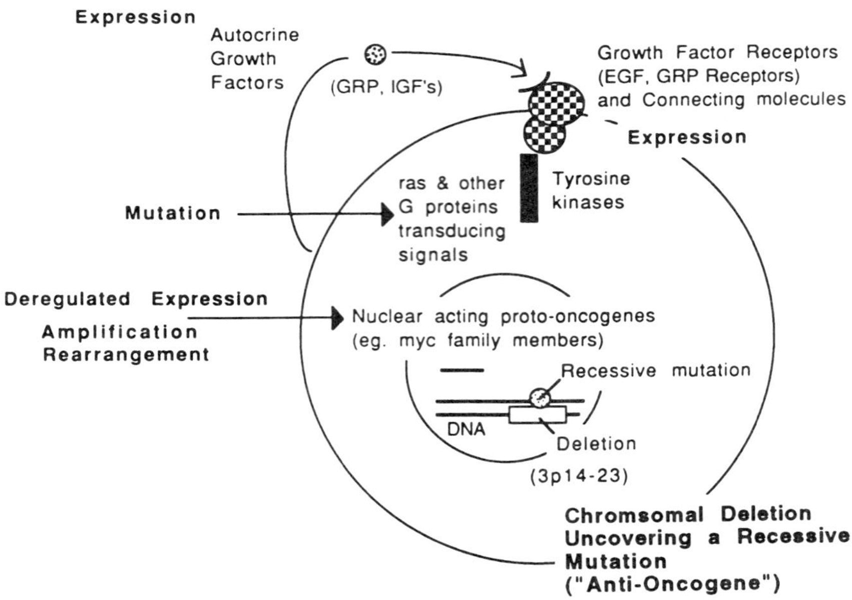

Figure 4 Molecular mechanisms involved in the pathogenesis of lung cancer. (From Ref. 148.)

inherited mutation, perhaps in the undeleted 3p14-23 chromosome region or elsewhere, could be the "lung cancer susceptibility gene." These questions will remain unanswered until careful linkage analysis in lung cancer families is performed.

Future prevention and treatment of lung cancer will depend on a better understanding of the cellular and molecular events that occur in its pathogenesis. Widespread screening of cigarette smokers or those involved in high-risk lung cancer occupations in improbable at present unless a valid, reproducible genetic marker or indicator is identified. Furthermore, such screening would raise many ethical questions; cigarette smoking, for instance, is associated with many other lethal conditions, and, in addition, the assignment of an individual to a low-risk group would not preclude him or her from developing lung cancer. Treatment of lung cancer may in the future involve a number of different modalities primarily involving inhibition of the deregulated expression of various oncogenes and growth factors. Anti–growth factor trials are already in progress (290). The introduction of normal copies of tumor-suppressor genes through gene therapy or the replacement of aberrant or absent gene products would also seen to be logical therapeutic interventions (291). In the future, prevention of lung cancer through smoking cessation programs and limitation to exposure to other potent lung carcinogens will still remain the best solution to the major cause of cancer-related mortality in the United States.

Acknowledgments

We thank David G. Thomassen for manuscript review and Sally Goehring for manuscript preparation.

References

1. Watkins, D. J. G. (1904). A family tree bearing upon the question of the inheritance of cancer. *Br. Med. J.* 1:190.
2. Shields, P. G., and Harris, C. C. (1991). Molecular epidemiology and the genetics of environmental cancer. *JAMA* 266:681–687.
3. Malkin, D., Li F. P., Strong, L. C., Fraumeni, J. F., Nelson, C. E., Kim, D. H., Kassel, J., Gryka, M. A., Bischoff, F. Z., Tainsky, M. A., and Friend S. H. (1990). Germ-line p53 mutations in a familial syndrome of breast cancer, sarcomas, and other neoplasms. *Science* 250:1233–1238.
4. Srivastaza, S., Zou, V., Pirollo, K., Blattner, W., Chang, E. H. (1990). Germ-line transmission of a mutated p53 gene in a cancer-prone family with Li-Fraumeni syndrome. *Nature* 348:747–749.
5. Knudson, A. G. (1971). Mutation and cancer: Statistical study of retinoblastoma. *Proc. Natl. Acad. Sci. USA* 68:820–823.

6. Friend, S. H., Bernards, R., Rogelj, S., Weinberg, R. A., Rapaport, J. M., Albert, D. M., and Dryja, T. P. (1986). A human DNA segment with properties of the gene that predisposes to retinoblastoma and osteosarcoma. *Nature* 323:643–646.
7. U.S. Department of Health and Human Services. (1990). The health benefits of smoking cessation. DHHS Publication No (CDC) 90-8416. U.S. Department of Health and Human Services, Public Health Service, Centers for Disease Control, Center for Chronic Disease Prevention and Health Promotion, Office on Smoking and Health.
8. Peto, J. (1980). Genetic predisposition to cancer. In: *Cancer Incidence in Defined Populations*. Edited by J. Cairns, J. Lyon, and M. Skolnick. Cold Spring Harbor, NY, Cold Spring Harbor Laboratory, pp. 203–213.
9. Tokuhata, G. K., and Lilienfeld, A. M. (1963). Familial aggregation of lung cancer among hospital patients. *Public Health Rep.* 78:277–283.
10. Tokuhata, G. K. (1964). Familial factors in human lung cancer and smoking. *Am. J. Public Health* 54:24–32.
11. Ooi, W., Elston, R., Chen, V., Bailey-Wilson, J., and Rothschild, H. (1986). Increased familial risk for lung cancer. *J. Natl. Cancer Inst.* 76:217–222.
12. Lynch, H., Kimberling, W., Markvicka, S., Biscone, K., Lynch, J., Whorton, E., and Mailliard, J. (1986). Genetics and smoking-associated cancers: A study of 485 families. *Cancer* 57:1640–1646.
13. Samet, J., Humble, C., and Pathak, D. (1986). Personal and family history of respiratory disease and lung cancer risk. *Am. Rev. Respir. Dis.* 134:466–470.
14. Shaw, G. L., Falk, R. T., Dickle, L. W., Mason, T. J., and Buffler, P. A. (1991). Lung cancer risk associated with cancer in relatives. *J. Clin. Epidemiol.* 44:429–437.
15. Sellers, T. A., Ooi, W. L., Elston, R. C., Chen V. W., Bailey-Wilson, J. E., and Rothschild, H. (1987). Increased familial risk for non-lung cancer among relatives of lung cancer patients. *Am. J. Epidemiol.* 126:237–246.
16. Sellers, T. A., Bailey-Wilson, J. E., Elston, R. C., Wilson, A. F., Elston, Z., Ooi, W. L., and Rothschild, H. (1990). Evidence for mendelian inheritance in the pathogenesis of lung cancer. *J. Natl. Cancer Inst.* 82:1272–1279.
17. Horwitz, R. I., Smaldone, L. F., and Viscoli, C. M. (1988). An ecogenetic hypothesis for lung cancer in women. *Arch. Intern. Med.* 148:2609–2612.
18. Osann, K. E. (1991). Lung cancer in women: The importance of smoking, family history of cancer, and medical history of respiratory disease. *Cancer Res.* 51:4893–4897.
19. Sanders, B. M., Jay, M., Draper, G. J., and Roberts, E. M. (1989). Non-ocular cancer in relatives of retinoblastoma patients. *Br. J. Cancer* 60:358–365.
20. Strong, L. C., Herson, J., Haas, C., Elder, K., Chakraborty, R., Weiss, K. M., and Majumder, P. (1984). Cancer mortality in relatives of retinoblastoma patients. *J. Natl. Cancer Inst.* 73:303–311.
21. Brisman, R., Robinson Baker, R., Elkins, R., and Hartmann, W. H. (1967). Carcinoma of lung in four siblings. *Cancer* 20:2048–2053.
22. Swaye, P., Van Ordstrand, H. S., McCormack, L. J., Wolpaw, S. E. (1969). Familial hamman-rich syndrome. *Dis. Chest* 55:7–12.
23. Fraumeni, J. F., Wertelecki, W., Blattner, W. A., Jensen, R. D., and Leventhal, B. G.

(1975). Varied manifestations of a familial lymphoproliferative disorder. *Am. J. Med.* 59:145–151.

24. Mulvihill, J. J. (1976). Host factors in human lung tumors: An example of ecogenetics in oncology. *J. Natl. Cancer Inst.* 57:3–7.
25. Goffman, T. E., Hassinger, D. D., and Mulvihill, J. J. (1982). Familial respiratory tract cancer. Opportunities for research and prevention. *JAMA* 247:1020–1023.
26. Paul, S. M., Bacharach, B., and Geopp, C. (1987). A genetic influence on alveolar cell carcinoma. *J. Surg. Oncol.* 36:249–252.
27. Joishy, S. K., Cooper, R. A., and Rowley, P. T. (1977). Alveolar cell carcinoma in identical twins. *Ann. Int. Med.* 87:447–450.
28. Rohwedder, J. J., and Weatherbee, L. (1974). Multiple primary bronchogenic carcinoma with a review of the literature. *Am. Rev. Respir. Dis.* 109:435–445.
29. Martini, N., and Melamed, M. (1975). Multiple primary lung cancers. *J. Thor. Cardiovasc. Surg.* 70:606–612.
30. Johnson, B. E., Ihde, D. C., Matthews, M. J., Bunn, P. A., Zabell, A., Makuch, R. W., Johnston-Early, A., Cohen, M. H., Glatstein, E., and Minna, J. D. (1986). Non-small-cell lung cancer. Major cause of late mortality in patients with small cell lung cancer. *Am. J. Med.* 80:1103–1110.
31. Markman, M., Pavy, M., and Abeloff, M. (1982). Acute leukemia following intensive therapy for small-cell carcinoma of the lung. *Cancer* 50:672–675.
32. Boice, J. D., and Fraumeni, J. F. (1985). Second cancer following cancer of the respiratory system in Connecticut 1935-1982. *Natl. Cancer Inst. Monogr.* 68: 83–98.
33. Johnson, D., Porter, L., List, A., Hande, K., Hainsworth, J., and Greco, F. (1986). Acute nonlymphocytic leukemia after treatment of small cell lung cancer. *Am. J. Med.* 81:962–968.
34. Whang-Peng, J., Lee, E. C., Minna, J. D., Abeloff, M. D., Bradley, E. C., Young, R. C., and Longo, D. L. (1988). Deletion of 3(p14p23) in secondary erythroleukemia arising in long-term survivors of small cell lung cancer. *J. Natl. Cancer Inst.* 80:1253–1255.
35. Aird, I., Bentall, H. H., Mehigan, J. A., and Fraser Roberts, J. A. (1954). The blood groups in relation to peptic ulceration and carcinoma of colon, rectum, breast, and bronchus. *Br. Med. J.* :315–321.
36. McConnel, R. B., Clarke, C. A., and Downton, F. (1955). Blood groups in carcinoma of lung. *Br. Med. J.* :674.
37. Parker, G., and Walsh, R. J. (1958). Blood groups and disease. Carcinoma of various organs. *Med. J. Aust.* :835.
38. Rennie, H. M., and Haber, R. W. (1961). Blood groups in carcinoma of the lung. *Med. J. Aust.* :61.
39. Jakoubkova, J., and Majsky, A. (1965). Blood groups and neoplastic disease. *Neoplasma* 12:611.
40. Ashley, D. J. B. (1969). Blood groups and lung cancer. *J. Med. Genet.* 6:183–186.
41. Roberts, T. E., Hasleton, P., Swindell, R., and Lawson, R. (1988). Blood groups and lung cancer. *Br. J. Cancer* 58:278.
42. Roots, I., Drakoulis, N., Ploch, M., Heinemeyer, G., Loddenkemper, R., Minks, T.,

Nitz, M., Otte, F., and Koch, M. (1988). Debrisoquine hydroxylation phenotype, acetylation phenotype, and ABO blood groups as genetic host factors of lung cancer risk. *Klin. Wochenschr.* 66:87–97.
43. Lee, J. S., Ro, J. Y., Sahin, A. A., Hong, W. K., Brown, B. W., Mountain, C. F., and Hittelman, W. N. (1991). Expression of blood-group antigen A—a favorable prognostic factor in non-small-cell lung cancer. *N. Engl. J. Med.* 324:1084–1090.
44. Tongio, M. M., Kerschen, C., Pauli, G., Roeslin, N., Grange, D., and Mayer, S. (1982). HLA antigens and primary bronchial carcinoma. *Cancer* 49:2482–2488.
45. Markman, M., Braine, H. G., and Abeloff, M. D. (1984). Histocompatibility antigens in small cell carcinoma of the lung. *Cancer* 54:2943–2945.
46. Takasugi, M., Terasaki, P. I., Henderson, B., Mickey, M. R., Menck, H., and Thompson, R. (1973). HL-A antigens in solid tumors. *Cancer Res.* 33:648–650.
47. Sengar, D. P. S., McLeish, W. A., Stewart, T. H. M., and Harris, J. E. (1977). HLA antigens in bronchogenic carcinoma. *Oncology* 34:143–145.
48. Ford, C. H. J., Newman, C. E., and MacKintosh, P. (1981). HLA frequency and prognosis in lung cancer. *Br. J. Cancer* 43:610–614.
49. Dellon, A. L., Rogentin, G. N., and Chretien, P. B. (1975). Prolonged survival in bronchogenic carcinoma associated with HL-A antigens W-19 and HL-A5: A preliminary report. *J. Natl. Cancer Inst.* 54:1283–1286.
50. Rogentine, G. N., Dellon, A. L., and Chretien, P. B. (1977). Prolonged disease-free survival in bronchogenic carcinoma associated with HLA-Aw19 and HLA-B5. *Cancer* 39:2345–2347.
51. Weiss, G. B., Nawrocki, L. B., and Daniels, J. C. (1980). HLA type and survival in lung cancer. *Cancer* 46:38–40.
52. Svejgaard, A., Jersild, C., Nielsen, L. S., and Bodmar, W. F. (1974). HL-A antigens and disease: Statistical and genetical considerations. *Tissue Antigens* 4:95–105.
53. Law, M. R. (1990). Genetic predisposition to lung cancer. *Br. J. Cancer* 61: 195–206.
54. Phillips, D. H., Hewer, A., Martin, C. N., Colin Garner, R., and King, M. M. (1988). Correlation of DNA adduct levels in human lung with cigarette smoking. *Nature* 336:790–792.
55. Nebert, D. W. (1981). Possible clinical importance of genetic differences in drug metabolism. *Br. Med. J.* 283:537.
56. Miller, E. C. (1978). Some current perspectives on chemical carcinogenesis in humans and experimental animals: Presidential address. *Cancer Res.* 38:1479–1496.
57. Gelboin, H. V. (1980). Benzopyrene metabolism, activation and carcinogenesis: Role and regulation of mixed function oxidases and related enzymes. *Physiol. Rev.* 60:1107.
58. Conney, A. H. (1982). Induction of microsomal enzymes by foreign chemicals and carcinogenesis by polycyclic aromatic hydrocarbons: GHA Clowes Memorial Lecture. *Cancer Res.* 42:4875.
59. Pelkonen, D., and Nebert, D. W. (1982). Metabolism of polycyclic aromatic hydrocarbons: Etiologic role in carcinogenesis. *Pharmacol. Rev.* 34:189.
60. Ocraft, K. P., Muskett, J. M., and Brown, S. (1985). Localisation of the aryl

hydrocarbon hydroxylase gene to the 2q31-2pter of chromosome 2. *Ann. Hum. Genet.* 49:237.

61. Amsbaugh, S. C., Ding, J. H., Swan, D. C., Popescu, N. C., and Chen, Y. T. (1986). Expression and chromosomal localization of the cytochrome P-450 gene in human mitogen-stimulated lymphocytes. *Cancer Res.* 46:2423.
62. Shimada, T., Misono, K. S., and Guengerich, F. P. (1986). Human liver microsomal cytochrome P-450 mephenytoin 4-hydroxylase, a prototype of genetic polymorphism in oxidative drug metabolism. *J. Biol. Chem.* 261:909–921.
63. Atlas, S. A., Vesell, E. S., and Nebert, D. W. (1976). Genetic control of interindividual variations in the inducibility of aryl hydrocarbon hydroxylase in cultured human lymphocytes. *Cancer Res.* 36:4619–4630.
64. Okuda, T., Vesell, E. S., Plotkin, E., Tarone, R., Bast, R. C., and Gelboin, H. V. (1977). Interindividual and intraindividual variations in aryl hydrocarbon hydroxylase in monocytes from monozygotic and dizygotic twins. *Cancer Res.* 37:3904–3911.
65. Kellermann, G., Luyten-Kellermann, M., and Shaw, C. R. (1973). Genetic variation of aryl hydrocarbon hydroxylase in human lymphocytes. *Am. J. Hum. Genet.* 25: 327–331.
66. Trell, L., Korsgaard, R., Janzon, L., and Trell, E. (1985). Distribution and reproducibility of aryl hydrocarbon hydroxylase inducibility in a prospective population study of middle aged male smokers and non-smokers. *Cancer* 56:1988.
67. McLemore, T. L., Martin, R. R., Pickard, L. R., Springer, R. R. Wray, N. P., Toppell, K. L., Mattox, K. L., Guinn, G. A., Cantrell, E. T., and Busbee, D. L. (1978). Analysis of aryl hydrocarbon hydroxylase activity in human lung tissue, pulmonary macrophages, and blood lymphocytes. *Cancer* 41:2292–2300.
68. Kellermann, G., Shaw, C. R., and Luyten-Kellermann, M. (1973). Aryl hydrocarbon hydroxylase inducibility and bronchogenic carcinoma. *N. Engl. J. Med.* 289: 934–937.
69. Korsgaard, R., Stiksa, G., Simonsson, B. G., and Trell, E. (1977). Smoking habits and aryl hydrocarbon hydroxylase inducibility in patients with malignant tumors of the respiratory tract. *Scand. J. Respir. Dis.* (Suppl) 99:50.
70. Paigen, B., Gurtoo, H. L., Minowada, J., Houten, L., Vincent, R., Paigen, K., Parker, N. B., Ward, E., and Hayner, N. T. (1977). Questionable relation of aryl hydrocarbon hydroxylase to lung-cancer risk. *N. Engl. J. Med.* 297:346–350.
71. Lieberman, J. (1978). Aryl hydrocarbon hydroxylase in bronchogenic carcinoma. *N. Engl. J. Med.* 298:686–687.
72. Kouri, R. E., McKinney, C. E., Slomiany, O. R., Snodgrass, N. P., Wray, N. P., and McLemore, T. L. (1982). Positive correlation between high aryl hydrocarbon hydroxylase activity and primary lung cancer as analysed in cryopreserved lymphocytes. *Cancer Res.* 42:5030–5037.
73. Harris, C. C., Autrup, H., Stoner, G., Yang, S. K., Leutz, J. C., Gelboin, H. V., Selkirk, J. K., Connor, R. J., Barrett, L. A., Jones, R. T., McDowell, E., and Trump, B. F (1977). Metabolism of benzopyrene and 7, N12-dimethylbenzanthracene in cultured human bronchus and pancreatic duct. *Cancer Res.* 37:3349–3355.
74. Oesch, F., Schmassmann, H., Ohnhaus, E., Althaus, U., and Lorenz, J. (1980).

Mono-oxygenase, epoxide hydrolase, and glutathione-S-transferase activities in human lung. Variation between groups of bronchogenic carcinoma and non-cancer patients and interindividual differences. *Carcinogenesis* 1:827–835.

75. Karki, N. T., Pokela, R., Nuutinen, L., and Pelkonen, O. (1987). Aryl hydrocarbon hydroxylase in lymphocytes and lung tissue from lung cancer patients and controls. *Int. J. Cancer* 39:565–570.
76. Idle, J. R., Mahgoub, A., Angelo, M. M., Dring, L. G., Lancaster, R., and Smith, R. L. (1979). The metabolism of [^{14}C]-debrisoquine in man. *Br. J. Clin. Pharmacol.* 7:257.
77. Eichelbaum, M. (1984). Polymorphic drug oxidation in humans. *Fed. Proc.* :2298.
78. Steiner, E. Iselius, L., Alvan, G., Lindsten, J., and Sjoqvist, F. (1985). A family study of genetic and environmental factors determining polymorphic hydroxylation of debrisoquine. *Clin. Pharmacol. Ther.* 38:394.
79. Eichelbaum, M., Baur, M. P., Dengler, H. J., Osikowska-Evers, O., Tieves, G., Zekorn, C., and Rittner, C. (1987). Chromosomal assignment of human chromosome P-450 (debrisoquine/sparteine type) to chromosome 22. *Br. J. Clin. Pharmacol.* 23:455.
80. Gonzalez, F. J., Skoda, R. C., Kimura, S., Umeno, M. Zanger, U. M., Nebert, D. W., Gelboin, H. V., Hardwick, J. P., and Meyer, U. A. (1988). Characterization of the common genetic defect in humans deficient in debrisoquine metabolism. *Nature* 331:442–446.
81. Evans, D. A. P., Mahgoub, A., Sloan, T. P., Idle, J. R., and Smith, R. L. (1980). A family and population study of the genetic polymorphism of debrisoquine oxidation in a white British population. *J. Med. Genet.* 17:102–105.
82. Heim, M. H., and Meyer, U. A. (1990). Genotyping of poor metabolisers of debrisoquine by allele-specific PCR amplification. *Lancet* 336:529–532.
83. Law, M. R., Hetzel, M. R., and Idle, J. R. (1989). Debrisoquine metabolism and genetic predisposition to lung cancer. *Br. J. Cancer* 59:686–687.
84. Ayesh, R., Idle, J. R. Ritchie, J. C., Crothers, M. J., and Hetzel, M. R. (1984). Metabolic oxidation phenotypes as markers for susceptibility to lung cancer. *Nature* 312:169–170.
85. Caporaso, N., Hayes, R. B., Dosemeci, M., Hoover, R., Ayesh, R., Hetzel, M., and Idle, J. (1989). Lung cancer risk, occupational exposure, and the debrisoquine metabolic phenotype. *Cancer Res.* 49:3675–3679.
86. Caporaso, N. E., Tucker, M. A., Hoover, R. N., Hayes, R. B., Pickle, L. W., Issaq, H. J., Muschik, G. M., Green-Gallo, L., Buivys, D., Aisner, S., Resau, J. H., Trump, B. F., Tollerud, D., Weston, A., and Harris, C. C. (1990). Lung cancer and the debrisoquine metabolic phenotype. *J. Natl. Cancer Inst.* 82:1264–1272.
87. Speirs, C. J., Murray, S., Davies, D. S., Biola Mabadejie, A. F., and Boobis, A. R. (1990). Debrisoquine oxidation phenotype and susceptibility to lung cancer. *Br. J. Clin. Pharmacol.* 29:101–109.
88. Sugimura, H., Caporaso, N. E., Shaw, G. L., Modali, R. V., Gonzalez, F. J., Hoover, R. N., Resau, J. H., Trump, B. F., Weston, A., and Harris, C. C. (1990). Human debrisoquine hydroxylase gene polymorphisms in cancer patients and controls. *Carcinogenesis* 11:1527–1530.

89. Crespi, C. L., Penman, B. W., Gelboin, H. V., and Gonzalez, F. J. (1991). A tobacco smoke-derived nitrosamine, 4-(methylnitrosamino)-1-(3-pyridyl)-1-butonone, is activated by multiple human cytochrome P450s including the polymorphic human cytochrome P4502D6. *Carcinogenesis* 12:1197–1201.
90. Kawajiri, K., Nakachi, K., Imai, K., Yoshii, A., Shinoda, N., and Watanabe, J. (1990). Identification of genetically high risk individuals to lung cancer by DNA polymorphisms of the cytochrome P450IAI gene. *FEBS Lett.* 263:131–133.
91. Nakachi, K., Imai, K., Hayashi, S., Watanabe, J., and Kawajiri, K. (1991). Genetic susceptibility to squamous cell carcinoma of the lung in relation to cigarette smoking dose. *Cancer Res.* 51:5177–5180.
92. Seidegard, J., Pero, R. W., Miller, D. G., and Beattie, E. J. (1986). A glutathione transferase in human leukocytes as a marker for the susceptibility to lung cancer. *Carcinogenesis* 7:751–753.
93. Seidegard, J., Pero, R. W., Markowitz, M. M., Roush, G., Miller, D. G., and Beattie, E. J. (1990). Isoenzyme(s) of glutathione transferase (class Mu) as a marker for the susceptibility to lung cancer: a follow up study. *Carcinogenesis* 11:33–36.
94. Farber, E. (1984). The multistep nature of cancer development. *Cancer Res.* 44: 4217–4223.
95. Weinberg, R. A. (1989). Oncogenes, antioncogenes, and the molecular basis of multistep carcinogenesis. *Cancer Res.* 49:3713–3721.
96. Doll, R. (1971). The age distribution of cancer: Implications for models of carcinogenesis. *J. R. Stat. Soc.* A134:133–161.
97. Doll, R., and Peto, R. (1978). Cigarette smoking and bronchial carcinoma: Dose and time relationships among regular smokers and lifelong non-smokers. *J. Epidemiol. Commun. Health* 32:303–313.
98. Day, N. E. (1984). Epidemiological data and multistage carcinogenesis. In: *Models, Mechanisms and Etiology of Tumor Promotion*. Edited by M. Borzsonyl, K. Lapis, N. E. Day, and H. Yamasaki. Lyon, IARC, pp. 339–357.
99. Saccomanno, G., Archer, V. E., Auerbach, O., Saunders, R. P., and Brennan, L. M. (1974). Development of carcinoma of the lung as reflected in exfoliated cells. *Cancer* 31:256–270.
100. Viallet, J., and Minna, J. D. (1990). Dominant oncogenes and tumor suppressor genes in the pathogenesis of lung cancer. *Am. J. Respir. Cell Mol. Biol.* 2:225–232.
101. Volegstein, B., Fearon, E. R., Hamilton, S. R., Kern, S. E., Preisinger, A. C., Leppert, M., Nakamura, Y., White, R., Smits, A. M. M., and Bos, J. L. (1988). Genetic alterations during colorectal-tumor development. *N. Engl. J. Med.* 319: 525–532.
102. Fearon, E. R., and Vogelstein, B. (1990). A genetic model for colorectal tumorigenesis. *Cell* 61:759–767.
103. Blondal T., and Lindgren, A. (1982). Fluorescence cytophotometric measurements of nuclear DNA in adenocarcinoma of the lung: Relation of proliferative activity and DNA ploidy to prognosis. *Anal. Quant. Cytol.* 4:225–232.
104. Olszewski, W., Dazynbunrez, Z., Claps, M. L., and Melamed, M. (1982). Flow cytometry of lung carcinoma: A comparison of DNA stemline and cell cycle distribution with histology. *Anal. Quant. Cytol.* 4:90–98.

105. Bunn, P. A., Carney, D. N., Gazdar, A. F., Whang-Peng, J., and Matthews, M. J. (1983). Diagnostic and biological implications of flow cytometric DNA content analysis in lung cancer. *Cancer Res.* 43:5026–5032.
106. Sahin, A. A., Ro, J. Y., El-Naggar, A. K., Lee, J. S., Ayala, A. G., Teague, K., and Hong, W. K. (1990). Flow cytometric analysis of the DNA content of nonsmall cell lung cancer. *Cancer* 65:530–537.
107. Benfield, J. R., Wain, J. C., Derrick, M., Smith, S. S., Ohnuki, Y., Bates, S. E., Shively, J., Teplitz, R. L., and Hammond, W. G. (1988). Biochemical and cytogenetic studies of human lung cancers. *J. Thorac. Cardiovasc. Surg.* 96:840–848.
108. Tirindelli-Danesi, D., Teodori, L., Mauro, F., Modini, C., Botti, C., Cicconetti, F., and Stipa, S. (1987). Prognostic significance of flow cytometry in lung cancer: A 5-year study. *Cancer* 60:844–851.
109. Zimmerman, P. V., Hawson, G. A. T., Bint, M. H., and Parsons, P. G. (1987). Ploidy as a prognostic determinant in surgically treated lung cancer. *Lancet* 2:530–533.
110. Asamura, H., Nakajima, T., Mukai, K., and Shimosato, Y. (1989). Nuclear DNA content by cytofluorometry of stage 1 adenocarcinoma of the lung in relation to postoperative recurrence. *Chest* 96:312–318.
111. Miyamoto, H., Harada, M., Isobe, H., Akita, H. D., Haneda, H., Yamaguchi, E., Kuzumaki, N., and Kawakami, Y. (1991). Prognostic value of nuclear DNA content and expression of the ras oncogene product in lung cancer. *Cancer Res.* 51:6346–6350.
112. Whang-Peng, J., Bunna, P. A., Kao-Shan, C. S., Lee, E. C., Carney, D. N., Gazdar, A., and Minna, J. D. (1982). A nonrandom chromosomal abnormality, del 3p(14-23), in human small cell lung cancer (SCLC). *Cancer Genet. Cytogenet.* 6: 119–134.
113. Whang-Peng, J., Kao-Shan, C. S., Lee, E. C., Bunn, P. A., Carney, D. N., Gazdar, A. F., and Minna, J. D. (1982). Specific chromosome defect associated with human small-cell lung cancer: Deletion 3p(14-23). *Science* 215:181–182.
114. Wurster-Hill, D. H., Cannizzaro, L. A., Petengill, O. S., Sorenson, G. D., Cate, C. C., and Maurer, L. H. (1984). Cytogenetics of small cell carcinoma of the lung. *Cancer Genet. Cytogenet.* 13:303–330.
115. de Leij, L., Postmus, P. E., Buys, C. H. C. M., Elema, J., Ramaekers, F., Poppema, S., Brouwer, M., van der Veen, A. Y., Mesander, G., and The, T. H. (1985). Characterization of three new variant type cell lines derived from small cell carcinoma of the lung. *Cancer Res.* 45:6024–6033.
116. Falor, W. H., Ward-Skinner, R., and Wegryn, S. (1985). A 3p deletion in small cell lung carcinoma. *Cancer Genet. Cytogenet.* 16:175–177.
117. Whang-Peng, J., and Lee, E. C. (1985). Cytogenetics of human small cell lung cancer. *Recent Results Cancer Res.* 97:37.
118. Zech, L., Bergh, J., and Nilsson, K. (1985). Karotypic characterization of established cell lines and short-term cultures of human lung cancers. *Cancer Genet. Cytogenet.* 15:335.
119. Morstyn, G., Brown, J., Novak, U., Gardner, J., Bishop, J., and Garson, M. (1987). Heterogeneous cytogenetic abnormalities in small cell lung cancer cell lines. *Cancer Res.* 47:3322–3327.

120. Sozzi, G., Bertoglio, M. G., Borrello, M. G., Giani, S., Cilotti, S., Pierotti, M., and Della Porta, G. (1987). Chromosomal abnormalities in a primary small cell lung cancer. *Cancer Genet. Cytogenet.* 27:45–50.
121. Defusco, P. A., Frytak, S., Dahl, R. J., Weiland, L. H., Unni, K. K., and Dewald, G. W. (1989). Cytogenetic studies in 11 patients with small cell carcinoma of the lung. *Mayo Clin. Proc.* 64:168–176.
122. Brauch, H., Johnson, B., Hovis, J., Takahiko, Y., Gazdar, A., Pettengill, O. S., Graziano, S., Sorenson, G. D., Poiesz, B. J., Minna, J., Linehan, M., and Zbar, B. (1987). Molecular analysis of the short arm of chromosome 3 in small-cell and non-small-cell carcinoma of the lung. *N. Engl. J. Med.* 317:1109–1113.
123. Naylor, S. L., Johnson, B. E., Minna, J. D., and Sakaguchi, A. Y. (1987). Loss of heterozygosity of chromosome 3p markers in small cell lung cancer. *Nature* 329: 451–454.
124. Johnson, B. E., Sakaguchi, A. Y., Gazdar, A. F., Minna, J. D., Burch, D., Marshall, A., and Naylor, S. L. (1988). Restriction fragment length polymorphism studies show consistent loss of chromosome 3p alleles in small cell lung cancer patients' tumors. *J. Clin. Invest.* 82:502–507.
125. Miller, Y. E., Minna, J. D., and Gazdar, A. F. (1989). Lack of expression of aminoacylase-1 in small cell lung cancer. *J. Clin. Invest.* 83:2120–2124.
126. Kok, K., Osinga, J., Carritt, B., Davis, M. B., van der Hout, A. H., van der Veen, A. Y., Landsvater, R. M., de Leij, L. F. M. H., Berendsen, H. H., Postmus, P. E., Poppema, S., and Buys, C. H. C. M. (1987). Deletion of a DNA sequence at the chromosomal region 3p21 in all major types of lung cancer. *Nature* 330:578–581.
127. Grunberger, D., Perera, F. P., Mucha, J., Jaretzki, A., Carberry, D., Grimes, M., Mayer, J., and Weinstein, I. B. (1990). Restriction fragment length polymorphism of chromosome 3 (3p) and the epidermal growth factor receptor gene in human non-small cell lung carcinomas. *Cancer Lett.* 51:133–141.
128. Viegas-Pequignot, E., Flury-Herard, A., De Cremoux, H., Chlerq, C., Bignon, J., and Dutrillaux, B. (1990). Recurrent chromosome aberrations in human lung squamous cell carcinomas. *Cancer Genet. Cytogenet.* 49:37–49.
129. Fan, Y. S., and Li, P. (1987). Cytogenetic studies of four human lung adenocarcinoma cell lines. *Cancer Genet. Cytogenet.* 26:317–325.
130. Jin, Y., Mandahl, N., Heim, S., Schuller, H., and Mitelman, F. (1988). Isochromosomes i (8q) or i (9q) in three adenocarcinomas of the lung. *Cancer Genet. Cytogenet.* 33:11–17.
131. Buys, C. H. C. M., Kok, K., van der veen, A. Y., Carritt, B., Osinga, J., van der hout, A. H., Davis, M. B., De leij, L. F. M. H., Postmus, P. E., and Berendsen, H. H. (1988). A deletion at the short arm of chromosome 3 is common to all major types of lung cancer. *Lung Cancer* 4:121–127.
132. Zbar, B., Brauch, H., Talmadge, C., and Linehan, M. (1987). Loss of alleles of loci on the short arm of chromosome 3 in renal cell carcinoma. *Nature* 327:721–724.
133. Yokota, J., Wada, M., Shimosato, Y., Terada, M., and Sugimura, T. (1987). Loss of heterozygosity on chromosomes 3, 13, and 17 in small-cell carcinoma and on chromosome 3 in adenocarcinoma of the lung. *Proc. Natl. Acad. Sci.* 84:9252–9256.

134. Weston, A., Willey, J. C., Modali, R., Sugimura, H., McDowell, E. M., Resau, J., Light, B., Haugen, A., Mann, D. L., Trump, B. F., and Harris, C. C. (1989). Differential DNA sequence deletions from chromosomes 3, 11, 13, and 17 in squamous-cell carcinoma, large-cell carcinoma, and adenocarcinoma of the human lung. *Proc. Natl. Acad. Sci.* 86:5099–5103.
135. Skinner, M. A., Vollmer, R., Huper, G., Abbott, P., and Iglehart, J. D. (1990). Loss of heterozygosity for genes on 11p and the clinical course of patients with lung carcinoma. *Cancer Res.* 50:2303–2306.
136. Lee, J. S., Pathak, S., Hopwood, V., Tomasovic, B., Mullins, T. D., Baker, F. L., Spitzer, G., and Neidhart, J. A. (1987). Involvement of chromosome 7 in primary lung tumor and nonmalignant normal lung tissue. *Cancer Res.* 47:6349–6352.
137. Miura, I., Resau, J., Tomiyasu, T., and Testa, J. R. (1990). Isochromosome (8q) in four patients with adenocarcinoma of the lung. *Cancer Genet. Cytogenet.* 48:203–207.
138. Liang, J. C., Kurzrock, R., Gutterman, J. U., and Gallick, G. E. (1986). Trisomy 12 correlates with elevated expression of $p21^{ras}$ in a human adenosquamous carcinoma of the lung. *Cancer Genet. Cytogenet.* 23:183–188.
139. Yunis, J. J. (1983). The chromosomal basis of human neoplasia. *Science* 221:227–236.
140. Yunis, J. J., and Soreng, A. L. (1984). Constitutive fragile sites and cancer. *Science* 226:1199–1204.
141. Hecht, F., and Sutherland, G. R. (1984). Fragile sites and cancer breakpoints. *Cancer Genet. Cytogenet.* 12:179–181.
142. Kao-shan, C., Fine, R. L., Whang-Peng, J., Lee, E. C., and Chubner, B. A. (1987). Increased fragile sites and sister chromatid exchanges in bone marrow and peripheral blood of young cigarette smokers. *Cancer Res.* 47:6278–6282.
143. Liu, C., Wang, G., and Li, P. (1989). The expression frequency of common fragile sites and genetic susceptibility to lung cancers. *Cancer Genet. Cytogenet.* 42: 107–114.
144. Gordon, H. (1985). Oncogenes. *Mayo Clin. Proc.* 60:697–713.
145. Bishop, J. M. (1987). The molecular genetics of cancer. *Science* 235:305–311.
146. Friend, S. H., Dryja, T. P., and Weinberg, R. A. (1988). Oncogenes and tumor-suppressing genes. *N. Engl. J. Med.* 318:618–622.
147. Bishop, J. M. (1991). Molecular themes in oncogenesis. *Cell* 64:235–248.
148. Birrer, M. J., and Minna, J. D. (1988). Molecular genetics of lung cancer. *Semin. Oncol.* 15:226–235.
149. Birrer, M. J., and Minna, J. D. (1989). Genetic changes in the pathogenesis of lung cancer. *Ann. Rev. Med.* 40:305–317.
150. Minna, J. D. (1989). Genetic events in the pathogenesis of lung cancer. *Chest* 96: 17S–23S.
151. Slebos, R. J. C., and Rodenhuis, S. (1989). The molecular genetics of human lung cancer. *Eur. Respir. J.* 2:461–469.
152. Klein, G. (1987). The approaching era of the tumor suppressor genes. *Science* 238: 1539–1545.
153. Sager, R. (1989). Tumor suppressor genes: The puzzle and the promise. *Science* 246: 1406–1412.
154. Sikora K., and Ong, G. (1990). Cancer genes. *Thorax* 45:409–413.

155. Stanbridge, E. J. (1990). Human tumor suppressor genes. *Annu. Rev. Genet.* 24: 615–657.
156. Hollingsworth, R. E., and Lee, W. (1991). Tumor suppressor genes: New prospects for cancer research. *J. Natl. Cancer Inst.* 83:91–96.
157. Marshall, C. J. (1991). Tumor suppressor genes. *Cell* 64:313–326.
158. Zimmerman, K. A., Yancopoulos, G. D., Collum, R. G., Smith, R. K., Kohl, N. E., Denis, K. A., Nau, M. M., Witte, O. N., Toran-Allerand, D., Gee, C. E., Minna, J. D., and Alt, F. W. (1986). Differential expression of myc family genes during murine development. *Nature* 319:780–783.
159. Saksela, K. (1990). myc genes and their deregulation in lung cancer. *J. Cell Biochem.* 42:153–180.
160. Battey, J., Moulding, C., Taub, R., Murphy, W., Stewart, T., Potter, H., Lenoir, G., and Leder, P. (1983). The human c-myc oncogene: Structural consequences of translocation into the IgH locus in Burkitt lymphoma. *Cell* 34:779–787.
161. Nau, M. M., Brooks, B. J., Battey, J., Sausville, E., Gazdar, A. F., Kirsch, I. R., McBride, O. W., Bertness, V., Hollis, G. F., and Minna, J. D. (1985). L-myc, a new myc-related gene amplified and expressed in human small cell lung cancer. *Nature* 318:69–73.
162. Stanton, L. W., Schwab, M., and Bishop, J. M. (1986). Nucleotide sequence of the human N-myc gene. *Proc. Natl. Acad. Sci. USA* 83 1772–1776.
163. Krystal, G., Birrer, M., Way, J., Nau, M., Sausville, E., Thompson, C., Minna, J., and Battey, J. (1988). Multiple mechanisms for transcriptional regulation of the myc gene family in small-cell lung cancer. *Mol. Cell Biol.* 8:3373–3381.
164. Land, H. L., Parada, L., and Weinberg, R. (1983). Tumorigenic conversion of primary embryo fibroblast requires at least two cooperating oncogenes. *Nature* 304: 596–602.
165. Yancopoulos, G., Nisen, P., Tesfaye, A., Kohl, N., Goldfarb, M., and Alt, F. (1985). N-myc can cooperate with ras to transform normal cells in culture. *Proc. Natl. Acad. Sci. USA* 82:5455–5459.
166. Birrer, M. J., Segal, S., DeGreve, J., Kaye, F., Sausville, E. A., and Minna, J. D. (1988). L-myc cooperates with ras to transform primary rat embryo fibroblasts. *Mol. Cell Biol* 8:2668–2673.
167. Cole, M. (1986). The myc oncogene: Its role in transformation and differentiation. *Annu. Rev. Genet.* 20:361–384.
168. Little, C. D., Nau, M. M., Carney, D. N., Gazdar, A. F., and Minna, J. D. (1983). Amplification and expression of the c-myc oncogene in human lung cancer cell lines. *Nature* 306:194–196.
169. Carney, D. N., Gazdar, A. F., Bepler, G., Guccion, J. G., Marangos, P. J., Moody, T. W., Zweig, M. H., and Minna, J. D. (1985). Establishment and identification of small cell lung cancer cell lines having classic and variant features. *Cancer Res.* 45: 2913–2923.
170. Gazdar, A. F., Carney, D. N., Nau, M. M., and Minna, J. D. (1985). Characterization of variant subclasses of cell lines derived from small cell lung cancer having distinctive biochemical, morphological, and growth properties. *Cancer Res.* 45: 2924–2930.

171. Johnson, B. E., Battey, J., Linnoila, I., Becker, K. L., Makuch, R. W., Snider, R. H., Carney, D. N., and Minna, J. D. (1986). Changes in the phenotype of human small cell lung cancer cell lines after transfection and expression of the c-myc proto-oncogene. *J. Clin. Invest.* 78:525–532.
172. Nau, M. M., Carney, D. N., Battey, J., Johnson, B., Little, C., Gazdar, A., and Minna, J. D. (1984). Amplification, expression and rearrangement of c-myc and N-myc oncogenes in human lung cancer. *Curr. Top. Microbiol. Immunol.* 113: 172–177.
173. Saksela, K., Bergh, J., Lehto, V., Nilsson, K., and Alitalo, K. (1985). Amplification of the c-myc oncogene in a subpopulation of human small cell lung cancer. *Cancer Res.* 45:1823–1827.
174. Seifter, E. J., Sausville, E. A., and Battey, J. (1986). Comparison of amplified and unamplified c-myc gene structure and expression in human small cell lung carcinoma cell lines. *Cancer Res.* 46:2050–2055.
175. Yoshimoto, K., Hirohashi, S., and Sekiya, T. (1986). Increased expression of the c-myc gene without gene amplification in human lung cancer and colon cancer cell lines. *Jpn. J. Cancer* 77:540–545.
176. Kiefer, P. E., Bepler, G., Kubasch, M., and Haveman, K. (1987). Amplification and expression of protooncogenes in human small cell lung cancer cell lines. *Cancer Res.* 47:6236–6242.
177. Takahashi, T., Obuta, Y., Skido, Y., Hida, T., Ueda, R., Watanabe, H., Ariyoshi, Y., Sugiera, T., and Takahashi, T. (1989). Expression and amplification of myc gene family in small cell lung cancer and its relation to biological characteristics. *Cancer Res.* 49:2683–2688.
178. Brooks, B. J., Battey, J., Nau, M. M., Gazdar, A. F., and Minna, J. D. (1987). Amplification and expression of the myc gene in small-cell lung cancer. *Adv. Viral Oncol.* 7:155–172.
179. Wong, A. J., Ruppert, J. M., Eggleston, J., Hamilton, S. R., Baylin, S. B., and Vogelstein, B. (1986). Gene amplification of c-myc and N-myc in small cell carcinoma of the lung. *Science* 233:461–463.
180. Morstyn, G., Brown, J., Novak, U., Gardner, J., Bishop, J., and Garson, M. (1987). Heterogeneous cytogenetic abnormalities in small cell lung cancer cell lines. *Cancer Res.* 47:3322–3327.
181. Johnson, B. E., Inde, D. C., Makuch, R. W., Gazdar, A. F., Carney, D. N., Oie, H., Russell, E., Nau, M. M., and Minna, J. D. (1987). myc family oncogene amplification in tumor cell lines established from small cell lung cancer patients and its relationship to clinical status and course. *J. Clin. Invest.* 79:1629–1634.
182. Nau, M. M., Brooks, B. J., Carney, D. N., Gazdar, A. F., Battey, J. F., Sausville, E. A., and Minna, J. D. (1986). Human small-cell lung cancers show amplification and expression of the N-myc gene. *Proc. Natl. Acad. Sci. USA* 83:1092–1096.
183. Kawashima, K., Shikawa, H., Imoto, K., Izawa, M., Naruke, T., Okabayashi, K., and Nishimura, S. (1988). Close correlation between restriction fragment length polymorphism of the L-myc gene and metastasis of human lung cancer to the lymph nodes and other organs. *Proc. Natl. Acad. Sci. USA* 85:2353–2356.
184. Tamai, S., Sugimura, H., Caporaso, N. E., Resau, J. H., Trump, B. F., Weston, A.,

and Harris, C. C. (1990). Restriction fragment length polymorphism analysis of the L-myc gene locus in a case-control study of lung cancer. *Int. J. Cancer* 46:411–415.

185. Slebos, R. J. C., Evers, S. G., Wagenaar, S. S., and Rodenhuis, S. (1989). Cellular protooncogenes are infrequently amplified in untreated nonsmall cell lung cancer. *Br. J. Cancer* 59:76–80.

186. Barbacid, M. (1987). ras genes. *Annu. Rev. Biochem.* 56:779–827.

187. McGrath, J. P., Capon, D. J., Goeddel, D. V., and Levinson, A. D. (1984). Comparative biochemical properties of normal and activated human ras p21 protein. *Nature* 310:644–649.

188. Mabry, M., Nakagawa, T., Baylin, S., Pettengill, O., Sorenson, G., and Nelkin, B. (1989). Insertion of the v-Ha-ras oncogene induces differentiation of calcitonin-producing human small cell lung cancer. *J. Clin. Invest.* 84:194–199.

189. Mabry, M., Nakagawa, T., Nelkin, B. D., McDowell, E., Gesell, M., Eggleston, J. C., Casero, R. A., and Baylin, S. B. (1988). v-Ha-ras oncogene insertion: A model for tumor progression of human small cell lung cancer. *Proc. Natl. Acad. Sci. USA* 85:6523–6527.

190. Capon, D. J, Seeburgh, P. H., McGrath, J. P., Hayflick, J. S., Edman, U., Levinson, A. D., and Goeddel, D. V. (1983). Activation of Ki-ras 2 gene in human colon and lung carcinomas by two different point mutations. *Nature* 304:507–513.

191. Santos, E., Martin-Zanca, D., Reddy, E. P., Pierotti, M. A., Porta, G. D., and Barbacid, M. (1984). Malignant activation of a K-ras oncogene in lung carcinoma but not in normal tissue of the same patient. *Science* 223:661–664.

192. Nakano, H., Yamamotto, F., Neville, C., Evans, D., Mizuno, T., and Perucho, M. (1984). Isolation of transforming sequences of two human lung carcinomas. Structural and functional analysis of the activated c-k-ras oncogenes. *Proc. Natl. Acad. Sci. USA* 81:71–75.

193. Heighway, J., and Hasleton, P. S. (1986). c-ki-ras amplification in human lung cancer. *Br. J. Cancer* 53:285–287.

194. Rodenhuis, D., van de Wetering, M. L., Mooi, W. J., Evers, S. G., van Zandwijk, N., and Bos, J. L. (1987). Mutational activation of the K-ras oncogene. A possible pathogenic factor in adenocarcinoma of the lung. *N. Engl. J. Med.* 317:929–935.

195. Rodenhuis, S., Slebos, R. J. C., Boot, A. J. M., Evers, S. G., Mooi, W. J., Wagenaar, S. S., van Bodegom, P. C., and Bos, J. L. (1988). Incidence and possible clinical significance of K-ras oncogene activation in adenocarcinoma of the human lung. *Cancer Res.* 48:5738–5741.

196. Slebos, R. J. C., Kibbelaar, R. E., Dalesio, O, Kooistra, A., Stam, J., Meijer, C. J. L. M., Wagenaar, S. S., Vanderschueren, R. G. J. R. A., van Zandwijk, N., Mooi, W. J., Bos, J. L., and Rodenhuis, S. (1990). K-ras oncogene activation as a prognostic marker in adenocarcinoma of the lung. *N. Engl. J. Med.* 323:561–565.

197. Slebos, R. J. C., Hruban, R. H., Dalesio, O., Mooi, W. J., Offerhaus, G. J. A., and Rodenhuis, S. (1991). Relationship between k-ras oncogene activation and smoking in adenocarcinoma of the human lung. *J. Natl. Cancer Inst.* 83:1024–1027.

198. Heighway, J., Thatcher, N., Cerny, T., and Hasleton, P. S. (1986). Genetic predisposition to human lung cancer. *Br. J. Cancer* 53:453–457.

199. Sugimura, H., Caporaso, N. E., Modali, R. V., Hoover, R. N., Resau, J. H., Trump,

B. F., Lonergan, J. A., Krontiris, T. G., Mann, D. L., Weston, A., and Harris, C. C. (1990). Association of rare alleles of the Harvey ras protooncogene locus with lung cancer. *Cancer Res.* 50:1857–1862.

200. Shiraishi, M., Morinaga, S., Noguchi, M., Shimosato, Y., and Sekiya, T. (1987). Loss of genes on the short arm of chromosome 11 in human lung carcinomas. *Jpn. J. Cancer* 78:1302–1308.

201. Reeve, A., Housiaux, R., Gardner, R., Chewings, W., Grindley, R., and Millow, L. (1984). Loss of a harvey ras allele in sporadic Wilms' tumor. *Nature* 309:174–176.

202. Imer, J., and Wasylyk, B. (1989). AP-1, a composite transcription factor implicated in abnormal growth control. *Prog. Growth Factor Res.* 1:69–77.

203. Bohmann, D., Bos, T., Admon, A., Nishimura, T., Vogt, P., and Tijan, R. (1987). Human protooncogene c-jun encodes a DNA binding protein with structural and functional properties of transcription factor AP-1. *Science* 238:1386–1392.

204. Haluska, F., Huebner, K., Isobe, M., Nishimura, T., Croce, C., and Vogt, P. (1988). Localization of the human JUN protooncogene to chromosome region 1p31-32. *Proc. Natl. Acad. Sci. USA* 85:2215–2218.

205. Schutte, J., Minna, J., and Birrer, M. (1989). Deregulated expression of human c-jun transforms primary rat embryo cells in cooperation with an activated c-HA-ras gene and transforms Rat-la cells as a single gene. *Proc. Natl. Acad. Sci. USA* 86:2257–2261.

206. Schütte, J., Nau, M., Birrer, M., Thomas, F., Gazdar, A., and Minna, J. D. (1988). Constitutive expression of multiple mRNA forms of the c-jun oncogene in human lung cancer cell lines. *Proc. Am. Assoc. Cancer Res.* 29:455.

207. Rapp, U. R., Goldsborough, M. D., Mark, G. E., Bonner, T. I., Groffen, J., Reynolds, F. H., and Stephenson, J. R. (1983). Structure and biological activity of v-raf, a unique oncogene transduced by a retrovirus. *Proc. Natl. Acad. Sci. USA* 80:4218–4222.

208. Havemann, K., Kiefer, P., Haeder, M., Hartough, G., Heimann, B., Moelling, K., and Bepler, G. (1988). Oncogene expression in the spectrum of pulmonary carcinoma. *Lung Cancer* 4:155–161.

209. Rapp, U. R., Huleihel, M., Dawson, T., Linnoila, I., Minna, J. D., Heidecker, G., Cleveland, J. L., Beck, T., Forchhammer, J., and Storm, S. M. (1988). Role of raf oncogenes in lung carcinogenesis. *Lung Cancer* 4:162–167.

210. Bonner, T., O'Brien, S. J., Nash, W. G., Rapp, U. R., Morton, C. C., and Leder, P. (1984). The human homologs of the raf (mil) oncogene are located on human chromosomes 3 and 4. *Science* 223:71–74.

211. Sithanandum, G., Heidecker, G., Beck, T., Minna, J. D., Zbar, B., and Rapp, U. R. (1989). Loss of heterozygosity at the c-raf-1 locus and analysis of c-raf protein in small-cell lung carcinoma. *Mol. Diagn. Hum. Cancer* 7:171–175.

212. Pfeifer, A. M. A., Mark, G. E., Malan-Shibley, L., Graziano, S., Amstad, P., and Harris, C. C. (1989). Cooperation of c-raf-1 and c-myc protooncogenes in the neoplastic transformation of simian virus 40 large tumor antigen-immortalized human bronchial epithelial cells. *Proc. Natl. Acad. Sci. USA* 86:10075–10079.

213. Pfeifer, A. M. A., Jones, R. T., Bowden, P. E., Mann, D. Spillare, E., Klein-Szanto, A. J. P., Trump, B. F., and Harris, C. C. (1991). Human bronchial epithelial cells

transformed by the c-raf-1 and c-myc protooncogenes induce multidifferentiated carcinomas in nude mice: A model for lung carcinogenesis. *Cancer Res.* 51:3793–3801.

214. Reddel, R. R., Ke, Y., Kaighn, E., Malan-Shibley, L., Lechner, J. F., Rhim, J. S., and Harris, C. C. (1988). Human bronchial epithelial cells neoplastically transformed by v-ki-ras: Altered response to inducers of terminal squamous differentiation. *Oncogene Res.* 3:401–408.

215. Amstad, P., Reddel, R. R., Pfeifer, A., Malan-Shibley, L., Mark, G. E., and Harris, C. C. (1988). Neoplastic transformation of a human bronchial epithelium cell line by a recombinant retrovirus encoding viral harvey ras. *Mol. Carcinog.* 1:151.

216. Griffin, C. A., and Baylin, S. B. (1985). Expression of the c-myb oncogene in human small cell lung carcinoma. *Cancer Res.* 45:272–275.

217. Cline, M. J., and Battifora, H. (1987). Abnormalities of protooncogenes in non-small cell lung cancer. Correlations with tumor type and clinical characteristics. *Cancer* 60:2669–2674.

218. Sakiyama, S., Nakamura, Y., and Yasuda, S. (1986). Expression of epidermal growth factor receptor gene in cultured human lung cancer cells. *Jpn. J. Cancer Res.* 77:965–969.

219. Shiraishi, M., Noguchi, M., Shimosato, Y., and Sekiya, T. (1989). Amplification of protooncogenes in surgical specimens of human lung carcinomas. *Cancer Res.* 49: 6474–6479.

220. Coussens, L., Yan-Feng, T. L., Chen, Y. L. E., Gray, A., McGrath, J., Seeburg, P. H., Libermann, T. A., Schlessinger, J., Franke, U., Levinson, A., and Ullrich, A. (1985) Tyrosine kinase receptor with extensive homology to EGF receptor shares chromosomal location with neu oncogene. *Science* 230:1132–1139.

221. Bargmann, C. I., Hung, M. C., and Weinberg, R. A. (1986). The neu oncogene encodes an epidermal growth factor receptor related protein. *Nature* 319:226–230.

222. Kern, J. A., Schwartz, D. A., Nordberg, J. E., Weiner, D. B., Greene, M. I., Torney, L., and Robinson, R. A. (1990). $p185^{neu}$ expression in human lung adenocarcinoma predicts shortened survival. *Cancer Res.* 50:5184–5191.

223. Schneider, P. M., Hung, M., Chiocca, S. M., Manning, J., Zhao, X., Fang, K., and Roth, J. A. (1989). Differential expression of the c-erbβ-2 gene in human small cell and non-small cell lung cancer. *Cancer Res.* 49:4968–4971

224. Knudson, A. G., Meadows, A. T., Nichols, W. W., and Hill, R. (1976). Chromosomal deletion and retinoblastoma. *N. Engl. J. Med.* 295:1120–1123.

225. Benedict, W. F., Murphree, A. L., Banerjee, A., Spina, C. A., Sparkes, M. C., and Sparkes, R. S. (1983). Patient with 13 chromosome detection: Evidence that the retinoblastoma gene is a recessive cancer gene. *Science* 219:973–975.

226. Fung, Y., Murphree, A. L., T'Ang, A., Qian, J., Hinrichs, S. H., and Benedict, W. F. (1987). Structural evidence for the authenticity of the human retinoblastoma susceptibility gene. *Science* 236:1657.

227. Lee, W. H., Bookstein, R., Hong, F., Young, L., Shew, J., and Lee, E. (1987). Human retinoblastoma susceptibility gene: cloning, identification, and sequence. *Science* 235:1394.

228. Francke, U. (1976). Retinoblastoma and chromosome 13. *Cytogenet. Cell Genet.* 16:131–134.

229. Sparkes, R. S., Sparkes, M. C., Wilson, M. G., Towner, J. W., Benedict, W. F., Murphree, A. L., and Yunis, J. J. (1980). Regional assignment of genes for human esterase D and retinoblastoma to chromosome band 13q14. *Science* 208:1042–1044.
230. Friend, S. H., Bernards, R., Rogelj, S., Weinberg, R. A., Rapaport, J. M., Albert, D. M., and Dryja, T. P. (1986). A human DNA segment with properties of the gene that predisposes to retinoblastoma and osteosarcoma. *Nature* 323:643–646.
231. Huang, H. S., Yee, J., Shew, J., Chen, P., Bookstein, R., Friedmann, T., Lee, E. Y. P., and Lee, W. (1988). Suppression of the neoplastic phenotype by replacement of the rb gene in human cancer cells. *Science* 242:1563–1566.
232. Harbour, J. W., Lai, S., Whang-Peng, J., Gazdar, A. F., Minna, J. D., and Kaye, F. J. (1988). Abnormalities in structure and expression of the human retinoblastoma gene in SCLC. *Science* 241:353–357.
233. Horowitz, J., Park, S., Bogenmann, E., Cheng, J., Yandell, D. W., Kaye, F. J., Minna, J. D., Dryja, T. P., and Weinberg, R. A. (1990). Frequent inactivation of the retinoblastoma anti-oncogene is restricted to a subset of human tumor cells. *Proc. Natl. Acad. Sci. USA* 87:2775–2779.
234. Yokota, J., Akiyama, T., Fung, Y. T., Benedict, W. F., Namba, Y., Hanaoka, M., Wada, M., Terasaki, T., Shimosato, Y., Sugimura, T., and Terada, M. (1988). Altered expression of the retinoblastoma (RB) gene in small-cell carcinoma of the lung. *Oncogene* 3:471–475.
235. Hensel, C. H., Hsieh, C., Gazdar, A. F., Johnson, B. E., Sakaguchi, A. Y., Naylor, S. L., Lee, W., and Lee E. Y. P. (1990). Altered structure and expression of the human retinoblastoma susceptibility gene in small cell lung cancer. *Cancer Res.* 50: 3067–3072.
236. Rygaard, K., Sorenson, G. D., Pettengill, O. S., Cate, C. C., Spang-Thomsen, M. (1990). Abnormalities in structure and expression of the retinoblastoma gene in small cell lung cancer cell lines and xenografts in nude mice. *Cancer Res.* 50:5312–5317.
237. Miller, C., Mohandas, T., Wolf, D., Prokocimer, M., Rotter, V., Phillip Koeffler, H. (1986). Human p53 gene localized to short arm of chromosome 17. *Nature* 319: 783–784.
238. Parada, L. F., Land, H., Weinberg, R. A., Wolf, D., and Rotter, W. (1984). Cooperation between gene encoding p53 tumour antigen and ras in cellular transformation. *Nature* 312:649–651.
239. Eliyahu, D., Raz, A., Gruss, P., Givol, D., and Oren, M. (1984). Participation of p53 cellular tumour antigen in transformation of normal embryonic cells. *Nature* 312: 646–649.
240. Finlay, C. A., Hinds, P. W., and Levine, A. J. (1989). The p53 proto-oncogene can act as a suppressor of transformation. *Cell* 57:1083–1093.
241. Baker, J. J., Markowitz, S., Feuron, E. R., Wilson, J. K. U., and Vogelstein, B. (1990). Suppression of human colorectal carcinoma cell growth by wild-type p53. *Science* 249:912–915.
242. Chen, P., Chen, Y., Bookstein, R., and Lee, W. (1990). Genetic mechanisms of tumor suppression by the human p53 gene. *Science* 250:1576–1580.

243. Lane, D. P., and Benchimol, S. (1990). p53: Oncogene or anti-oncogene? *Genes Develop.* 4:1–8.
244. Levin, A. J., Momand, J., Finlay, C. A. (1991). The p53 tumour suppressor gene. *Nature* 351:453–456.
245. Lane, D. P., and Crawford, L. V. (1979). T antigen is bound to a host protein in SV40-transformed cells. *Nature* 278:261–263.
246. Linzer, D. J. H., and Levine, A. J. (1979). Characterization of a 54k dalton cellular SV40 tumor antigen present in SV40-transformed cells and uninfected embryonal carcinoma cells. *Cell* 17:43–52.
247. Takahashi, T., Nau, M. N., Chiba, I., Birrer, M. J., Rosenberg, R. K., Vinocour, M., Levitt, M., Pass, H., Gazdar, A. F., and Minna, J. D. (1989). p53: A frequent target for genetic abnormalities in lung cancer. *Science* 246:491–494.
248. Chiba, I., Takahashi, T., Nau, M. N., D'Amico, D., Cariel, D. T., Mitsudomi, T., Buchhagen, D. L., Carbone, D., Piantadosi, S., Koga, H., Reissman, P. T., Salmon, D. J., Carmack Holmes, E., and Minna, J. D. (1990). Mutations in the p53 gene are frequent in primary, resected non-small cell lung cancer. *Oncogene* 5:1603–1610.
249. Nigro, J. M., Baker, S. J., Preisinger, A. C., Miburn, Jessup, J., Hostetler, R., Cleary, K., Bigner, S. H., Davidson, N., Baylin, S., Devilee, P., Glover, T., Collins, F. S., Weston, A., Modali, R., Harris, C. C., and Vogelstein, B. (1989). Mutations in the p53 gene occur in diverse human tumour types. *Nature* 342:705–708.
250. Takahashi, T., D'Amico, D., Chiba, I., Buchhagen, D. L., and Minna, J. D. (1990). Identification of intronic point mutations as an alternative mechanism for p53 inactivation in lung cancer. *J. Clin. Invest.* 86:363–369.
251. Hollstein, M., Sidransky, D., Vogelstein, B., Harris, C. C. (1991). p53 mutations in human cancers. *Science* 253:49–53.
252. Lehman, T. A., Bennett, W. P., Metcalf, R. A., Welsh, J. A., Ecker, J., Modali, R. V., Ullrich, S., Romano, J. W., Appella, E., Testa, J. R., Gerwin, B. I., and Harris, C. C. (1991). p53 mutations, ras mutations, and p53-heat shock 70 protein complexes in human lung carcinoma cell lines. *Cancer Res.* 51:4090–4096.
253. LaForgia, S., Morse, B., Levy, J., Barnea, G., Cannizzaro, L. A., Li, F., Nowell, P. C., Boghosian-sell, L., Glick, J., Weston, A., Harris, C. C., Drabkin, H., Patterson, D., Croce, C. M., Schlessinger, J., and Huebner, K. (1991). Receptor protein-tyrosine phosphatase γ is a candidate tumor suppressor gene at human chromosome region 3p21. *Proc. Natl. Acad. Sci. USA* 88:5036–5040.
254. Hunter, T. (1989). Protein-tyrosine phosphatases: The other side of the coin. *Cell* 58:1013–1016.
255. Fischer, E. H., Charbonneau, H., and Tonks, N. K. (1991). Protein tyrosine phosphatases: A diverse family of intracellular and transmembrane enzymes. *Science* 253:401–406.
256. Weinberger, C., Thompson, C. C., Ong, E. S., Lebo, R., Gruol, D. J., and Evans, R. M. (1986). The c-erb-A gene encodes a thyroid hormone receptor. *Nature* 324: 641–646.
257. Dobrovic, A., Houle, B., Belouchi, A., and Bradley, W. E. C (1988). erb-A-related sequence coding for DNA-binding hormone receptor localized to chromosome 3p21-3p25 and deleted in small cell lung carcinoma. *Cancer Res.* 48:682–685.

258. Drabkin, H., Kao, F., Hartz, J., Hart, I., Gazdar, A., Weinberger, C., Evans, R., and Gerber, M. (1988). Localization of human ERBA2 to the 3p21→3p24.1 region of chromosome 3 and variable deletion in small cell lung cancer. *Proc. Natl. Acad. Sci. USA* 85:9258–9262.
259. de The, H., Marchio, A., Tiollais, P., and Dejean, A. (1987). A novel steroid thyroid hormone receptor-related gene inappropriately expressed in human hepatocellular carcinoma. *Nature* 330:667–670.
260. Haber, D. A., Buckler, A. J., Glaser, T., Call, K. M., Pelletier, J., Sohn, R. L., Douglass, E. C., and Housman, D. E. (1990). An internal deletion within a 11p13 zincfinger gene contributes to the development of Wilms' tumor. *Cell* 61:1257–1269.
261. Marshall, C. J. (1991). Tumor suppressor genes. *Cell* 64:313–326.
262. Sporn, M. B., and Roberts, A. B. (1985). Autocrine growth factors and cancer. *Nature* 313:745–747.
263. Walsh, J. H., Karnes, W. E., Cuttitta, F., and Walker, A. (1991). Autocrine growth factors and solid tumor malignancy. *West. J. Med.* 155:152–163.
264. Simms, E., Gazdar, A. F., Abrams, P. G., and Minna, J. D. (1980). Growth of human small cell (oat cell) carcinoma of the lung in serum-free growth factor-supplemented medium. *Cancer Res.* 40:4356–4363.
265. Carney, D. N., Bunn, P. A., Gazdar, A. F., Pagan, J. A., and Minna, J. D. (1981). Selective growth in serum free hormone-supplemented medium of tumor cells obtained by biopsy from patients with small cell carcinoma of the lung. *Proc. Natl. Acad. Sci. USA* 78:3185–3189.
266. Moody, T. W., Pert, C. B., Gazdar, A. F., Carney, D. N., and Minna, J. D. (1981). High levels of intracellular bombesin characterize human small-cell lung carcinoma. *Science* 241:1246–1248.
267. Sherwin, S. A., Minna, J. D., Gazdar, A. F., and Todoro, G. J. (1981). Expression of epidermal and nerve growth factor receptors and soft agar growth factor production by human lung cancer cells. *Cancer Res.* 41:3538–3542.
268. Erisman, M. D., Linnoila, R. I., Hernandez, O., Di Augustine, R. P., and Lazarus, L. H. (1982). Human lung small-cell carcinoma contains bombesin. *Proc. Natl. Acad. Sci. USA* 79:2379–2383.
269. Cuttitta, F., Carney, D. N., Mulshine, J., Moody, T. W., Fedorko, J., Fischler, A., and Minna, J. D. (1985). Bombesin-like peptides can function as autocrine growth factors in human small-cell lung cancer. *Nature* 316:823–826.
270. Sausville, E. A., Lebacq-Verheyden, A., Spindel, E. R., Cuttitta, F., Gazdar, A. F., and Battey, J. F. (1986). Expression of the gastrin-releasing peptide gene in human small cell lung cancer. *J. Biol. Chem.* 261:2451–2457.
271. Carney, D. N., Cuttitta, F., Moody, T. W., and Minna, J. D. (1987). Selective stimulation of small cell lung cancer clonal growth by bombesin and gastrin-releasing peptide. *Cancer Res.* 47:821–825.
272. Moody, T. W., Carney, D. N., Cuttitta, F., Quattrocchi, K., and Minna, J. D. (1985). High affinity receptors for bombesin/GRP-like peptides on human small cell lung cancer. *Life Sci.* 37:105–113.
273. Weber, S., Zuckerman, J. E., Bostwick, D. G., Bensch, K. G., Sikic, B. I., and

Raffin, T. A. (1985). Gastrin releasing peptide is a selective mitogen for small cell lung carcinoma in vitro. *J. Clin. Invest.* 75:306–309.

274. Minna, J. D., Battey, J. F., Brooks, B. J., Cuttitta, F., Gazdar, A. F., Johnson, B. E., Ihde, D. C., Lebacq-Verheyden, A., Mulshine, J., Nau, M. M., Oie, H. K., Sausville, E. A., Seifter, E., and Vinocour, M. (1986). Molecular genetic analysis reveals chromosomal deletion, gene amplification, and autocrine growth factor production in the pathogenesis of human lung cancer. *Cold Spring Harbor Symp. Quant. Biol.* LI:843–853.
275. Gaudino, G., Cirillo, D., Naldini, L, Rossino, P., and Comoglio, P. M. (1988). Activation of the protein-tyrosine kinase associated with the bombesin receptor complex in small cell lung carcinoma. *Proc. Natl. Acad. Sci. USA* 85:2166–2170.
276. Hirsch, F. R., Holst, J. J., Spang-Thomsen, M., and Larsson, L. (1990). Immunocytochemical demonstration of bombesin immunoreactivity in small cell carcinoma of the lung. A methodological study and review of the literature. *Lung Cancer* 6: 1–8.
277. Aguayo, S., Kane, M., Schwarz, M., King, T., Grauer, L., Dienhart, D., Bunn, P. A., and Miller Y. E. (1987). Bombesin like immunoreactivity in bronchoalveolar lavage from smokers and interstitial lung disease. *Clin. Res.* 35:530A.
278. Willey, J., Lechner, J., and Harris, C. C. (1984). Bombesin and the C-terminal tetradecapeptide of gastrin-releasing peptide are growth factors for normal human bronchial epithelial cells. *Exp. Cell Res.* 153:245–248.
279. Gusterson, B., Cowley, G., Smith, J. A., and Ozanne, B. (1984). Cellular localisation of human epidermal growth factor receptor. *Cell Biol. Int. Rep.* 8:649.
280. Kasselberg, A. G., Orth, D. N., Gray, M. E., and Stahlmann, M. T. (1985). Immunocytochemical localisation of human epidermal growth factor/urogastrone in several human tissues. *J. Histochem. Cytochem.* 33:315.
281. Cerny, T., Barnes, D. M., Hasleton, P., Barber, P. V., Healy, K., Gullick, W., and Thatcher, N. (1986). Expression of epidermal growth factor receptor (EGF-R) in human lung tumours. *Br. J. Cancer.* 54:265–269.
282. Hendler, F. J., and Ozanne, B. W. (1984). Human squamous cell lung cancers express increased epidermal growth factor receptors. *J. Clin. Invest.* 74:647–651.
283. Gamou, S., Hunts, J., Harigai, H., Hirohashi, S., Shimosato, Y., Pastan, I., and Shimuzu, N. (1987). Molecular evidence for the lack of epidermal growth factor receptor gene expression in small cell lung carcinoma cells. *Cancer Res.* 47:2668–2673.
284. Dazzi, H., Hasleton, P. S., Thatcher, N., Barnes, D M., Wilkes, S., Swindell, R., and Lawson, R. A. M. (1989). Expression of epidermal growth factor receptor (EGF-R) in non-small cell lung cancer. Use of archival tissue and correlation of EGF-R with histology, tumor size, node status and survival. *Br. J. Cancer* 59: 746–749.
285. Betsholtz, C., Bergh, J., Bywater, M., Pettersson, M., Johnsson, A., Heldin, C., Ohlsson, R., Knott, T. J., Scott, J., Bell, G. I., and Westermark, B. (1987). Expression of multiple growth factors in human lung cancer cell line. *Int. J. Cancer* 39:502–507.

286. Nakanishi, Y., Mulshine, J. L., Kasprzyk, P. G., Natale, R. B., Maneckjee, R., Avis, I., Treston, A. M., Gazdar, A. F., Minna, J. D., and Cuttitta, F. (1988). Insulin-like growth factor-1 can mediate autocrine proliferation of human small cell lung cancer cell line in vitro. *J. Clin. Invest.* 82:354–359.
287. Vostrejs, M., Moran, P. L., and Seligman, P. A. (1988). Transferrin synthesis by small cell lung cancer acts as an autocrine regulator of cellular proliferation. *J. Clin. Invest.* 82:331–339.
288. Bliss, D. P., Battey, J. F., Linnoila, R. I., Birrer, M. J., Gazdar, A. F., and Johnson, B. E. (1990). Expression of the atrial nutriuretic factor gene in small cell lung cancer tumors and tumor cell lines. *J. Natl. Cancer Inst.* 82:305–310.
289. Maneckjee, R., and Minna, J. D. (1990). Opioid and nicotine receptors affect growth regulation of human lung cancer cell lines. *Proc. Natl. Acad. Sci. USA* 87:3294–3298.
290. Avis, I. L., Kovacs, T. O. G., Kasprzyk, P. G., Treston, A. M., Bartholomew, R., Walsh, J. H., Cuttitta, F., and Mulshine, J. L. (1991). Preclinical evaluation of an antiautocrine growth factor monoclonal antibody for treatment of patients with small-cell lung cancer. *J. Natl. Cancer Inst.* 83:1470–1476.
291. Sager, R. (1986). Genetic suppression of tumor formation: A new frontier in cancer research. *Cancer Res.* 46:1573–1580.

15

Other Host Factors and Lung Cancer Susceptibility

MELVYN S. TOCKMAN

The Johns Hopkins University School of Hygiene and Public Health
Baltimore, Maryland

Altered susceptibility marks the potential for an accentuated host response (29), whereby subgroups of otherwise similarly exposed individuals show an enhanced probability of disease (e.g., lung cancer). Sometimes the altered susceptibility is inborn. Most genetic abnormalities associated with human lung cancer, however, are somatic mutations acquired by the cells of the pulmonary epithelium. Nevertheless, several lines of evidence are suggestive of an inborn predisposition to lung cancer (43). First-degree relatives of lung cancer patients are found to have a 2.4-fold risk of developing lung cancer, independent of personal cigarette smoking habits (49). Inheritance of a recessive tumor-suppressor gene heterozygosity at 11p has been associated with non–small-cell lung cancer (23). Certain metabolic phenotypes may enhance cytochrome pathway oxidation of procarcinogen metabolites (8) or modify the repair rate of injured (i.e., adducted) DNA (6). Other signs of altered host susceptibility are less clearly genetic. Reports linking lung cancer susceptibility to fibrotic and chronic obstructive pulmonary disease (COPD) have appeared in the literature with increasing frequency. This chapter will explore some of the experimental and epidemiological studies that suggest that these host factors and their underlying mechanisms contribute to the risk for lung cancer.

I. Inflammation/Scarring and Growth Factor Expression

Hogg has proposed reclassifying interstitial lung disease based upon the cause of the inflammatory fibrotic reaction (25). Three pathogenetic categories are included in his proposed classification; the first two are fibrotic reactions due to (nongranulomatous and granulomatous) chronic inflammatory responses, while the third comprises a local fibrotic reaction to neoplastic cells. Both nongranulomatous and granulomatous fibrotic reactions in the pulmonary parenchyma have been reported to show an increased association with lung cancer and will be discussed below. Fibrosis of the parenchymal interstitium is most likely to be associated with the development of adenomatous malignant changes resulting from proliferation of alveolar Type II pneumocytes (58). This contrasts with the inflammatory response of the epithelium lining the larger bronchi, which is more likely to undergo squamous metaplasia. Hogg's third category of interstitial lung disease, attributed to the neoplastic process, credits the desmoplastic reaction within the interstitial space to the proliferation of neoplastic cells (25). The possibility of common proliferation mechanisms between inflammatory and neoplastic responses becomes comprehensible after considering some of the recent laboratory observations (described below).

A. Epidemiological Studies

Silicosis

Occupational exposure to crystalline silica increasingly has been linked to elevation of human lung cancer risk in studies from around the world (1,9,34,37, 41,42,50,65). Yet, substantial methodological limitations of these studies have led reviewers to conclude that data demonstrating a definite causal link are not yet available (1,50). While laboratory data provide a plausible mechanism for linkage of fibrosis and lung cancer, epidemiological data suggest that if it exists, the excess lung cancer risk associated with crystalline silica exposure is small (risk ratio of approximately 2.0), and crystalline silica shows far greater potential to cause lung fibrosis than to induce lung cancer.

In 1982, two reports suggested that there may be an excess lung cancer risk among silicotics (16,17). The following year, the International Agency for Research on Cancer (IARC) convened a meeting of investigators with the goal of "coordinating studies to improve understanding of the potential carcinogenic risk from exposure to silica, with particular attention being paid to exposure to silica in the working environment in the absence of other agents known to be carcinogenic for the lung" (30). The results of these studies were assembled into a monograph by IARC in 1989–90 to communicate the state of the epidemiological information linking silica dust exposure with lung cancer risk. Introducing the IARC volume, Simonato and Saracci report (56):

> Our present knowledge of the potential carcinogenic effect of silica dust is characterized by three main findings: (i) silica is carcinogenic in experimental systems (30); (ii) lung cancer risk is increased among workers exposed to silica and not exclusively among those exposed to known carcinogens; (iii) when investigated separately, the lung cancer risk is concentrated among the subpopulation of exposed workers who develop silicosis.

Additional reports have continued to appear following the IARC monograph. Attempting to avoid confounding from other carcinogenic exposures (e.g., cigarette smoking and known occupational carcinogens), Amandus and Costello estimated the lung cancer mortality risks of 9912 white male metal ore miners (369 silicotics and 9543 nonsilicotics) interviewed and radiographed during employment between 1959–61 at 38 U.S. underground mines and followed from 1959 and 1975 (1). They observed a nonsignificant trend toward excess lung cancer mortality in silicotics compared to nonsilicotics after cigarette smoking habit, years spent underground, and low radon exposure had been considered.

In Koskela's study (34), the standardized lung cancer mortality of granite workers was 1.56–2.26 times greater than that of the general population. This cohort of Finnish granite workers, identified between 1940 and 1971 and followed through 1985, had been exposed to "pure" silica, with no significant exposure to radon, asbestos, or polycyclic aromatic hydrocarbons. Smoking data were available for 75%. Yet while sufficient periods of exposure and follow-up were observed for both silicosis and lung cancer to have developed, only three patients with cancer also had pulmonary silicosis.

In the Mehnert et al. study of slate quarry workers (41), the study population demonstrated an elevated mortality from nonmalignant respiratory diseases, primarily silicosis. The standardized lung cancer mortality among silicotics was somewhat greater than among nonsilicotics, but the confidence interval of neither group excluded a chance association. While the data are consistent with a fibrosis-induced amplification of lung cancer risk, the excess lung cancer among silicotics in this study might have been confounded by higher levels of exposure and a lack of information on smoking.

Lagorio et al. (37) conducted a case-referent study of ceramic workers, exposed to "pure" silica dust in the manufacture of sanitary ware and crockery. In this study, 72 lung cancer deaths (validated from hospital records) and 319 referents (matched by age at death and year of death) were drawn from the 1968–1984 municipal registries of a small Italian town in which a high proportion of the male population was employed in the ceramic industry. Silicotics were identified from the records of the Italian Institute for Compensation for Occupational Diseases. Work and smoking histories were obtained from next-of-kin interviews. The Mantel-Haenszel rate ratio among silicotics (3.9, 95% CI = 1.8–8.3) significantly exceeded that among nonsilicotic ceramic workers (1.4, 95% CI = 0.7–2.8). Yet, while the overall excess lung cancer risk among silicotics was significant, all of this excess was due to the cigarette smoking silicotics; no lung cancer excess was present among nonsmoking silicotics.

In their extensive review, Pairon et al. of Inserm (50) separately summarized epidemiological studies which, according to their authors, showed a carcinogenic (positive) effect of silica and those which did not. These reviewers identified 19 positive studies, of which 7 specifically reported an excess lung cancer risk among silicotic participants, and 18 negative studies, 5 of which found no excess lung cancer risk among silicotics patients. This review summarized the present uncertainty by an equivocal conclusion (50):

> In our opinion, studies published to date do not justify the classification of BPC (bronchopulmonary cancer) as an occupational disease linked to silica exposure. On the other hand, patients suffering from pneumoconiosis are probably at an increased risk of BPC, even if exposure to silica is not the only aetiological factor.

Asbestosis

Kipen et al. (33) note that the first reports of an association of asbestosis and lung cancer date from 1935. Subsequently, Doll found that asbestos-exposed workers who developed interstitial fibrosis (asbestosis) more frequently went on to develop lung cancer than those who did not (15). Since that time, additional studies have supported the consideration that development of interstitial fibrosis is a necessary step in the development of asbestos-related pulmonary cancers; i.e., they are scar carcinomas. In one of the early reports to describe the clinical/pathological presentation of asbestos-related lung cancer, Kannerstein and Churg (31) describe the predominance of asbestos-related cancer in the lower lobes, similar to the location of the interstitial fibrosis of asbestosis rather than the upper lobes of cigarette-associated lung cancer (7). Further, the increased proportion of adenocarcinoma associated with asbestos exposure may be related to the proliferation of Type II pneumocytes in the parenchyma, rather than the squamous metaplasia of the more proximal bronchi.

As part of their continuing cohort mortality study of 17,800 members of the insulation workers' union (International Association of Heat and Frost Insulators and Asbestos Workers, AFL-CIO, CLC), Kipen et al. examined 138 cases (of 450 pathologically confirmed lung cancer deaths) with adequate radiographs and nonmalignant pulmonary tissue to assess the presence or absence of diffuse interstitial pulmonary fibrosis (33). These investigators found that parenchymal fibrosis was present in all those with lung cancer whose pulmonary tissues were microscopically examined. Newhouse et al. found that among a British cohort of asbestos textile workers and laggers. 90% of those who died with lung cancer had histological evidence of asbestosis (48).

Hughes and Weill conducted a prospective mortality study of 839 men employed in the manufacture of asbestos cement products (28). Defining asbestosis by the presence of ≥1/0 ILO radiographic lesions, these investigators report a fourfold excess risk of lung cancer among workers with these radiographic changes, and no excess risk among those without opacities even though the levels of reported asbestos exposure were similar. While radiographs which are negative for evidence of asbestosis, do not exclude the presence of histological interstitial pulmonary fibrosis (33), these observations are consistent with the view that asbestos becomes a lung carcinogen through its ability to induce fibrotic proliferation (28).

Tuberculosis

Hogg relates two dominant factors for the production of granulomatous inflammation (25). First, the alveolar macrophage must be unable to completely digest or engulf the inflammatory stimulus, and second, lymphocyte effector cells must initiate a cell-mediated inflammatory response. Infection with bacteria (i.e., tuberculosis) and fungi exemplify this response. Given that excess lung cancer risk follows nongranulomatous interstitial fibrosis (described above), it is reasonable to consider the evidence that granulomatous fibrosis also may precede an elevated lung cancer risk.

Richardson et al. (53) conducted a cross-sectional study among 359 lung cancer patients (cases) and 450 patients with cancers of breast, colon, uterus, and prostate (controls). The presence of tuberculous scarring was assessed radiographically (53). These investigators found the frequency of tuberculous scars of the lung to be significantly higher for lung carcinomas than for the other carcinomas, with an age-adjusted odds ratio of 1.70 (95% CI = 1.47–1.96).

A population-based case-control study of lung cancer and prior tuberculosis infection was conducted in Shanghai by Zheng et al. (67). They identified 1405 lung cancer patients from the Shanghai Cancer Registry and 1495 controls from sex- and age-stratified random sampling of the general population of the Shanghai urban area. From interviews conducted among all living cases and controls, information was collected regarding prior lung diseases (including TB) and cigarette smoking. Among males, prior TB infection was reported by 26% of the cases and 20% of the controls, while 12% and 8%, respectively, reported prior TB infection among the females. After adjustment for smoking, age, sex, education, and occupation, the odds ratio was 1.5 (95% CI = 1.2–1.8). For those with a TB history within 20 years, the lung cancer risk was higher for adenocarcinoma than for squamous/oat cell cancers, with most of the tumors arising in peripheral locations. This study took great pains to avoid selection, misclassification, and recall biases. In a subsequent study of lung cancer among women in two industrial cities of northeast China (Shenyang and Harbin), this team of investigators found an increased risk of lung cancer associated with prior (4–10 years) diagnosis of TB (66).

Howe et al. (27) followed a large cohort of patients assembled from the Canadian National Tuberculosis Register (n = 64,037), comparing their standardized proportionate mortality to that of the Canadian population. These investigators found a significant elevation of lung cancer risk for both males (SPMR 1.5, 95% CI = 1.21–1.47) and females (SPMR 1.5, 95% CI = 1.11–1.98). A considerably smaller study of the Hawaii State Tuberculosis Branch patient records showed that among never-smoking women, prior tuberculosis infection was associated with an elevated lung cancer risk (OR 8.2, 95% CI = 1.3–54.4) (24). Several older studies, perhaps due to few expected cases or lack of cigarette smoking information, showed a positive trend which, nevertheless, fell short of a significant association of lung cancer with prior tuberculosis scarring (21,60).

B. Experimental Studies

Kuschner, in a discussion of the relevance of animal studies to the evaluation of human lung cancer risk has considered that fibers (e.g., asbestos) may lead to the development of lung cancer by way of interstitial fibrosis (36). Pathologists, according to Kuschner, have "been impressed" by the continuity of change from the epithelial proliferative change that accompanies interstitial fibrosis to the type II cellular proliferation and subsequent cancer. Wagner et al. (63) report a series of experiments in which SPF Wistar rats were exposed by inhalation to dust clouds of the UICC asbestos standard reference samples for periods of between 1 day and 2 years. These investigators standardized for survival time to determine whether there was any relationship between the grade of asbestosis and the presence of lung tumors. All tumors were peripheral, appearing to arise from the region of the respiratory bronchioles in which the asbestos fiber had accumulated. Accumulations of type II epithelial cells that proliferated in the alveoli of the respiratory bronchioles were associated with adenomata. Squamous carcinomata originated from foci of squamous metaplasia occurring in the asbestotic lesions in the more proximal respiratory bronchioles. Regardless of lung cancer cell type, animals with lung tumors had significantly more asbestosis than those without tumors (63). Similar results have been reported by Davis and Cowie (13). These investigators also report a significant relationship between the extent of pulmonary fibrosis and the development of pulmonary tumors. They found that pulmonary tumors usually developed from areas of adenomatoid change and advanced fibrosis (13).

Until recently, there has been little insight into the mechanism that might link inflammatory repair of "chronic injury" to cancer. Antoniades et al. have demonstrated the reversible, simultaneous expression of a potent mitogen, c-sis/platelet-derived growth factor (PDGF)-2, and its receptor in skin epithelial cells of injured swine (4). While neither PDGF nor PDGF receptor is expressed normally by uninjured epithelial cells, their reversible expression was correlated with the stage of acute tissue repair—maximal during initial repair, and suppressed by the time of complete reepithelialization. In contrast, lung epithelial cells subject to the chronic inflammation of idiopathic pulmonary fibrosis were found by these investigators to sustain an elevated expression of the c-*sis*/PDGF-2 proto-oncogene and its mitogenic protein product, without evidence of PDGF receptor mRNA or PDGF receptor protein (2). These investigators hypothesize that the lack of PDGF receptor expression in IPF may be critical to distinguish the mechanisms underlying chronic inflammation from that of lung cancer. Unregulated PDGF expression in IPF may lead to paracrine (adjacent cell) stimulation resulting in fibroblast proliferation and collagen production. In extending their observations to lung cancer, Antoniades et al. found that the malignant epithelial cells of patients with primary lung cancer express both the c-*sis*/PDGF-2 mRNA and the PDGF-receptor mRNA along with their protein products (3). It is reasonable to suspect that the coexpression of both PDGF and its receptor in lung cancer epithelial cells may result in autocrine (same cell) stimulation and unregulated growth. The sequence of steps that IPF cells must undergo to express the PDGF receptor and thus progress from inflammation to lung cancer remains to be described.

In addition to PDGF, other growth factors including transforming growth factors α and β_1 (TGF-α and TGF-β_1) autoregulate the expression of their mRNAs, leading to an increased secretion of respective effector peptides (32). Growth factors alter the balance of gene transcription and peptide expression which signals growing cells toward either terminal differentiation or proliferation. These growth factor responses might be amplified during tumor promotion to effect or inhibit the proliferation of malignant cells, Masui et al. (40) have shown that TGF-β_1, one of the constituents of human platelets, inhibits the growth of cultured normal human bronchial epithelial cells by inhibiting DNA synthesis while acting as a potent inducer of squamous differentiation in this culture system. In contrast, these investigators showed that TGF-β_1 showed little growth factor (i.e., growth inhibitory) activity for existing cancer (human lung carcinoma cell lines). Kim et al. (32) have demonstrated that TGF-β_1 autoinduction is mediated by binding of the AP-1 complex, a complex of the *jun* and *fos* oncoproteins. By reversibly binding to DNA, the AP-1 complex switches between the transcription of proteins that code for either proliferation or differentiation (51). Whether lowered TGF-β_1 expression participates in a transformation from inflammatory epithelial cell proliferation to neoplasia and whether this expression is modified by the expression of c-*sis*/PDGF-2 or its receptor remain unknown.

II. Obstruction

As long as 25 years ago, studies had shown that bullous emphysema was found with greater frequency on radiographs in patients with lung cancer than in hospitalized controls (5,18). Cohen had presented evidence that impairment of pulmonary function, even in the absence of cigarette smoking, is associated with an increased risk for lung cancer (10). She found that first-degree relatives of patients with lung cancer had significantly higher rates of impaired ventilation than did similar relatives of patients with no pulmonary conditions, after adjustment for smoking, age, sex, race, socioeconomic status, or a variety of genetic markers. More recently, prospective follow-up has shown a high incidence of lung cancer in patients with chronic obstructive pulmonary disease (12,35,38,57,61). A molecular explanation may exist for the association of ventilatory obstruction and lung cancer susceptibility. Retinol (vitamin A) has been associated with normal differentiation of epithelial cells (11), protection against chronic bronchitis and emphysema (44,45,62), and prevention of cancer in animals (47,59) and in human experimental studies (26).

A. Epidemiological Studies

Following 835 chronic obstructive pulmonary disease (COPD) patients from the Bellevue Emphysema Clinic (New York), Davis (12) observed an elevated incidence of lung cancer (11.6 per 1000 person years). She surmised that the epithelial injury resulting from COPD placed the obstructed patients at risk of lung cancer. Skillrud and colleagues (57) followed 113 patients with impaired ventilation and 113 controls (matched for amount smoked, age, and occupation). After 10 years of follow-up, these investigators found that the cumulative probability for the development of lung cancer was 8.8% (9 patients) among those with obstruction and 2.0% (2 patients) among those with normal pulmonary function, resulting in a 4.4-fold greater risk for lung cancer among those with obstruction.

Tockman et al. (61) examined the risk for developing lung cancer among patients with chronic obstructive lung disease who participated in the Intermittent Positive Pressure Breathing (IPPB) Trial (n = 676) and participants in the Johns Hopkins Lung Project (JHLP), one of the three Cooperative Early Lung Cancer Detection Programs of the National Cancer Institute (n = 3728). These investigators noted that the IPPB Trial participants with a forced expiratory volume of less than 60% of predicted had a 4.85-fold excess risk of lung cancer, while the lesser obstructed participants in the JHLP with impaired pulmonary function had a 2.7-fold increased risk. The risk for lung cancer increased linearly, in proportion to the degree of airways obstruction. Among cigarette smokers, the presence of airways obstruction was more an indicator for the subsequent development of lung cancer than was age or the level of smoking.

Kuller et al. (35) found that for 6075 cigarette-smoking men with acceptable tracings participating in the Multiple Risk Factor Intervention Trial (MRFIT), the FEV_1 (adjusted for age, height, number of cigarettes smoked, and thiocyanate levels) was an independent predictor of lung cancer mortality over 7.5 years of follow-up. As described above, the relationship was found to be linear, with lung cancer incidence rates (per 1000 person-years) that increased from 0.43 (among those in the highest FEV_1 quintile) to 3.02 in the lowest FEV_1 quintile. Although adjusting for cigarette smoking simultaneously in a variety of ways, including number of cigarettes smoked, age at onset of smoking, and thiocyanate levels, these investigators nevertheless maintain that "the most plausible hypothesis" is that FEV_1 is a better measure of exposure to carcinogens in cigarette smoke than the usual history of smoking exposure.

In the largest study of COPD and subsequent lung cancer, Lange et al. (38) reported their 10-year follow-up of 13,946 randomly selected participants in the Copenhagen City Heart Study. In this study, the 225 subjects who died from lung cancer were primarily older, male smokers. After adjustment for age, sex, and pack-years of smoking, these investigators found an increasing susceptibility to lung cancer with ventilatory obstruction measured either as (adjusted) FEV_1% predicted or as (adjusted) FEV_1/FVC. Compared to participants with FEV_1% predicted $\geq 80\%$, those with values between 40 and 79 and $<40\%$ had excess lung cancer mortalities of 2.1- and 3.9-fold, respectively.

Early reports suggested that impairment of carcinogen clearance or a combination of predisposing epithelial tissue injury followed by carcinogen exposure was responsible for the COPD-associated increase in lung cancer susceptibility (10,57). Tockman et al. (61) point out, however, that causal explanations that require an obstructive lesion to precede the development of the neoplasm do not account for the similar age distributions in patients with airways obstruction and lung cancer. It is estimated that for both chronic obstructive pulmonary disease and lung cancer, a 15- to 20-year latent period must pass from the time of exposure until clinical manifestations of either illness cause a patient to seek medical help. Given the prolonged latency required for both diseases, the initiation of lung cancer and the initiation of airways obstruction would have to occur at approximately the same time, and probably long before substantial airways obstruction would have influenced the development of lung cancer.

As an alternative, these investigators suggest that rather than differences in exposure, the lowered, smoking-adjusted FEV_1 represents a marker of altered host susceptibility due to an error in a molecular mechanism common to both the processes of inflammatory injury and carcinogenesis (61). The recent review of de Luca (14) describing the hormonelike role of retinoids and the report of Schule et al. (55) characterizing retinoic acid as a negative regulator of AP-1–responsive genes may provide insight into a common molecular mechanism underlying both pulmonary inflammatory injury and neoplasia.

Yet, while vitamin A and its synthetic analogs have inhibited the occurrence of induced tumors and have reversed metaplastic changes in experimental animals, most epidemiological studies based on dietary questionnaires or blood measurement have failed to observe this association (64). The role of retinoids in human chemoprevention has been recently enhanced by the report of Hong et al. (26), which reported that daily treatment with high doses of isotretinoin is effective in preventing second primary tumors in patients who have been treated for squamous cell respiratory tract cancers of the head and neck, although it does not prevent recurrences of the original tumor.

B. Experimental Studies

Deficiency of vitamin A has long been known to cause squamous metaplasia and keratinization of columnar epithelia (14). Retinoids control epithelial differentiation and may prevent alterations caused by exposure to chemical carcinogens, observations that led Sporn et al. to propose the concept of chemoprevention (59). Through chemoprevention, retinoic acid or similar compounds might prevent epithelial tumorigenesis by reversing the initiation or promotion stages of carcinogenesis. These stages may be reflected morphologically by squamous metaplasia, considered an early lesion along the path toward tumor formation (54).

Retinoids exert their effects on epithelial cells via nuclear receptors, analogous to those of steroids, but often with opposite effect (14). For example, vitamin A deficiency induces basal cells to form a continuous layer over the basement membrane making a transition from pseudostratified to stratified epithelium. This stratification is followed by gradual keratinization of the epithelium. Similar changes are seen under the influence of hydrocortisone (46).

Retinoids are known to be inhibitors of cell growth (22). Retinoic acid exerts its biological effects by acting through two classes of intracellular proteins, including the retinoic acid receptors (RARs) (RARα, -β, and, -γ) and the retinoid X receptors (RXRs), both of which are members of the steroid receptor superfamily. RARs but not RXR are able to repress AP-1–mediated induction of gene expression, by inhibiting the binding of AP-1 to DNA (55). By reversibly binding to DNA, the AP-1 complex effects the transcription of proteins which code for either proliferation or differentiation (51). Retinol levels and retinol transport are carefully regulated in the plasma. Retinol-binding protein (RBP), the retinol carrier in blood, is a 21-kd peptide (19). This molecule is synthesized in the liver and secreted into the bloodstream, where it complexes with *trans*-thyretin (55 kda), minimizing its loss by glomerular filtration. While the mechanism of cellular retinol uptake and release is poorly understood, if retinol is protected from the tissue dehydrogenase that would convert it to retinoic acid (52), it may be recycled. Most plasma retinol that leaves the blood returns to the circulation, and this cycle is repeated on average seven to nine times (20). Retinoic acid can also be generated directly from β-carotene and, depending on the availability of carotenoids, retinol recycling may be a prominent feature of retinoid homeostasis (52). Factors that affect retinol homeostasis, including recycling and derivation from β-carotene, may underlie the inconsistent epidemiological associations of dietary or plasma levels of retinol and lung cancer susceptibility described earlier.

While these mechanisms are speculative, they are consistent with the data and suggest that it may be possible to identify those smokers at highest risk for lung cancer by detecting the presence of ventilatory obstruction and that chemoprevention of lung cancer with vitamin A, its synthetic analogs or β-carotene may eventually be possible.

III. Metabolic Phenotype and DNA Repair

Caporaso and colleagues compared the abilities of 245 lung cancer patients and 234 controls (with COPD) to metabolize debrisoquine, an antihypertensive drug (8). These investigators found that after similar doses of the drug, extensive metabolizers excrete up to several hundred times more of the urinary metabolite 4-hydroxy-debrisoquine than do poor metabolizers. Debrisoquine phenotypes are defined by the metabolic ratio (MR) of debrisoquine to its chief metabolite recovered in an aliquot of an 8-h urine sample. Deficient metabolism is inherited as an autosomal recessive. This study demonstrated Hardy-Weinberg equilibrium conditions in the controls, while the lung cancer case group contained an excess of extensive metabolizers. Patients who metabolize the drug extensively were at about eight times greater risk of getting lung cancer than were patients who metabolize the drug poorly or moderately. The key metabolic step is an oxidation performed by P450-2D6 cytochrome. Since 90% of the U.S. population are estimated to be extensive or moderate metabolizers of debrisoquine, an advantage would accrue to the 10% of the population who metabolize debrisoquine poorly and thus would be at lower risk of lung cancer.

An assay for measuring nucleotide excision repair of UV- and chemically induced DNA damage has been reported by Athas et al. (6) These investigators transfected damaged, nonreplicating, recombinant plasmid DNA harboring a chloramphenicol acetyltransferase (*cat*) reporter gene into peripheral blood lymphocytes. Excision repair of the damaged bacterial *cat* gene was monitored as a function of time. While this assay has been validated by discriminating the reduced DNA repair ability of xeroderma pigmentosum patients from that of controls, there is clear potential to explore DNA repair as a component of lung cancer susceptibility.

The utility of lung cancer susceptibility markers awaits scientific validation. Clinically, markers of enhanced lung cancer susceptibility may have a role in focusing smoking cessation efforts. Furthermore, markers of susceptibility can be combined with markers of early lung cancer during studies of the validity of population lung cancer screening. This dual-phase strategy, whereby a simple, highly sensitive, but not necessarily specific initial (susceptibility) screen might be followed by a more specific, confirmatory test, has been recently suggested as most suitable for the vast population at risk of lung cancer (39).

References

1. Amandus, H., and Costello, J. (1991). Silicosis and lung cancer in U.S. metal miners. *Arch. Environ. Health* 46:82–89.
2. Antoniades, H. N., Bravo, M. A., Avila, R. E., Galanopoulos, T., Neville-Golden, J., Maxwell, M., and Selman, M. (1990). Platelet-derived growth factor in idiopathic pulmonary fibrosis. *J. Clin. Invest* 86:1055–1064.
3. Antoniades, H. H., Galanopoulos, T., Neville-Golden, J., and O'Hara, C. J. (1992). Malignant epithelial cells in primary human lung carcinomas coexpress in vivo platelet-derived growth factor (PDGF) and PDGF receptor mRNAs and their protein products. *Proc. Natl. Acad. Sci. USA* 89:3942–3946.
4. Antoniades, H. N., Galanopoulos, T., Neville-Golden, J., Kiristy, C. P., and Lynch, S. E. (1991). Injury induces in vivo expression of platelet-derived growth factor (PDGF) and PDGF receptor mRNAs in skin epithelial cells and PDGF mRNA in connective tissue fibroblasts. *Proc. Natl. Acad. Sci. USA* 84:565–569.
5. Aronberg, D. J., Sagel, S. S., LeFrak, S., Kuhn, C., and Susman, N. (1980). Lung carcinoma associated with bullous lung disease in young men. *AJR* 134:249–252.
6. Athas, W. F., Hedayati, M. A., Matanoski, G. M., Farmer, E. R., and Grossman, L. (1991). Development and field-test validation of an assay for DNA repair in circulating human lymphocytes. *Cancer Res.* 51:5786–5793.
7. Byers, T. E., Vena, J. E., and Rzepka, T. F. (1984). Predilection of lung cancer for the upper lobes: An epidemiologic inquiry. *J. Natl. Cancer Inst.* 72:1271–1275.
8. Caporaso, N., Pickle, L. W., Bale, S., Ayesh, R., Hetzel, M., and Idle, J. (1989). The distribution of debrisoquine metabolic phenotypes and implications for the suggested association with lung cancer risk. *Genet. Epidemiol.* 6:517–524.
9. Chiyotani, K., Saito, K., Okubo, T., and Takahashi, K. (1990). Lung cancer risk among pneumoconiosis patients in Japan, with special reference to silicotics. In *Occupational Exposure to Silica and Cancer Risk*. Edited by L. Simonato, A. C. Fletcher, R. Saracci, and T. L. Thomas. Lyon, International Agency for Research on Cancer, pp. 95–104.
10. Cohen, B. H. (1980). Chronic obstructive pulmonary disease: A challenge in genetic epidemiology. *Am. J. Epidemiol.* 112:274–288.
11. Committee on Diet, Nutrition, and Cancer, National Research Council. (1982). *Diet, Nutrition, and Cancer*. Washington DC, National Academy Press, pp. 138–144.
12. Davis, A. L. (1976). Bronchogenic carcinoma in chronic obstructive pulmonary disease. *JAMA* 235:621–622.
13. Davis, J. M. G., and Cowie, H. A. (1990). The relationship between fibrosis and cancer in experimental animals exposed to asbestos and other fibers. *Environ. Health Perspect.* 88:305–309.
14. de Luca, L. M. (1991). Retinoids and their receptors in differentiation, embryogenesis, and neoplasia. *FASEB J* 5:2924–2933.

15. Doll, R. (1955). Mortality from lung cancer in asbestos workers. *Br. J. Ind. Med.* 12: 81–86.
16. Finkelstein, M., Kusiak, R., and Suranyi, G. (1982). Mortality among miners receiving workmen's compensation for silicosis in Ontario: 1940–1975. *J. Occup. Med.* 24:663–667.
17. Goldsmith, D. F., Guidotti, T. L., and Johnston, D. R. (1982). Does occupational exposure to silica cause lung cancer? *Am. J. Ind. Med.* 3:423–440.
18. Goldstein, M. J., Snider, G. L., Liberson, M., and Poske, R. M. (1968). Bronchogenic carcinoma and giant bullous disease. *Am. Rev. Respir. Dis.* 97:1062–1070.
19. Goodman, D. S. (1984). Plasma retinol binding protein. In *The Retinoids*. Edited by M. B. Sporn, A. B. Roberts, and D. S. Goodman. Orlando, FL, Academic Press, pp. 41–88.
20. Green, M. H., Green, J. B., and Lewis, K. C. (1987). Variation in retinol utilization rate with vitamin A status in the rat. *J. Nutr.* 117:694–703.
21. Hammond, E. C., Selikoff, I. J., and Robitzek, E. H. (1967). Isoniazid therapy in relation to later occurrence of cancer in adults and in infants. *Br. Med. J.* 2: 792–795.
22. Haussler, M., Sidell, N., Kelly, M., Donaldson, C., Altman, A., and Mangelsdorf, D. (1983). Specific high-affinity binding and biologic action of retinoic acid in human neuroblastoma cell lines. *Proc. Natl. Acad. Sci. USA* 80:5525–5529.
23. Heighway, J., Thatcher, N., Cerny, T., and Hasleton, P. S. (1986). Genetic predisposition to human lung cancer. *Br. J. Cancer* 53:453–457.
24. Hinds, M. W., Cohen, H. I., and Kolonel, L. N. (1982). Tuberculosis and lung cancer risk in nonsmoking women. *Am. Rev. Respir. Dis.* 125:776–778.
25. Hogg, J. C. (1991). Chronic interstitial lung disease of unknown cause: A new classification based on pathogenesis. *Am. J. Roentgenol.* 156:225–233.
26. Hong, W. K., Lippman, S. M., Itri, L. M., Karp, D. D., Lee, J. S., Byers, R. M., Schantz, S. P., Kramer, A. M., Lotan, R., Peters, L. J., et al (1990). Prevention of second primary tumors with isotretinoin in squamous-cell carcinoma of the head and neck. *N. Engl. J. Med.* 323:795–801.
27. Howe, G. R., Lindsay, J., Coppock, E., and Miller, A. B. (1979). Isoniazid exposure in relation to cancer incidence and mortality in a cohort of tuberculosis patients. *Int. J. Epidemiol.* 8:305–312.
28. Hughes, J. M., and Weill, H. (1991). Asbestosis as a precursor of asbestos related lung cancer: Results of a prospective mortality study. *Br. J. Ind. Med.* 48:229–233.
29. Hulka, B. S., and Wilcosky, T. (1988). Biological markers in epidemiologic research. *Arch. Environ. Health* 43:83–89.
30. IARC. (1987). *IARC Monographs on the Evaluation of the Carcinogenic Risk of Chemicals to Humans*, Vol. 42, *Silica and Some Silicates*. Lyon, International Agency for Research on Cancer, pp. 39–143.
31. Kannerstein, M., and Churg, J. (1972). The pathology of carcinoma of the lung associated with asbestos exposure. *Cancer* 30:14–21.
32. Kim, S. J., Angel, P., Lafyatis, R., Hattori, K., Kim, K. Y., Sporn, M. B., Karin, M., and Roberts, A. B. (1990). Autoinduction of transforming growth factor b1 is mediated by the AP-1 complex. *Mol. Cell Biol.* 10:1492–1497.

33. Kipen, H. M., Lilis, R., Suzuki, Y., Valciukas, J. A., and Selikoff, I. J. (1987). Pulmonary fibrosis in asbestos insulation workers with lung cancer: A radiological and histopathological evaluation. *Br. J. Ind. Med.* 44:96–100.
34. Koskela, R. S., Klockars, M., Jarvinen, E., Rossi, A., and Kolari, P. J. (1990). Cancer mortality of granite workers 1940–1985. In *Occupational Exposure to Silica and Cancer Risk*. Edited by L. Simonato, A. C. Fletcher, R. Saracci, and T. L. Thomas. Lyon, International Agency for Research on Cancer, pp. 43–53.
35. Kuller, L. H., Ockene, J., Meilahn, E., and Svendsen, K. H. (1990). Relation of forced expiratory volume in one second (FEV_1) to lung cancer mortality in the Multiple Risk Factor Intervention Trial (MRFIT). *Am. J. Epidemiol.* 132: 265–274.
36. Kuschner, M. (1992). Animal models in the assessment of fiber carcinogenesis. In *Relevance of Animal Studies to the Evaluation of Human Cancer Risk*. New York, Wiley-Liss, Inc., pp. 71–77.
37. Lagorio, S., Forastiere, F., Michelozzi, P., Cavariani, F., Perucci, C. A., and Axelson, O. (1990). A case-referent study on lung cancer mortality among ceramic workers. In *Occupational Exposure to Silica and Cancer Risk*. Edited by L. Simonato, A. C. Fletcher, R. Saracci, and T. L. Thomas. Lyon, International Agency for Research on Cancer, pp. 21–28.
38. Lange, P., Nyboe, J., Appleyard, M., Jensen, G., and Schnohr, P. (1990). Ventilatory function and chronic mucus hypersecretion as predictors of death from lung cancer. *Am. Rev. Respir. Dis.* 141:613–617.
39. Makuch, R. W., and Muenz, L. R. (1987). Evaluating the adequacy of tumor markers to discriminate among distinct populations. *Semin. Oncol.* 14:89–101.
40. Masui, T., Wakefield, L. M., Lechner, J. F., La Veck, M. A., Sporn, M. B., and Harris, C. C. (1986). Type B transforming growth factor is the primary differentiation-inducing serum factor for normal human bronchial epithelial cells. *Proc. Natl. Acad. Sci. USA* 83:2438–2442.
41. Mehnert, W. H., Staneczek, W., Mohner, M., Konetzke, G., Muller, W., Ahlendorf, W., Beck, B., Winkelmann, R., and Simonato, L. (1990). A mortality study of a cohort of slate quarry workers in the German Democratic Republic. In *Occupational Exposure to Silica and Cancer Risk*. Edited by L. Simonato, A. C. Fletcher, R. Saracci, and T. L. Thomas. Lyon, International Agency for Research on Cancer, pp. 55–64.
42. Merlo, F., Doria, M., Fontana, L., Ceppi, M., Chesi, E., and Santi, L. (1990). Mortality from specific causes among silicotic subjects: A historical prospective study. In *Occupational Exposure to Silica and Cancer Risk*. Edited by L. Simonato, A. C. Fletcher, R. Saracci, and T. L. Thomas. Lyon, International Agency for Research on Cancer, pp. 105–111.
43. Minna, J. D., Pass, H., Glatstein, E., and Ihde, D. C. (1989). Cancer of the lung. In *Cancer: Principles & Practice of Oncology*, third edition. Edited by V. T. DeVita, S. Hellman, and S. A. Rosenberg. Philadelphia, J.B. Lippincott, Co., pp. 591–705.
44. Morabia, A., Menkes, M. J. S., Comstock, G. W., and Tockman, M. S. (1990). Serum retinol and airway obstruction. *Am. J. Epidemiol.* 132:77–82.
45. Morabia, A., Sorenson, A., Kumanyika, S. K., Abbey, H., Cohen, B. H., and Chee,

E. (1989). Vitamin A, cigarette smoking, and airway obstruction. *Am. Rev. Respir. Dis.* 140:1312–1314.

46. Mossman, B. T., Ley, B. W., and Craighead, J. E. (1976). Squamous metaplasia of the tracheal epithelium in organ culture. I. Effects of hydrocortisone and beta-retinyl acetate. *Exp. Mol. Pathol.* 24:405–414.
47. Nettesheim, P., and Williams, M. L. (1976). The influence of vitamin A on the susceptibility of the rat lung to 3-methylcholanthrene. *Int. J. Cancer* 17:351–357.
48. Newhouse, M., Berry, G., and Wagner, J. C. (1985). Mortality of factory workers in east London 1933–80. *Br. J. Ind. Med.* 42:4–11.
49. Ooi, W. L., Elston, R. C., Chen, V. W., Bailey-Wilson, J. E., and Rothschild, H. (1986). Increased familial risk for lung cancer. *J. Natl. Cancer Inst.* 76:217–222.
50. Pairon, J. C., Brochard, P., Jaurand, M. C., and Bignon, J. (1991). Silica and lung cancer: A controversial issue. *Eur. Respir. J.* 4:730–744.
51. Ponta, H., Cato, A. C., and Herrlich, P. (1992). Interference of pathway specific transcription factors. *Biochim. Biophys. Acta* 1129:255–261.
52. Posch, K. C., Enright, W. J., and Napoli, J. L. (1989). Retinoic acid synthesis by cytosol from the alcohol dehydrogenase negative deermouse. *Arch. Biochem. Biophys.* 274:171–178.
53. Richardson, S., Hirsch, A., Ruffie, P., and Bickel, M. (1987). Relationship between tuberculous scar and carcinomas of the lung. *Eur. J. Radiol.* 7:163–164.
54. Saccomanno, G., Archer, V. E., Auerbach, O., Saunders, R. P., and Brennan, L. M. (1974). Development of carcinomas of the lung as reflected in exfoliated cells. *Cancer* 33:256–270.
55. Schule, R., Rangarajan, P., Yang, N., Kliewer, S., Ransone, L. J., Bolado, J., Verma, I. M., and Evans, R. M. (1991). Retinoic acid is a negative regulator of AP-1-responsive genes. *Proc. Natl. Acad. Sci. USA* 88:6092–6096.
56. Simonato, L., and Saracci, R. (1990). Epidemiological aspects of the relationship between exposure to silica dust and lung cancer. In *Occupational Exposure to Silica and Cancer Risk.* Edited by L. Simonato, A. C. Fletcher, R. Saracci, and T. L. Thomas. Lyon, International Agency for Research on Cancer, pp. 1–5.
57. Skillrud, D. M., Offord, K. P., and Miller, R. D. (1986). Higher risk of lung cancer in chronic obstructive pulmonary disease. *Ann. Intern. Med.* 105:503–507.
58. Spencer, H. (1982). Lung scar cancer. In *Morphogenesis of Lung Cancer.* Edited by Y. Shimosato, M. R. Melamed, P. Nettesheim. Boca Raton, FL, CRC Press, pp. 111–120.
59. Sporn, M. B., Dunlop, N. M., Newton, D. L., and Smith, J. M. (1976). Prevention of chemical carcinogenesis by vitamin A and its synthetic analogs (retinoids). *Fed. Proc.* 35:1332–1338.
60. Stott, H., Peto, J., Stephens, R., Fox, W., Sutherland, I., Foster-Carter, A. F., Teare, H. D., and Fenning, J. (1976). An assessment of the carcinogenicity of isoniazid in patients with pulmonary tuberculosis. Tubercle 57:1–15.
61. Tockman, M. S., Anthonisen, N. R., Wright, E. C., and Donithan, M. G. (1987). Airways obstruction and the risk for lung cancer. *Ann. Intern. Med.* 106:512–518.
62. Tockman, M. S., Khoury, M. J., and Cohen, B. H. (1986). Milk drinking and possible protection of the respiratory epithelium. *J. Chron. Dis.* 39:207–209.

63. Wagner, J. C., Berry, G., Skidmore, J. W., and Timbrell, V. (1974). The effects of the inhalation of asbestos in rats. *Br. J. Cancer* 29:252–269.
64. Willett, W. C. (1990). Vitamin A and lung cancer. *Nutr. Rev.* 48:201–211.
65. Winter, P. D., Gardner, M. J., Fletcher, A. C., and Jones, R. D. (1990). A mortality follow-up study of pottery workers: Preliminary findings on lung cancer. In *Occupational Exposure to Silica and Cancer Risk*. Edited by L. Simonato, A. C. Fletcher, R. Saracci, and T. L. Thomas. Lyon, International Agency for Research on Cancer, pp. 83–94.
66. Wu-Williams, A. H., Dai, X. D., Blot, W., Xu, Z. Y., Sun, X. W., Xiao, H. P., Stone, B. J., Yu, S. F., Feng, Y. P., Ershow, A. G., Sun, J., Fraumeni, J. F., Jr., and Henderson, B. E. (1990). Lung cancer among women in north-east China. *Br. J. Cancer* 62:982 –987.
67. Zheng, W., Blot, W. J., Liao, M. L., Wang, Z. X., Levin, L. I., Zhao, J. J., Fraumeni, J. F., Jr., and Gao, Y. T. (1987). Lung cancer and prior tuberculosis infection in Shanghai. *Br. J. Cancer* 56:501–504.

16

Lung Cancer Cell Type and Occupational Exposure

ANDREW CHURG

University of British Columbia
Vancouver, British Columbia, Canada

I. Introduction

The notion that occupational agents induce histologically specific types of lung cancer is an attractive one, both from the point of view of epidemiologic investigation and from the advantage to be gained in attributing an individual case of cancer to a particular exposure. Certainly claims that certain occupations are associated with particular types of lung cancer abound in the literature. Unfortunately, the pathologic diagnosis of lung cancer, which to the epidemiologist or clinician may appear as transparent as a report bearing the diagnosis "poorly differentiated squamous carcinoma," is in practice bedeviled by a host of factors both intrinsic to the pathologist and beyond his or her control (Table 1). Moreover there are a host of epidemiological variables such as age, sex, year of diagnosis, and, most important, smoking status (see Table 1), all of which affect cell type and are thus potential confounders (often in complicated ways), and few of which are properly dealt with in most studies of occupational exposure and lung cancer histology.

This chapter considers very briefly the pathologic diagnosis of lung cancer, current notions of the histogenesis of lung cancer, the numerous factors that affect accurate histologic diagnosis and that affect cell type, and reports of histologic

Table 1 Factors Affecting the Histologic Type and Pathologic Diagnosis of Lung Cancer

Pathologic Diagnostic Factors	Epidemiologic Factors
Classification definitions	Age
Nature of diagnostic specimen	Sex
Tumor heterogeneity	Smoking
Tumor differentiation	Race
Effects of therapy	Country of residence
Diagnostic techniques	Secular trends
Intra/Inter observer variability	Occupation

diagnosis in specific occupational groups. This topic has been previously reviewed by Ives et al. (1), and the reader is referred to that paper for further comments on the (sometimes differing) general approach and specific details of the problem.

II. Histologic Classification of Lung Cancer

Strictly speaking, the term "lung cancer" should include all of the myriad types of malignancies arising in the lung (see Ref. 2); in practice it is usually restricted to so-called "bronchogenic" carcinomas, a term that is, strictly speaking, inaccurate, but useful because it denotes four major histopathlogic types of carcinoma (Tables 2 and 3) that are extremely common and generally associated with cigarette smoking. Compared to bronchogenic carcinomas, all other primary lung cancers are rare in both relative and absolute terms; since none of these uncommon lesions has any known epidemiological association (occupational or otherwise), they will be ignored here.

Table 2 Revised World Health Organization Classification of Lung Cancer

Squamous carcinoma	Adenocarcinoma
Well differentiated	Acinar type
Moderately differentiated	Papillary type
Poorly differentiated	Bronchioloalveolar
Small-cell carcinoma	Solid carcinoma with mucus production
Oat cell type	Large-cell carcinoma
Intermediate cell type	Giant cell carcinoma
Combined types	Clear cell carcinoma

Source: Ref. 3.

Table 3 Simplified Classification of Bronchogenic Carcinoma Using Only Major Cell Types

Squamous cell carcinoma	Adenocarcinoma
Small-cell carcinoma	Large-cell carcinoma

As is true for any type of tumor, there is no universally accepted pathologic classification scheme for lung cancer. One current widely accepted one is that proposed by the World Health Organization (WHO) (3), shown in Table 2. Examples of other fairly similar systems can be found in Refs. 2 and 4. All have in common the use of four main categories: squamous carcinoma, small-cell carcinoma, adenocarcinoma, and large-cell carcinoma (see Table 3). These major categories in theory have strict definitions: squamous carcinomas show keratin formation and/or intercellular bridges. Adenocarcinomas form glands and/or secrete mucin. Small-cell carcinomas are composed of cells somewhat larger than a lymphocyte with high nuclear:cytoplasmic ratios, very finely divided chromatin, and inconspicuous nucleoli; by electron microscopy they usually contain neurosecretory granules (5), although the definition is not based on ultrastructural features. Large-cell carcinomas show no differentiating features by light microscopy, but by electron microscopy most are quite evidently very poorly differentiated squamous cell or adenocarcinomas (6,7). In practice (see below), adherence to these definitions is often difficult and commonly idiosyncratic.

Examples of the results obtained using the basic four-category scheme are shown in Table 4. Factors accounting for some of the very evident variations will be discussed below.

All of these classification systems also employ subcategories under each

Table 4 Frequency (%) of the Major Cell Types in Various Series

	Reference						
Cell type	8	9	10	11	12	13	13
Squamous cell	35	38	33	71	33	71	32
Small-cell	25	20	22	12	16	9	27
Adeno	25	26	28	9	45	12	32
Large-cell	14	9	17	7	6	8	14
Source[a]	M	M	M	S	S	S	S

[a]M = mixed autopsy and surgical; A = autopsy only; S = surgical only.

main heading (e.g., Table 2), but here they differ in both the way in which the subcategories are defined (grade of differentiation vs. some other pattern matching scheme) and in the very nature of the lesions included. For example, the classification system used by the Working Party for Therapy of Lung Cancer (WPL) subdivides adenocarcinomas into well, moderately, and poorly differentiated, whereas the WHO (see Table 2) subclassifies adenocarcinomas as acinar, papillary, bronchioloalveolar, or solid with mucus production. The potential for confusion is obvious, and the use of these categories by individual pathologists is often totally arbitrary (see below).

III. Histogenesis of Lung Cancer

The histogenesis of lung cancer, both in terms of the sequence of pathologic appearances leading to the development of a tumor and in terms of the cell of origin of such tumors, has been and continues to be controversial. The former issue is somewhat more clear. Cytologic studies, particularly those carried out by Saccomanno and colleagues on uranium miners (14), have shown that individuals developing invasive carcinomas first have squamous metaplasia of the normally columnar bronchial epithelium, and then the appearance of progressively more dysplastic squamous cells, eventually leading to lesions classified as squamous carcinoma in situ. Equivalent features can be seen in histologic sections if extensive sampling is done: for example, Auerbach et al. (15) sectioned the entire bronchial tree from lung specimens from uranium miners and found that squamous carcinoma in situ was present in the bronchial epithelium in more than 90% and was commonly multifocal. These studies have also made clear the fact that development of invasive carcinoma is relatively slow; with each stage (mild dysplasia, moderate dysplasia, severe dysplasia, carcinoma in situ) lasting on average 2–5 years before progression (14).

The precursor lesion(s) for nonsquamous carcinomas is uncertain. There is no defined in situ histologic lesion of small-cell carcinoma; rather, small-cell carcinoma appears to arise in a setting of squamous dysplasia and squamous carcinoma in situ, at least in uranium miners (14,16), suggesting that small-cell carcinoma is derived from dysplastic squamous cells. Similarly, there is no defined in situ lesion for adenocarcinoma in the bronchial epithelium, and central adenocarcinomas may also arise from squamous dysplasia (16).

Peripheral adenocarcinomas are often said to be associated with scars, and one can sometimes find dysplastic columnar epithelium overlying peripheral scars; however, the current consensus is that most of the scarring seen with peripheral tumors is a desmoplastic response to the tumor rather than a precursor of malignancy (17,18). Recently Miller (19) has proposed that some adenocarcinomas may arise as multifocal, microscopic, cytologically bland proliferations of cells resembling those seen in bronchioloalveolar carcinomas, proliferations not associated with scars. The one setting in which scarring really is associated with an increased risk of carcinoma is that of the diffuse fibrosis seen in usual interstitial pneumonia (fibrosing alveolitis) and asbestosis, but in both these circumstances the incidence of all histologic types of lung cancer and not only adenocarcinomas is increased (20 and see below).

The cell of origin of bronchogenic carcinomas remains in dispute. Small-cell carcinoma in particular has been a contentious issue; these tumors were originally thought to be either sarcomas or lymphomas, and were only recognized as carcinomas through the descriptions of Barnard (21). With the electron microscopic discovery that small-cell carcinomas contained neurosecretory granules (5) and thus resembled (and presumably were derived from) the neuroendocrine cells normally present in the bronchial tree, the issue of a distinct cell of origin for these tumors once again arose. Pearce supported this idea by including the neuroendocrine cells of the bronchus among the cells thought to be derived by migration from the neural crest during embryogenesis (22). However, current studies based both on biochemical parameters and direct observation of developmental chimeras have shown that neuroendocrine cells develop in situ in the bronchial tree (23–25).

The comments just made apply to the origin of normal neuroendocrine cells, but taking this one step further, the idea that small-cell carcinomas actually do derive from a cell showing neuroendocrine differentiation is most likely also incorrect. As noted above, small-cell carcinomas appear in a setting of squamous dysplasia; moreover, as detailed below, combinations of small-cell carcinoma with squamous or adenocarcinoma, or transformation of small-cell carcinoma into squamous or adenocarcinoma over time, is reasonably common, an event difficult to explain if small-cell carcinoma is derived from a cell committed to neuroendocrine differentiation.

The occurrence of tumors showing combinations of squamous and adenocarcinoma, or transformation over time from one to the other, also argue against the origin of either squamous or adenocarcinoma from a specifically differentiated cell in the bronchus. A more reasonable and widely accepted explanation is that all three types of tumor (large-cell carcinoma being treated here as merely very poorly differentiated squamous or adenocarcinoma) derive from a stem cell intrinsic to the bronchial epithelium (26).

Just what cell that might be is as yet uncertain, and there are two schools of thought: (1) all of the specialized types of cell normally seen in the bronchial epithelium, and by implication all of the common types of carcinoma, arise by differentiation of basal cells; or (2) bronchial secretory cells are actually the progenitors of both more specialized cells and of basal cells (for a recent review see Ref. 26). Modern data, particularly data derived from studies using isolated cell fractions, indicate that the first theory is probably correct in the large airways (26). It is particularly interesting that in such experiments isolated basal cells can give rise not only to differentiated bronchial epithelium, including secretory and ciliated cells, but also to metaplastic squamous cells under certain conditions, especially vitamin A deficiency (26).

The situation in the bronchioles and the lung periphery appears to be different. Cell fractionation experiments indicate that the Clara cells of the smallest airways can act as stem cells (26), and a few tumors with apparent Clara cell differentiation have been reported (27). Also there are occasional adenocarcinomas (mostly bronchioloalveolar carcinomas) that secrete surfactant apoprotein and are thus presumed to be derived from the type II cells of the alveolus (28). Nonetheless, routine light microscopy as well as electron microscopy and immunohistochemical examination suggest that most peripheral carcinomas are derived from bronchial stem cells much in the manner of central tumors (27,28).

IV. Factors Affecting the Histologic Classification of Lung Cancer

As shown in Table 1, histologic type of lung cancer is influenced by a variety of factors intrinsic to the process of pathologic diagnosis. When attempting to consider the effects of occupation on lung cancer type, the effects of a variety of other epidemiological variables that appear to affect cell type must also be accounted for.

A. Factors Intrinsic to the Process of Pathologic Diagnosis

Epidemiological studies that investigate the relationship of lung cancer cell type and other factors are by definition no better than the underlying pathologic diagnosis. Table 1 lists some of the factors that may affect the pathologic diagnosis of lung cancer. Probably the most basic is the choice of classification scheme. Although many investigators who publish in this area currently use the four basic categories shown in Table 3, this has not always been true, even in the recent past (see below). When one comes to the level of daily pathologic practice, there is an even greater chance that some nonstandard scheme is used. Thus it is not uncommon to see pathology reports bearing the terms "undifferentiated" or "poorly differentiated" carcinoma, or "pleomorphic" carcinoma. In some instances the specimen is such that no legitimate diagnosis beyond "non–small-cell carcinoma" can be rendered.

While the major classification categories are reasonably well defined (except for large-cell carcinoma, which has a negative definition and tends to be a repository for all tumors not easily classified) (29), the subcategories shown in Table 2 generally are not. In particular, the histologic distinctions between well, moderately, and poorly differentiated squamous or adenocarcinoma are totally arbitrary choices by the reviewing pathologist. This problem is worse than it might appear at first glance because most lung cancers are quite heterogeneous in histologic appearance (29), and mixtures of grade (for example, part poorly differentiated adenocarcinoma and part moderately or well-differentiated adenocarcinoma) are the rule rather than the exception. There are no accepted guidelines for classifying tumors with mixed grades; some pathologists would diagnose to match the worst differentiated area on the grounds that the more anaplastic areas of tumor determine behavior; others would pick the majority pattern for determining diagnosis.

The problems of classification are compounded by the tendency of lung cancers to show not only grades of differentiation within a single cell type, but mixtures of cell types. Because small-cell carcinoma is treated quite differently from all other carcinomas, the issue of mixed cell type has received a great deal of attention in recent years. Mixed small-cell and non–small-cell carcinomas have been found in 10–24% of autopsy cases (30–33). Even more intriguing is the fact that 5–10% of cases reported as pure small-cell at biopsy have had only non–small-cell features at autopsy (31,32). Mixtures of squamous and adenocarcinoma also occur. The overall frequency of combined cell types is uncertain: Yesner (29) reported combinations in only 2% of 10,000 cases, and Whitwell (35) found combined histologic features in 6% of 1900 cases. However, Roggli et al. (36) reported a study of 100 consecutive cases in which the whole tumor or at least 10 blocks were examined. They found that only 34% of the tumors were homogeneous in regard to major classification group, 21% showed minor subtype mixtures, and a remarkable 45% showed mixtures of the major classification groups. The interested reader is referred to the particularly useful discussion provided by Roggli et al. (36) on this issue.

The reported distribution of lung cancer cell types also varies with the type of specimen examined. Since small-cell carcinomas are not usually resected, series using surgical resections tend to show lower frequencies of small-cell carcinoma than biopsy (or cytology) or autopsy series. Peripheral tumors, many of which are adenocarcinomas, tend to present more often at a time when they are still resectable compared to central tumors. Table 5, which contains cell type frequencies determined by review by one pathologist from the same cases examined in surgical and then autopsy specimens, illustrates this point. Additional detailed examples can be found in Refs. 1 and 2.

It is believed that radiation and chemotherapy have an effect on cell type, particularly small-cell carcinoma (31). Radiation definitely produces giant cells in quite ordinary squamous and adenocarcinomas; such tumors are often misdiagnosed as giant cell carcinoma (a variant of large-cell carcinoma), and even the experienced pathologist may not be able to determine whether such a tumor was initially a squamous or an adenocarcinoma.

Finally one must consider variations related to the choice of diagnostic technique. Standard classification schemes are based entirely on light microscopy.

Table 5 Lung Cancer Cell Type (as % of Total) in Autopsy and Surgical Specimens from the Same Set of Patients

Cell type	Surgical	Autopsy
Squamous cell	48	35
Small-cell	19	23
Adeno	16	26
Large-cell	16	15

Even something as simple as the routine addition of a special stain for mucin will tend to change the distribution of tumors, since many tumors will show focal mucin production if enough sections are prepared (2,37). Academic pathologists put a great deal of effort into examining tumors with newer techniques such as electron microscopy and immunohistochemistry. Such investigations have produced further subclassifications (for example, the various types of adenocarcinoma proposed in Refs. 38 and 39). The recognition of the neuroendocrine nature of small-cell carcinoma stems largely from the electron microscopic observation that they produce neurosecretory granules (5). Immunohistochemical studies of intermediate filaments may eventually provide much greater accuracy in separating the various cell types. But the problem from the point of view of epidemiological investigation is that these techniques are not and cannot be applied in every case, and there is no agreement about how to interpret the results.

As a practical matter, any attempt to use histopathologic classification of lung cancer in epidemiological studies must, at present, be confined to light microscopic observations, must use a very standard classification scheme, and must have every case reviewed by the same pathologist. Even this approach is extraordinarily limited, as can be seen from three published samples. Feinstein et al. (40) reported a study in which five experienced pathologists classified 50 different tumors. For well-differentiated squamous and adenocarcinomas, a consensus was reached in about 95% of cases. However, the rate of disagreement rose to about 25% of readings for cases labeled by the majority as small-cell carcinoma or large-cell carcinoma, and to around 40% for cases labeled by the majority as poorly differentiated squamous or poorly differentiated adenocarcinomas. Yesner et al. (41) performed a similar type of study and found that only 10% of large-cell carcinomas, 43% of poorly differentiated adenocarcinomas, 47% of poorly differentiated squamous carcinomas, and 34% of intermediate type small-cell carcinomas were universally agreed on by a panel. More recently, Stanley and Matthews had three pathologists review nearly 500 cases using the

WPL classification (42): They obtained agreement on the *major* classification category in only 67% of cases. The poorly differentiated squamous and adenocarcinomas, small-cell carcinomas, and large-cell carcinomas continued to be major areas of disagreement.

These observations suggest that, for accurate classification of lung cancer, one should use only the four major categories of tumor, and for really accurate classification, only well-differentiated tumors. However, given that a very large fraction of lung cancers are poorly differentiated, the latter suggestion will probably reduce the number of available cases to an unusable value. Considering, as will become evident, that most series of workers with occupational exposure are fairly small to begin with, and that in most instances there is not an overwhelming preponderance of one cell type, one must accept the possibility that an equally competent pathologist(s) could review the same material and come to a completely different conclusion about dominant cell type. This limitation must be kept in mind in considering reports of specific associations between cell type and any epidemiological variable.

B. Epidemiological Factors Other Than Occupation That Affect Lung Cancer Histology

Epidemiological factors other than occupation that affect cell type will only be touched on here, more to point out the importance of accounting for these potential confounders in any study of lung cancer cell type and occupation than to discuss them in detail, but most are covered in other chapters in this volume. Of these factors, the most basic is the presence or absence of a cigarette-smoking history. Kreyberg (43) originally suggested that only squamous and small-cell carcinoma were associated with cigarette smoking, but all recent studies indicate that the vast majority of adenocarcinomas also arise in cigarette smokers and that a cigarette smoke dose-tumor incidence relationship can usually be demonstrated (9,44–51). To cite just one example, Geddes et al. (44) histologically typed a series of nearly 300 lung cancers. Overall, 98% of the tumors occurred in smokers; 100% of small-cell carcinomas, 98% of squamous cell carcinomas, and 96% of adenocarcinomas were associated with smoking. However, in never smokers there is very clearly a preponderance of adenocarcinomas, accounting for as many as 75% of lung cancers in never-smoking women, and somewhat fewer in men (45,47,51).

The effect of sex and secular trends on lung cancer histopathology are frequently overlooked, and textbooks for medical students still list squamous cell carcinoma as the most common cell type. This claim was certainly true 30 or 40 years ago, but starting in the 1960s there was a progressive decrease in the frequency of squamous carcinoma and a progressive increase in the frequency of adenocarcinoma (9,45,48). For example, Vincent et al. (9) found on review of more than 1400 lung cancers in men that in 1963 adenocarcinomas accounted for approximately 13% of the total and squamous cell carcinomas for about 45%; by 1974 squamous carcinomas had dropped to some 30% of all cases and adenocarcinomas had risen to about 35%. A similar but less dramatic effect (because adenocarcinomas have always been common) was seen for women. More recent studies (45,48,52) confirm that this trend has continued into the 1980s.

Age influences both the incidence of lung cancer and the reported distribution of histologic types. Most lung cancers arise in persons older than 50, particularly individuals aged 50–70. It appears that, for both men and women, squamous cell carcinoma increases in frequency with age at diagnosis, whereas small-cell carcinomas decrease with age (45,53).

Country of residence affects lung cancer histology. Adenocarcinomas, for example, appear to be much more frequent in the Orient than in Europe or North America (54). Even given the same geographic location, race (or country of origin) may be important. For example, among women living in Hawaii, those of Japanese or Chinese descent showed a preponderance of adenocarcinomas during a period in which women of Hawaiian descent had mainly squamous and small-cell carcinomas (55). Wynder and Covey found that adenocarcinomas were more common in Jews than non-Jews in North America (45). However, it is unclear to what extent the confounding effect of cigarette smoke has been considered in these reports.

V. Exposure to Specific Occupational Agents

The remainder of this chapter considers the issue of occupation and lung cancer cell type for a number of substances generally accepted to cause lung cancer in humans. Several studies (49,50,53,56) consider the issue of the histology of lung cancer in very broad occupational groups, such a blue collar vs. white collar; for example, Vena et al. (50) claimed that all types of occupational exposure were associated with an increased risk of squamous carcinoma and also an increased risk of adenocarcinoma in light smokers, but no increased risk of small-cell carcinoma. Studies of this type are difficult to reconcile with reports on specific occupations that fail to show differences in cell type.

Only studies on specific exposures, which provide a breakdown by histologic type of lung cancer, and which use a reasonably modern classification system, are considered below. The reader interested in the older literature is referred to Hueper (57), who summarizes much of the data before 1965.

The values reported in the tables below are breakdowns by percent of total; where the numbers add up to less than 100%, the remaining tumors were either not classified or were classified in some nonstandard way ("pleomorphic, undifferentiated," etc.).

A. Arsenic

Most reports of arsenic exposure have come from smelter workers. Table 6 lists five such reports. These studies suffer from poor control of a number of factors including age, smoking history, and a very large proportion of tumors labeled as poorly differentiated squamous. Given the nonreproducibility of the latter diagnosis (see above), the accuracy of these studies is dubious. Moreover, they come to diametrically opposite conclusions, with one report (60) finding an excess of adenocarcinoma, one report an excess of squamous carcinoma (59), and one report an excess of squamous carcinoma and small-cell carcinoma in nonsmokers but not in smokers (62).

The older literature, summarized by Hueper (57), is difficult to interpret because of the classification scheme used, but the reported figures for 47 cases from several series are 40% squamous cell carcinoma, 9% adenocarcinoma, and 51% "round cell and anaplastic" carcinoma (?small-cell). Hueper concludes that these values do not differ from a comparison series of smokers.

Table 6 Arsenic-Exposed Smelter Workers (Values as Percent of Total)

	Cell type					
	Squamous	Small-	Adeno-	Large-	N	Ref.
Smelter workers	61	20	9	9	54	58[a]
Controls	60	24	7	7	45	
Smelter workers	44	33	11	0	18	59[b]
Controls	0	33	50	0	6	
Smelter workers	31	24	38	7	42	60[c]
Controls	47	14	12	19	42	
Smelter workers	65	9	9	3	32	61[d]
Smelter-nonsmoker	60	30	10	0	10	62[e]
Control-nonsmoker	28	22	33	11	18	
Smelter-smoker	41	33	15	7	18	
Control-smoker	49	33	9	5	118	

[a]Large number with unknown smoking history. Large number poorly differentiated squamous.
[b]Most tumors called poorly or undifferentiated. Authors conclude that numbers are insufficient.
[c]Specimen types matched. Virtually all smokers. Well matched for age. Excess of adenocarcinoma claimed.
[d]Controls are cancer registry values grouped as Kreyberg I and II. Disagreement among reviewing pathologists about diagnosis in 5 of 18 reviewed cases.
[e]Substantial age differences among groups. Lack of detailed smoking data. Many poorly differentiated squamous.

Overall there is little convincing evidence that arsenic exposure in smelters produces a specific type of carcinoma.

B. Chromium and Nickel Compounds

Few studies have provided data on histologic type of lung cancer arising in workers exposed to chromium or nickel compounds (Table 7). Taken at face value, these studies appear to suggest that there is an excess of squamous carcinoma in these workers, but in fact most of the studies have no associated control group and are essentially uninterpretable. Abe et al. (63) concluded that small-cell carcinoma was associated with low smoking levels and short latency, and that different parts of the manufacturing process and different valencies of chromium had different carcinogenic potential. Given that the diagnoses were apparently unreviewed and given the size of the group even claimed to be pathologically classifiable (N = 18), these conclusions must be treated with caution.

Hueper (57) presented summary data for 123 chromate-exposed cases through about 1965 and found 37% squamous carcinoma, 9% adenocarcinoma, and 54% "round cell, anaplastic, and undifferentiated" carcinoma, values he believes are no different from pure smoking-induced tumors. Of 11 tumors thought to be related to nickel compounds, Hueper lists 64% as squamous carcinoma, 9% as adenocarcinoma, and 27% as (probably) small-cell carcinoma.

As is true of arsenic, there is little reason to be believe that chromium and nickel compounds cause specific types of lung cancer.

Table 7 Chromium and Nickel Workers (Values as Percent of Total)

	Cell type					
	Squamous	Small-	Adeno-	Large-	N	Ref.
Chromium	65	25	0	0	20	63[a]
Exposed smokers	83	17	0	0	12	64[b]
Control smokers	65	25	10	0	20	
Exposed nonsmokers	60	0	40	0	5	
Control nonsmokers	0	0	100	0	2	
Chromium	88	0	12	0	8	65[c]

[a]No control group. 10% unclassified tumors. All smokers.
[b]Some unclassified. Mostly smokers. Nonsmoker numbers too small for definitive conclusion.
[c]Very small group. No controls. No pathology review. Average age = 46.

C. Chloromethyl Ether

Chloromethyl ether exposure presents probably the strongest and most consistent case for development of a specific type of lung cancer, namely small-cell carcinoma, with a specific occupational exposure. As shown in Table 8, most studies, despite variability in the nature of the specimen, show a greater than 60% incidence of small-cell carcinoma in these workers. Even if the large proportion of unclassified tumors in some studies (67,68) were to turn out to be all of some other specific type, small-cell carcinoma would still predominate. This situation is one instance in which the universal lack of control groups, although unfortunate, does not appear to vitiate the results. Of particular additional note in these reports are the relatively young age of the patients, the fairly common development of small-cell carcinoma in nonsmokers [(70) otherwise an extremely rare event], and the overall high incidence of carcinoma in nonsmokers (70). All of these features argue that chloromethyl ether produces a very specific type of lung cancer.

D. Asbestos

Much of the current interest in the relationship of specific cancer types and occupation stems from claims that asbestos exposure is associated with adenocarcinoma of the lung (57,71). The study of Whitwell et al. (71) is frequently cited in this regard, and perhaps no other report better illustrates the importance of proper control selection, since the claimed relative increase in adenocarcinoma in Whitwell's study depends entirely on which of his control groups one uses. In fact the best matched control group does not differ from the asbestos exposed group in a statistically significant fashion.

Compared to most other specific exposures, there are a relatively large

Table 8 Chloromethyl Ether Workers (Values as Percent of Total)

	Cell type					
	Squamous	Small-	Adeno-	Large-	N	Ref.
No control group	7	86	0	0	14	66
No control group. 60% unclassified tumors	0	20	20	0	5	47
No control group. 37% unclassified tumors	0	63	0	0	8	68
No control group	0	80	0	20	5	69
No control group. High cancer rate (21%) in nonsmokers	4	68	18	7	28	70

number of studies on workers with asbestos exposure. These studies suffer from many of the same problems described above for arsenic, metals, and chloromethyl ether, including lack of control populations and lack of detailed smoking and age data. Table 9 shows only studies that have internal control populations (see Refs. 72 and 73 for data on reports without internal controls). One additional study of interest is that of Blot et al. (see Ref. 1). This is based on death certificates; even if the specific cell types listed on the death certificates are accurate (the pathologic diagnoses are apparently unreviewed), the vast majority of cases are simply labeled as carcinoma without histologic type. This point emphasizes the inadequacy of death certificates in investigating pathologic variables.

The whole asbestos issue is confounded by the presence or absence of asbestosis, since there is a growing consensus that the risk of lung cancer is probably only increased in asbestos workers who have asbestosis (74,75). If this concept is correct, then studies reporting workers without asbestosis or workers with and without asbestosis presumably include a large number of purely smoking-induced tumors. Taken as a whole, current studies are certainly in accord with this idea, since there appears at present to be no consistent change in cell type between asbestos-exposed workers without asbestosis and nonexposed workers

Table 9 Asbestos Workers Without Asbestosis or Mixtures of Asbestotic and Nonasbestotic Workers (Values as Percent of Total)

	Cell type					
	Squamous	Small-	Adeno-	Large-	N	Ref.
Exposed	28	28	28	15	39	77[a]
Control	28	33	21	19	43	
Exposed	23	28	35	0	93	71[b]
Control	18	40	30	0	96	
Exposed	53	45	2	0	49	76[c]
Control	69	24	7	0	112	
Exposed	50	25	15	10	193	78[d]
Control	52	16	19	14	648	
All Exposed	46	20	20	2	46	75[e]
All Control	33	20	27	14	234	

[a]No smoking match. Cases of asbestosis included but not separated.
[b]No smoking match. Use of different internal controls yields different results. Mixed asbestotic and nonasbestotic Many unclassified.
[c]Sequential surgical specimens. Control group older by 10 years.
[d]Surgical and autopsy series including many insulators, some of whom are probably asbestotics.
[e]Includes asbestotics and nonasbestotics. Good specimen type match. 25% with poor smoking histories.

(see Table 9), although individual reports demonstrate inconsistent increases in squamous (76) and small-cell (77) carcinoma.

Hueper (57) summarized the older literature in regard to workers with asbestosis. Of 104 reported cases, he classifies 43% as squamous cell, 38% as round cell (presumably meant here as small-cell), and 18% as adenocarcinoma. Hueper comments that this latter figure appears to represent an increase in adenocarcinoma, but this claim is based on a single comparison series taken from the United States (test cases come from several different countries), and there is no information on the smoking or age distribution of this series. Females make up a disproportionate number of cases of asbestotics in Hueper's summary (17%) compared to their general prevalence in series of smokers from this time period, and the apparent excess in adenocarcinoma may be entirely related to sex distribution.

More recent studies examining cases with documented asbestosis generally suffer from poor design (Table 10). For example, the review by Hasan et al. (80) has very few cases and no controls; the values found are not particularly discrepant from what might be expected over the same time period in ordinary smokers (see comments on secular trends, above), particularly if females are included in their data. In a considerably older series, Whitwell et al. (71) used cases going back to 1962, and found that 38% of those with severe asbestosis had adenocarcinoma, while only 25% of those with no or mild asbestosis had adenocarcinoma, but the difference is not statistically significant. Hourihane and McCaughey (81) furnished data on males and females. In the women 70% of the cases were adenocarcinomas, but 6 of 7 cases developed in nonsmokers, and a value of 70% adenocarcinomas in nonsmoking women is probably to be expected in the general population. Four of the male cases also occurred in nonsmokers.

Table 10 Asbestos Workers with Asbestosis (Values as Percent of Total)

	Cell type					
	Squamous	Small-	Adeno-	Large-	N	Ref.
Severe asbestosis	19	28	38	0	58	71
Mild or no asbestosis	29	25	25	0	28	
	33	17	50	0	12	80[a]
Males	29	18	35	0	17	81[b]
Females	20	10	70	0	10	
Asbestosis	45	30	10	15	20	76
No asbestosis	46	12	27	12	26	

[a]No controls, no smoking data. No data on sex breakdown.

[b]Many nonsmokers (especially females). Mean age 55 for females, 58 for males.

Baker et al. (76) specifically compared 20 workers with asbestosis to 26 with asbestos exposure and no evidence of asbestosis. There appeared to be excesses of small-cell carcinoma in the asbestotics and adenocarcinomas in the nonasbestotics, but the differences were only marginally significant.

The question of cell type and asbestos exposure is also potentially confounded by the apparently synergistic interaction of smoke and asbestos in producing bronchogenic carcinoma (82,83). However, the published data are largely derived from smokers, and there is insufficient information to comment on histologic changes between smokers and nonsmokers. At present there are no hard data to support a claim of specific associations for cell type and asbestos exposure, whether or not asbestosis is present.

E. Radon

Except for coal mining, where ventilation levels have always been kept relatively high to prevent explosions, underground mining of any sort may lead to an increase in lung cancer caused by exposure to radon and radon daughters (84). Although this fact is widely accepted (for a review of 21 series of underground miners see Ref. 84), the question of radiation and cell type is confused. In part this problem stems from older studies (Table 11) (85) in which matching for age and smoking was poor and there was dispute about diagnoses (see particularly the comments of Ives et al. (1) in this regard) but in part is probably also an effect of time since first exposure (84). As well, synergism with cigarette smoke appears to increase the incidence of bronchogenic carcinoma in radiation-exposed workers (84,86); to what extent changes in the type of tumor caused by cigarette smoke itself in the whole population over time (see above) confound the issue is unclear. However, the work of Samet et al. (87) has shown that uranium miners with no or low smoking histories also experience increases in lung cancer incidence, so that an independent effect of radiation is clear.

Table 11 Representative Data for Uranium Miners in the 1960s (Values as Percent of Total)

	Cell type				
	Squamous	Small-	Adeno-	Large-	N
Exposed 40–200 WLM	43	36	14	7	14
Control	64	21	7	7	14
Exposed 2500–9700 WLM	20	77	0	0	30
Control	53	10	10	10	30

WLM = Exposure measured in Working Level Months
Source: Ref. 85.

Table 11 shows data from one of the original studies by Saccomanno and colleagues (85) of Colorado uranium miners. Although there is an apparent dramatic increase in small-cell carcinoma at both low and high radiation exposure levels (and those in between) (85), the patients with 2500–9700 WLM are more than 12 years younger than the controls, on average, and smoked an average of 12 pack-years less. The matching in the intermediate exposure categories is also disparate, although the 40–200 WLM group is well matched to controls. But even given the usual increase in squamous carcinomas and decrease in small-cell carcinomas with age (see above), it is hard to believe that poor matching accounts for all of the differences; indeed, the finding of any group of pure cigarette smokers in whom 77% of lung cancers were small-cell carcinomas would be extraordinary! Moreover, subsequent work by the same group showed that small-cell carcinoma was also increased in nonsmokers (90).

Further clarification of the situation has been produced by the realization that the dramatic relative increase in small-cell carcinomas was masking the presence of an absolute increase in squamous and adenocarcinomas as well (88). A similar increase in both squamous and small-cell carcinoma was also reported by Horacek et al. (89) (it is worth pointing out that 54% of the tumors in this series were small-cell carcinomas).

Further useful information in this regard can be obtained by tabulating studies of miners where the original data are presented for smokers and nonsmokers (Table 12). A follow-up study of 383 uranium miners was reported in 1988 by Saccomanno and colleagues (90) and is discussed by Archer (84). This study included both the original group discussed above and workers with considerably lower exposure. As shown in Table 12, the relative proportion of cell types had

Table 12 Cell Type in Studies Reporting Smoking and Nonsmoking Miners (Values as Percent of Total)

	Cell type					
	Squamous	Small-	Adeno-	Large-	N	Ref.
Smoking miners	36	32	13	12	356	90
Nonsmoking miners	40	24	12	20	25	
Smoking miners	50	33	8	8	12	91
Nonsmoking miners	25	38	25	12	8	
Smoking miners	0	100	0	0	2	92
Nonsmoking miners	23	62	15	0	13	
Smoking miners	28	72	0	NU	32	93
Nonsmoking miners	25	75	0	NU	4	

NU = category not used for classification.

changed considerably (unfortunately, no control group is provided). Butler et al. (91) and Gottlieb and Husen (92) examined Navajo uranium miners, many of whom were either low or nonsmokers, and found that small-cell carcinoma was clearly increased in the nonsmokers (Table 12). Similarly, Edling (93) found a high incidence of small-cell carcinoma in nonsmoking iron ore miners, although here the total numbers were small and the smokers also showed a preponderance of small-cell carcinomas.

Although Saccomanno et al. (90) concluded that small-cell carcinoma particularly developed in those with high exposure and in nonsmokers, Archer (84) proposed that the major effect is a temporal one, with small-cell carcinoma having a short latency and squamous cell carcinoma a much longer latency. Alternately Samet and colleagues (91,94) suggested that small-cell carcinoma is definitely increased in both smokers and nonsmokers as a result of radon exposure, but that smoking may hide the increase by leading to the development of all the other cell types.

F. Miscellaneous Suspected Carcinogens

Aside from the specific exposures listed above, a number of other agents are suspected to be human lung carcinogens, and for some of these substances individual studies examining the question of cell type exist. Smith and Suzuki (95) reviewed a series of workers with beryllium exposure. They found that 47% of cases in the exposed group were adenocarcinoma compared to only 10% in the controls; however, 60% of the control cases were labeled small-cell carcinoma. Moreover, a very large fraction of the specimens were not reviewed by a pathologist. This fact and the peculiar distribution seen in the control series suggest serious misclassification error. Waxweiler et al. (96) reported a group of workers with vinyl chloride exposure; the only apparent major difference was a finding of 30% large-cell carcinoma in the exposed cases compared to 10% in the controls. Given the known lack of pathologic uniformity in diagnosing large-cell carcinoma (see above), it is likely that no real differences exist between the groups. Yamada (97) studied a group of workers who made mustard gas; 5 of 11 cases were labeled squamous cell carcinoma and the rest undifferentiated carcinoma. Vallyathan et al. (98) studied 171 autopsy specimens from coal miners, a group for which an increase in lung cancer is far from clear; there were no differences between the miners and a set of matched smokers.

VI. Conclusions

This chapter has emphasized the facts that most histologic types of bronchogenic carcinomas are closely related tumors that probably arise from the same stem cell and that accurate histologic diagnosis, even in terms of major type divisions, remains a difficult problem confounded by both marked interobserver variability and intrinsic tumor heterogeneity. Moreover, a number of important epidemiological variables aside from occupation have distinct effects on lung cancer cell type. In this circumstance it is perhaps wishful thinking to assume that one can account for all confounders in such a way as to sort out the specific associations of lung cancer cell type and occupation.

Certainly there is little in the literature to support such associations on a broad scale. In my opinion the majority of reports cited in this review have failed to find anything other than random variations in cell type, and even where particular associations are postulated, the study design is usually obviously flawed. Alternately, what appears to be a reasonably carefully prepared study is contradicted by an equally good study of a similar occupational exposure. Even using the simple criterion of consistency of effect and ignoring internal defects in each report, for most occupational exposures there is no obvious cell type predominance; rather most occupational agents that increase the incidence of carcinoma appear to increase of of all cell types.

Two exceptions to this rule stand out. One is the rather dramatic and consistent finding of small-cell carcinomas as the majority of tumors in workers with exposure to chloromethyl ether. This association is particularly interesting because it occurs in both smokers and nonsmokers, the latter a group in which small-cell carcinoma is rare. A somewhat similar, but not as clear-cut, conclusion applies to radiation (radon) exposure in underground miners. These observations, if confirmed, imply that some very specific occupational carcinogens can affect tumor differentiation in such a way as to cause very specific types of neoplasms, but clearly this is an unusual rather than a common effect.

Acknowledgment

Supported by a grant from the National Cancer Institute of Canada.

References

1. Ives, J. C., Buffler, P. A., and Greenberg, S. D. (1983). Environmental associations and histopathologic patterns of carcinoma of the lung: the challenge and dillemma in epidemiologic studies. *Am. Rev. Respir. Dis.* 128:195–209.
2. Churg, A. (1988). Tumors of the lung. In *Pathology of the Lung*. Edited by W. M. Thurlbeck. New York, Thieme Medical Publishers, pp. 311–424.
3. World Health Organization. (1982). The World Health Organization histological typing of lung tumours. *Am. J. Clin. Pathol.* 77:123–129.
4. Hammar, S. P. (1988). Common neoplasms. In *Pulmonary Pathology*. Edited by D. H. Dail and S. P. Hammar. New York, Springer-Verlag, pp. 727–846.

5. Bensch, K. G., Corrin, B., Pariente, R., and Spencer, H. (1968). Oat-cell carcinoma of the lung. Its origin and relationship to bronchial carcinoid. *Cancer* 22:1163–1172.
6. Churg, A. (1978). The fine structure of large cell undifferentiated carcinoma of the lung: Evidence for its relationship to squamous cell carcinoma and adenocarcinoma. *Human Pathol.* 9:143–156.
7. Horie, A., and Ohta, M. (1981). Ultrastructural features of large cell carcinoma of the lung with reference to the prognosis in patients. *Human Pathol.* 12:423–432.
8. Auerbach, O., Garfinkel, L., and Parks, U. R. (1975). Histologic type of lung cancer in relation to smoking habits, year of diagnosis and sites of metastases. *Chest* 67: 382–388.
9. Vincent, R. G., Pickren, J. W., Lane, W. W., Bross, I., Takita, H., Gutierrez, A., and Rzepka, T. (1977). The changing histopathology of lung cancer. A review of 1682 cases. *Cancer* 99:1647–1655.
10. Cox, J., and Yesner, R. (1979). Adenocarcinoma of the lung: Recent results from the Veterans Administration Lung Group. *Am. Rev. Respir. Dis.* 120:1025–1029.
11. Hinson, K. F. W., Miller, A. B., and Tall, R. (1975). An assessment of the world health organization classification of the histologic typing of lung tumors applied to biopsy and resected material. *Cancer* 35:399–405.
12. Melamed, M., Flehinger, B., Zaman, M. B., Heelen, R. T., Perchick, W. A., and Martini, N. (1984). Screening for early lung cancer: Results of the Memorial Sloan-Kettering Study in New York. *Chest* 86:44–53.
13. Healy, T. M. (1980). The pathology of carcinoma of the lung: The pattern over 15 years. *Ir. J. Med. Sci.* 149:91–94.
14. Saccomanno, G., Archer, V. E., Auerbach, R., Saunders, P., and Brennan, L. M. (1974). Development of carcinoma of the lung as reflected in exfoliated cells. *Cancer* 34:256–270.
15. Auerbach, O., Saccomanno, G., Kuschner, M., Brown, R. D., and Garfinkel, L. (1978). Histologic findings in the tracheobronchial tree of uranium miners and non-miners with lung cancer. *Cancer* 42:483–489.
16. Auerbach, O. (1980). Natural history of carcinoma of the lung. In *Pulmonary Disease and Disorders*. Edited by A. P. Fishman. New York, McGraw-Hill, pp. 1388–1396.
17. Cagle, P. T., Cohle, S. D., and Greenberg, S. D. (1985). Natural history of pulmonary scar carcinomas. *Cancer* 56:2031–2035.
18. Barksy, S. H., Huang, S. J., and Bhuta, S. (1986). The extracellular matrix of pulmonary scar carcinomas is suggestive of a desmoplastic origin. *Am. J. Pathol.* 124: 412–419.
19. Miller, R. R. (1990). Bronchioloalveolar cell adenoma. *Am. J. Surg. Pathol.* 14: 904–912.
20. Turner-Warwick, M., Lebowitz, M., Burrows, B., and Johnson, A. (1980). Cytogenic fibrosing alveolitis and lung cancer. *Thorax* 35:496–499.
21. Barnard, W. G. (1926). Nature of oat-celled sarcoma of mediastinum. *J. Pathol.* 29:241–249.
22. Pearce, A. G. E. (1969). The cytochemistry and ultrastructure of polypeptide hormone-producing cells of the APUD series and the embryologic, physiologic, and pathologic implications of the concept. *J. Histochem. Cytochem.* 17:303–314.

23. Ledourain, N., and Teillet, M. A. (1973). The migration of neural crest cells to the digestive tract in avian embryo. *J. Embryol. Expt. Morphol.* 30:31–38.
24. Tischler, A. S. (1978). Small cell carcinoma of the lung. Cellular origin and relationship to other neoplasms. *Semin. Oncol.* 5:244–250.
25. Sidhu, G. S. (1979). The endodermal origin of digestive and respiratory tract APUD cells-histopathologic evidence and a review of the literature. *Am. J. Pathol.* 96:5–13.
26. Nettesheim, P., Jetten, A. M., Inayama, Y., Brody, A. R., George, M. A., Gilmore, L. B., Gray, T., and Hook, G. E. R. (1990). Pathways of differentiation of airway epithelial cells. *Environ. Health Perspect.* 85:317–329.
27. Sidhu, G. S., and Forrester, E. M. (1977). Glycogen rich clara cell-type bronchiolo-alveolar carcinoma. *Cancer* 40:2209–2214.
28. Singh, G., Katyal, S. L., and Torikata, C. (1981). Carcinoma of type II pneumocytes. *Am. J. Pathol.* 102:195–201.
29. Yesner, R. (1973). Observer variability and reliability in lung cancer diagnosis. *Cancer Chemo. Rep.* 4(Part 3):55–60.
30. Adelstein, D. J., Tomashefski, J. F., Snow, N. J., Horrigan, J. P., and Hines, J. D. (1986). Mixed small cell and nonsmall cell lung cancer. *Chest* 89:699–704.
31. Abeloff, M. D., Eggleston, J. C., and Mendelsohn, G. (1979) Changes in morphologic and biochemical characteristics of small cell carcinoma of the lung. *Am. J. Med.* 66:757–763.
32. Matthews, M. J. (1979). Effects of therapy on the morphology and behavior of small cell carcinoma of the lung. In *Lung Cancer: Progress in Therapeutic Research*. Edited by F. Muggia and M. Rozencweig. New York, Raven Press, p. 155.
33. Brereton, H. D., Matthews, M. M., Costa, J., Kent, C. H., and Johnson, R. E. (1978). Mixed anaplastic small-cell and squamous-cell carcinoma of the lung. *Ann. Intern. Med.* 88:805–811.
34. Yesner, R. (1978). The spectrum of lung cancer and ectopic hormones. *Pathol. Ann.* 13(Pt 2):217–240.
35. Whitwell, F. (1961). The histopathology of lung cancer in Liverpool: The specificity of the histological cell types of lung cancer. *Br. J. Cancer* 15:440–459.
36. Roggli, V. L., Vollmer, R. T., Greenberg, S. D., McGavran, M. H., Spjut, H. J., and Yesner, R. (1985). Lung cancer heterogeneity. *Human Pathol.* 16:569–579.
37. Kreyberg, L. (1971). Comments on the histological typing lung tumors. *Acta Pathol. Scand.* 79:409–422.
38. Kimula, Y. (1978). A histochemical and ultrastructural study of adenocarcinoma of the lung. *Am. J. Surg. Pathol.* 2:253–264.
39. Herrera, G. A., Alexander, C. B., and deMoraes, H. P. (1983). Ultrastructural subtypes of pulmonary adenocarcinoma. *Chest* 84:581–586
40. Feinstein, A. R., Gelfman, N. A., and Yesner, R. (1970). Observer variability in the histopathologic diagnosis of lung cancer. *Am. Rev. Respir. Dis.* 101:671–684.
41. Yesner, R., Gerstl, B., and Auerbach, O. (1965). Application of the World Health Organization classification of lung carcinoma to biopsy material. *Ann. Thorac. Surg.* 1:33–49.
42. Stanley, K. E., and Matthews, M. J. (1981). Analysis of a pathology review of patients with lung tumors. *JNCI* 66:989–992.

43. Kreyberg, L. (1961). Relationship of different histological lung tumor groups to tobacco smoking. *Br. J. Cancer* 15:51–58.
44. Geddes, M., Buiatti, E., Seniori, C. A., and Santucci, M. (1984). Cell type distribution in histological spectrum of primary lung cancer. *Tumori* 70:255–260.
45. Wynder, E. L., and Covey, L. (1987). Epidemiologic patterns in lung cancer by histologic type. *Eur. J. Cancer Clin. Oncol.* 10:1491–1496.
46. Valaitis, J., Warren, S., and Gable, D. (1981). Increasing incidence of adenocarcinoma of the lung. *Cancer* 47:1042–1046.
47. Brownson, R. C., Reif, J. S., Keefe, T. J., Ferguson, S. W., and Pritzl, J. A. (1987). Risk factors for adenocarcinoma of the lung. *Am. J. Epidemiol.* 125:25–34.
48. Dodds, L., Davis, S., and Polissar, L. (1986). A population-based study of lung cancer incidence trends by histologic type, 1974-81. *JNCI* 76:21–29.
49. Stayner, L. T., and Wegman, D. H. (1983). Smoking, occupation, and histopathology of lung cancer: A case-control study with the use of the Third National Cancer Survey. *JNCI* 70:421–426.
50. Vena, J. E., Byers, T. E., Cookfair, D., and Swanson, M. (1985). Occupation and lung cancer risk. An analysis by histologic subtypes. *Cancer* 56:910–917.
51. Rosenow, E. C., and Carr, D. T. (1979). Bronchogenic carcinoma. *CA* 29:233–245.
52. Wu, A. H., Henderson, B. E., Thomas, D. C., and Mack, T. M. (1986). Secular trends in histologic types of lung cancer. *JNCI* 77:53–56.
53. Sanila, R. J., Karjalainen, S., Oksanen, H. M., Hakulinen, T. R., and Teppo, L. H. I. (1990). Relationship between occupation and lung cancer as analyzed by age and histologic type. *Cancer* 65:1651–1656.
54. Belcher, J. R. (1971). World-wide differences in the sex ratio of bronchial carcinoma. *Br. J. Dis. Chest* 65:205–221.
55. Hinds, M. W., Stemmerman, G. N., Yang, H. Y., Kolonel, L. N., Lee, J., and Wagner, E. (1981). Differences in lung cancer risk from smoking among Japanese, Chinese, and Hawaiian women in Hawaii. *Int. J. Cancer* 27:297–302.
56. Wegman, D. H., and Peters, J. M. (1978). Oat cell lung cancer in selected occupations. *J. Occ. Med.* 20:793–796.
57. Hueper, W. C. (1966). *Occupational and Environmental Cancers of the Respiratory System*. Berlin, Springer-Verlag.
58. Newman, J. A., Archer, V. E., Saccomanno, G., Kuschner, M., Auerbach, O., Grondahl, R. D., and Wilson, J. C. (1976). Histologic types of bronchogenic carcinoma among members of copper-mining and smelting communities. *Ann. NY Acad. Sci.* 271:260–268.
59. Axelson, O., Dahlgren, E., Jansson, C. D., and Rehnlung, S. O. (1978). Arsenic exposure and mortality: A case-referent study from a Swedish copper smelter. *Br. J. Ind. Med.* 35:8–15.
60. Wicks, M. J., Archer, V. E., Auerbach, O., and Kuschner, M. (1981). Arsenic exposure in a copper smelter as related to histologic type of lung cancer. *Am. J. Ind. Med.* 2:25–31.
61. Tokudome, S., Haratake, J., Horie, A., et al. (1988). Histologic types of lung cancer among male Japanese copper smelter workers. *Am. J. Ind. Med.* 14:137–143.
62. Pershagen, G., Bergman, F., Klominek, J., Damber, L., and Wall, S. (1987).

Histological types of lung cancer among smelter workers exposed to arsenic. *Br. J. Ind. Med.* 44:454–458.
63. Abe, S., Ohsaki, Y., Kimura, K., Tsuenta, Y., Mkaimi, H., and Murao, M. (1982). Chromate lung cancer with special reference to its cell type and relation to the manufacturing process. *Cancer* 49:783–787.
64. Kreyberg, L. (1978). Lung cancer in workers in a nickel refinery. *Br. J. Ind. Med.* 35:109–116.
65. Uyama, T., Monden, Y., Tsuyuguchi, M., Harada, K., Kimura, S., and Taniki, T. (1980). Lung cancer in chromate workers: High-risk group for multiple lung cancer. *J. Surg. Oncol.* 41:213–218.
66. Figueroa, W. G., Raszkowski, R., and Weiss, W. (1973). Lung cancer in chloromethyl ether workers. *N. Engl. J. Med.* 288:1096–1097.
67. Sakabe, H. (1973). Lung cancer due to exposure to bis(chloromethyl)ether. *Ind. Health* 11:145.
68. Theiss, A. M., Hay, W., and Zeller, E. (1973). Toxicology of bis(chloromethyl) ether-carcinogenicity in man. *Zen Arbeitsmed.* 23:97–102.
69. Lemen, R. A., Johnson, W. M., Wagoner, J. K., Archer, V. E., and Saccomanno, G. (1976). Cytologic observations and cancer incidence following exposure to BCME. *Ann. NY Acad. Sci.* 271:71–80.
70. Weiss, W., and Boucot, K. R. (1975). The respiratory effects of chloromethylether. *JAMA* 234:1139–1142.
71. Whitwell, F., Scott, J., and Grimshaw, M. (1977). Relationship between occupations and asbestos-fibre content of the lungs in patients with pleural mesothelioma, lung cancer, and other diseases. *Thorax* 32:377–386.
72. Churg, A. (1985). Lung cancer cell type and asbestos exposure. *JAMA* 253:2984–2985.
73. Davies, C. A., Landau, S. P., and Goldsmith, C. (1988). Lung cancer cell type and mining exposure. *S. Afr. Med. J.* 74:607–610.
74. Hughes, J. R., and Weill, H. (1991). Asbestosis as a precursor of asbestos-related lung cancer. *Br. J. Ind. Med.* 48:229–233.
75. Sluis-Cremer, G. K., and Bezuidenhout, B. N. (1989). Relation between asbestosis and bronchial cancer in amphibole asbestos miners. *Br. J. Ind. Med.* 46:537–540.
76. Baker, J. E., Reutens, D. C., Graham, D. F., Sterrett, G. F., Musk, A. W., Hobbs, M. S., Armstrong, B. K., and de Klerk, N. H. (1986). Morphology of bronchogenic carcinoma in workers formerly exposed to crocidolite at Wittenoom Gorge in Western Australia. *Int. J. Cancer* 37:547–550.
77. Martischnig, K. M., Newell, D. J., Barnsley, W. C., Cowan, W. K., Feinman, E. L., and Oliver, E. (1977). Unsuspected exposure to asbestos and bronchogenic carcinoma. *Br. Med. J.* 1:746–749.
78. Kannerstein, M., and Churg, J. (1972). Pathology of carcinoma of the lung associated with asbestos exposure. *Cancer* 30:14–21.
79. Auerbach, O., Garfinkel, L., Parks, V. R., Conston, A. S., Galdi, V. A., and Joubert, L. (1984). Histologic type of lung cancer and asbestos exposure. *Cancer* 54:3017–3021.
80. Hasan, F. M., Nash, G., and Kazemi, H. (1978). Asbestos exposure and related neoplasia. *Am. J. Med.* 65:649–654.

81. Hourihane, D. O. B., and McCaughey, W. T. E. (1966). Pathological aspects of asbestosis. *Postgrad. Med. J.* 42:613–622.
82. McDonald, J. C. (1980). Asbestos-related disease: An epidemiologic review. In *Biological Effects of Mineral Fibers*. Edited by J. C. Wagner. Lyon, IARC, pp. 587–602.
83. Hammond, E. C., Selikoff, I. J., and Seidman, H. (1979). Asbestos exposure, cigarette smoking, and death rates. *Ann. NY Acad. Sci.* 330:473–491.
84. Archer, V. E. (1988). Lung cancer risks of underground miners: cohort and case-control studies. *Yale J. Biol. Med.* 61:183–193.
85. Saccomanno, G., Archer, V. E., Auerbach, O., Kuschner, M., Saunders, P., and Klein, M. G. (1971). Histologic types of lung cancer among uranium miners. *Cancer* 27:515–523.
86. Damber, L., and Larsson, L. G. (1982). Combined effects of mining and smoking in the causation of lung carcinoma. *Acta Radiol. Oncol.* 21:305–313.
87. Samet, J. M., Kutvirt, D. M., Waxweiler, R. J., and Key, C. R. (1984). Uranium mining and lung cancer in Navajo men. *N. Engl. J. Med.* 310:1481–1484.
88. Archer, V. E., Saccomanno, G., and Jones, J. H. (1974). Frequency of different histologic types of bronchogenic carcinoma as related to radiation exposure. *Cancer* 34:2056–2060.
89. Horacek, J., Placek, V., and Sevc, J. (1977). Histologic types of bronchogenic cancer in relation to different conditions of radiation exposure. *Cancer* 40:832–835.
90. Saccomanno, G., Huth, G. C., Auerbach, O., and Luschner, M. (1988). Relationship of radioactive radon daughters and cigarette smoking in the genesis of lung cancer in uranium miners. *Cancer* 62:1402–1408.
91. Butler, C., Samet, J. M., Black, W. C., Key, C. R., and Kutvirt, D. M. (1986). Histopathologic findings of lung cancer in Navajo men: Relationship to uranium mining. *Health Phys.* 51:365–368.
92. Gottlieb, L. S., and Husen, L. A. (1982). Lung cancer among Navajo uranium miners. *Chest* 81:449–452.
93. Edling, C. (1982). Lung cancer and smoking in a group of iron ore miners. *Am. J. Ind. Med.* 3:191–199.
94. Samet, J. M. (1989). Radon and lung cancer. *JNCI* 81:745–757.
95. Smith, A. B., and Suzuki, Y. (1980). Histopathologic classification of bronchogenic carcinomas among a cohort of workers occupationally exposed to beryllium. *Environ. Res.* 21:10–14.
96. Waxweiler, R. J., Smith, A. H., Falk, H., and Tyroler, H. A. (1981). Excess lung cancer risk in a synthetic chemicals plant. *Environ. Health Perspect.* Oct:159–165.
97. Yamada, A. (1963). On the late injuries following occupational inhalation of mustard gas, with special references to carcinoma of the respiratory tract. *Acta Pathol. Jpn.* 13:131–155.
98. Vallyathan, V., Green, F. H., Rodman, N. F., Boyd, C. B., and Althouse, R. (1985). Lung carcinoma by histologic type in coal miners. *Arch. Pathol. Lab. Med.* 109: 419–423.

17

Reducing Lung Cancer Through Smoking Prevention and Control

DONALD R. SHOPLAND and MARIANNE HAENLEIN

National Cancer Institute
National Institutes of Health
Bethesda, Maryland

I. Introduction

While tobacco use in the United States predates the arrival of Columbus and the early settlers, large-scale consumption of manufactured cigarettes was not common in this country until well after the beginning of the twentieth century. Some 20 to 30 years following the rapid increase in cigarette consumption, lung cancer deaths began their parallel rise (Fig. 1) (1). This dramatic change in personal behavior has had a profound effect on the health status of the country and represents one of the more interesting, if not tragic, public health stories of this century.

In this chapter, we will briefly characterize these historical changes in tobacco use patterns in the U.S. population and describe how tobacco control research and public health efforts have evolved in parallel to epidemiological evidence linking smoking and early cancer mortality. More important, we will describe in detail the significant change in National Cancer Institute (NCI) program direction, which occurred in the mid-1980s, and how results from NCI's smoking prevention and cessation intervention trials are now aggressively being applied in an effort to significantly reduce lung and other cancers caused by tobacco use.

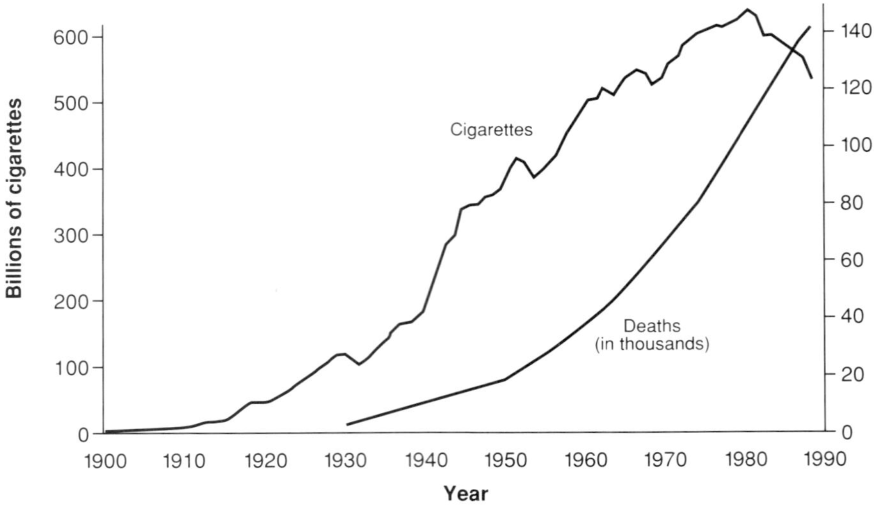

Figure 1 Cigarette consumption and lung cancer deaths in the United States, 1900–1989. (From Ref. 1.)

II. A Brief Historical Perspective

Despite extensive efforts to reduce tobacco use during the last half of this century and some reduction in tobacco consumption, total per capita consumption of tobacco remains significantly elevated. Changes in tobacco consumption patterns are also reflected in the type of tobacco and the manner in which tobacco has been consumed over the century (Fig. 2).

In 1900, for example, manufactured cigarettes accounted for only 0.16 pounds of the approximately 7.5 pounds of tobacco consumed annually per adult, while over 4 pounds was consumed in the form of spitting tobacco (both chewing tobacco and snuff) (2). By contrast, in 1991 manufactured cigarettes accounted for 90% of the 5.4 total pounds of tobacco consumed annually per adult (3).

Consumption of machine-manufactured cigarettes began to increase significantly following the introduction of Camel cigarettes in 1913, the first modern blended cigarette using milder flue-cured tobaccos, which enabled the user to obtain nicotine directly and more efficiently through inhalation. Camel was also the first truly nonregional cigarette and was launched with a then massive $1.5 million national advertising and promotional campaign (4). Other national brands such as Lucky Strike and Chesterfield soon followed with national advertising campaigns, and cigarette consumption accelerated. By the mid-1930s mass-produced cigarettes accounted for more than half of all tobacco consumed per

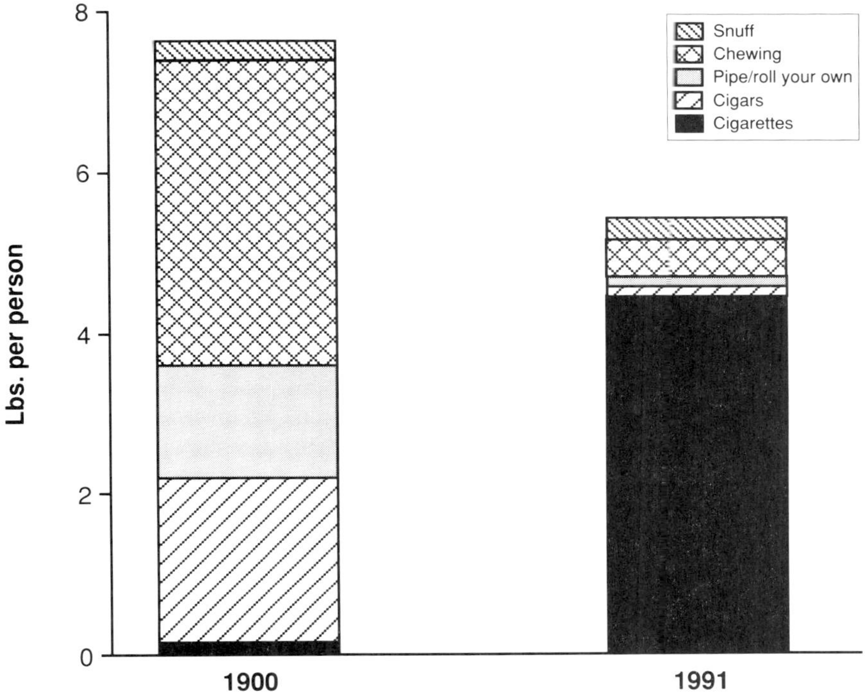

Figure 2 Per capita consumption of tobacco among adults, by major product category, United States, 1900 and 1991. Values expressed as unstemmed processing weight in pounds per adult, 18 years and older. (From Refs. 2 and 3.)

adult, and in the early 1950s consumption peaked at nearly 13 pounds of tobacco per capita, with manufactured cigarettes accounting for 10.4 pounds of this total (2).

Thus, in the span of less than a generation, the spittoon was replaced with the ashtray, and as a consequence the health of the country was altered in a way few could have predicted. As noted previously, however, the impact of this change on the public health did not become apparent for several decades. In fact, it was not until some 20–30 years following this dramatic increase in cigarette consumption that lung cancer deaths began to increase. Initially lung cancer was thought to be almost exclusively a male problem, as comparatively few women were diagnosed with the disease (5). It became clear only much later that the gender differences in lung cancer incidence could be almost entirely accounted for by differences in lifetime exposure to cigarette smoking within various age groups of men and women (6). The parallel relationship between trends in lung cancer and smoking behavior, regardless of gender, is strikingly apparent when smoking prevalence and lung cancer are examined across successive birth cohorts of men and women.

The first major development in the modern history of the investigation of the effects of smoking on health occurred in 1950 with publication of four retrospective studies on smoking habits among lung cancer patients and controls (7–10). At that time, the question was "Are smokers more likely to get lung cancer than nonsmokers?" Although many epidemiologists were satisfied that the answer was yes, other investigators turned to prospective studies in an effort to confirm these findings.

The prospective studies of Hammond and Horn in the United States (11,12) and Doll and Hill in the United Kingdom (13) clearly demonstrated that individuals who smoked were at significantly increased risk for lung cancer mortality. This elevation in risk was almost entirely confined to those who smoked cigarettes and, together with evidence for a gradient according to the amount smoked, provided strong support for a direct casual association between smoking and lung cancer.

Results from subsequently published prospective and retrospective studies both confirmed and extended these early findings to include a host of other chronic and debilitating diseases including associations between smoking and at least nine major sites of cancer (14). In addition to the causal relationship between cigarette consumption and lung cancer, smoking is now firmly established as a cause for cancers of the larynx, oral cavity, esophagus, and bladder, and it contributes to an elevation in the death rates for cancers of the kidney, stomach, and pancreas in both men and women and cervical cancer in women (15).

A clear dose-response relationship for each of these sites also has been established, whether measured by number of cigarettes smoked daily, a younger age of initiation, or total duration of the behavior (14). Smoking cessation results in some amelioration of risk, although the degree of excess risk among former smokers is strongly dependent on total prior exposure to cigarette smoke, number of years since quitting smoking, and the health status of the individual at the time of cessation (16).

While approximately 22% of all cancer deaths in women are directly related to cigarette smoking, the smoking of cigarettes, pipes, and cigars accounts for nearly 45% of all cancer deaths among men (15). The most recent estimate of the total cancer burden attributable to the inhalation of tobacco smoke in the United States is in excess of 175,000 cancer deaths annually (15).

The enormity of this public health problem is further exacerbated by the dismal survival rates for several cancers associated with smoking. The lung cancer survival rate is extremely poor and has changed little in absolute terms over the past 30 years. Today only about 11% of all patients diagnosed with lung cancer can expect to live more than 5 years (17). Lung cancer is now the leading cause of cancer mortality for both men and women in the United States, responsible for nearly 30% of all cancer deaths annually; lung cancer's share of total cancer mortality is increasing, and lung cancer recently displaced coronary heart disease as the single leading cause of excess mortality among smokers in the United States (15).

These somber statistics add to the growing recognition of the importance of both preventing smoking uptake among adolescents as well as getting adults to quit the behavior before significant health problems develop.

III. Efforts to Control Tobacco Use in the United States

The remainder of this chapter synthesizes what has been learned over the past 40 years of efforts to control tobacco use and is largely based on information summarized in the National Cancer Institute's first Smoking and Tobacco Control Monograph *Strategies to Control Tobacco Use in the United States: A Blueprint for Public Health Action in the 1990's* (18).

As with most successful public health efforts, the current state-of-the-science in the control of tobacco use is built on a broad base of scientific investigation as well as equally important practical, trial-and-error experience from both successful and unsuccessful programs that have evolved in parallel with our scientific knowledge. Frequently it is this operational experience with what works or does not work in real-life settings that forms the core of interventions tested in controlled intervention trials. It should come also as no surprise that current concepts about effective approaches for controlling tobacco use have posed significant challenges both in terms of the scientific tools needed to evaluate them and the data needed to establish definitive proof of their impact.

A. Information-Based Approaches

The clear identification of cigarette smoking as a major health risk, beginning in the 1950s, led almost immediately to efforts to inform the public. It was believed that information about the health risks imposed by cigarette smoking would "speak for themselves" and that smokers would stop their unhealthy habit and others would not start. Figure 3 shows the changes in per capita cigarette consumption during this century and illustrates the relationship between such changes and information campaigns designed to communicate the risks of smoking. Cigarette consumption declined with each of three major events:

1. The first significant decline was observed in the early 1950s following publication of the first scientific studies linking smoking to lung cancer among males.
2. A smaller but still significant downturn in consumption occurred in 1964 when the first report of the Surgeon General was published identifying smoking as a major overall health risk linking smoking to a

number of diseases in addition to lung cancer (19). This downturn was very short-lived, and by the following year consumption had again increased.

3. The third notable decline occurred in the late 1960s when antismoking messages for broadcast media were mandated by the Federal Communications Commission in order to counterbalance paid cigarette advertisements (20). When cigarette advertising in electronic media was banned by Congress in 1970, mandated antismoking spots virtually disappeared and per capita consumption again increased.

Health risk information is often downplayed as a means of influencing behavior, but information about the risks of smoking has provided much of the motivational substrate for changes in smoking both for the individual and the population (18). While these early information campaigns clearly had the intended effect, i.e., a change in smoking behavior, in and of themselves, they were unable to sustain these effects as each decline in per capita consumption was followed by a subsequent rise.

While it would appear that the impact of these campaigns was limited in their ability to sustain large-scale behavior change, an examination of changes in smoking rates within specific age and gender cohorts permits a better understanding of how individual campaigns affected smoking behavior of different groups of smokers at different points in time. The four cohorts cited in Figures 4 and 5

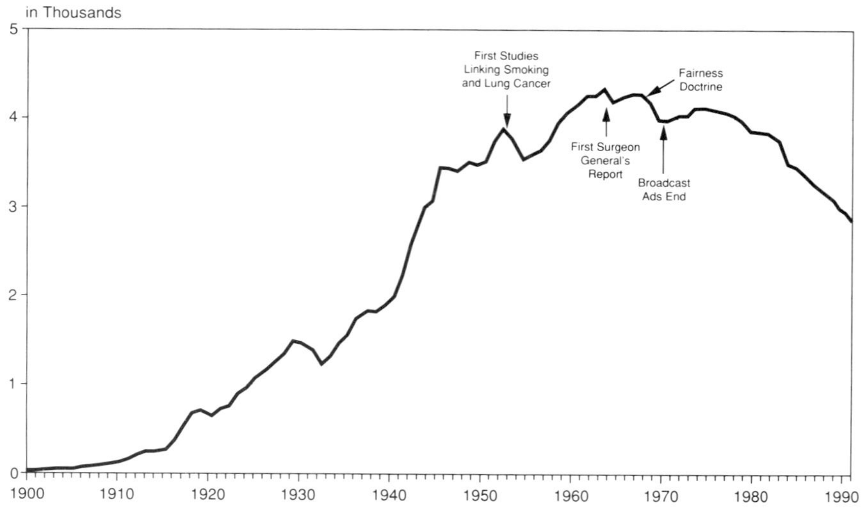

Figure 3 Per capita consumption of cigarettes among adults, 18 years and older, United States, 1900 to 1990. (From Refs. 1, 18.)

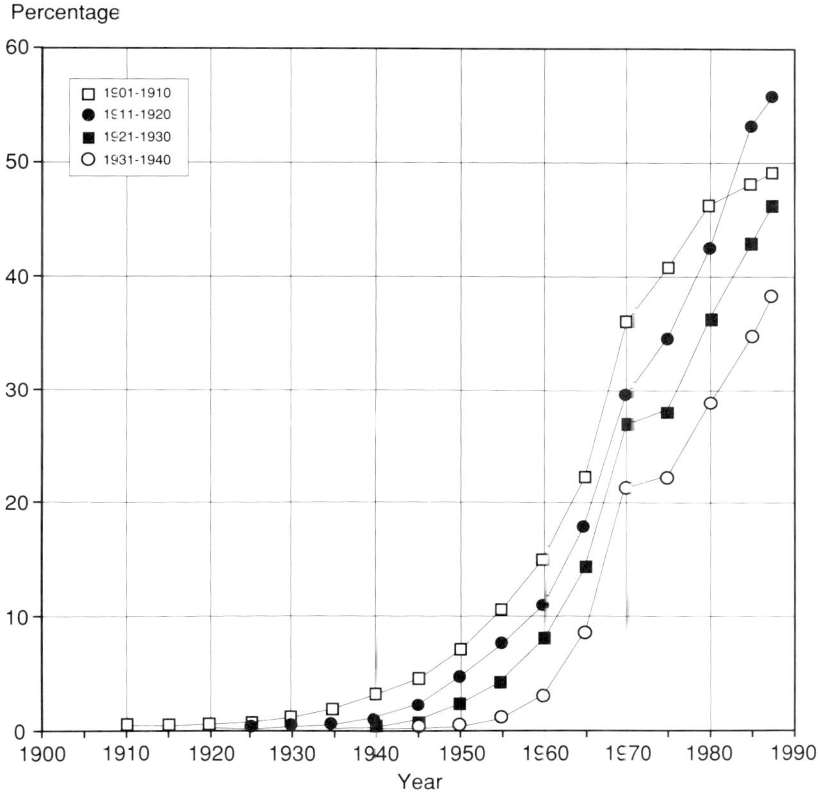

Figure 4 Percentage of former smokers among white males, born from 1901 to 1940 (through 1987). (From Ref. 18.)

(1901–10, 1911–20, 1921–30, 1931–40) were chosen because those born later would not have fully completed initiation of smoking at the time of the first campaigns in the early 1950s.

These figures show the percentage of former smokers in white versus black males, plotted by age-cohort and calendar year. Among white men the percentage of former smokers begins to rise earlier and is more pronounced than that observed among blacks. In white males a sharp upturn is seen to occur in the early 1950s and accelerates during the late 1960s. For black men the prevalence of former smokers is virtually zero during the entire decade of the 1950s but begins to increase before the end of the 1960s.

This difference is even more evident when the fraction of smokers who have quit during each 5-year period is examined by calendar year (Figs. 6 and 7). While

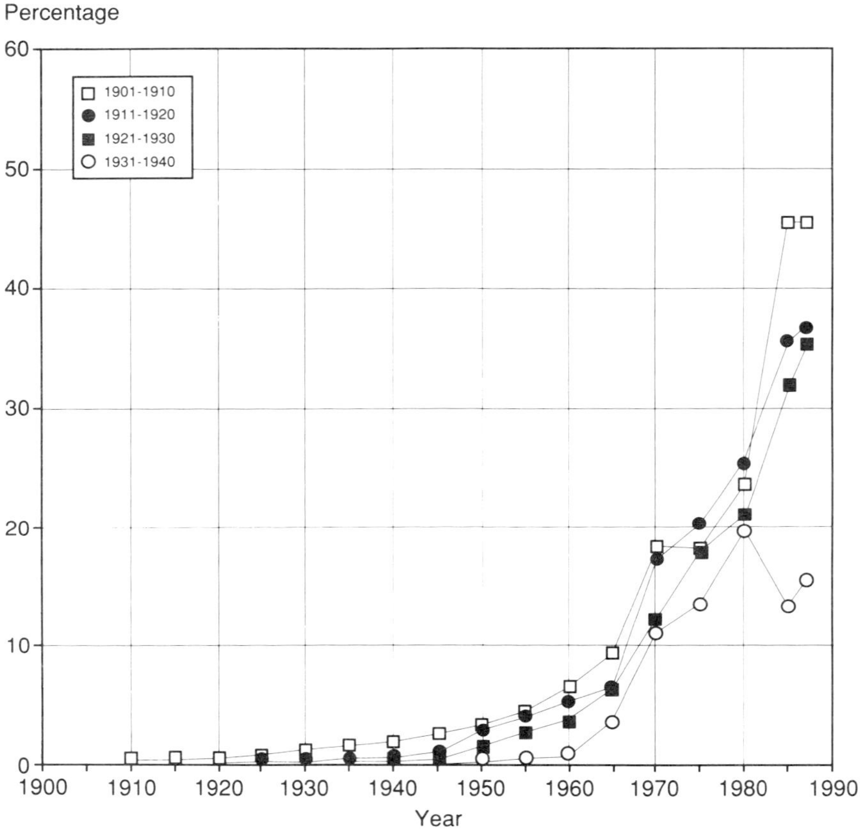

Figure 5 Percentage of former smokers among black males, born 1901–1940 (through 1987). (From Ref. 18.)

both black and white men show substantial change in prevalence during the period of counteradvertising that occurred in the late 1960s and early 1970s, only white men demonstrated a significant change in behavior during the initial wave of public information dissemination about the health risks of smoking that occurred in the early 1950s. The question of racial differences in both the source and timing of information transfer can be explored through comparisons of the same 5-year quit rates among white women. Figure 8 clearly shows that white women exhibit a pattern that more closely approximates black men than white men, suggesting that the absence of an effect in black men in response to the early information campaigns is not solely a racial phenomenon.

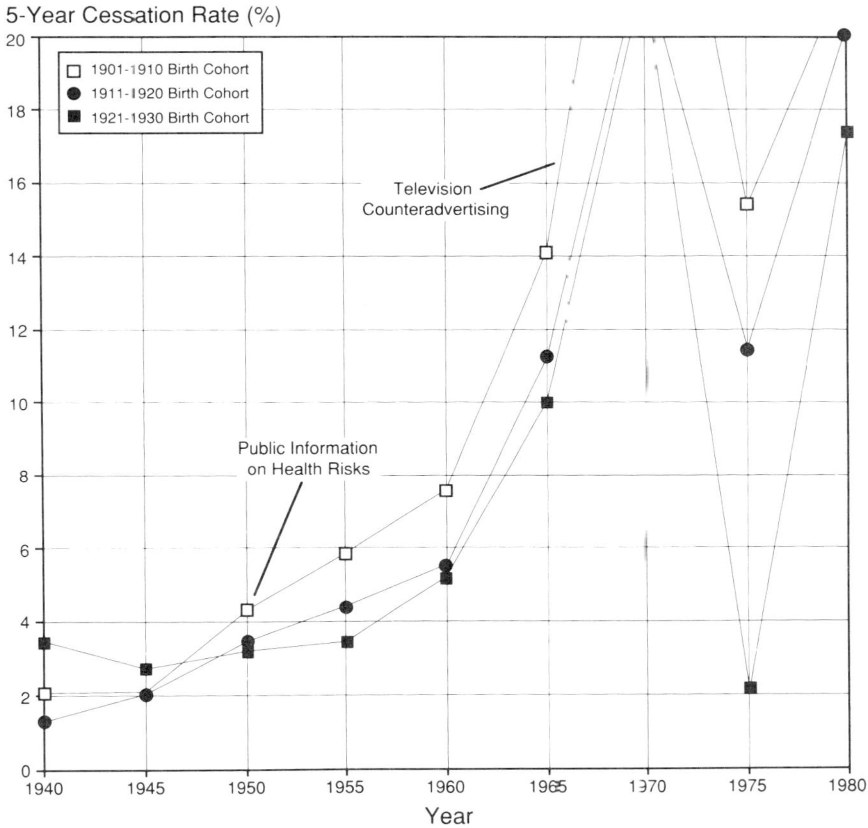

Figure 6 Percentage of white male current smokers quitting over 5-year intervals. Select cohorts born 1901–1930. (From Ref. 18.)

While the data show that only white male smokers reacted to the first wave of public information in the 1950s—most likely because all of the early studies linking smoking and lung cancer were conducted among white men—the counteradvertising campaigns of the late 1960s produced a greater level of cessation across all the major demographic groups. These latter campaigns were more intensive and utilized broader themes and issues, thereby appealing to a more diverse audience. Further, the counteradvertising campaigns used far-reaching electronic media—primarily television—while those of the early 1950s relied almost exclusively on print media.

These patterns reflect an important criteria for the effectiveness of informa-

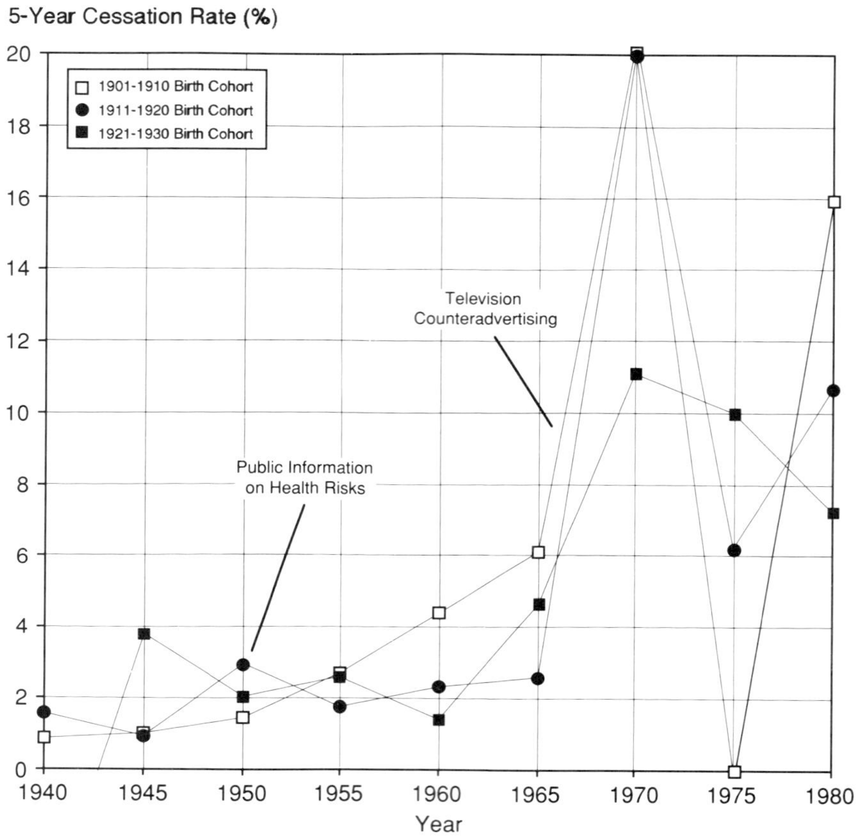

Figure 7 Percentage of black male current smokers quitting over 5-year intervals. Select cohorts born 1901–1930. (From Ref. 18.)

tional campaigns in changing public behavior. It must be clear to the target audience that the information being presented relates to them. Because the early studies of the health effects of tobacco use focused on white males, little information was available that would enable either black males or women to personalize the health message. The evidence presented in the first Surgeon General's report, on the other hand, reflected a growing body of scientific information, which demonstrated that the adverse consequences of smoking were not limited to only white males but had implications across various demographic groups. The counteradvertising campaigns of the late 1960s and early 1970s were much more intense than previous campaigns and used more socially directed themes and

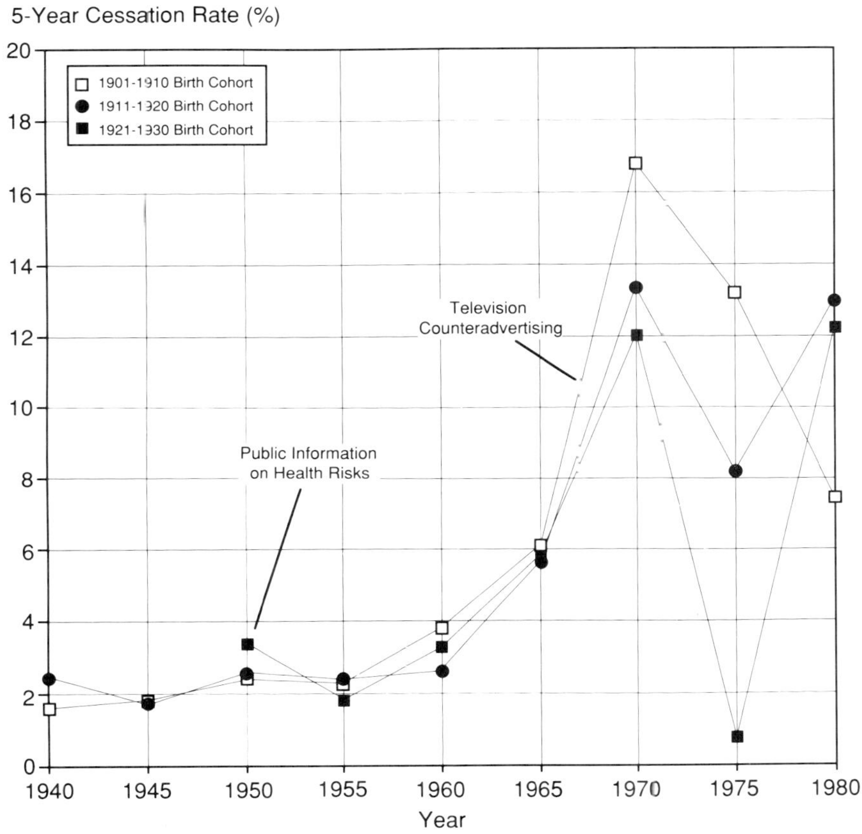

Figure 8 Percentage of white female current smokers quitting over 5-year intervals. Select cohorts born 1901–1930. (From Ref. 18.)

messages that appealed to a broader, more diverse audience. When Congress banned cigarette advertising on radio and television in 1970, cessation rates plummeted following the removal of mandated antitobacco advertisements (20,21).

Taken together, national consumption data and cohort data reveal an important effect of these early informational campaigns on smoking patterns in the United States. Awareness of the harmful effects of tobacco use are now widely known and accepted. In recent surveys, an overwhelming percentage of the general population agree that smoking is hazardous, and a clear majority of smokers agree that smoking is harmful and further recognize that it is harming them as individuals (22).

B. Influence of Tobacco Industry

The question as to why initial reductions in cigarette consumption were not maintained can be explained. Following each such campaign, consumption data rebounded and cessation rates revealed a similar rebound pattern. This is due, in part, to unique counterforces present in society coupled with the recognition that use of tobacco is addictive for the majority of users (23). In contrast to most public health issues, messages about the health consequences of tobacco use were being directly and aggressively countered by the tobacco industry (24,25).

Immediately upon the earliest announcements of the adverse health effects of tobacco use, the industry countered with opposing information that not only introduced elements of doubt in the public's mind but attacked the credibility of the sources of this information. Simultaneously, they initiated efforts to "improve" their product in relation to the health issue (18). The industry launched a series of efforts to modify cigarettes, first adding filters and later making changes in cigarette design which artificially manipulated tar and nicotine levels.

In the mid-1950s filters were aggressively portrayed in advertising as acting as a screen against the adverse effects of cigarette smoke (26), and the reduction in tar content was intended to imply a direct elimination of any serious carcinogenic effects (25). Market share of filtered cigarettes increased from less than 1% at the beginning of the 1950s to over half the market by the end of the decade (25). Today, virtually the entire domestic cigarette market is comprised of filtered brands (3). Similarly, only 3% of the U.S. cigarette market in 1970 was made up of brands yielding less than 15 mg tar, but by 1980 the proportion had increased to 45% (25).

C. Individual Approaches

Given the limited success of these early efforts, public health officials began to focus on the individual. Research and public health efforts were launched to explore strategies for empowering individuals to overcome their desire to smoke. Programs focused on developing coping strategies, identifying triggers, setting goals, and self-reinforcement for success (27,28). In a parallel effort, research was conducted to identify the factors contributing to individual differences in the initiation, maintenance, and cessation of smoking. Differences were identified in the smoking patterns of various groups, the motivations to quit, the factors contributing to relapse, and, perhaps most importantly, differences in the efficacy of various cessation approaches were linked to different stages in a change process (1).

A broader focus on the general public came into the picture only in relation to efforts to recruit individuals into cessation programs and to expand the reach of these programs. Thus, both print and electronic media were used to advertise the availability of cessation programs and self-help materials and to provide information about the hazards of smoking (29).

However, information began to emerge that cast doubt on the ability of individual-centered approaches to remedy what was in effect a national problem. A significantly large proportion of those smokers who do successfully quit, and an equally large proportion of those who attempt to quit but fail, indicate a clear preference to quit on their own, with very few using formal or clinic-based cessation approaches (30).

Further, research evidence suggests that the success of clinic-based approaches is positively correlated with the intensity of the program (29). As program intensity rises, unfortunately, so too does cost, while participation rates decline. At a time when insurance reimbursements for formal cessation programs remain spotty and health care costs are skyrocketing, such costs pose a formidable barrier to the widespread use of these strategies.

Perhaps most important to the development of a national smoking control strategy was the realization that the social environment plays a critical role in support of an individual's attempt to quit smoking and an equally important role in affecting initiation of smoking among children (18). With this realization, both research and public health efforts began to focus on efforts to better understand the environmental factors that influence individual smoking behavior and to evaluate their potential in smoking control.

D. Environmental Approaches

In general, the environmental factors explored in relation to smoking control can be grouped into those that impact access to tobacco and those designed to directly impact the social acceptability of tobacco use. Factors shown to reduce tobacco consumption by creating barriers to access include increasing cost and policy restrictions to regulate where and when tobacco can be consumed, limiting access for minors, and mandating education about the health effects of tobacco (31). Factors shown to directly impact the acceptability of tobacco use include a variety of strategies for disseminating information about the growing body of scientific evidence concerning the effects of both direct and indirect exposure tobacco smoke as well as policies restricting advertising and requiring warning labels on tobacco products (18).

Increasing the cost of cigarettes has been accomplished primarily through adding excise and sales taxes to the product. These increases generally result in rather immediate and dramatic decreases in consumption (32), however, not unlike the effects of informational campaigns, the effects of increased cost can be relatively short-lived. Evidence from the recent 25 cent cigarette tax in California provides further support for this concern. Immediately following the implementation of the tax, the drop in per capita consumption attributable to the tax was 5%. A survey of smokers in the state conducted a year and a half after the tax indicated that while about half of the pretax smokers tried to quit around the time of the tax, compared to only one third in the rest of the nation, there was no difference in the proportion of California smokers in this survey who were nonsmokers at 3 months compared to the reset of the nation's smokers (33).

Implementation of policies, on the other hand, can have significant long-term effects on smoking behavior even when their immediate effect is small (21). The vast majority of clean indoor air policies have restricted the locations in which smoking is permitted. Clean indoor air legislation as well as worksite policies gained support with the 1986 Surgeon General's report on the health consequences of environmental tobacco smoke (34). In 1970, fewer than 15 states had any legislation regulating smoking in public places, and all were classified as nominal. By 1987, the number of states with such legislation had risen to over 40, and of these only 6 were classified a nominal (21). A similar trend at the local level was also identified with only a handful of local smoking ordinances enacted prior to 1980, but by the end of the decade, over 500 such laws had been passed at the local level (35). For both state and local ordinances, the trend was clearly toward more and more restrictive clean indoor air legislation (36).

Legislation limiting access to minors also has represented an important environmental smoking control strategy, addressing the critical need to reduce the number of individuals initiating the habit. Other policies include prohibiting smoking in schools, mandating school curricula on the health effects of tobacco, and banning the promotional distribution of cigarettes to minors. These prevention efforts have focused primarily on youth because the majority of smokers begin smoking before age 20. In fact, the majority initiate the habit before the age when the purchase of cigarettes is legal (usually age 18) in most states (21); studies have consistently revealed that underage children can easily purchase cigarettes with essentially no barrier to the purchase of cigarettes from vending machines (37). This may change with the recent passage of the Synar amendment (Public Law 102-321), which will require each state to adopt age 18 as the legal age of purchase for tobacco and require enforcement of this provision or lose some portion of federal funding under the Alcohol Drug Abuse and Mental Health Administration block grant program (38).

Congressional laws and regulatory processes that affect cigarette advertising, including mandated rotating warning labels on cigarette packages and in advertising, are of limited impact in the context of competing tobacco industry cues (18). Laws banning direct electronic media advertising for cigarettes (1970) and smokeless tobacco (1986) may play some role in smoking and tobacco use control, however, the tobacco industry continues to spend billions of dollars annually (39,40) to advertise through the print media as well as through direct sponsorship of sport and entertainment events, such as the Virginia Slims Tennis

Tournament, Winston sponsorship of World Cup soccer. Marlboro auto races, rock concerts, art festivals, and even educational events such as the Philip Morris national Bill of Rights tour (41).

E. Integrated Approaches

With a clearer understanding of at least some of the individual and environmental factors that influence smoking initiation, maintenance, and cessation, efforts were launched to integrate the roles of the individual and the environment in smoking control and to simultaneously enhance environmental cues that would discourage smoking and increase the ability of the individual to control his or her behavior in relation to smoking. Both the individual and the environment were recognized to be dynamic, and smoking cessation was now understood to be a cyclic process (42). This cyclic pattern accounts for differences in the needs of smokers at different stages of the change process. Initially, smokers may not even think about quitting (precontemplation); they may be triggered to consider quitting (contemplation), perhaps by an increase in the cigarette tax, an informational campaign or physician reminder; they might then move on to make a quit attempt (action), perhaps using self-help material or a cessation program; and finally, they may slip (relapse) or continue cessation (maintenance). As many as one third of current smokers attempt to quit each year, about 90% percent fail (22), and may cycle back into the process at any stage. While much has been learned about both the individual and environmental cues for smoking and the process of change, this transition in the process from a quit attempt to abstinence is thought by many to remain one of the most significant gaps in our knowledge of tobacco control.

IV. The National Cancer Institute's Smoking and Tobacco Control Program

In the early 1980s NCI undertook a major research and planning effort to identify effective smoking intervention approaches that would reduce tobacco use prevalence nationally and, in turn, result in a decrease in the incidence and mortality of cancer caused by or related to smoking and use of other tobacco products (1). This initiative marked the beginning of what is now known as the Smoking and Tobacco Control Program (STCP).

To achieve the goals of a decrease in tobacco-related cancer morbidity and mortality, the STCP incorporated program components that addressed the full spectrum of disease prevention and control. These components included: (1) basic research relating tobacco use to cancer and addressing socio-behavioral aspects of tobacco use; (2) surveillance to monitor and assess patterns and trends of tobacco use as well as progress in preventing and controlling such use; (3) intervention research to identify approaches to reduce the incidence and/or prevalence of smoking and tobacco use; and (4) research applications and information dissemination to ensure the synthesis of available information on smoking prevention and cessation, the development of messages and materials specifically designed to encourage smoking prevention and cessation among individuals at risk for cancer, the communication of specific smoking control messages, and the dissemination of materials and programs to reduce cigarette smoking.

A. Phases of Cancer Control Research

To aid in establishing program priorities for the Smoking and Tobacco Control Program, the NCI implemented a system of research program logic that stressed an orderly sequence of phases through which all cancer control research would be guided (Fig. 9). As with all of NCI's prevention and control efforts, the logic of the cancer control phases is used to determine the nature of study readiness. This logic is comprised of five sequential phases that emphasize an orderly progression of activity from basic investigations to large-scale demonstration projects and national dissemination, and it outlines a time line for the implementation of each phase of activity. At each transition from one phase to the next lies decision points with operational criteria to determine if research outcomes from a previous phase warrant proceeding further to the next phase.

The STCP intervention efforts primarily reflect phase III and IV intervention trials, although a few involved phase II study components that preceded the development and testing of specific intervention methods. The STCP's most recent activities focused on the dissemination and public health application of the results of these efforts, reflecting the initiation of phase V demonstration and implementation studies.

Sixty intervention trials in 9 separate focus areas constituted the original STCP core (Fig. 10). Three of the focus areas reflect efforts to develop intervention approaches within specified channels, including physician/dentist-delivered, self-help, and mass media channels. The remaining six focus areas involve the development of strategies targeting specific populations. Brief descriptions of these intervention research and public health demonstration efforts are provided below.

B. Intervention Channels

Intervention research efforts focusing on specific channels for reducing smoking prevalence and initiation reflect a range of approaches, from physician and dentist interventions that rely on one-on-one counseling opportunities from health providers, to self-help/minimal interventions that involve only minimal contact with smokers, to mass-media based interventions utilizing print and/or electronic media containing messages about smoking cessation and prevention. These approaches differ both in the amount of intensive contact with smokers (or potential smokers) as well as the number of individuals reached by any given intervention dose.

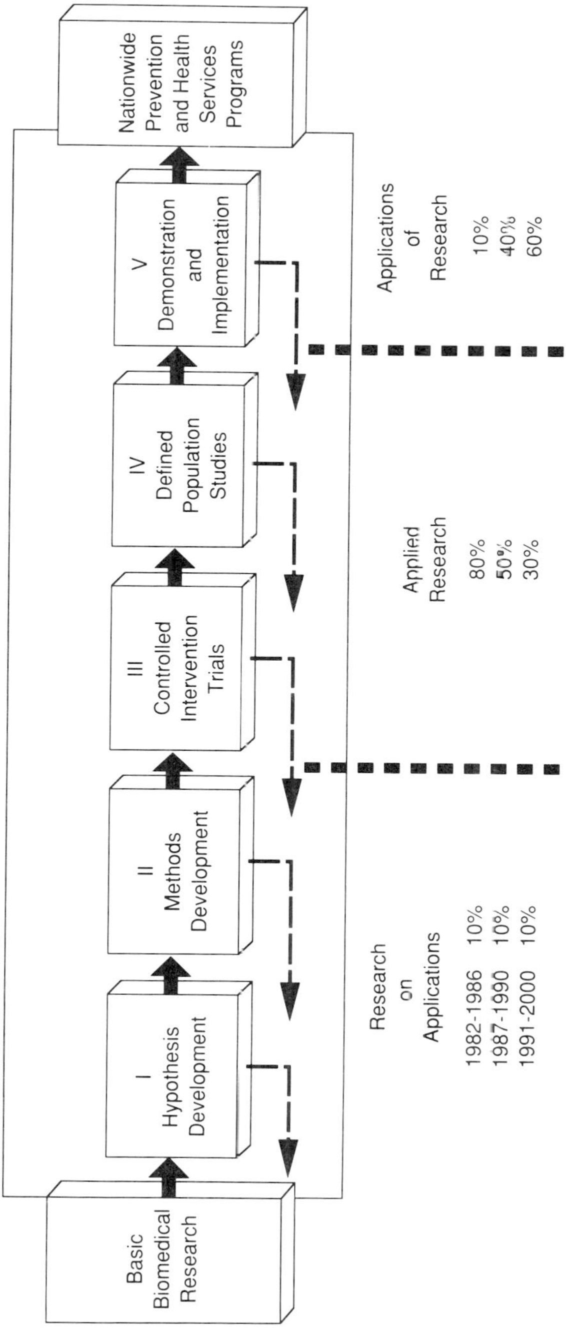

Figure 9 Cancer control phases applied to smoking and tobacco control research. (From Refs. 1, 18.)

Goal: To develop and evaluate interventions to aid in either stopping or preventing tobacco use.

Number of Trials (1983-1987): 60

Intervention Areas	Number of Trials
School-Based Interventions	10
Self-Help Strategies	7
Physician/Dentist Interventions	6
Mass Media Interventions	5
Interventions in Black Populations	8
Interventions in Hispanic Populations	3
Interventions in Populations of Women	5
Control of Smokeless Tobacco Use	5
Heavy Smoker Interventions	11
Total	**60**

Figure 10 Smoking and tobacco intervention trials of the National Cancer Institute, 1983–1987.

C. Interventions Targeting Special Populations

The second strategy in the STCP's efforts to develop intervention approaches focused on identifying and intervening with target populations in which the greatest tobacco-related cancer prevention and control gains can be expected. These target populations include adolescents, blacks, Hispanics, women, and smokeless tobacco users. They represent groups with (1) higher incidence and/or prevalence of smoking and tobacco use; (2) higher prevalence of combined exposure to tobacco and other known carcinogens; and (3) higher dosage of exposure to tobacco-related cancers (currently or potentially).

D. The Community Intervention Trial for Smoking Cessation

Building on the research base established in the phase II and III trials, NCI launched the Community Intervention Trial for Smoking Cessation (COMMIT) in 1987. COMMIT is the largest smoking intervention trial in the world, involving directly or indirectly nearly 2 million people in the testing of a community-based intervention protocol that can be disseminated nationwide to meet NCI's year 2000 objective to reduce smoking prevalence (43). Heavy smokers (25 or more cigarettes per day) are emphasized due to their greater cancer risk and their difficulty in quitting.

The trial design includes 11 pairs of communities in North America that were matched in size, demographics, and location. Following the baseline survey, one community from each pair was selected randomly in May 1988 as the intervention site.

The primary hypothesis being tested is that the implementation of a defined intervention protocol, delivered through multiple community groups and organizations and using limited resources, will result in a quit rate among heavy smokers at least 10 percentage points greater than that observed in the comparison community. The COMMIT interventions will build on, coordinate, and facilitate community smoking control activities. Results from the STCP trials have defined numerous strategies for inclusion in COMMIT. Trial investigators evaluated the STCP trial results, scientific literature, and other data sources to define a protocol of 40 required interventions. In the 11 sites, the 4-year intervention effort will involve more than 1000 doctors, 700 dentists, 1400 worksites, 1000 community organizations, 250 media outlets, 400 schools, and 60 cessation service providers.

V. Public Health Applications

A. Building Tobacco Control Capacity Among State and Local Health Departments

In the mid-1980s NCI initiated several broad efforts designed to assist state and local health agencies in developing the technical capacity to plan for and deliver state-of-the-science cancer prevention and control interventions and, later, under a second program, to work in partnership with state health agencies to build the institutional infrastructures necessary to support, maintain, and enhance ongoing cancer control efforts. Although these programs are focused broadly on cancer control, major components of many of the projects within each program address tobacco control specifically.

The first program, entitled Technical Development in Health Agencies, encouraged knowledge and skill development among health department staff through the implementation of intervention programs in cancer control. Nine grants were awarded in 1986 under this program and, of these, eight conducted tobacco use reduction activities. These ranged from conducting surveillance activities to monitoring smoking prevalence, to implementing school-based tobacco prevention programs in cooperation with the ACS, to conducting mass media campaigns. These grants demonstrated the complexity of the multilevel process of developing the technical capacity for planning, implementing, and evaluating cancer prevention and control programs and highlighted some of the factors that contribute to successful program implementation. These included organizational commitment, availability of appropriate data, availability of trained staff, establishment of linkages with state and community agencies, establishment of a plan for achieving stated objectives, access to cancer and health experts, an informed legislature, the ability to obtain necessary funding, and diffusion of cancer prevention and control efforts.

The second program launched by NCI in 1987 was the Data-Based Intervention Research (DBIR) program. The DBIR program again focused broadly on cancer prevention and control and sought not only to build technical capacity for the delivery of cancer prevention and control interventions, but to establish the institutional infrastructures necessary to support, maintain, and enhance ongoing cancer control efforts. Currently 21 states and the District of Columbia are funded under the DBIR program. Each state in the program conducts four phases of activity: (1) identification and analysis of data relevant to cancer control planning; (2) use of analyzed data to establish a state cancer control plan as well as an intervention plan for specific, high priority interventions; (3) implementation of selected high priority interventions; and (4) evaluation.

While seven states remain in the planning phases, 12 of the remaining 15 are implementing tobacco control interventions. These interventions have included surveillance activities to monitor smoking trends, information synthesis activities to identify regionally available tobacco control resources, implementation of school-based curriculum programs, prenatal smoking cessation interventions in local health clinics, mass media campaigns, and a variety of educational efforts for state and local policymakers. Results from these intervention efforts are expected to be available in 1993.

In addition to the specific NCI phase IV and V research contributions of these tobacco-related interventions, the DBIR program has contributed significantly to tobacco control efforts through a unique emphasis on the provision of state-based data on cancer and cancer-related issues to legislators, policymakers, and the general public. Through these efforts, public interest has been stimulated and policy action has resulted. Consistent with the lessons from NCI's phase III and IV research efforts and ongoing phase V efforts, these programs address the full spectrum of combined social and individual change required to meet the cancer control challenges of the future.

Information dissemination efforts to ensure the synthesis of available information on smoking prevention and cessation and its dissemination and use to reduce smoking prevalence are critical to the achievement of the goal to reduce tobacco-related cancer incidence and mortality. One of the major barriers in the effort to control smoking behavior in the U.S. population over the past 25 years has been the lack of a systematic plan to make practical use of available smoking control technology. Thus, several efforts have been undertaken by the NCI in this area, including the development of consensus documents that synthesize the results of the intervention research trials, development of comprehensive smoking prevention and control standards, development of state tobacco prevention and control plans, production of smoking and tobacco use control monographs, and establishment of several target group networks (1).

Over the past decade a substantial body of intervention research has emerged demonstrating the efficacy of a wide range of smoking prevention and cessation approaches. Data from these trials and from the lessons gained from our contextual understanding of social factors that have influenced smoking behavior in this century (18) have provided the NCI with the recognition that comprehensive public health strategies to reduce smoking are now required if we are to reduce smoking rates to less than 15% nationally by the end of this decade. Several of NCI's most aggressive efforts are discussed below.

B. The American Stop Smoking Intervention Study for Cancer Prevention

In 1987 the STCP staff began to develop a concept for a large-scale demonstration project (phase V) which would systematically and comprehensively apply the current state-of-the-art in smoking control technology. Comprehensive strategies are characterized by the delivery of persistent and inescapable messages to quit, or to not start smoking, coupled with continuously available support for individual cessation attempts, provided through multiple channels and reinforced by environmental and economic incentives to not smoke.

This strategy has provided the foundation for the largest, most comprehensive smoking control project every undertaken—the American Stop Smoking Intervention Study for Cancer Prevention (ASSIST) (44). ASSIST is a cooperative project representing the combined resources of the NCI, the national and local offices of the American Cancer Society, and state and local health departments. Project funding started in October 1991 and is currently being conducted in 17 states (Fig. 11), with a combined population of 90 million Americans.

The ASSIST framework incorporates a three-axes model, consisting of target populations, intervention channels, and interventions (Fig. 12). The model organizes the multiple and diverse activities of a comprehensive smoking control initiative:

Target Populations (axis 1) can include youth, ethnic minorities, blue-collar workers, individuals with less education, women, or other populations with relatively high smoking rates or which have been slow to change their behavior.

Channels (axis 2) are the organizational structures or mechanisms by which specific intervention activities will reach targeted groups. In ASSIST, five major channels are envisioned as the primary means for contacts with smokers and potential smokers.

Interventions (axis 3) are the instruments for producing change, both for the individual and the larger community environment that will affect broader behavior change in various populations. In ASSIST, interventions will take the form of direct contacts with individuals and groups through a

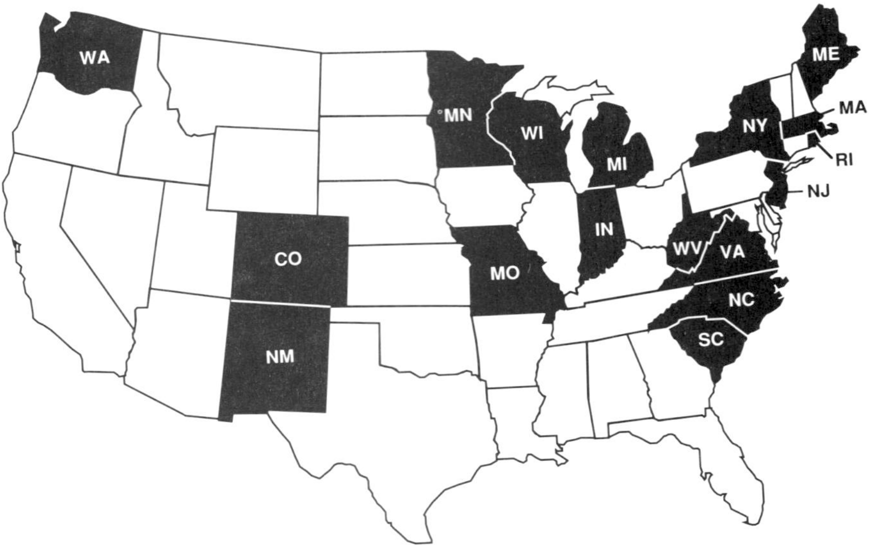

Figure 11 Location of states participating in ASSIST. (From Ref. 18.)

variety of program services, while media and tobacco control policies are expected to create broader social change and increase demand for intervention services.

ASSIST will be implemented in two phases. Phase 1, the planning period, started in October 1991 and will last 2 years. During this phase each funded state health department will establish tobacco control coalitions and perform a detailed site analysis by thoroughly surveying its region to determine the current status of tobacco control and to assess needs. Based on findings in their site analysis, each state tobacco control coalition will then develop a comprehensive tobacco prevention and control plan for their entire state. In phase 2, the intervention phase, the comprehensive plan will be implemented. Phase 2 will last 5 years, ending in September 1998. Examples of phase 2 activities include implementation of smoking control policies and delivery of smoking cessation and prevention services. Intervention activities will include such things as protection of nonsmokers from tobacco smoke through restrictions of smoking in various public settings, placement of tobacco use prevention programs and curricula in schools, training of health care professionals to deliver cessation advice, use of media to more aggressively cover smoking as a community issue, and interventions for worksites.

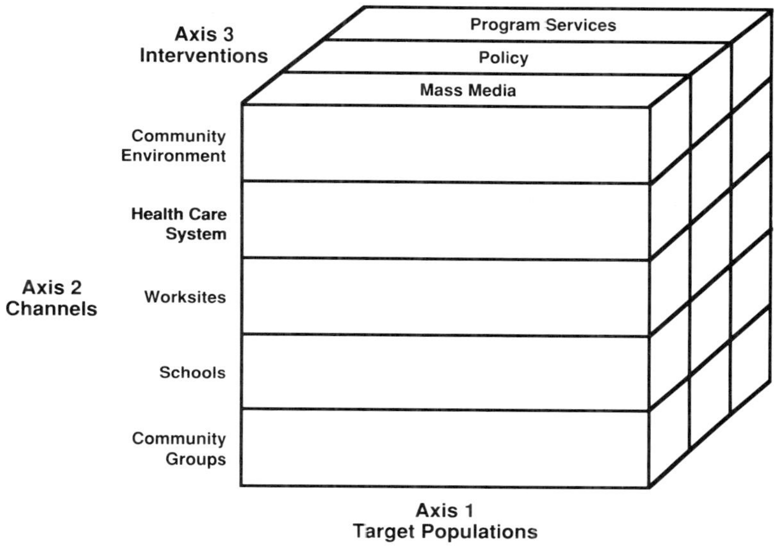

Figure 12 ASSIST project conceptual framework. (From Ref. 18.)

A major emphasis of ASSIST is the targeting of interventions to populations or groups classified as high risk either due to their continued high prevalence rates or particularly susceptible to the effects of smoking Based on current projections, ASSIST will result in more than 4.5 million additional adults quitting, and 2 million adolescents will be prevented from becoming addicted. Should these goals be realized, 1.2 million premature deaths (lifetime risk) will be averted due to ASSIST, including hundreds of thousands of deaths from lung and other cancers caused by tobacco use.

C. National Training Program for Clinicians

NCI has initiated steps to build national training programs based upon the consensus documents developed from the intervention research trials (45). Pioneering this effort are the train-the-trainers programs: one for physicians and another for oral health professionals (46). Three levels of training are now available. The first is a simple grand rounds presentation, lasting 45–60 min. The second is a longer workshop lasting about 3 h. This format is much preferred to the shorter session, given the variety of skills that physicians need to learn to treat smokers effectively, but reality and feasibility will dictate the preferred approaches.

The third level of training is paramount to the STCP training strategy: the training of trainers. Physicians are recruited and trained to conduct the 1- and 3-h sessions. These physicians are recruited from organizations that have a commitment to the prevention of cancer and also have the ability to reach large numbers of practicing physicians.

To date more than 40,000 physicians and 15,000 oral health professionals have been trained in the NCI protocol. A national target to train a total of 100,000 physicians and 50,000 dentists and other oral health professionals by the middle of this decade has been set.

VI. Summary

Although tobacco use has a long history in America, the practice of inhaling cigarette smoke is a phenomenon of the twentieth century. Twenty-five years after the widespread adoption and use of machine-manufactured cigarettes, first by men and later women, lung cancer deaths and death rates began to rise precipitously. Today, lung cancer is the leading cause of cancer mortality among both men and women and is projected to kill over 150,000 Americans this year alone (47).

Substantial progress, however, has been made in the United States to reduce cigarette smoking over the past three decades in an effort to reduce lung and other cancers caused by smoking (48). Overall, the prevalence of smoking is now at its lowest level since 1955 when the first large-scale study of tobacco use patterns was conducted in the United States (49). Among men, smoking is probably at its lowest point since before World War I; smoking prevalence is declining among women but these changes have occurred more recently, and the rate of decline is not as steep as that observed among men. Among more contemporary age cohorts of both men and women, however, virtually no differences with respect to their smoking behavior are currently evident, and smoking among all the major demographic groups continues to decline (50).

Despite these encouraging trends, however, the absolute number of cigarette smokers has not changed appreciably compared to 30 years ago; nearly 50 million Americans still consider themselves regular smokers. Further, smoking rates among teens, the replacement smokers for those adults who either quit smoking or die prematurely due to their behavior, has declined only marginally during the past 10 years, and nearly 3000 new teens take up the deadly addiction each and every day in the United States (51). Unless comprehensive and sustained efforts to control smoking are undertaken soon, lung cancer and other chronic diseases related to smoking will continue to exact a heavy toll on the public health of this country for decades to come.

By the beginning of the 1980s the National Cancer Institute recognized that if progress to eliminate or substantially reduce smoking and the diseases associated with that behavior were to be fully realized, new approaches to smoking prevention and cessation would be required. Consequently, NCI embarked on an aggressive program of research and public health efforts to reduce smoking through its Smoking and Tobacco Control Program. Following nearly 10 years of research, during which time the institute funded more than 60 prevention and cessation intervention trials ($300 million), the STCP is now applying the most promising of this technology in an attempt to accelerate the current downward trend in smoking prevalence.

A key component to this national strategy is the realization that comprehensive, community-based intervention efforts are now required if we are to have any chance of reaching the national health goals for smoking by the turn of the century (52). In the NCI model, comprehensive efforts stress public health policy interventions capable of influencing the larger social environment, while simultaneously offering prevention and cessation services to smokers and potential smokers.

This model will be aggressively implemented and tested in ASSIST, the American Stop Smoking Intervention Study for Smoking Prevention, the largest, most comprehensive health promotion project to reduce smoking ever undertaken in the United States. ASSIST, which began in October 1991, involves the NCI, the national and local offices of the American Cancer Society, and health departments in 17 states. The project will reach an estimated 90 million people including millions of children and adolescents over the next 7 years. If the goal of a 43% reduction in smoking prevalence is achieved, ASSIST will have prevented 2 million youths from taking up the addiction while assisting 4.5 million adults to quit. Should these goals be realized, 1.2 million premature deaths will be averted, including between 400,000 and 500,000 lung cancer deaths.

References

1. National Cancer Institute. (1990). Smoking, Tobacco and Cancer Program Status Report 1985–1989. NIH Publication No. 90-3107. U.S. Department of Health and Human Services, National Institutes of Health, National Cancer Institute, Bethesda, MD.
2. Milmore, B. K., and Conover, A. G. (1956). Tobacco consumption in the United States, 1880–1955. In *Tobacco Smoking Patterns in the United States*. Edited by W. Haenszel, M. B. Shimkin, and H. P. Miller. U.S. Department of Health, Education and Welfare, National Institutes of Health, National Cancer Institute, Public Health Monograph No. 45, Bethesda, MD, pp. 107–111.
3. U.S. Department of Agriculture. Tobacco Outlook and Situation Report. U.S. Department of Agriculture, Economic Research Service, Apr 1992.
4. Smith, J. W. (1990). *Smoke Signals. Cigarettes, Advertising and the American Way of Life*. Chapel Hill, University of North Carolina Press.
5. U.S. Department of Health and Human Services. (1980). *The Health Consequences of Smoking for Women*. A Report of the Surgeon General. U. S. Department of Health

and Human Services, Public Health Service, Office of the Assistant Secretary for Health, Office on Smoking and Health, Washington, D.C.

6. Harris, J. E. (1983). Cigarette smoking among successive birth cohorts of men and women in the United States during 1900–1980. *JNCI* 71:473–479.
7. Wynder, E. L., and Graham, E. A. (1950). Tobacco smoking as a possible etiologic factor in bronchiogenic carcinoma. A study of six hundred and eighty-four proved cases. *JAMA* 143:329–336.
8. Doll, R., and Hill, A. B. (1950). Smoking and carcinoma of the lung. Preliminary report. *BMJ* 2:739–748.
9. Levine, M. L., Goldstein, H., and Gerhardt, P. R. (1950). Cancer and tobacco smoking. A preliminary report. *JAMA* 143:336–338.
10. Schrek, R., Baker, L. A., Ballard, G. P., and Dolgoff, S. (1950). Tobacco smoking as an etiologic factor in disease. I. Cancer. *Cancer Res.* 10:49–58.
11. Hammond, E. C., and Horn, D. (1954). The relationship between human smoking habits and death rates. *JAMA* 155:1316–1328.
12. Hammond, E. C., and Horn, D. (1958). Smoking and death rates—report on forty-four months of followup of 187,783 men. I. Total mortality. *JAMA* 166:1159–1172.
13. Doll, R., and Hill, A. B (1964). Mortality in relation to smoking: Ten years' observation of British doctors. *BMJ* 1:1399–1410.
14. U.S. Department of Health and Human Services. (1982). *The Health Consequences of Smoking: Cancer*. A report of the Surgeon General, 1982. DHHS Publication (PHS) 82-50179. U.S. Department of Health and Human Services, Public Health Service, Office of the Assistant Secretary for Health, Office on Smoking and Health, Washington, D.C.
15. Shopland, D. R., Eyre, H. J., and Pechacek, T. F. (1991). Smoking attributed cancer mortality in 1991: Is lung cancer now the leading cause of death among smokers in the United States? *JNCI* 83:1142–1148.
16. Shopland, D. R. (1990). Changes in tobacco consumption and lung cancer risk. Evidence from studies of individuals. In *Evaluating the Effectiveness of Primary Prevention of Cancer*. IARC Scientific Publication No. 103, Lyon, France, pp. 77–91.
17. Boring, C. C., Squires, T. S., and Tong, T. (1991). Cancer statistics, 1991. *CA* 41:19–36.
18. National Cancer Institute. (1991). *Strategies to Control Tobacco Use in the United States: A Blueprint for Public Health Action in the 1990's*. Smoking and Tobacco Control Monographs. NIH Publication No. 92-3316. U.S. Department of Health and Human Services, Public Health Service, National Institutes of Health, National Cancer Institute, Bethesda, MD.
19. U.S. Department of Health, Education and Welfare. (1964). *Smoking and Health*. Report of the Advisory Committee to the Surgeon General of the Public Health Service. PHS Publication No. 1103. U.S. Department of Health, Education and Welfare, Public Health Service, Washington, D.C.
20. Warner, K. E. (1989). Effects of the anti-smoking campaign: An update. *AJPH* 79: 144–151.
21. U.S. Department of Health and Human Services. (1989). *Reducing the Health Consequences of Smoking: 25 Years of Progress*. A Report of the Surgeon General,

1989. DHHS Publication No. (CDC) 89-8411. U.S. Department of Health and Human Services, Public Health Service, Centers for Disease Control, Washington, D.C.

22. Pierce, J., and Hatziandreu, E. (1989). *Report of the 1986 Adult Use of Tobacco Survey*. Publication No. 10491. U.S. Department of Health and Human Services, Public Health Service, Centers for Disease Control, Rockville, MD.
23. U.S. Department of Health and Human Services. (1988). *The Health Consequences of Smoking: Nicotine Addiction*. A Report of the Surgeon General—1988. DHHS Publication (CDC) 88-8406. U.S. Department of Health and Human Services, Public Health Service, Office on Smoking and Health, Washington, D.C.
24. Wagner, S. (1971). *Cigarette Country. Tobacco in American History and Politics*. New York, Praeger Publishers.
25. Whelan, E. M. (1984). *A Smoking Gun. How the Tobacco Industry Gets Away with Murder*. Philadelphia, George F. Stickley Co.
26. False and Misleading Advertising (Filter-tip Cigarettes). Hearings Before a Subcommittee on the Committee on Government Operations. House of Representatives, 85th Congress, 1st Session, July 18–19; 23–26, 1957.
27. Schwartz, J. L. (1969). A critical review and evaluation of smoking control methods. *Public Health Rep.* 84:483–506.
28. Schwartz, J. L. (1992). Methods of smoking cessation. *Med. Clin. North Am.* 76: 451–476.
29. Schwartz, J. L. (1987). *Review and Evaluation of Smoking Cessation Methods: The United States and Canada, 1978–1985*. NIH Publication No. 87-2940. U.S. Department of Health and Human Services, Public Health Service, National Institutes of Health, National Cancer Institute, Bethesda, MD.
30. Fiore, M. C., Novotny, T. E., Pierce, J. P., Giovino, G. A., Hatziandreu, E. S., Newcomb, P. A., Surawicz, T. S., and Davis, R. M. (1990). Methods used to quit smoking in the United States. Do cessation programs help? *JAMA* 263:2760–2765.
31. Bierer, M. F., and Rigotti, N. A. (1992). Public policy for the control of tobacco related disease. *Med. Clin. North Am.* 76:515–539.
32. Peterson, D. E., Zeger, S. L., Remington, P. L., and Anderson, H. A. (1992). The effect of state cigarette tax increases on cigarette sales, 1955 to 1988. *AJPH* 82:94–96.
33. Burns, D. M., and Pierce, J. P. (1992). Tobacco Use in California 1990–1991. Sacramento, California Department of Health Services.
34. U.S. Department of Health and Human Services. (1986). *The Health Consequences of Involuntary Smoking*. A Report of the Surgeon General, 1986. DHHS Publication No. (CDC)87-8398. U.S. Department of Health and Human Services, Public Health Service, Center for Disease Control, Office on Smoking and Health, Washington, D.C.
35. National Cancer Institute. (1989). *Major Local Smoking Ordinances in the United States*. A detailed matrix of the provisions of workplace, restaurant, and public places smoking ordinances. NIH Publication No. 90-479. U.S. Department of Health and Human Services, National Institutes of Health, National Cancer Institute, Bethesda, MD.
36. National Cancer Institute. (1993). *Major Local Tobacco Control Ordinances in the*

United States. Smoking and Tobacco Control Monograph No. 3. U.S. Department of Health and Human Services, Public Health Service, National Institutes of Health, Bethesda, MD, National Cancer Institute, in press.

37. Forester, J. L, Hourigan, M., and McGovern, P. (1992). Availability of cigarettes to underage youth in three communities. *Prev. Med.* 21:320–328.
38. Giovino, G. A., Eriksen, M. P., and McKenna, J. W. (1992). The vital diversity of tobacco control research. *AJPH* 82:1203–1205.
39. Davis, R. M. (1987). Current trends in cigarette advertising and marketing. *N. Engl. J. Med.* 316:725–732.
40. Federal Trade Commission. (1992). Report to Congress for 1990. Pursuant to the Federal Cigarette Labeling and Advertising Act. U.S. Federal Trade Commission, Washington, D.C.
41. Blum, A., (1991). The Marlboro grand prix. *N. Engl. J. Med.* 324:913–917.
42. Prochaska, J. O., and DiClemente, C. C. (1986). Toward a comprehensive model of change. In *Treating Addictive Behaviors*. Edited by W. Miller and N. Heather. New York, Academic Press, 1986.
43. COMMIT Research Group. (1991). Community Intervention Trial for Smoking Cessation (COMMIT): Summary of design and intervention. *JNCI* 83:1620–1628.
44. McKenna, J., and Carbone, E. (1989). Huge tobacco control project begun by NCI, ACS. *JNCI* 81:93–94.
45. Glynn, T. J., Manley, M. W., and Pechacek, T. F. (1990). Physician-initiated smoking cessation program: The National Cancer Institute Trials. In *Advances in Cancer Control: Screening and Prevention Research*. New York, Wiley-Liss, pp. 11–25.
46. Manley, M., Epps, R. P., Husten, C., Glynn, T., and Shopland, D. (1991). Clinical interventions in tobacco control. *JAMA* 266:3172–3173.
47. American Cancer Society. (1992). *Cancer Facts and Figures—1992*. Atlanta, American Cancer Society.
48. Shopland, D. R., Pechacek, T. F., and Cullen, J. W. (1990). Toward a tobacco-free society. *Sem. Oncol.* 17:402–412.
49. Haenszel, W., Shimkin, M. B., and Miller, H. P., eds. (1956). *Tobacco Smoking Patterns in the United States*. Public Health Monograph No. 45. U.S. Department of Health, Education and Welfare, National Institutes of Health, National Cancer Institute, Bethesda, MD.
50. MMWR (1992). Cigarette smoking among adults—US, 1990. *MMWR* 41:354–355, 361–362.
51. Broder, S. (1992). Cigarette advertising and corporate responsibility. *JAMA* 268: 782–783.
52. U.S. Department of Health and Human Services. (1991). *Healthy People 2000: National Health Promotion and Disease Prevention Objectives*. PHS Publication No. 91-50213. U.S. Department of Health and Human Services, Public Health Service, Office of the Assistant Secretary for Health, Office of Disease Prevention and Health Promotion, Washington, D.C.

18

Interactions of Tobacco Smoking with Other Causes of Lung Cancer

RODOLFO SARACCI and PAOLO BOFFETTA

International Agency for Research on Cancer
Lyon, France

I. Tobacco Smoking as a Confounder or Effect Modifier

The well-recognized and dominant role of tobacco smoking in lung cancer causation in economically developed countries, and its increasing impact in developing countries, often leads to the contention that no investigation of other environmental agents can now be unbiased and informative without explicitly considering the role played by tobacco smoking as well. This view is only partly correct. There is no question that, for example, a well-designed epidemiological study aimed at clarifying the possible carcinogenic role for the lung of an airborne workplace pollutant should include, if feasible, an assessment of the workers' smoking habits. Still, if information on tobacco smoking is not obtainable, as is often the case when workers have been first enrolled many years previously and then followed up to the present day, the results of recording lung cancer occurrence may be interpretable even in the absence of smoking habit histories. In fact, it has been shown by simple algebraic arguments (1,2) and empirically confirmed by systematically studying occupational groups, taking their smoking habits into account or not (3), that an increased risk of lung cancer, if appreciable (say two-fold or more), observed in the workers exposed to the pollutant, compared to unexposed workers comparable in age and sex, cannot solely be explained by the unmeasured tobacco consumption, unless an extreme and unrealistic imbalance in smoking habits between exposed workers and unexposed subjects occurs, causing a substantial degree of the type of bias known in epidemiology as *confounding*. Thus, it would be reasonable in such a case to relate the increase in risk, at least in part, to the pollutant (or, more generally, to the workplace, if other pollutants are also present). Whether, however, it may be related to the pollutant(s) alone or to the pollutant(s) jointly acting with tobacco smoking is a different issue, of *interaction* of environmental agents with tobacco smoking or, stated differently, of tobacco smoking and environmental agents reciprocally modifying their effects on cancer risk. Among pathogenic agents, tobacco smoking is one for which epidemiology has provided a comparatively large set of data on the interactions with other exogenous agents in the causation, and in the protection against causation, of cancer, in particular lung cancer. In this chapter, after providing the necessary definitions pertinent to interactions, in elementary formal terms, we review in some detail these sets of data, pointing out in the final section some general public health implications.

II. Measuring Interactions

The question of how to define and measure "interaction," extensively studied in epidemiology in the last two decades, can be traced back to at least 1962, when Cornfield (4) first introduced a function (the multiple logistic) in his analysis of the factors related to the occurrence of coronary heart disease in the Framingham Heart Study. This analysis offered a model and a scale of measurement on which the presence or absence of interaction may be assessed. In 1968 Selikoff and coworkers (5) showed that the combined exposure to tobacco smoking and to asbestos in insulation workers was associated with a lung cancer risk far exceeding that expected from the separate exposure to each of these agents, indicating the occurrence of an interaction between the two agents. Since this seminal study, the asbestos/tobacco smoking/lung cancer topic has often been quoted in methodological discussions of interactions as exemplary and based on relatively abundant data.

For the present review, interaction is described and measured, calculating separately for each study considered the following estimates (6):

Relative risks (*RRs*) for lung cancer in subjects exposed to an environmental agent (e.g., asbestos) relative to the unexposed, separately for smokers and nonsmokers. Here, "relative risk" broadly includes the estimates found in the epidemiological literature as risk ratios, odds ratios, rate ratios, and (standardized) mortality ratios. The RRs are derived by categorizing the published data for both smoking and the other agent dichotomously and by contrasting smokers exposed to the agent with smokers unexposed and nonsmokers exposed with nonsmokers unexposed. It is important to note that constancy of these relative risks in smokers and nonsmokers implies a multiplicative relation, while values lower in smokers than in nonsmokers imply a less than multiplicative relation, including the additive or less than additive.

Absolute interaction magnitude, as derived from the statistical model most closely describing the relation between the observed RRs among subjects exposed to smoking alone (R_s), to the agent alone (R_o), or to both agents (R_{so}), all RRs here being calculated taking the subjects not exposed to either agent as reference.

A zero difference between the observed value of R_{so} and the value of $R_s + R_o - 1$ defines zero interaction (i.e., simple additive relation or model: $R_{so} = R_s + R_o - 1$), a value smaller than zero defines a negative interaction (antagonism), and a value greater than zero defines a positive interaction (synergism) (7,8).

A particular case of the latter is the multiplicative model, in which $R_{so} = R_s \cdot R_o \geqslant R_s + R_o - 1$ (for any R_s and $R_o \geqslant 1$). The absolute interaction magnitude, as approximately reconstructed from the figures available in the published papers, is classified with reference to the additive (A) and multiplicative (M) models as follows: less than additive ($<A$), for R_{so} below -25% of A; near additive ($\sim A$), for R_{so} within $\pm 25\%$ of A; additive (A) for R_{so} within $\pm 10\%$ of A; intermediate (I), for R_{so} above 25% of A but below 25% of M; near multiplicative ($\sim M$), for R_{so} within $\pm 25\%$ of M; multiplicative (M), for R_{so} within $\pm 10\%$ of M; and more than multiplicative ($>M$), for R_{so} above 25% of M.

Relative interaction magnitude expressed as percent of the excess risk due to interaction (PERDI) and classified in four intervals: <25, 25–49, 50–74, and ⩾75. This percent of the total excess over simple additivity of effects is given by $100 \times (R_{so} - R_s - R_o + 1)/(R_{so} - 1)$ and provides an intuitive expression of the contribution specifically due to the interaction (8,9) relative to the total excess risk (or excess incidence) due to the joint exposure to tobacco smoking and to another agent. This fraction, as discussed in the final section of this chapter, is most relevant from a practical, preventive viewpoint.

In this review, the statistical variability of the absolute and relative measures of interaction has not been considered systematically. However, the reader should bear in mind that the measures in interaction are subject to very large imprecision, since the small number of lung cancers among nonsmokers exposed to the different risk factors strongly reduces the power of the relevant studies. Even in the case of several studies showing a similar pattern of interaction (as in the case of arsenic, see Section III.C), the data available are not sufficient to formally reject alternative models.

In addition, one has to take into account the fact that exposure to both smoking and the other factor can be (and in fact frequently is) subject to misclassification, which will result in biased estimates of R_s and R_o. With respect to the measure of interaction, one should in theory distinguish between the situation in which the misclassification in one exposure (e.g., smoking) is nondifferential with respect to the other exposure (i.e., smokers and nonsmokers will be misclassified irrespective of their exposure to the other agent) and the situation in which there is a differential misclassification among the two exposures (i.e., smokers exposed to asbestos tend to be misclassified differently from unexposed smokers). It should be noted that it is not relevant in this context whether the misclassification of each exposure is in itself differential or nondifferential (i.e., whether, in a case-control study, cases and controls are or are not equally misclassified with respect to their smoking habits). In the case of differential misclassification between the two exposures, both the absolute and the relative measures of the association can be biased, and the direction of the bias (i.e., toward either a more than multiplicative or a less than additive pattern) will depend on the degree of misclassification across the various strata of combined exposure to smoking and the other factor. In the case of nondifferential misclassification, the effect on the measures of interaction will be limited, and it will hardly cause a change in the categories used in this review for both the absolute interaction and the PERDI (unless the degree of misclassification should be high). In practice, however, hardly any data are available to investigate the existence and the degree of such misclassification.

III. Interactions of Tobacco Smoking

A. Asbestos

The interaction between tobacco smoking and asbestos exposure has been investigated in detail in a number of epidemiological studies, which are summarized in Table 1. Most of these studies have been previously reviewed (6), and the evidence available at that time indicated an interaction in the multiplicative region, although there was not a fully uniform pattern across studies. In particular, an additive interaction was observed among Canadian chrysotile miners and millers (10–12), while Australian underground crocidolite miners exhibited a more than multiplicative interaction (13). Workers in manufacturing exposed to amosite or a combination of amosite, chrysotile, and crocidolite also showed variations in the size of the observed interaction (14–17). On the contrary, studies on insulators (18–21) and case-control studies investigating any type of asbestos exposure (22–24) appeared to follow more uniformly a multiplicative pattern.

A recent case-control analysis nested in the cohort of Australian crocidolite miners (25) confirmed the pattern of more than multiplicative interaction that had been previously found. A study on Norwegian maintenance workers exposed to asbestos (26) found a more than multiplicative interaction, based on nine lung cancer deaths among exposed persons and no death among unexposed. In a recently published study from China on workers exposed to asbestos in various manufacturing industries, a multiplicative interaction was detected (27).

The previous review by Saracci on the interaction between asbestos exposure and tobacco smoking concluded that a variable pattern of interaction had been observed; explanations cited for the variation included the possibility that asbestos and smoking act each at several stages of the carcinogenic process as well as differences in the biological effect of different types of asbestos fibers (6). The investigations published since then tend to confirm these conclusions.

B. Radon and Other Sources of Ionizing Radiation

The interaction between radon exposure and tobacco smoking has been investigated among uranium miners, mainly from the United States, and nonuranium miners, mainly from Sweden. The studies are summarized in Table 2.

Several reports have been published on the follow-up of the cohort of miners in the Colorado Plateau of the United States. The RRs of three different periods of follow-up (28–30) are similar in smokers and nonsmokers; these data appear to conform well to a multiplicative interaction, with a large percentage of the total excess of lung cancer being attributable to the interaction effect. A recent analysis of data from another population of U.S. uranium miners did not find a statistically significant departure from a multiplicative interaction, thus confirming the previous results (31). Similarly, in two cohort studies of Ontario uranium miners, there was no (statistically significant) departure from a multiplicative model of interaction (32,33). It should be kept in mind, however, that in the descriptive terms used in this review, lack of statistically significant departure from the multiplicative model may correspond to patterns of interaction in the greater than multiplicative or intermediate ranges. The U.S. Committee on the Biological Effects of Ionizing Radiation conducted detailed analyses of the studies available up to 1988 and concluded that although most studies supported a multiplicative model of interaction between radon exposure and tobacco smoking, a submultiplicative model may provide a more accurate description (34).

Studies on nonuranium miners exposed to radon present a less consistent pattern. An early study on iron miners from Sweden showed an additive effect (35), while two more recent studies, which included a fraction of the follow-up experience of the previous cohort, indicated a multiplicative effect (36,37). Two further twin studies on Swedish iron miners indicated an interaction intermediate between additive and multiplicative, with a higher RR among nonsmokers than among smokers (38,39). A study on Swedish zinc-lead miners presented RRs for smokers four times smaller than those for nonsmokers, suggesting a less than additive interaction (antagonism) (40). A cohort study of niobium miners from Norway suggested a more than multiplicative interaction between mining employment and heavy tobacco smoking (41). However, no firm conclusion can be drawn from the last two studies, which were based on only 27 and nine lung cancer deaths, respectively. A further study on fluorspar miners from Canada presented very similar RRs for smokers and nonsmokers, thus suggesting a multiplicative interaction (42).

Table 1 Studies on the Interaction Between Tobacco Smoking and Asbestos in the Causation of Lung Cancer

Author(s), design, location, years of observation, exposure	Exposure assessment		No. of cases	No. of Co[a]	RR[b]		Interaction[c]		Notes
	Smoking	Asbestos			Smokers	Nonsmk.	Absolute	PERDI	
Berry et al. (14), cohort, UK, 1960–70, mixed asbestos factory	D, O	D	27 Ma 15 Fe	12.0 Ma 2.1 Fe	2.3 7.4	 5.0	[>M] [>M]	[50–74] [≥75]	Assuming $R_s = 10$
Selikoff & Hammond (18), cohort, New Jersey, 1963–74, chrysotile and amosite in insulation	P	D	45	7.6	[6.0]	[0]	[>M]	[≥75]	Assuming $R_s = 10$
Martischnig et al. (22), ca-co, UK, 1973–74, any asbestos exposure	R	R	201	201	[3.2]	1.1	>M	≥75	
Blot et al. (19), ca-co, 1970–76, shipyard exposures	R, O	R, O	458	553	[1.6]	[1.3]	~M	<25	
Hammond et al. (20), cohort, US & Canada, 1967–76, chrysotile and amosite in insulation	P	D	272	51.7	[5.3]	[5.7]	M	50–75	
Selikoff et al. (15), cohort, US, 1961–77, amosite factory	P	D	50	9.8	4.7	25	I	25–49	
Blot et al. (21), ca-co, US, 1972–76, shipyard exposures	O	O	319	341	[1.6]	[1.9]	~M	25–49	
Pastorino et al. (23), ca-co, Italy, 1976–79, any asbestos exposure	R	R	204	211	[1.8]	[2.8]	I	25–49	
Acheson et al. (16), cohort, UK, 1947–80, amosite factory	D	D	23	14.5	[1.6]	[2.0]	[~M]	[25–49]	Assuming $R_s = 10$
Liddell et al. (12), ca-co in cohort, Canada, 1950–75, chrysotile mining & milling	O, P	D	223	715	[1.7]	[3.0]	~A	<25	

Baker (13), cohort, Australia, 1944–81, crocidilite mining & milling	P	D	62	29	[5.0]	0.7	>M	≥75	
Hilt et al. (26), cohort, Norway, 1966–73, maintenance workers exposed to asbestos	P	D	9	A	[4.3]	0	>M	≥75	
Berry et al. (17), cohort, UK, 1971–80, mixed asbestos factory	P	D	53 Ma 13 Fe	26.0 Ma 2.6 Fe	2.0 4.3	6.3 12.5	[A] [I]	[0] [≤25]	Assuming $R_s = 10$
Kjuus et al. (24), ca-co, Norway 1979–83, any asbestos exposure	R	R	176	176	[2.1]	[2.4]	~M	25–49	
de Klerk et al. (25), ca-co in cohort, Australia, 1979–86, crocidolite miners	P	D	40	1799	2.6	1.9	>M	50–74	Based on crude analysis Exposure to ≥10g/ml y vs. lower exposure
Cheng & Kong (27), cohort, China, 1972–87, mixed asbestos factories	D	D	21	6.7	1.6	1.6	M	25–49	

[a]Controls or number of expected cases.
[b]Relative risk due to asbestos exposure. Numbers in brackets are reconstructed from published data.
[c]For definitions of categories of absolute magnitude of interaction, see text (Section II). Numbers in brackets are based on an assumption of relative risk due to smoking (R_s).
ca-co, case-control study; P, exposure information collected prospectively from study subjects; R, exposure information collected retrospectively from study subjects; O, exposure information collected from informants other than study subjects, e.g., relatives; D, exposure information collected from documents; Ma, males; Fe, females; NA, not available; A, additive; M, multiplicative; I, intermediate; PERDI, percent excess risk due to interaction; R_s, relative risk due to smoking; ppd, pack per day; py, pack-year.

Table 2 Studies on the Interaction Between Tobacco Smoking and Radon Exposure in the Causation of Lung Cancer

Author(s), design, location, years of observation	Radon exposure		No. of cases	No. of Co[a]	Radon exposure	RR[b]		Interaction[c]		Notes
	Smoking	Radon				Smokers	Nonsmk.	Absolute	PERDI	
Archer et al. (28), cohort, US, mid-1950–74	P	D	76	NA	Uranium mining	[6.5]	[6.9]	M	50–74	
Axelson & Sundell (40), ca-co, Sweden, 1957–76	D, O	D	27	171	Lead-zinc mining	14.9	58.1	<A	0	
Lundin et al. (29), cohort, US, 1950–68	P	D	57	16.2	Uranium mining	3.5	3.8	M	50–74	
Damber & Larsson (36), ca-co, Sweden, 1972–77	R, O	R, O	589 456	582 899	Iron mining	[2.7] [2.2]	2.4 7.0	~M ~A	50–74 <25	
Edling (38), ca-co, Sweden, 1957–77	O	D	44	44	Iron mining	[15]	[38]	[I]	[25–49]	Assuming $R_s = 10$
Edling & Axelson (39), ca-co, Sweden, 1957–77	O	D	28	28	Iron mining	[11]	[27]	[I]	[25–49]	Assuming $R_s = 10$
Whittemore & McMillan (30), ca-co in cohort, US, mid-1950–77	P	D	194	776	Uranium mining	[19.1]	[18.2]	M	≥75	
Radford & St. Clair Renard (35), cohort, Sweden, 1951–76	O	D	50	12.8	Iron mining	2.9	10.0	~A	<25	
Damber & Larsson (37), ca-co, Sweden, 1972–82	R, O	R, O	69 60	67 118	Iron mining	[5.5] [3.1]	5.5 3.6	M ~M	50–74 50–74	

Solli et al. (41), cohort, Norway, 1953–81	R	R	12	3.0	Niobium mining	8.0	[2.4]	[>M]	[≥75]	Assuming R_s = 10. Smokers classified as ≤27 py vs. >27 py
Morrison et al. (42), cohort, Canada, 1950–84	D	P	113	NA	Unit WLM in fluorspar mining	1.005	1.004	[M]	—	Assuming R_s = 10
Qiao et al. (43), ca-co in cohort, China, 1985	R	R, D	107	107	90–414 WLM	—	8.8	~M	50.74	Smokers classified as 0.84 pipe-year vs. >186 pipe-years
					≥415 WLM	—	19.4	<A	—	
Lubin et al.(44), ca-co, China, 1981–84	R	R, D	74	74	≥100 WLM	[8.7]	[6.0]	>M	25–49	Unadjusted analysis
					100–399 WLM	[9.2]	[2.0]	>M	≥75	
					≥400 WLM	[8.3]	[18.0]	<A	50–74	
Chen et al. (45) cohort, China, 1970–82	R, O	R, O, D	29	8.0	Underground hematite mining	2.6	0.6	>M	≥75	

[a]Controls or number of expected cases.

[b]Relative risk due to radon exposure. Numbers in brackets are reconstructed from published data.

[c]For definitions of categories of absolute magnitude of interaction, see text (Section II). Numbers in brackets are based on an assumption of relative risk due to smoking (R_s).

ca-co, case-control study; P, exposure information collected prospectively from study subjects; R, exposure information collected retrospectively from study subjects; O, exposure information collected from informants other than study subjects, e.g., relatives; D, exposure information collected from documents; NA, not available; A, additive; M, multiplicative; I, intermediate; PERDI, percent excess risk due to interaction; py, pack-year; R_s, relative risk due to smoking; WLM, working level-months.

Two studies on lung cancer among tin miners are available from China (43,44). In both cases, analyses by different levels of radon exposure are presented, and in both studies a multiplicative or more than multiplicative interaction is shown up to the level of about 400 working level-months (WLM), while above that level the RRs are higher among nonsmokers than among smokers, leading to a less than additive effect. A further study on hematite miners from China found a more than multiplicative effect between tobacco smoking and underground mining (45).

In conclusion, the studies on the interaction between radon exposure and tobacco smoking indicate a multiplicative (or submultiplicative) effect among uranium miners, but a very inconsistent pattern among other miners, ranging from less than additive (antagonism) to more than multiplicative. The results of the Chinese studies on tin miners are particularly interesting because they suggest a different pattern of interaction at high levels of radon exposure (above 400 WLMs) as compared to lower levels (there were, however, only 14 lung cancer deaths among nonsmokers in the higher category of exposure). Qualitative differences in the mining situations, such as dustiness, may affect the actual radiation dose to the lungs and therefore explain the variability in results in different groups of miners.

A cohort and a case-control study have been carried out on atomic bomb survivors (46,47). They provide limited information on the interaction with tobacco smoking, which seems to follow an additive pattern: RRs for exposure to ⩾100 rads compared to <10 rads were 1.5 in smokers and 2.3 in nonsmokers (46).

C. Arsenic

Six epidemiological investigations have provided data on the interaction between occupational exposure to arsenic and tobacco smoking (48–53). They are summarized in Table 3. A study analyzed the mortality of Chinese tin miners exposed to arsenic (51): in that study, the main use of tobacco was in water pipes; the remaining studies investigated lung cancer among miners in Sweden, the United States, or Japan. It should be noted that the study by Järup and Pershagen (53) is an extension of a previous investigation (49).

A multiplicative interaction was found in the earlier Swedish study (49) while, in the first cohort study from the United States, there was a suggestion of an interaction in the intermediate range, but detailed data were not reported (48), and the second U.S. cohort study found an additive interaction (50). In a further case-cohort study from the United States, based on workers at eight copper smelters, including those previously studied (48,50), the interaction term between tobacco smoking and arsenic exposure was found not to be significant, indicating lack of departure from the multiplicative model (detailed data, however, were not presented) (54). The recent study from Sweden analyzed in great detail the interaction between cumulative exposure and intensity of exposure to arsenic and tobacco smoking among copper smelters (53). Overall, the interaction was additive at low exposure levels (below 100 mg/m^3/year) and intermediate at higher levels. In a cohort of arsenic miners from Japan, with certified arsenic poisoning, a supramultiplicative interaction has been suggested on the basis of seven cases among smokers and one among nonsmokers (52). Finally, the case-control study among Chinese tin miners found an additive interaction between estimated arsenic exposure (upper vs. lower tertile) and water pipe smoking (upper vs. lower tertile; there was no pure nonsmoking category) (51).

Although only limited data are available on the interaction between arsenic exposure and tobacco smoking, most of the studies point toward a less than multiplicative interaction. The multiplicative interaction found in the early Swedish report (49) was contradicted by the later report from the same study, which was based on a more detailed assessment of arsenic exposure and on a longer follow-up (53). However, none of the available studies rejected the multiplicative model at the level of conventional statistical significance.

D. Crystalline Silica

Nine epidemiological studies have provided results useful to quantitatively assess the interaction between exposure to silica and tobacco smoking (Table 4): a case-control study on Italian ceramic workers (55), two case-control studies on silica-exposed workers from Italy and Canada (56,57), two cohorts of silicotics from Japan and the United States (58,59), three occupational cohorts of U.S. metal miners, South African gold miners, and granite workers from Singapore, respectively (60–62), and a necropsy case-control study from South Africa (63). In six of these studies (55,58,59,61–63) the RR for smoking (R_s) was not presented and was assumed to be equal to 10 (similar results on interaction are obtained by assuming $R_s = 5$ or $R_s = 20$).

The results of these studies are not consistent two of them found a nearly additive interaction between silicotic status and tobacco smoking (56,59), while the study among silicotic gold miners from South Africa (60) as well as the two cohorts of silicotics (58,61) and the cohort of Singapore granite workers (62) found a more than multiplicative interaction between cumulative dust exposure or silicotic status and tobacco smoking. The study on French Canadians exposed to silica excluded lung adenocarcinomas and showed an intermediate interaction (57). In addition, the study by Mastrangelo and co-workers (56) found a less than additive interaction between silica exposure and tobacco smoking in nonsilicotic workers exposed to silica, as did the South African study on silicosis at necropsy (63), and a nearly multiplicative interaction was found among Italian ceramic workers (55).

Although most of the available studies point toward a less than multiplicative interaction between silica exposure and tobacco smoking, the pattern emerging from this review is not consistent. One problem complicating, even more than for the other agents, the study of the interactions of crystalline silica with tobacco

Table 3 Studies on the Interaction Between Tobacco Smoking and Arsenic Exposure in the Causation of Lung Cancer

Author(s), design, location, years of observation	Exposure assessment		No. of cases	No. of Co[a]	Arsenic exposure	RR[b]		Interactions[c]		Notes
	Smoking	Arsenic				Smokers	Nonsmk.	Absolute	PERDI	
Pinto et al. (48), cohort, US, 1949–73	R, O	D	32	10.5	Copper smelter pensioners	2.9	5.1	[I]	[50–74]	Assuming R_s = 10
Pershagen et al. (49), ca-co in cohort, Sweden, 1928–77	O	D	76	152	Smelter workers exposed to arsenic	2.9	3.0	M	50–74	
Welch et al. (50), cohort, US, 1963–78	R, O	D	80	25.5	Copper smelters exposure ⩾500 μg/m³ vs. <500 μg/m³	2.2	3.9	A	0	Multiplicative interaction if reference category <100 μg/m³
Taylor et al. (51), ca-co, China 1971–84	R	D	107	107	Tin miners: cumulative arsenic exposure; highest vs. lowest tertile	[3.5]	5.0	~A	0	Upper vs. lower tertile of pipe tobacco smoking; prevalent cases

Tsuda et al. (52), cohort, Japan, 1972–89	NA	D	8	1.4	Employment in arsenic mine	12.5	2.6	[>M]	[25–49]	Assuming R_s = 10
Järup & Pershagen (53), ca-co in cohort, Sweden, 1928–87	O	D	107	214	Cumulative exposure among copper smelters					Similar results using intensity of exposure; includes data from Pershagen et al. (1981)
					0.25–14.9 μg/m³/yr	—	0.8	A	<25	
					15–99 μg/m³/yr	—	2.8	~A	<25	
					⩾100 μg/m³/yr	—	7.1	I	50–74	

[a]Controls or number of expected cases.

[b]Relative risk due to arsenic exposure. Numbers in brackets are reconstructed from published data.

[c]For definitions of categories of absolute magnitude of interaction, see text (Section II). Numbers in brackets are based on an assumption of relative risk due to smoking (R_s).

ca-co, case-control study; P, exposure information collected prospectively from study subjects; R, exposure information collected retrospectively from study subjects; O, exposure information collected from informants other than study subjects, e.g., relatives; D, exposure information extracted from documents; NA, not available; A, additive; M, multiplicative; I, intermediate; R_s, relative risk due to smoking; PERDI, percent excess risk due to interaction.

Table 4 Studies on the Interaction Between Tobacco Smoking and Silica Exposure in the Causation of Lung Cancer

Author(s), design, location, years of observation	Exposure assessment		No. of cases	No. of Co[a]	Silica exposure	RR[b]		Interaction[c]		Notes
	Smoking	Silica				Smokers	Nonsmk.	Absolute	PERDI	
Forastiere et al. (55), ca-co, Italy, 1968–84	O	O	72	314	Ceramic workers	[4.1]	[1.5]	~M	25–49	Assuming $R_s = 10$
					Ceramic w. with silicosis	[1.8]	[0]	[>M]	[50–74]	
Mastrangelo et al. (56), ca-co, Italy, 1978–80	D	D	309	309	Silica exposure without silicosis	[0.9]	1.3	~A	0	Unadjusted analysis
					Silicosis	[1.7]	5.3	~A	<25	
Hessel et al. (63), ca-co autopsy study, South Africa, 1975–79	D	D	231	218	Hilar gland silicosis	0.7	1.1	[<A]	[0]	Smokers of ≥21 cpd vs. nonsmokers. Assuming $R_s =$ 10
					Parenchymal silicosis	0.9	1.6	[<A]	[0]	
Siemiatycki et al. (57), ca-co, Montreal, French Canadians, 1979–85	R	R	479	NA	Substantial silica exposure estimated from job titles	[1.5]	2.6	I	25–49	Adenocarcinoma excluded
Chiyotani et al. (58), cohort, Japan 1979–83	D	D	60	12.5	Pneumoconiosis patients	6.1	1.8	[>M]	[≥75]	58% silicotics Assuming $R_s = 10$

Amandus & Costello (59), cohort, US, 1959–75, metal miners	D	D	132	108	Silicosis	[1.3]	[2.2]	~A	<25	Assuming R_s = 10
					Silicosis, low radon mines	1.7	5.1	[~A]	[<25]	
Hnizdo & Sluis-Cremer (60), cohort, South Africa, 1968–86, silicotics gold miners	P, D	D	77	NA	31+ dust particles-yrs vs. ≤30	[1.9]	[1.4]	>M	25–49	Smokers of 26+ py vs. smokers of ≤25 py
Amandus et al. (61), cohort, US, 1970–83	D	D	33	12.9	Silicosis	3.4	1.7	[>M]	[50–74]	Assuming R_s = 10
Chia et al. (62), cohort, Singapore, 1970–84, granite workers	D	D	9	4.5	Silicosis	2.2	1.3	[>M]	[50–74]	Assuming R_s = 10

[a]Controls or number of expected cases.

[b]Relative risk due to silica exposure. Numbers in brackets are reconstructed from published data.

[c]For definitions of categories of absolute magnitude of interaction, see text (Section II). Numbers in brackets are based on the assumption of relative risk due to smoking = 10.

ca-co, case-control study; P, exposure information collected prospectively from study subjects; R, exposure information collected retrospectively from study subjects; O, exposure information collected from informants other than study subjects, e.g., relatives; D, exposure information collected from existing documents; NA, not available; A, additive; M, multiplicative; I, intermediate; PERDI, percent excess risk due to interaction; py, pack-year; R_s, relative risk due to smoking.

cpd, cigarette per day.

smoking arises from the fact that in some investigations silicosis is used as a surrogate marker for exposure to silica. Neither these investigations nor those, more straightforwardly interpretable, involving nonsilicotic subjects provide clear evidence for the carcinogenicity of crystalline silica [the evidence was evaluated as "limited" by the International Agency for Research on Cancer (64)] or for the role that tobacco smoking may play in it. Given these limitations, no conclusion can be drawn at present on the model of interaction between tobacco smoking and silica exposure.

E. Other Occupational Exposures

Two studies are available on the interaction between occupational exposure to nickel in the smelting and refining of nickel-containing ores and tobacco smoking: they concur in showing an additive pattern of interaction (65,66).

In the only study of workers exposed to chloromethylethers that analyzed lung cancer according to smoking habits, the RR was lower in smokers than in nonsmokers (3.5, based on five deaths, and 168, based on six deaths, respectively), suggesting a less than additive interaction (antagonism) (67,68).

F. Dietary Factors

A number of studies (summarized in Table 5) have presented results in sufficient detail to allow an analysis of the interaction between tobacco smoking and diet. The dietary factors analyzed differed across these studies. Frequency of consumption of green-yellow vegetables or fresh fruit was considered in five studies (69–73), while five studies took into account vitamin A or β-carotene intake (74–78), and one study measured cholesterol and high-fat food intake (79,80). Two additional studies presented results according to serum β-carotene level, a variable that is indirectly related to dietary habits (81,82). The RRs reported here are those for the subjects with lower consumptions of a dietary component, presumptively protective, versus the subjects with higher consumptions, the exact categorizations of the subjects varying from study to study, as shown in Table 5.

A multiplicative interaction was found with fruit consumption in the cohort study on California Seventh-Day Adventists (73) and with vegetable consumption in the Japanese women studied by Hirayama (69) and among the subjects of the Italian study by Pisani and coworkers (71). A case-control study from New Jersey (70) found a more than multiplicative interaction with vegetable intake. These results are confirmed by a recent study on the effect of diet among nonsmoking U.S. women, which suggested a very strong association between vegetable consumption and lung cancer risk (RR, 0.2 for the highest quartile compared to the lowest quartile) (83). In contrast, the study from New York State (72) found an intermediate interaction between tobacco smoking and fruit and vegetable intake, and the interaction was slightly lower than additive among men enrolled in the Japanese cohort (69). A possible explanation of the discrepancy is the prevalence of smoking, which is much lower among Seventh-Day Adventists and

Table 5 Studies on the Interaction Between Tobacco Smoking and Dietary Factors in the Causation of Lung Cancer

Author(s), design, location, years of observation, exposure	Smoking	Diet	No. of cases	No. of Co[a]	Categories of exposure		RR[b]		Interaction[c]		Notes
							Smokers	Nonsmk.	Absolute	PERDI	
Hirayama (69), cohort, 1965–75, Japan, green-yellow vegetables intake	P	P	611 Ma 196 Fe	NA NA	Rare or no vs. daily consumption	Ma Fe	[1.2] [1.8]	[2.2] [1.4]	A ~M	0 25–49	
Pisani et al. (71), ca-co, Italy, 1979–80, green leaf vegetable intake	R	R	417	849	7+/wk vs. never		1.3	1.4	[M]	[<25]	Assuming R_s = 10
Ziegler et al. (70), ca-co, New Jersey, 1980–81, vegetable intake	R	R	763	900	Lowest vs. highest quartile		1.8	0.3	[>M]	[50–75]	Assuming R_s – 10
Byers et al. (72), ca-co, New York State 1980–84, vit A intake from fruits & vegetables	R	R	296 Ma	587 Ma	Lowest vs. highest quartile	Ma	1.3	1.9	[I]	[<25]	Smokers of 40+ pys vs. nonsmokers; assuming R_s = 20; no risk with vit A among Fe
Fraser et al. (73), cohort, California, 7th Day Adventists, 1977–82, frequency of fruit consumption	P	P	52	NA	<3 times/wk vs. ≥2 times/d		[4.5]	[3.6]	M	50–75	Based on unadjusted analysis

Table 5 Continued

Author(s), design, location, years of observation, exposure	Smoking	Diet	No. of cases	No. of Co[a]	Categories of exposure		RR[b]		Interaction[c]		Notes
							Smokers	Nonsmk.	Absolute	PERDI	
Bjelke (74), cohort, Norway, 1964–73, vit A intake	P	P	53	NA	Intake below or above median		[2.5]	[0.9]	>M	50–74	
Mettlin et al. (75), ca-co, US, 1957–65, vit A intake	R	R	292	801	75,000–124,000 IU vs. ⩾12,500 IU		[1.6]	[1.5]	~M	25–49	Smoking classified as ⩽1 ppd & >1 ppd
					<75,000 IU vs. ⩾12,500 IU		[2.4]	[1.4]	>M	50–74	
Kvale et al. (77), cohort, Norway, 1964–78, vit A intake	P	P	168	NA	Intake below vs. above median	all	[1.3]	[1.1]	~M	<25	
						SSC	[1.6]	[4.3]	I	<25	
Shekelle et al. (76), cohort, US, 1957–78, β carotene intake	P	P	33	NA	Intake below vs. above median		[3.0]	[3.4]	~M	25–49	Unadjusted analysis
LeMarchand et al. (78), ca-co, Hawaii, 1983–85, β carotene intake	R, O	R, O	230 Ma 102 Fe	597 Ma 268 Fe	Lowest vs. highest tertile	Ma	1.6	1.9	[~M]	[25–49]	Assuming R_s = 10
						Fe	2.4	1.4	[A]	[<25]	

Goodman et al. (79,80), ca-co, Hawaii, 1983–85, cholesterol and high fat food intake	R, O	R, O	326	865	Cholesterol intake above vs. below median		[3.8]	1.5	>M	≥75	Smoking classified as ≤40 pys vs. 71+ pys
					Dairy food intake above vs. below median		[9.6]	8.6	M	50–75	
					Sausage intake above vs. below median		[3.3]	1.2	>M	50–74	
Nomura et al. (81), ca-co in cohort, Japan, 1971–84, serum β carotene level	P	P	74	302	22.1–40.5 μg/dl vs. ≥41 μg/dl		—	1.1	>M	≥75	Smoking classified as <1 ppd vs. nonsmokers
					≤22.0 μg/dl vs. ≥41 μg/dl		—	2.6	>M	50–74	
Pastorino et al. (82), ca-co, Italy, serum β carotene level	R	R	47 Fe	159 Fe	Lowest vs. highest tertile	Fe	2.4	8.9	[I]	[<25]	Assuming R_s = 10

[a]Controls or number of expected cases.

[b]Relative risk due to dietary factor. Numbers in brackets are reconstructed from published data.

[c]For definitions of categories of absolute magnitude of interaction, see text (Section II). Numbers in brackets are based on an assumption of relative risk due to smoking (R_s).

ca-co, case-control study; P, exposure information collected prospectively from study subjects; R, exposure information collected retrospectively from study subjects; O, exposure information collected from informants other than study subjects, e.g., relatives; Ma, males; Fe, females; NA, not available; A, additive; M, multiplicative; I, intermediate; PERDI, percent excess risk due to interaction; SSC, squamous and small-cell carcinomas; R_s, relative risk due to smoking; ppd, pack per day; py, pack-year.

Japanese women than in the other populations that were studied. Although the available data are insufficient to draw a final conclusion with respect to the interaction between fruit or vegetable intake and tobacco smoking, they strongly point toward a multiplicative or even more than multiplicative pattern, suggesting independence of effect of tobacco smoking and factors related to fruit and vegetable consumption in the causation of lung cancer. The PERDI ranges from 0 (in the men of only one study) to 75%, indicating that the protective effect of consuming vegetables and fruits may involve a nonnegligible component arising from the removal of the adverse interaction between smoking and low intakes of fruits and vegetables.

A multiplicative or more than multiplicative interaction between vitamin A (or β-carotene) intake and tobacco smoking has been shown by all relevant studies with the exception of the women enrolled in the study from Hawaii (78). The PERDI varies between 20 and 69%, and this variability may reflect the different categories of tobacco smoking and vitamin A intake used in the different analyses. In the only study in which more than two levels of vitamin A intake were considered, there was a suggestion of an inverse relation between strength of interaction and vitamin A intake (75). The only study that presented results by histology suggested a weaker role for interaction with vitamin A intake for squamous and small-cell lung carcinomas than for the other histological types (77). A more than multiplicative interaction was shown by the only investigation on cholesterol intake, with the PERDI as high as 75% (79), and was confirmed by a subsequent analysis on dairy food and sausage consumption (80). However, this study was restricted to smokers, so the results are based on the comparison of light (up to 40 pack-years) and heavy (more than 70 pack-years) smokers. The two studies analyzing tobacco smoking and serum β-carotene levels showed contrasting results, since a very strong interaction with more than two-thirds of excess risk due to the interaction was detected in a Japanese study (81), while a less than multiplicative interaction was found in a small Italian investigation (82).

The available evidence strongly points to a multiplicative or more than multiplicative interaction between tobacco smoking and vitamin A or β-carotene intake in the causation of lung cancer in humans. The data on hand are insufficient to reach any conclusion with respect to other dietary components as well as serum β-carotene levels.

G. Other and Mixed Exposures

Little information is available for other exposures that are known or suspected risk factors of lung cancer. The relevant studies are briefly reviewed in this section, but no conclusions can be drawn at present for any of them. Interaction is particularly difficult for complex mixtures, such as "occupations" or air pollution, in which the individual carcinogenic agents are unknown.

A case-control study from California analyzed the risk of lung cancer with respect to tobacco smoking and family history of any type of cancer (84). The latter variable was not associated with lung cancer risk among nonsmokers (RR, 0.7), but among smokers of 20 or more cigarettes per day the risk of lung cancer was much stronger in subjects with a family history of cancer (RR, 47.4) than in subjects without it (RR, 8.9).

The population-based case-control studies from two Norwegian counties that provided information on smoking and asbestos exposure also presented data on the interaction between tobacco smoking and exposure for at least 3 years to seven possible or definite lung carcinogens, including asbestos (85). The interaction seemed to be nearly multiplicative, with a PERDI equal to 59% (based on the unadjusted analysis). A further analysis, based on exposure to the seven agents above as well as to 15 occupational exposures not considered to be carcinogenic, found an intermediate interaction with tobacco smoking (PERDI, 45%). A case-control study from Japan reported an additive interaction between tobacco smoking and employment in ironworks (detailed data, however, were not presented) (86).

A number of epidemiological studies have provided data on the interaction between urban air pollution and tobacco smoking. They gave somewhat inconsistent results as to the type of interaction with tobacco smoking. Some studies provided evidence of a combined effect exceeding an additive effect and often compatible with a multiplicative interaction (87–91). Other studies were more consistent with an additive effect (92–94). In most of the studies, urban/rural differences in lung cancer rates were more pronounced or only seen among smokers. A positive interaction between urban air pollution and smoking may contribute to these results (95).

IV. Implications for Public Health

No uniform conclusion emerges from this review that can be generally applied to tobacco smoking interaction with environmental agents that are widely different: from Tables 1–5 the reader can glean an overall view of the spectrum of variability in absolute size and, more important, in the relative contributions that the interactive effect makes to the total effect of the two agents. However, some implications, relevant from a public health and preventive viewpoint, can be drawn.

First, it is important not to view the different degrees of interaction (less than additive, additive, etc.) as necessarily reflecting different underlying biological mechanisms. Siemiatycki and Thomas (96) have shown that even when they restricted their analysis within the boundaries of multistage carcinogenesis, both additive and multiplicative relations could derive from carcinogenic processes that are independent in a biological sense and, conversely, that additive and multiplicative relations can arise from processes that imply biological interactions. If one takes a broader view, a multiplicative relation can well describe data presumably disparate in their biological genesis, as of lung cancer previously illustrated, of noninfectious pulmonary diseases in smokers and nonsmokers (20,97), and of coronary heart disease associated with tobacco smoking, cholesterol levels, and blood pressure (4,98). Thus, it appears that while the incompatibility of predictions derived from mechanistic models with observed data is a strong element against the implied mechanisms, compatibility is at most a moderate element of support.

Second, when a positive interaction (synergism) occurs between tobacco smoking and another agent, there is an expanded possibility of preventive control, since the fraction of the total excess risk specifically due to interaction can be removed or reduced by eliminating or decreasing either exposure. Paradoxically, as always happens when more than one choice is available, this may lead to diversity of opinions on what priority and importance should be given to the different courses of action: for instance, for a population of asbestos workers should one put more effort into removing exposure to asbestos *or* to tobacco smoking? Critical in making the decision is how much the fraction of the excess risk is due to interaction in comparison with the separate effects of each individual exposure and with the sum total of the effects. If this fraction is substantial, the choice between different preventive approaches may become a practical issue. Table 6 shows selected values of the RRs due to two carcinogenic agents (one of which can be assumed to be tobacco smoking) and, under the hypothesis of multiplicative interaction, the PERDI. Generally, it can be stated from Table 6 that if the RR for one of the two agents is 2 or less, it is unlikely that the interaction can account for more than half the total excess risk, and indeed it can account for substantially less, unless the RR for the other agent, which could in turn be a combination of interacting agents, is well above 10. For example, if one takes a

Table 6 Percent Excess Risk due to Interaction (PERDI) Between Two Agents, *a* and *b*, Under the Multiplicative Hypothesis and Different Values of Relative Risks

	Relative risk (*a*)			
Relative risk (*b*)	1.3	2	5	10
1.3	13	19	22	23
2		33	44	47
5			67	73
10				82

RR of, say, 1.3 for the occurrence of lung cancer due to regular exposure to environmental tobacco smoke in a workplace where an occupational pollutant by itself increases the risk by a factor of 2, and the two agents act multiplicatively, less than 20% of the excess risk will be due to the interaction. From a practical viewpoint, the two agents can be regarded roughly as behaving as additive, with complete prevention entailing the removal of both. Even smaller interactive effects, and smaller PERDI, would occur in the presence of a less than multiplicative interaction.

A third point of public health import is that a more than multiplicative interaction is a necessary, although not sufficient, condition for an agent interacting with tobacco smoking to be noncarcinogenic in the absence of smoking. Evidence for or against this hypothesis can be sought indirectly by investigating whether the data depart in a statistically significant way from a multiplicative condition or, directly, by examining whether among nonsmokers the risk of lung cancer in subjects exposed to the environmental agent is or is not equal to the risk in unexposed subjects. Given, however, the low frequency of lung cancer among nonsmokers, the latter (direct) evidence may be difficult to determine: for instance, in some of the studies previously reviewed there is, apparently, no difference in risk between subjects exposed and unexposed to the environmental agent, but because of the very small number of cases of lung cancer, the power of these studies to detect a difference is low and no firm conclusion can be drawn. Conclusions, however, may be possible when this type of limited direct evidence is combined with the indirect one, derived from the examination of the departure of the data from a multiplicative model and with consideration of other relevant biological data. A combination of evidence was used to show that asbestos is capable of producing lung cancer even in the absence of tobacco smoking (99). The practical relevant consequence of demonstrating that an agent interacting with tobacco smoking is not carcinogenic in the absence of smoking would be that exposure to the agent alone does not increase lung cancer risk; this demonstration cannot be made, within the limitations of the currently available data, for any of the environmental agents reviewed in this chapter.

A fourth point of public health relevance arises from a number of exposures, briefly reviewed in Section III.G, for which both the issue of whether they do increase the risk of cancer in humans and the existence and degree of an interaction with tobacco smoking are still clouded. These ill-defined interactions of tobacco smoking cover some agents widely distributed, such as "general (urban) air pollution" (95,100), or "occupation" (85), not further specified, in the genesis of lung cancer. Difficulty in disentangling the separate and joint effects arises in part because the exposure to some of these interacting agents can be defined only in nonspecific terms, for example, "general air pollution," which is a highly complex mixture of variable composition.

From a practical viewpoint, one may regard as reasonably clear the case for an effect of some of these agents (e.g., air pollution) and as essentially unclear the respective contributions of tobacco smoking and the agent to the effect. Lacking better knowledge and unequivocal evidence of a more than multiplicative interaction, one may have to act on the assumption that both tobacco smoking and the agent are independently capable of increasing cancer risk.

Fifth and finally, the presence of interaction complicates the determination of the probability that an exposure has been the cause of an individual case of lung cancer, an issue of obvious relevance, not so much in public health as in an insurance context and in liability and compensation cases. Formal procedures of calculation for this purpose have been developed, which require, however, a critical appreciation of their probabilistic as well as empirical bases (see, for example, 101,102).

References

1. Cornfield, J., Haenszel, W., Hammond, E. C., et al. (1959). Smoking and lung cancer: recent evidence and a discussion of some questions. *JNCI* 22:173–203.
2. Axelson, O. (1978). Aspects of confounding in occupational health epidemiology. *Scand. J. Work Environ. Health* 4:85–89.
3. Hrubec, Z., Blair, A. E., Rogot, E., et al. (1992). *Mortality Risks by Occupation Among U.S. Veterans of Known Smoking Status*. 1954–1980. Vol. 1. NIH Publication No. 92-3407. U.S. Department of Health and Human Services.
4. Cornfield, J. (1962). Joint dependence on risk of coronary heart disease on serum cholesterol and systolic blood pressure: a discriminant function analysis. *Fed. Proc.* 21(Suppl 11):58–61.
5. Selikoff, I. J., Hammond, E. C., and Churg, J. (1968). Asbestos exposure, smoking, and neoplasia. *JAMA* 204:104–110.
6. Saracci, R. (1987). The interactions of tobacco smoking and other agents in cancer etiology. *Epidemiol. Rev.* 9:175–193.
7. Saracci, R. (1980). Interaction and synergism. *Am. J. Epidemiol.* 112:465–466.
8. Rothman, K. J. (1976). The estimation of synergy or antagonism. *Am. J. Epidemiol.* 103:506–511.
9. Walker, A. M. (1981). Proportion of disease attributable to the combined effect of two factors. *Int. J. Epidemiol.* 10:81–85.
10. McDonald, J. C., Liddell, F. D. K., Gibbs, G. W., et al. (1980). Dust exposure and mortality in chrysotile mining 1910–75. *Br. J. Indust. Med.* 37:11–24.
11. Thomas, D. C. (1983). Statistical methods for analyzing effects of temporal patterns of exposure on cancer risks. *Scand. J. Work Environ. Health* 9:353–366.
12. Liddell, F. D. K., Thomas, D. C., Gibbs, J. W., et al. (1984). Fibre exposure and mortality from pneumoconiosis, respiratory and abdominal malignancies in chrysotile production in Quebec, 1926–75. *Singapore Ann. Acad. Med.* 13(Suppl 2): 340–344.
13. Baker, J. E. (1985). Lung cancer incidence amongst previous employees of an

asbestos mine in relationship to crocidolite exposure and tobacco smoking. Ph.D. thesis, University of Western Australia, Perth.

14. Berry, G., Newhouse, M. L., and Turok, M. (1972) Combined effect of asbestos exposure and smoking on mortality from lung cancer in factory workers. *Lancet* 2: 476–479.
15. Selikoff, I. J., Seidman, H., and Hammond, E. C. (1980). Mortality effects of cigarette smoking among amosite asbestos factory workers. *JNCI* 65:507–513.
16. Acheson, E. D., Gardner, J. M., Winter, P. D., et al. (1984). Cancer in a factory using amosite asbestos. *Int. J. Epidemiol.* 13:3–10.
17. Berry, G., Newhouse, M. L., and Antonis, P. (1985). Combined effect of asbestos and smoking on mortality from lung cancer and mesothelioma in factory workers. *Br. J. Indust. Med.* 42:12–18.
18. Selikoff, I. J., and Hammond, E. D. (1975). Multiple risk factors in environmental cancer. In *Persons at High Risk of Cancer*. Edited by J. Fraumeni. New York, Academic Press, pp. 467–483.
19. Blot, W. J., Harrington, J. M., Toledo, A., et al. (1978). Lung cancer after employment in shipyards during World War II. *N. Engl. J. Med.* 299:620–624.
20. Hammond, E. C., Selikoff, I. J., and Seidman, H. (1979). Asbestos exposure, cigarette smoking and death rates. *Ann. NY Acad. Sci.* 330:473–490.
21. Blot, W. J., Morris, L. E., Stroube, R., et al. (1980). Lung and laryngeal cancer in relation to shipyard employment in coastal Virginia. *JNCI* 65:571–575.
22. Martischnig, K. M., Newell, D. J., Barnsley, W. C., et al. (1977). Unsuspected exposure to asbestos and bronchogenic carcinoma. *Br. Med. J.* 1:746–749.
23. Pastorino, U., Berrino, F., Gervasio, A., et al. (1984). Proportion of lung cancers due to occupational exposure. *Int. J. Cancer* 33:231–237.
24. Kjuus, H., Skjaerven, R., Langård, S., et al. (1986). A case-referent study of lung cancer, occupational exposures and smoking. 2. Role of asbestos exposure. *Scand. J. Work Environ. Health* 12:203–209.
25. de Klerk, N. H., Musk, A. W., Armstrong, B. K., et al. (1991). Smoking, exposure to crocidolite, and the incidence of lung cancer and asbestosis. *Br. J. Indust. Med.* 48:412–417.
26. Hilt, B., Langård, S., Andersen, A., et al. (1985). Asbestos exposure, smoking habits, and cancer incidence among production and maintenance workers in an electrochemical plant. *Am. J. Indust. Med.* 8:565–577.
27. Cheng, W. N., and Kong, J. (1992). A retrospective mortality cohort study of chrysotile asbestos products workers in Tianjin 1972–1987. *Environ. Res.* 59: 271–278.
28. Archer, V. E., Gillam, D., and Wagoner, J. K. (1976). Respiratory disease mortality among uranium miners. *Ann. NY Acad. Sci.* 271:280–293.
29. Lundin, F. E., Jr., Archer, V. E., and Wagoner, J. K. (1979). An exposure-time response model for lung cancer mortality in uranium miners: effects of radiation exposure, age and cigarette smoking. In *Energy and Health*. Edited by N. E. Breslow and A. S. Whittemore. SIAM-SIMS Conference serial no. 6, Philadelphia.
30. Whittemore, A. S., and McMillan, A. (1983). Lung cancer mortality among US uranium miners: a reappraisal. *JNCI* 71:489–499.

31. Samet, J. M., Pathak, D. R., Morgan, M. V., et al. (1991). Lung cancer mortality and exposure to Rn progeny in a cohort of New Mexico underground uranium miners. *Health Phys.* 61:745–752.
32. Muller, J., Kusiak, R., and Ritchie, A. C. (1989). Factors modifying lung cancer risk in Ontario uranium miners 1955–1981. Ontario Ministry of Labour.
33. L'Abbé, K. A., Howe, G. R., Burch, J. D., et al. (1991). Radon exposure, cigarette smoking, and other mining experience in the Beaverlodge uranium miners cohort. *Health Phys.* 60:489–495.
34. Committee on the Biological Effects of Ionizing Radiations. (1988). *Health Risks of Radon and Other Internally Deposited Alpha-Emitters*. BEIR IV. Washington, D. C., National Academy Press, pp. 504–563.
35. Radford, E. P., and St. Clair Renard, K. G. (1984). Lung cancer in Swedish iron miners exposed to low doses of radon daughters. *N. Engl. J. Med.* 310:1485–1494.
36. Damber, L., and Larsson, L. G. (1982). Combined effects of mining and smoking in the causation of lung carcinoma: a case-control study in northern Sweden. *Acta Radiol. Oncol.* 21:305–313.
37. Damber, L., and Larsson, L. G. (1985). Underground mining, smoking, and lung cancer: a case-control study in the iron ore municipalities of northern Sweden. *JNCI* 74:1207–1213.
38. Edling, C. (1982). Lung cancer and smoking in a group of iron ore miners. *Am. J. Indust. Med.* 3:191–199.
39. Edling, C., and Axelson, O. (1983). Quantitative aspects of radon daughter exposure and lung cancer in underground miners. *Br. J. Indust. Med.* 40:182–187.
40. Axelson, O., and Sundell, L. (1978). Mining, lung cancer and smoking. *Scand. J. Work Environ. Health* 4:46–52.
41. Solli, H. M., Andersen, A., Stranden, E., et al. (1985). Cancer incidence among workers exposed to radon and thoron daughters at a niobium mine. *Scand. J. Work Environ. Health* 11:7–13.
42. Morrison, H. I., Semenciw, M., Mao, Y., et al. (1988). Cancer mortality among a group of fluorspar miners exposed to radon progeny. *Am. J. Epidemiol.* 128:1266–1275.
43. Qiao, Y. L., Taylor, P. R., Yao, S. X., et al. (1989). Relation of radon exposure and tobacco use to lung cancer among tin miners in Yunnan Province, China. *Am. J. Indust. Med.* 16:511–521.
44. Lubin, J. H., Qiao, Y. L., Taylor, P. R., et al. (1990). Quantitative evaluation of the radon and lung cancer association in a case control study of Chinese tin miners. *Cancer Res.* 50:174–180.
45. Chen, S. Y., Hayes, R. B., Liang, S. R., et al. (1990). Mortality experience of haematite mine workers in China. *Br. J. Indust. Med.* 47:175–181.
46. Prentice, R. L., Yoshimoto, Y., and Mason, M. W. (1983). Relationship of cigarette smoking and radiation exposure to cancer mortality in Hiroshima and Nagasaki. *JNCI* 70:611–622.
47. Blot, W. J., Akiba, S., and Kato, H. (1984). Ionizing radiation and lung cancer: a review including preliminary results from a case-control study among A-bomb survivors. In *Atomic Bomb Survivor Data: Utilization and Analysis*. Edited by R. L. Prentice and D. J. Thompson. SIAM-SIMS Conference serial no. 10. Philadelphia.

48. Pinto, S. S., Henderson, V., and Enterline, P. E. (1978). Mortality experience of arsenic-exposed workers. *Arch. Environ. Health* 33:325–331.
49. Pershagen, G., Wall, S., Taube, A., et al. (1981). On the interaction between occupational arsenic exposure and smoking and its relationship to lung cancer. *Scand. J. Work Environ. Health* 7:302–309.
50. Welch, K., Higgins, I., Oh, M., et al. (1982). Arsenic exposure, smoking, and respiratory cancer in copper smelter workers. *Arch. Environ. Health* 37:325–335.
51. Taylor, P. R., Qiao, Y. L., Schatzkin, A., et al. (1989). Relation of arsenic exposure to lung cancer among tin miners in Yunnan Province, China. *Br. J. Indust. Med.* 46:881–886.
52. Tsuda, T., Nagira, T., Yamamoto, M., et al. (1990). An epidemiological study on cancer in certified arsenic poisoning patients in Toroku. *Indust. Health* 28:53–62.
53. Järup, L., and Pershagen, G. (1991) Arsenic exposure, smoking, and lung cancer in smelter workers—a case-control study. *Am. J. Epidemiol.* 134:545–551.
54. Enterline, P. E., Marsh, G. M., Esmen, N. A., et al. (1987). Some effects of cigarette smoking, arsenic, and SO_2 on mortality among US copper smelter workers. *J. Occup. Med.* 29:831–838.
55. Forastiere, F., Laborio, S., Michelozzi, P., et al. (1986). Silica, silicosis and lung cancer among ceramic workers: a case-referent study. *Am. J. Indust. Med.* 10: 363–370.
56. Mastrangelo, G., Zambon, P., Simonato, L., et al. (1988). A case-referent study investigating the relationship between exposure to silica dust and lung cancer. *Arch. Occup. Environ. Health* 60:299–302.
57. Siemiatycki, J., Gérin, M., Dewar, R., et al. (1990). Silica and cancer associations from a multicancer occupational exposure case-referent study. In *Occupational Exposure to Silica and Cancer Risk*. Edited by L. Simonato, A. C. Fletcher, R. Saracci, et al. IARC Scientific Publication no. 97. Lyon, International Agency for Research on Cancer, pp. 29–42.
58. Chiyotani, K., Saito, K., Okubo, T., et al. (1990). Lung cancer risk among pneumoconiosis patients in Japan, with special reference to silicotics. In *Occupational Exposure to Silica and Cancer Risk*. Edited by L. Simonato, A. C. Fletcher, R. Saracci, et al. IARC Scientific Publication no. 97. Lyon, International Agency for Research on Cancer, pp. 95–104.
59. Amandus, H., and Costello, J. (1991). Silicosis and lung cancer in U.S. metal miners. *Arch. Environ. Health* 46:82–89.
60. Hnizdo, E., and Sluis-Cremer, G. K. (1991). Silica exposure, silicosis, and lung cancer: a mortality study of South African gold miners. *Br. J. Indust. Med.* 48:53–60.
61. Amandus, H. E., Shy, C., Wing, S., et al. (1991). Silicosis and lung cancer in North Carolina dusty trades workers. *Am. J. Indust. Med.* 20:57–70.
62. Chia, S. E., Chia, K. S., Phoon, W. H., et al. (1991). Silicosis and lung cancer among Chinese granite workers. *Scand. J. Work Environ. Health* 17:170–174.
63. Hessel, P. A., Sluis-Cremer, G. K., and Hnizdo, E. (1990). Silica exposure, silicosis, and lung cancer: a necropsy study. *Br. J. Indust. Med.* 47:4–9.
64. IARC (1987). Silica. In IARC Monographs on the Evaluation of Carcinogenic Risks to Humans. Vol. 42, *Silica and Some Silicates*. Lyon, International Agency for Research on Cancer, pp. 38–143.

65. Lessard, R., Reed, D., Maheux, B., et al. (1978). Lung cancer in New Caledonia, a nickel smelting island. *J. Occup. Med.* 20:815–817.
66. Magnus, K., Andersen, A., and Høgetveit, A. C. (1982). Cancer of the respiratory organs among workers at a nickel refinery in Norway. Second report. *Int. J. Cancer* 30:681–685.
67. Weiss, W. (1980). The cigarette factor in lung cancer due to chloromethylethers. *J. Occup. Med.* 22:527–529.
68. Steenland, K., and Thun, M. (1986). Interaction between tobacco smoking and occupational exposures in the causation of lung cancer. *J. Occup. Med.* 28:110–118.
69. Hirayama, T. (1979). Diet and cancer. *Nutr. Cancer* 1:67–81.
70. Ziegler, R. G., Mason, T. J., Stemhagen, A., et al. (1986). Carotenoid intake, vegetables, and the risk of lung cancer among white men in New Jersey. *Am. J. Epidemiol.* 123:1080–1093.
71. Pisani, P., Berrino, F., Macaluso, M., et al. (1986). Carrots, green vegetables and lung cancer: a case-control study. *Int. J. Epidemiol.* 15:463–468.
72. Byers, T. E., Graham, S., Haughey, B. P., et al. (1987). Diet and lung cancer risk: findings from the Western New York diet study. *Am. J. Epidemiol.* 125:351–363.
73. Fraser, G. E., Beeson, W. L., and Phillips, R. L. (1991). Diet and lung cancer in California Seventh-Day Adventists. *Am. J. Epidemiol.* 133:683–693.
74. Bjelke, J. (1975). Dietary vitamin A and human lung cancer. *Int. J. Cancer* 15: 561–565.
75. Mettlin, C., Graham, S., and Swanson, M. (1979). Vitamin A and lung cancer. *JNCI* 62:1435–1438.
76. Shekelle, R. B., Lepper, M., Liu, S., et al. (1981). Dietary vitamin A and risk of cancer in the Western Electric study. *Lancet* 2:1185–1191.
77. Kvåle, G., Bjelke, E., and Gart, J. J. (1983). Dietary habits and lung cancer risk. *Int. J. Cancer* 31:397–405.
78. Le Marchand, L., Yoshizawa, C. N., Kolonel, L. N., et al. (1989). Vegetable consumption and lung cancer risk: a population-based case-control study in Hawaii. *JNCI* 81:1158–1164.
79. Goodman, M. T., Kolonel, L. N., Yoshizawa, C. N., et al. (1988). The effect of dietary cholesterol and fat on the risk of lung cancer in Hawaii. *Am. J. Epidemiol.* 128:1241–1255.
80. Goodman, M. T., Hankin, J. H., Wilkens, L. R., et al. (1992). High-fat foods and the risk of lung cancer. *Epidemiology* 3:288–299.
81. Nomura, A. M. Y., Stemmermann, G. N., Heilbrun, L. K., et al. (1985). Serum vitamin levels and the risk of cancer of specific sites in men of Japanese ancestry in Hawaii. *Cancer Res.* 45:2369–2372.
82. Pastorino, U., Pisani, P., Berrino, F., et al. (1987). Vitamin A and female lung cancer: a case-control study on plasma and diet. *Nutr. Cancer* 10:171–179.
83. Candelora, E. C., Stockwell, H. G., Armstrong, A. W., et al. (1992). Dietary intake and risk of lung cancer in women who never smoked. *Nutr. Cancer* 17:263–270.
84. Osann, K. E. (1991). Lung cancer in women: the importance of smoking, family history of cancer, and medical history of respiratory disease. *Cancer Res.* 51:4893–4897.

85. Kvåle, G., Bjelke, E., and Heuch, I. (1986). Occupational exposure and lung cancer risk. *Int. J. Cancer* 37:185–193.
86. Yamaguchi, N., Kido, M., Hoshuyama, T., et al. (1992). A case-control study on occupational lung cancer risks in an industrialized city of Japan. *Jpn. J. Cancer Res.* 83:134–140.
87. Dean, G. (1966). Lung cancer and bronchitis in Northern Ireland. *Br. Med. J.* 1: 1506–1514.
88. Haenszel, W., Loveland, D. B., and Sirken, M. G. (1962). Lung-cancer mortality as related to residence and smoking histories: white males. *JNCI* 28:947–1001.
89. Vena, J. E. (1982). Air pollution as a risk factor in lung cancer. *Am. J. Epidemiol.* 116:42–56.
90. Jedrychowski, W., Becher, H., Wahrendorf, J., et al. (1990). Case-control study of lung cancer with special reference to the effect of air pollution in Poland. *J. Epidemiol. Commun. Health* 44:114–120.
91. Katsouyanni, K., Trichopoulos, D., Kalandidi, A., et al. (1991). A case-control study of air pollution and tobacco smoking in lung cancer among women in Athens. *Prev. Med.* 20:271–278.
92. Buell, P., Dunn, J. E., and Breslow, L. (1967). Cancer of the lung and Los Angeles type air pollution. *Cancer* 20:2139–2147.
93. Stocks, P., and Campbell, J. (1955). Lung cancer death rates among nonsmokers and pipe and cigarette smokers. *Br. Med. J.* 2:923–929
94. Haenszel, W., and Taeuber, K. E. (1964). Lung-cancer mortality as related to residence and smoking histories: white females. *JNCI* 32:803–838.
95. Pershagen, G., and Simonato, L. (1983). Epidemiological evidence on outdoor air pollution and cancer. In *Indoor and Outdoor Air Pollution and Human Cancer*. Edited by L. Tomatis. European School of Oncology Monograph Series. Berlin, Springer, pp. 135–148.
96. Siemiatycki, J., and Thomas, D. C. (1981). Biological models and statistical interactions: an example from multistage carcinogenesis. *Int. J. Epidemiol.* 10: 383–387.
97. Frank, A. L. (1979). Public health significance of smoking-asbestos interactions. *Ann. NY Acad. Sci.* 330:791–794.
98. Gordon, T. (1974). Hazards in the use of the logistic function with special reference to data from prospective cardiovascular studies. *J. Chronic Dis.* 27:97–102.
99. Saracci, R. (1977). Asbestos and lung cancer: an analysis of the epidemiological evidence on the asbestos-smoking interaction. *Int. J. Cancer* 20:323–331.
100. Committee on the Epidemiology of Air Pollutants. (1985). *Epidemiology and Air Pollution*. Washington, D. C., National Academy Press.
101. Jablon, S. (1985). The probability of causation: an approach to the problem of toxic torts, especially with respect to exposures to ionizing radiation. In *Epidemiology and Quantitation of Environmental Risk in Humans from Radiation and Other Agents*. Edited by A. Castellani. London, Plenum Press, pp. 47–62.
102. Checkoway, H., Pearce, N. E., and Crawford-Brown, D. J. (1989). *Research Methods in Occupational Epidemiology*. New York, Oxford University Press, pp. 291–332.

AUTHOR INDEX

Italic numbers give the page on which the complete reference is listed.

A

B

D

F

G

H

K

L

N

Q

R

T

W

X

Y

SUBJECT INDEX

B

C

D

N

O

P

R

S

T

U

V

W